PHYSICAL THERAPY CASE FILES®
Pediatrics

Eric S. Pelletier, PT, DPT, PCS
Assistant Professor
Department of Physical Therapy
Samson College of Health Sciences
University of the Sciences
Philadelphia, Pennsylvania

Series Editor: Erin E. Jobst, PT, PhD
Associate Professor
School of Physical Therapy
College of Health Professions
Pacific University
Hillsboro, Oregon

Mc
Graw
Hill
Education

New York   Chicago   San Francisco   Athens   London   Madrid   Mexico City
Milan   New Delhi   Singapore   Sydney   Toronto

Physical Therapy Case Files®: Pediatrics

1 2 3 4 5 6 7 8 9 0   DOC/DOC   19 18 17 16 15

ISBN 978-0-07-179568-5
MHID 0-07-179568-5

Notice

Medicine is an ever-changing science. As new research and clinical experience broaden our knowledge, changes in treatment and drug therapy are required. The authors and the publisher of this work have checked with sources believed to be reliable in their efforts to provide information that is complete and generally in accord with the standard accepted at the time of publication. However, in view of the possibility of human error or changes in medical sciences, neither the editors nor the publisher nor any other party who has been involved in the preparation or publication of this work warrants that the information contained herein is in every respect accurate or complete, and they disclaim all responsibility for any errors or omissions or for the results obtained from use of the information contained in this work. Readers are encouraged to confirm the information contained herein with other sources. For example and in particular, readers are advised to check the product information sheet included in the package of each drug they plan to administer to be certain that the information contained in this work is accurate and that changes have not been made in the recommended dose or in the contraindications for administration. This recommendation is of particular importance in connection with new or infrequently used drugs.

This book was set in Adobe Jenson Pro by Cenveo® Publisher Services.
The editors were Catherine A. Johnson and Christina M. Thomas.
The production supervisor was Catherine H. Saggese.
Project management was provided by Anubhooti Saxena, Cenveo Publisher Services.
RR Donnelley was the printer and binder.

Library of Congress Cataloging-in-Publication Data

Physical therapy case files. Pediatrics / [edited by] Eric S. Pelletier.
    p. ; cm.
Pediatrics
Includes bibliographical references and index.
ISBN 978-0-07-179568-5 (pbk.)—ISBN 0-07-179568-5
I. Pelletier, Eric S., editor.   II. Title: Pediatrics.
[DNLM: 1. Physical Therapy Modalities—Case Reports. 2. Adolescent. 3. Child. 4. Infant.
5. Needs Assessment—Case Reports. WB 460]
RJ53.P5
615.8'20832—dc23
                           2015020577

CONTENTS

Ryan Borck, PT, DPT
Physical Therapist
ATI Physical Therapy
Hinsdale, Illinois

Chad Cherny, PT, DPT, SCS, CSCS
Physical Therapist
Sports Medicine Biodynamics Center
Division of Occupational and Physical Therapy
Cincinnati Children's Hospital Medical Center
Cincinnati, Ohio

Colleen Patricia Coulter, PT, DPT, PhD, PCS
Physical Therapist IV, Team Leader Limb Deficiency Program
Clinical Coordinator APTA Pediatric Residency Program
Prosthetics and Orthotics Department
Children's Healthcare of Atlanta
Atlanta, Georgia

Christine A. Cronin, PT, DPT, PCS, MBA, MS
Associate Professor
Department of Rehabilitation and Movement Sciences
School of Health Related Professions
Rutgers, The State University of New Jersey
Newark, New Jersey

Maureen Donohoe, PT, DPT, PCS
Physical Therapist
Nemours Alfred I. DuPont Hospital for Children
Wilmington, Delaware

Beth Ennis, PT, EdD, PCS, ATP
Associate Professor
Bellarmine University
Louisville, Kentucky

Katherine Fash, PT, DPT
Team Leader
The Children's Hospital of Philadelphia
Philadelphia, Pennsylvania

Alyson Filipa, PT, DPT, MS, SCS, CSCS
Physical Therapist II
Division of Occupational Therapy and Physical Therapy
Cincinnati Children's Hospital Medical Center
Cincinnati, Ohio

Megan L. Freeland, PT, DPT, PCS
Director of Clinical Education
Assistant Professor
Doctor of Physical Therapy Program
School of Health Professions
Long Island University
Brooklyn, New York

Brian Giavedoni MBA, CP/L
Supervisor of Prosthetics
Assistant Supervisor, Orthotics and Prosthetics
Children's Healthcare of Atlanta
Atlanta, Georgia

Meri Goehring, PT, PhD, GCS
Associate Professor
Department of Physical Therapy
College of Health Professions
Grand Valley State University
Grand Rapids, Michigan

Rebecca Grant, PT, DPT, PCS
Children's Healthcare of Atlanta
Atlanta, Georgia

Phyllis L. Guarrera-Bowlby, PT, EdD, PCS
Associate Professor
Department of Rehabilitation and Movement Sciences
School of Health Related Professions
Rutgers, The State University of New Jersey
Newark, New Jersey

Dana Robinson Johnson, PT, DPT
Senior Physical Therapist
Shriners Hospitals for Children® – Philadelphia
Philadelphia, Pennsylvania

Barb Kellar, PT, MS, DPT
Physical Therapist
Chalfont, Pennsylvania

Lisa K. Kenyon, PT, DPT, PhD, PCS
Associate Professor
Department of Physical Therapy
Grand Valley State University
Grand Rapids, Michigan

Jessica Laniak, PT, DPT, OCS
Nemours Alfred I. duPont Hospital for Children
Wilmington, Delaware

David John Lorello, PT, DPT
Maricopa Integrated Health System
Arizona Burn Center
Phoenix, Arizona

Kathy Martin, PT, DHS
Professor and DPT Program Director
Krannert School of Physical Therapy
University of Indianapolis
Indianapolis, Indiana

Sarah Martyn, DPT
Good Shepherd Penn Partners at Penn Comprehensive Hemophilia
    and Thrombosis Program
Philadelphia, Pennsylvania

Paula G. Melson, PT, DPT, MMS
Rehabilitation Coordinator for Rheumatology
Division of Occupational and Physical Therapy
Cincinnati Children's Hospital Medical Center
Cincinnati, Ohio

Nisha Narula Pagan, PT, DPT, NCS, PCS
Owner, Whole Hearted Pediatric Physical Therapy
Long Beach, California

Mark V. Paterno, PT, PhD, MBA, SCS, ATC
Acting Scientific Director
Division of Occupational Therapy and Physical Therapy
Associate Professor
Division of Sports Medicine
Cincinnati Children's Hospital Medical Center
Cincinnati, Ohio

Ellen Rae Rosevear, OTR/L, MS
Mary Free Bed Rehabilitation Hospital
Grand Rapids, Michigan

Anastasiya Ruiz, MSPT, CIMI
Advanced Clinician I, Inpatient Rehabilitation Services
Pennsylvania Hospital/Good Shepherd Penn Partners
Philadelphia, Pennsylvania

Stephanie F. Sabo, PT, MPT
Physical Therapist II
Division of Occupational and Physical Therapy
Cincinnati Children's Hospital Medical Center
Cincinnati, Ohio

Kimberly A. Scharff, PT, DPT, PCS
Shriners Hospitals for Children® – Philadelphia
Philadelphia, Pennsylvania

Britta Schasberger, PT, EdD
Assistant Professor
Department of Physical Therapy
Samson College of Health Studies
University of the Sciences
Philadelphia, Pennsylvania

Wendy Webb Schoenewald, PT, OCS
Owner, WWS Physical Therapy and Vestibular Rehabilitation
Doylestown, Pennsylvania

Sarah Stewart, PT, PCS
Children's Healthcare of Atlanta
Atlanta, Georgia

Amanda Stoltz, PT, DPT
Physical Therapist
Shriners Hospitals for Children®
Portland, Oregon

Anne K. Swisher, PT, PhD, CCS
Professor
Division of Physical Therapy
West Virginia University
Morgantown, West Virginia

Kimberly D. Ward, PT, DPT, PCS, MPH
Assistant Professor
Department of Physical Therapy
Samson College of Health Sciences
University of the Sciences
Philadelphia, Pennsylvania

ACKNOWLEDGMENTS

Editing a text is not a solitary experience. There are many people to thank for bringing *Physical Therapy Case Files: Pediatrics* to fruition. I am indebted to Erin Jobst, Series Editor, for her patience, sense of humor, honesty, and encouragement throughout this process. Her vision and leadership is evident in all of the books within this series. I thank her for believing in me to bring this valuable resource to the students and clinicians of pediatric physical therapy.

The contributors of the cases have made this book the valuable resource that it is. From the first moment of recruitment to the final editorial suggestions, you all remained patient and you all persevered. Thank you for sharing your knowledge, clinical and academic expertise, time, and your love of helping children reach their full potential. Your contributions will influence many students and clinicians and impact the lives of the children they treat.

To the children and families I have had the honor of treating and to the students I have had the pleasure of teaching, thank you. Learning is a two-way street and I only hope you have learned from me half as much as I have learned from you.

A special thank you goes out to my favorite physical therapist, my wife Heather, for being my biggest supporter. With your love and encouragement, I find that anything is possible. To my children, Evan and Cameron, keep dreaming big and taking chances, I love you both so much more than you know. You have both made me a better pediatric physical therapist and I am so proud to be your dad.

Eric S. Pelletier, PT, DPT, PCS

As the physical therapy profession continues to evolve and advance as a doctoring profession, so does the rigor of the entry-level physical therapist education. Students must master fundamental foundation courses while integrating an understanding of new research in all areas of physical therapy. Evidence-based practice is the use of current best evidence in conjunction with the expertise of the clinician and the specific values and circumstances of the patient in making decisions regarding assessment and treatment. Evidence-based practice is a major emphasis in both physical therapy education and practice. However, the most challenging task for students is making the transition from didactic classroom-based knowledge to its application in developing a physical therapy diagnosis and implementing appropriate evidence-based interventions. Ideally, instructors who are experienced and knowledgeable in every diagnosis and treatment approach could guide students at the "bedside" and students would supplement this training by self-directed independent reading. While there is certainly no substitute for clinical education, it is rare for clinical rotations to cover the scope of each physical therapy setting. In addition, it is not always possible for clinical instructors to be able to take the time necessary to guide students through the application of evidence-based tests and measures and interventions. Perhaps an effective alternative approach is teaching by using clinical case studies designed with a structured clinical approach to diagnosis and treatment. At the time of writing the *Physical Therapy Case Files* series, there were no physical therapy textbooks that contain case studies that utilize and reference current literature to support an illustrated examination or treatment. In my own teaching, I have designed case scenarios based on personal patient care experiences, those experiences shared with me by my colleagues, and searches through dozens of textbooks and websites to find a case study illustrating a particular concept. There are two problems with this approach. First, neither my own nor my colleagues' experiences cover the vast diversity of patient diagnoses, examinations, and interventions. Second, designing a case scenario that is not based on personal patient care experience or expertise takes an overwhelming amount of time. In my experience, detailed case studies that incorporate application of the best evidence are difficult to design "on the fly" in the classroom. The twofold goal of the *Physical Therapy Case Files* series is to provide resources that contain multiple real-life case studies within an individual physical therapy practice area that will minimize the need for physical therapy educators to create their own scenarios and maximize the students' ability to implement evidence into the care of individual patients.

The cases within each book in the *Physical Therapy Case Files* series are organized for the reader to either read the book from "front to back" or to randomly select scenarios based on current interest. A list of cases by case number and by alphabetical listing by health condition is included in Section III to enable the reader to review his or her knowledge in a specific area. Sometimes a case scenario may include a more abbreviated explanation of a specific health condition or clinical test than was provided in another case. In this situation, the reader will be referred to the case with the more thorough explanation.

Every case follows an organized and well thought-out format using familiar language from both the World Health Organization's International Classification of Functioning, Disability, and Health (ICF) framework[1] and the American Physical Therapy Association's *Guide to Physical Therapist Practice*.[2] To limit redundancy and length of each case, we intentionally did not present the ICF framework or the *Guide's* Preferred Practice Patterns within each case. However, the section titles and the language used throughout each case were chosen to guide the reader through the evaluation, goal-setting, and intervention process and how clinical reasoning can be used to enhance an individual's activities and participation.

The front page of each case begins with a patient encounter followed by a series of open-ended questions. The discussion following the case is organized into *seven* sections:

1. **Key Definitions** provide terminology pertinent to the reader's understanding of the case; **Objectives** list the instructional and/or terminal behavioral objectives that summarize the knowledge, skills, or attitudes the reader should be able to demonstrate after reading the case; **PT Considerations** provides a summary of the physical therapy plan of care, goals, interventions, precautions, and potential complications for the physical therapy management of the individual presented in the case.

2. **Understanding the Health Condition** presents an abbreviated explanation of the medical diagnosis. The intent of this section is not to be comprehensive. The etiology, pathogenesis, risk factors, epidemiology, and medical management of the condition are presented in enough detail to provide background and context for the reader.

3. **Physical Therapy Patient/Client Management** provides a summary of the role of the physical therapist in the patient's care. This section may elaborate on how the physical therapist's role augments and/or overlaps with those of other healthcare practitioners involved in the patient's care, as well as any referrals to additional healthcare practitioners that the physical therapist should provide.

4. **Examination, Evaluation, and Diagnosis** guides the reader how to: organize and interpret information gathered from the chart review (in inpatient cases), appreciate adverse drug reactions that may affect patient presentation, and structure the subjective evaluation and physical examination. Not every assessment tool and special test that could possibly be done with the patient is included. For each outcome measure or special test presented, the reliability, validity, sensitivity, and specificity are discussed. When available, a minimal clinically important difference (MCID) for an outcome measure is presented because it helps the clinician to determine the "the minimal level of change required in response to an intervention before the outcome would be considered worthwhile in terms of a patient/client's function or quality of life."[3]

5. **Plan of Care and Interventions** elaborates on a few physical therapy interventions for the patient's condition. The advantage of this section and the previous section is that each case does *not* exhaustively present every outcome measure,

special test, or therapeutic intervention that *could be* performed. Rather, only selected outcome measures or examination techniques and interventions are chosen. This is done to simulate a real-life patient interaction in which the physical therapist uses his or her clinical reasoning to determine the *most appropriate* tests and interventions to utilize with that patient during that episode of care. For each intervention that is chosen, the evidence to support its use with individuals with the same diagnosis (or similar diagnosis, if no evidence exists to support its use in that particular patient population) is presented. To reduce redundancy, standard guidelines for aerobic and resistance exercise have not been included. Instead, the reader is referred to guidelines published by the American College of Sports Medicine,[4] Goodman and Fuller,[5] and Paz and West.[6] For particular case scenarios in which standard guidelines are deviated from, specific guidelines are included.

6. **Evidence-Based Clinical Recommendations** includes a minimum of three clinical recommendations for diagnostic tools and/or treatment interventions for the patient's condition. To improve the quality of each recommendation beyond the personal clinical experience of the contributing author, each recommendation is graded using the Strength of Recommendation Taxonomy (SORT).[7] There are over one hundred evidence-grading systems used to rate the quality of individual studies and the strength of recommendations based on a body of evidence.[8] The SORT system has been used by several medical journals including *American Family Physician*, *Journal of the American Board of Family Practice*, *Journal of Family Practice*, and *Sports Health*. We have also chosen to use the SORT system for two reasons: it is simple and its rankings are based on patient-oriented outcomes. The SORT system has only three levels of evidence: A, B, and C. Grade A recommendations are based on consistent, good-quality patient-oriented evidence (*e.g.*, systematic reviews, meta-analysis of high-quality studies, high-quality randomized controlled trials, high-quality diagnostic cohort studies). Grade B recommendations are based on inconsistent or limited-quality patient-oriented evidence (*e.g.*, systematic review or meta-analysis of lower-quality studies or studies with inconsistent findings). Grade C recommendations are based on consensus, disease-oriented evidence, usual practice, expert opinion, or case series (*e.g.*, consensus guidelines, disease-oriented evidence using only intermediate or physiologic outcomes). The contributing author of each case provided a grade based on the SORT guidelines for each recommendation or conclusion. The grade for each statement was reviewed and sometimes altered by the editors. Key phrases from each clinical recommendation are bolded within the case to enable the reader to easily locate where the cited evidence was presented.

7. **Comprehension Questions and Answers** includes two to four multiple-choice questions that reinforce the content or elaborate and introduce new, but related concepts to the patient's case. When appropriate, detailed explanations about why alternative choices would not be the best choice are also provided.

My hope is that these real-life case studies will be a new resource to facilitate the incorporation of evidence into everyday physical therapy practice in various settings and patient populations. With the persistent push for evidence-based healthcare to promote quality and effectiveness[9] and the advent of evidence-based reimbursement guidelines, case scenarios with evidence-based recommendations will be an added benefit as physical therapists continually face the threat of decreased reimbursement rates for their services and will need to demonstrate evidence supporting their services. I hope physical therapy educators, entry-level physical therapy students, practicing physical therapists, and professionals preparing for Board Certification in clinical specialty areas will find these books helpful to translate classroom-based knowledge to evidence-based assessments and interventions.

Erin E. Jobst, PT, PhD

1. World Health Organization. International Classification of Functioning, Disability and Health (ICF). Available at: http://www.who.int/classifications/icf/en/. Accessed August 7, 2012.
2. American Physical Therapy Association. *Guide to Physical Therapist Practice (Guide)*. Alexandria, VA: APTA; 1999.
3. Jewell DV. *Guide to Evidence-based Physical Therapy Practice*. Sudbury, MA: Jones and Barlett; 2008.
4. *ACSM's Guidelines for Exercise Testing and Prescription*. 8th ed. Wolters Kluwer/Lippincott Williams & Wilkins; 2010.
5. Goodman CC, Fuller KS. *Pathology: Implications for the Physical Therapist*. 3rd ed. Philadelphia, PA: W.B. Saunders Company; 2009.
6. Paz JC, West MP. *Acute Care Handbook for Physical Therapists*. 3rd ed. St. Louis, MO: Saunders Elsevier; 2009.
7. Ebell MH, Siwek J, Weiss BD, et al. Strength of Recommendation Taxonomy (SORT): A Patient-Centered Approach to Grading Evidence in the Medical Literature. *Am Fam Physician*. 2004;69: 548-56.
8. Systems to rate the strength of scientific evidence. Summary, evidence report/technology assessment: number 47. AHRQ publication no. 02-E015, March 2002. Available at: http://www.ahrq.gov/clinic/epcsums/strengthsum.htm. Accessed August 7, 2012.
9. Agency for Healthcare Research and Quality. Available at: www.ahrq.gov/clinic/epc/. Accessed August 7, 2012.

Introduction

The practice of pediatric physical therapy is multifaceted. Examining, evaluating, and planning care for children requires the ability to work not only with the child, but also with the child's caregivers. A physical therapist in a pediatric clinic could work with an infant, a toddler, a school-aged child, a pre-teen, and an adolescent all in one day. The variation in needs and challenges among the age groups is significant and navigating those challenges is never easy. It has been said that children are not small adults and they should not be treated as such. The treatment of pediatric clients has the potential to cross many areas of physical therapy care from orthopaedics to neuromuscular rehabilitation. From student physical therapists to pediatric clinical specialists, all clinicians working with children must navigate and integrate their knowledge of anatomy and physiology with concepts of growth and development and be able to cognitively meet each child where he or she is to achieve successful outcomes.

This book was developed to provide students and clinicians alike cases that navigate through some common (and not so common) pediatric diagnoses they may encounter in early intervention, school system, hospital, rehabilitation facility, or outpatient clinic. The cases will not exhaust all information about the diagnoses encountered, but rather give a snapshot of the presentation. Cases focus the reader's attention to the examination tools and interventions that seasoned clinicians choose in these populations. The contributors have provided evidence that supports the examination and intervention choices presented with the intent of illustrating their expert clinical decision making.

The 31 cases in this volume are not exhaustive of the pediatric clients that physical therapists may encounter in a given pediatric setting, but they range from neuromuscular developmental diagnoses to genetic disorders, musculoskeletal anomalies, and combinations of these areas. The cases also offer a glimpse into the varied environments that pediatric physical therapy is delivered. There are cases that discuss early intervention and school-based interventions, including a three-case series following a child with spastic diplegic cerebral palsy from early intervention services through her transition to adulthood (Cases 6-8). Other cases present interventions seen in inpatient units and outpatient care.

The goal of this book is to provide academic and clinical faculty, students, and novice to expert clinicians a resource for the interventions we use and a gateway for further exploration and development. I hope that we have met that mark. Please enjoy reading these cases and I hope the information inspires readers to reflect on their own clinical decision making and, in turn, helps all of the children we treat reach their maximum functional potential.

Listing of Cases

Listing by Case Number

Listing by Health Condition (Alphabetical)

Listing by Case Number

Listing by Health Condition (Alphabetical)

Thirty-One Case Scenarios

Brachial Plexus Palsy

Lisa K. Kenyon
Ellen Rae Rosevear

CASE 1

A 13-month-old boy was referred to an outpatient therapy clinic for management of concerns related to his obstetric brachial plexus palsy (OBPP). The child's medical history was obtained through an interview with his parents and a review of available records. The patient was born at full term following a pregnancy that was complicated by maternal diabetes. The forceps-assisted vaginal delivery was complicated by prolonged labor, fetal heart rate decelerations, and fetal shoulder dystocia. At birth, complete flaccidity and an absence of deep tendon and neonatal reflexes were noted in his right upper extremity (UE). A magnetic resonance imaging (MRI) study and computed tomography (CT) myelography performed at 3 months of age revealed an intact C5 nerve root and avulsion of C6 through T1 nerve roots. At 6 months of age, a nerve graft was performed. The parents report limited functional improvement since the nerve graft. They state that they are becoming increasingly concerned about their son's future and his ability to functionally use his right arm.

▸ How does the patient's age impact the choice of test and measures for children with OBPP?

▸ What factors are involved in determining if a child with OBPP is a candidate for surgical intervention?

▸ How might interventions change based on the child's age?

▸ What are the functional implications of OBPP as this child grows into adulthood?

KEY DEFINITIONS

ASYMMETRIC TONIC NECK REFLEX: Developmental reflex; as the baby's head is turned toward one side, the UE on that side extends and the UE on the opposite side flexes.

DEVELOPMENTAL REFLEXES: Involuntary responses that are also called primitive reflexes; in typically developing infants, these disappear or are inhibited during development.

MORO REFLEX: Developmental reflex that is observed in typically developing infants in response to a sudden loss of support at the head; in response to this loss of support, the typically developing infant symmetrically abducts both upper extremities and then symmetrically adducts both upper extremities.

PALMAR GRASP REFLEX: Developmental reflex observed in typically developing infants; when an object is placed in the infant's palm, the infant grasps the object.

TORTICOLLIS: See Case 17; unilateral shortening of the sternocleidomastoid muscle that causes the infant's head to be turned to one side and laterally flexed to the opposite side; may be congenital (infant is born with it) or may develop as a result of habitual positioning

Objectives

1. List maternal- and child-centered risk factors for OBPP.
2. Identify appropriate tests and measures to be used in the physical therapy examination of a child with OBPP.
3. Recognize factors involved in determining if a child with OBPP is a candidate for surgical intervention.
4. Identify appropriate outcomes and physical therapy interventions for a child with OBPP.
5. Consider the functional impact of OBPP as a child grows from infancy into adulthood.

Physical Therapy Considerations

PT considerations during management of a toddler who presents with an obstetric brachial plexus injury:

▶ **General physical therapy plan of care/goals:** Maintain or improve active and passive range of motion (ROM); encourage functional use of involved UE; improve sensory awareness; support motor and sensory recovery; maximize functional outcome and avoid further injury

▶ **Physical therapy interventions:** ROM (passive, active assisted, active) and strengthening exercises; functional UE activities (especially bimanual tasks); parent/child education related to joint alignment and extremity protection; neuromuscular electrical stimulation; biofeedback; splinting

▶ **Precautions during physical therapy**: Awareness of surgeon- and physician-specific protocols for activity restrictions; avoidance of overstretching; awareness of potential for decreased sensation in the involved UE; maintenance of appropriate biomechanical alignment of involved UE during weightbearing

▶ **Complications interfering with physical therapy**: Development of torticollis; decreased sensation, unstable joints, contractures, flaccidity, and/or neglect of involved UE

Understanding the Health Condition

The brachial plexus includes both motor and sensory nerves and is formed by the intercommunication of the five ventral rami or roots from cervical nerves C5 through C8 and the first thoracic nerve (T1; Fig. 1-1). These 5 roots merge to create 3 separate trunks: superior (upper C5-C6), middle (C7), and inferior (lower C8-T1). Each trunk then divides into 2 parts, forming 6 divisions classified as the anterior or posterior superior, middle, and inferior trunks. The 3 trunks regroup into 3 cords that are classified according to their relationship to the axillary artery. The posterior cord (C5-T1) comprises the posterior 3 trunk divisions. The lateral cord (C5-C7) is formed by the anterior divisions of the upper and middle trunks, and the medial cord (C8-T1) comprises the anterior division of the lower trunk. The nerves in the brachial plexus provide the motor and sensory innervation for

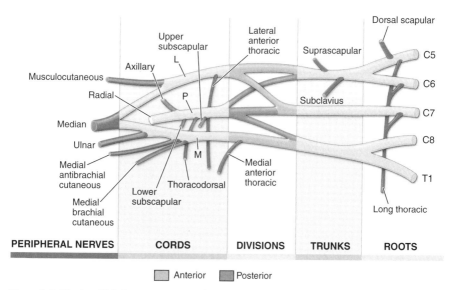

Figure 1-1. The brachial plexus comprised of the ventral rami or roots from cervical nerves C5 through C8 and the first thoracic nerve (T1). L, lateral; M, medial; P, posterior. (Reproduced with permission from Morton DA, Foreman K, Albertine KH. Chapter 29. Overview of the Upper Limb. In: Morton DA, Foreman K, Albertine KH. eds. *The Big Picture: Gross Anatomy*. New York, NY: McGraw-Hill; 2011. Figure 29-4.)

almost the entire UE. Notable exceptions include motor innervation of the trapezius and levator scapulae muscles and sensory innervation in the axilla.

OBPP most frequently occurs as the result of traction or stretching of the brachial plexus during a vaginal delivery. When the baby is in the typical head-down or vertex delivery position, forceful rotation or pulling on the head to deliver the shoulder may result in injury to the brachial plexus. Shoulder dystocia (difficult delivery of the shoulder) may also result in pulling on the nerves within the brachial plexus. The extent of injury in OBPP ranges from neuropraxia (temporary nerve conduction block due to stretching the nerves) to a complete avulsion in which the nerve root is forcefully torn away from the spinal cord.

Brachial plexus injuries are usually divided into 3 groups based on the portion of the brachial plexus involved: upper, lower, and total. Upper OBPP (often referred to as Erb's palsy) is the most common and involves the upper cervical nerves (C5-C6 and possibly C7).[1] An upper OBPP typically causes a child to maintain the involved UE in a stereotypical position classically called a "waiter's tip position": shoulder adduction and internal rotation with the elbow extended, forearm pronated, and wrist and fingers flexed. On occasion, the C4 nerve root and consequently the phrenic nerve may also be involved and can result in ipsilateral paralysis of the diaphragm. Lower OBPP is the least common type of OBPP and involves the lower portions of the brachial plexus (C7-T1).[1] Often known as Klumpke's palsy, lower OBPP results in intact proximal musculature at the shoulder and elbow, but paralysis of the wrist flexor and extensor muscles as well as the intrinsic muscles of the hand. Clinically, children with lower OBPPs hold the involved forearm in supination and demonstrate a poor grasp. Total OBPP injury (Erb-Klumpke palsy) involves the entire brachial plexus (C5-T1), resulting in total arm paralysis and loss of sensation. The degree of initial involvement in total OBPP injuries frequently diminishes over time with motor and sensory losses, eventually becoming more focused in areas innervated by the upper cervical roots. It is important to note that the pattern of motor and sensory loss in total OBPP injuries does not always fit into definitive categories, which may be related to the intercommunication and mixing of nerve roots in the brachial plexus. Although rare,[2] some children with brachial plexus injuries exhibit Horner syndrome, a condition that results from the loss of sympathetic nerve inputs provided through the T1 nerve root. Children with Horner syndrome may exhibit decreased sweating, abnormal pupillary contraction, and ptosis (droopy eyelid).

The incidence of OBPP varies from 0.15 to 2.54 per 1000 live births.[3] Risk factors include increased birth weight, shoulder dystocia, maternal diabetes, prolonged or difficult labor, breech delivery, and vacuum- or forceps-assisted delivery.[4,5] Although early studies reported rates of recovery as high as 92% in children with OBPP,[6-8] recent studies have suggested lower rates of full recovery ranging from 66% to 73%.[9-11] In a sample of 56 children with OBPP, Hoeksma et al.[9] found that 34% achieved full neurologic recovery within the first 3 weeks of life. An additional 32% achieved full neurologic recovery between 1.5 and 16 months of age (mean age of assessment 6.5 months). The remaining 34% had not achieved full recovery at 3 years of age. The authors reported that within this sample, the best predictors of a full neurologic recovery were recovery of shoulder external rotation and

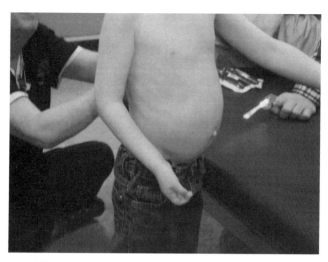

Figure 1-2. 4-year-old boy with right OBPP. Note the position of shoulder internal rotation and elbow flexion.

forearm supination. Prognosis for recovery could not be made based on an infant's initial presentation of symptoms (*e.g.*, Horner syndrome, total plexus involvement, phrenic nerve involvement) because an association between initial symptoms and total neurologic recovery was not found.[9]

Children with OBPP who do not achieve early and full recovery and those who never achieve full recovery may develop activity limitations that increase during childhood development. Children with OBPP may have difficulty reaching, grasping, and manipulating objects. These difficulties may increase as the child develops and is expected to add new skills and increase in independence. Bimanual skills and activities of daily living (ADLs) such as dressing, opening containers, and buttoning clothing may be especially challenging. Children with OBPP may also develop secondary impairments such as contractures and abnormal bone growth that may further impact functional use of the involved UE. Contracture development varies based on the child's specific pattern of motor loss. For example, a child with an upper brachial plexus (C5-C6) injury typically presents with contractures in shoulder adduction and internal rotation, forearm pronation, and either elbow extension or flexion depending on whether the triceps are innervated (Fig. 1-2). Although the development of bony deformities also depends on the pattern of motor loss, the majority of children with OBPP exhibit glenohumeral abnormalities.[12-14] Abnormal shortening of the clavicle and scapular abnormalities such as hypoplasia and malpositioning have been documented in children with OBPP (Fig. 1-3).[12,13] Compared to the uninvolved UE, bone mineral density is also decreased in the involved UE.[15]

In an attempt to maximize function, children with OBPP often exhibit atypical or abnormal muscle substitutions or other compensatory movement patterns based upon their available muscle innervation. For example, a child who has limited active ROM in overhead reach may use an increased lordosis to position the hand higher overhead (Fig. 1-4). Similarly, reaching patterns may lack variety and a child may

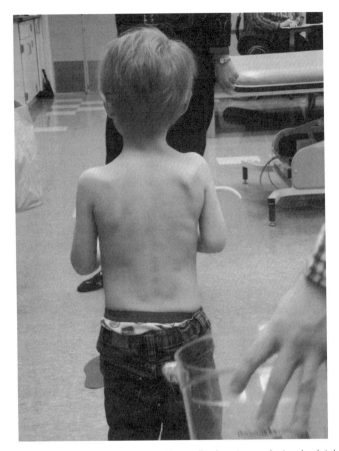

Figure 1-3. Note the scapular winging and shoulder girdle elevation on the involved right side.

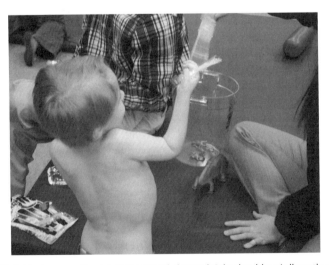

Figure 1-4. Note the increased lumbar lordosis and elevated right shoulder girdle as the child attempts to reach overhead with the involved right UE.

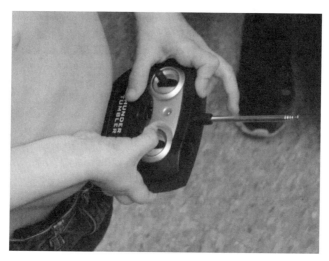

Figure 1-5. 4-year-old boy with right OBPP engaged in a bimanual task. Note the lack of refined grasp on the involved side.

perform all reaching tasks with the shoulder internally rotated, forearm pronated, and wrist flexed. Active forearm supination is often very difficult for children to achieve (Fig. 1-5). Because of a loss of sensation, some infants with OBPP will ignore or neglect the involved UE and may even develop self-injurious behaviors such as biting or pinching their involved arm. Some children may not be able to feel cuts, burns, or other injuries on the involved arm. During periods of nerve regeneration (whether occurring spontaneously or after a neurosurgical intervention), some children experience pain or hypersensitivity to touch prior to the restoration of normal sensation.[16] If neglect is severe and the child habitually turns the head away from the affected arm, a positional torticollis may develop.

Motor development may also be impacted in children with OBPP. Activities and mobility patterns in quadruped may be too difficult for some children and therefore may be skipped. Alternative forms of mobility such as scooting in sitting may be used or a child may just skip a floor mobility stage and go straight to walking. Children with OBPP also tend to perform movement transitions to their uninvolved side so they can maximally use their uninvolved UE to assist in these transitions. Protective reactions in sitting are often delayed or absent to the involved side. These factors combined with sensory losses in the involved UE may lead to the development of asymmetries in posture and movement.

For children who do not achieve early and full recovery, various neurosurgical interventions directed at ameliorating the primary insult may be considered. Neurosurgical options include nerve grafting, removal of scar tissue, and direct end-to-end anastomosis of nerve endings.[5,17,18] Traditionally, the primary determinant of the need for neurosurgical intervention was a lack of biceps function.[19] Later, studies that used a prediction model combining active movement scores of the elbow flexors and extensors, wrist and thumb extensors, and finger flexors and extensors were used to predict the need for neurosurgery.[6,7] Most recently, the best predictor of the need for neurosurgery has been identified as a lack of recovery in the shoulder external rotators and forearm supinators.[9]

Although opinions related to the timing and benefits of neurosurgical interventions vary,[5,17,18,20] it is generally agreed that children who have a total plexus injury plus Horner syndrome and who show no signs of recovery require neurosurgical repair in order to have any chance of an improved outcome.[3,17,20,21] It is also generally agreed that infants who demonstrate early and full recovery within 3 to 4 weeks of life are best managed conservatively and do not require neurosurgical interventions. Between these 2 extremes of recovery is what Bain et al.[20] refer to as the gray zone in which the necessity and timing of neurosurgical interventions is less clear. Because as many as 81% of children with OBPP fall within this gray zone at 1 month of age,[20] Bain et al.[20] created an algorithm to assist neurosurgeons with decision making for these children. The algorithm may be especially helpful given that the evidence related to the benefits of neurosurgical interventions versus nonoperative approaches is inconclusive for children with OBPP.[17]

Given the prevalence of UE contractures and other secondary orthopaedic impairments,[12-14] surgeries such as soft tissue releases, tendon transfers, and osteotomies are common in children with OBPP. While the timing of orthopaedic surgeries has been debated,[22-25] a recent study by Waters and Bae[26] found that in 23 young children with OBPP (average age 27 months) with mild-to-moderate glenohumeral dysplasia, tendon transfers at the rotator cuff combined with muscle lengthening procedures as indicated and open reduction of the glenohumeral joint improved shoulder function and promoted positive remodeling at the glenohumeral joint.

There are few studies examining the long-term impact of OBPP. Activities such as writing, performance of bimanual tasks, and participation in sports and leisure activities are difficult for children with OBPP.[27-29] In a study of 7- to 8-year-olds with a history of OBPP, a majority of the children preferred to use their uninvolved hand and greater than 45% complained of UE pain.[29] In a cohort of 70 individuals (7-20 years of age) with OBPP of varying degrees of severity, active shoulder ROM and hand function at age 5 years remained unchanged or improved during a follow-up 5 to 15 years later.[30] However, elbow function and active shoulder external rotation deteriorated over the course of the follow-up period.[30] A survey of adults with OBPP revealed that a majority of the respondents (average of 39.5 years) were still experiencing pain, impaired sensation, UE arthritis, and functional limitations that impeded ADLs.[31] Such studies suggest that **many children experience the impact of OBPP well into adulthood.**

Physical Therapy Patient/Client Management

The overall goals for the child with OBPP include encouraging functional use and improving active and passive ROM of the involved UE and promoting age-appropriate bimanual skills. For the current 13-month-old boy, bimanual tasks might include banging blocks, clapping, holding a large ball, donning and doffing socks, or holding a book. Based on the anticipated timeframe of nerve regeneration,[2,3,16] physical therapy interventions should also focus on supporting motor and sensory recovery until approximately 2 years of age.

Examination, Evaluation, and Diagnosis

A "rest" period of 7 to 10 days after birth is typically recommended for neonates with OBPP. This rest period allows for a reduction in the initial edema and hemorrhage of the affected nerves. During this time, any movement of the involved UE, including assessment of ROM, is prohibited. Therefore, the initial physical therapy examination is not conducted until after this rest period. A complete history must be obtained (birth, developmental, and medical) as well as current and past interventions related to the OBPP. Results of all medical tests such as MRIs, CTs, CT myelograms, and electromyography (EMG) should be gathered and reviewed. Other child-centered concerns should be explored, including the presence of pain or hypersensitivity in the involved UE.

Tests and measures should include age-appropriate examinations of pain, active and passive ROM, sensation, strength, motor function, and ADLs. In young infants, motor activity can be initially assessed through symmetrical assessment of developmental reflexes such as the Moro reflex, palmar grasp, and asymmetric tonic neck reflex. When moving the involved extremity, care must be taken to avoid aggressively stretching muscles or moving joints. Such activities may cause further damage to unstable joints. Motions of the involved limb should be assessed in a gravity-lessened position as well as in positions against gravity. Because visual estimates may not provide an accurate appraisal of active ROM in children with OBPP,[32] therapists should use tools such as the Active Movement Scale[33] to assess active motion in infants and young children such as the 13-month-old in this case. The Active Movement Scale[33] assesses 15 different motions of the involved UE and may be used with children with OBPP from birth to 4 years, 7 months of age. The 8-point ordinal scale ranges from a score of 0 (no contraction) to 7 (full motion against gravity) and does not require the child to perform tasks on demand. For older children, the Mallet Classification of Function in OBPP[34] is often used to measure and track motor recovery after a surgical intervention. In the Mallet Classification, the involved extremity is tested in 5 different movements: shoulder abduction, shoulder external rotation, placing the hand behind the head, placing the hand to the back, and bringing the hand to the mouth. Grades for each movement range from I (no active motion) to V (normal movement that is equal to the contralateral limb, if unaffected).

Sensation testing in any infant can be challenging. In the infant who has OBPP, the therapist must attempt to determine if there are areas of diminished or absent sensation in the involved arm. The Sensory Grading System for Children with Brachial Plexus Injury[16] can be used to provide general information about sensation in the involved UE. In this grading system, scores range from S0 (no reaction to painful or other stimuli) to S3 (apparently normal sensation). The skin wrinkle test[35] is another simple screen that can be used to assess the presence or absence of sensation at the palmar surface of the fingertips. Based on the premise that denervated skin does not wrinkle when soaked in water, the wrinkle test requires soaking the child's involved hand in warm water for 15 to 30 minutes and then checking for the presence of wrinkling. In an adaptation of the wrinkle test, the therapist can simply wrap the fingertips in a wet towel or other cloth for several minutes; this has been shown to be an effective alternative to prolonged soaking.[36] While the wrinkle test may help determine the presence of innervation to the skin, the presence of wrinkling does not correlate with the child's sensory function or discrimination.[35]

In 2013, Bialocerkowski et al.[37] conducted a systematic review to evaluate the psychometric properties of various outcome measures that have been used to quantify UE function in children with OBPP. The 3 tools with the most robust psychometric properties included the **Assisting Hand Assessment (AHA), the self-care domain of the Pediatric Evaluation of Disability Inventory (PEDI), and the Pediatric Outcomes Data Collection Instrument (PODCI).** The AHA was designed to evaluate a child's use of his involved hand for bimanual tasks during a 10- to 15-minute semi-structured play session.[38] Consisting of 22 items, the AHA is scored from video recordings of the play sessions and is intended for use with children ages 18 months to 12 years who have either OBPP or hemiplegic cerebral palsy.[38] The PEDI is a caregiver-report assessment that can be used as a normative measure in children ages 6 months to 7.5 years and as a criterion measure in children older than 7.5 years who have delays.[39] Although the self-care domain of the PEDI can differentiate between the reported self-care activities of children with OBPP who have different levels of involvement (upper, lower, or total plexus injuries),[40] the newer Pediatric Evaluation of Disability Inventory-Computer Adaptive Test (PEDI-CAT) was designed to be used with children who have any diagnosis or condition that impacts development or function.[41] The PEDI-CAT is administered via a computer software program and the item bank contains 276 activities and explores function in 4 domains: Daily Activities, Mobility, Social/Cognitive, and Responsibility.[41] The PEDI-CAT has adequate concurrent validity, reliability, and score distribution for use with children from birth through age 20 years.[41] The PODCI is a standardized outcome assessment for use with children younger than 19 years who have musculoskeletal conditions.[42] It provides a semi-quantitative patient and parent report of function and quality of life in the following 5 domains: transfers, UE function, ability to participate in sports, comfort or pain, and happiness. A global function score is derived from the first 4 domains.[42] Children with OBPP have reported lower PODCI scores in UE function, sports, and global function than their typically developing peers.[43] Given that the PODCI was developed primarily as an outcome measure for children undergoing orthopaedic surgery,[42] the PODCI may be the best tool to provide a preoperative baseline measure of function and to document postoperative functional gains for children with OBPP. Thus, this tool would not be appropriate for the current child who had a neurologic surgery (nerve graft) approximately 7 months prior to this therapy evaluation.

Although not specifically developed for use with children who have OBPP, normative developmental tests such as the Peabody Developmental Motor Scales, Second Edition (PDMS-2) may be helpful to monitor and track delays in gross or fine motor development. Designed to assess motor skills in children from birth through 5 years of age,[44] the PDMS-2 consists of a Gross Motor Scale and a Fine Motor Scale. Depending on the age of the child, the Gross Motor Scale consists of 3 of 4 subtests: Reflexes, Stationary, Locomotion, and Object Manipulation. The Fine Motor Scale consists of 2 subtests: Grasping and Visual-Motor Integration. Given that the toddler in this case is older than 12 months, the Stationary, Locomotion, and Object Manipulation subtests of the Gross Motor Scale and both subtests of the Fine Motor Scale could be administered.[44]

Plan of Care and Interventions

Precautions and contraindications for therapeutic interventions often vary among physicians and these may apply whether or not the child with OBPP has had a surgical intervention. As such, the physical therapist should verify if there are any precautions or contraindications regarding specific movements or UE weightbearing prior to initiating intervention. After the initial rest period of 7 to 10 days after birth, physical therapy interventions can typically commence safely. However, aggressive movements that force joints or overstretch the involved UE must be avoided because these may cause further damage. After the physical therapy examination has been completed, a home exercise program (HEP) should be initiated that includes appropriate ROM techniques for all UE joints at risk for contracture. The HEP should also emphasize precautions related to joint dislocation and subluxation. Murphy et al.[45] found that use of a digital video disc (DVD) increased compliance with a HEP over a 3-month period from a baseline of 74% without using the DVD to 96% when using the DVD. Although compliance at 12 months fell to 84%, the authors suggested that caregiver compliance with a HEP for children with OBPP may be improved using media such as a DVD.[45]

As the infant grows, interventions targeting activation of weak musculature during age-appropriate functional activities should be encouraged during therapy sessions as well as at home. Placing the infant in postures in which weak muscles are in a gravity-lessened position and using manual contacts to gently guide and direct movements may assist in strengthening. For example, the therapist could position the infant in sidelying on the uninvolved (left) side and strategically place toys in an area where the infant could easily reach the toys with the involved (right) UE. The therapist could then use manual contacts on the involved UE to help ensure that the infant's reaching pattern maximized use of weak musculature while discouraging unwanted motions such as internal rotation of the shoulder and pronation at the forearm. Recognizing that decreases in bone mineral density occur in the involved UE of children with OBPP, Ibrahim et al.[15] suggested that incorporation of weightbearing exercises into intervention programs of older children might be helpful in improving bone mineral density.

Other interventions to address UE contractures and improve function in children with an OBPP include **serial casting and splinting**. Ho et al.[46] found that serial casting and splinting of elbow contractures in children with OBPP was effective in reducing contractures. Maintenance of the treatment effect was dependent on patient age and compliance with follow-up preventive measures.[46] In children with OBPP who had previously undergone unsuccessful serial casting interventions, Basciani and Intiso[47] found that injections of botulinum toxin type-A followed by serial casting significantly improved active elbow extension at 12 months postinjection. DeMatteo et al.[48] further proposed that botulinum toxin type-A injections alone may provide an opportunity to facilitate motor learning through improved voluntary relaxation of antagonist muscles while allowing increased activity in muscles re-innervated either via spontaneous recovery or through a neurosurgical procedure such as a nerve graft.

Although early reports by Eng et al.[2] advocated the use of electrical stimulation in individuals with OBPP, few studies have explored this intervention. In a sample of 16 subjects with upper plexus injuries, Okafor et al.[49] randomly assigned infants to an electrical stimulation group or a conventional physical therapy group. At the end of a 6-week intervention period, the intervention group had statistically significant mean improvements in shoulder abduction, elbow flexion, wrist extension, and arm circumference. Given the small sample size (8 subjects in each group), further research is necessary to confirm these findings.

Evidence-Based Clinical Recommendations

SORT: Strength of Recommendation Taxonomy

A: Consistent, good-quality patient-oriented evidence
B: Inconsistent or limited-quality patient-oriented evidence
C: Consensus, disease-oriented evidence, usual practice, expert opinion, or case series

1. Children with obstetric brachial plexus palsy may experience the impact of the condition well into adulthood. **Grade A**

2. The tools with the most robust psychometric properties for quantifying UE function in children with OBPP are the Assisting Hand Assessment (AHA), the self-care domain of the Pediatric Evaluation of Disability Inventory (PEDI), and the Pediatric Outcomes Data Collection Instrument (PODCI). **Grade A**

3. Serial casting, splinting, and injection of botulinum toxin-A improve contractures and function in the affected upper extremity of children with OBPP. **Grade B**

COMPREHENSION QUESTIONS

1.1 Which of the following nerve segments is most frequently injured in obstetric brachial plexus palsy?
   A. C4-C5
   B. C5-C6
   C. C7-C8
   D. C8-T1

1.2 Which of the following conditions is a risk factor for obstetric brachial plexus palsy?
   A. Decreased birth weight
   B. Maternal hypoglycemia
   C. Premature birth
   D. Shoulder dystocia

1.3 The Assisting Hand Assessment is intended for use with children in which of the following age ranges?

A. 6 months to 7.5 years

B. 18 months to 12 years

C. Birth to 5 years

D. Birth to 19 years

ANSWERS

1.1 **B.** Obstetric brachial plexus palsy typically involves the upper plexus, which consists of C5-C6 nerve roots.

1.2 **D.** Shoulder dystocia, or difficult delivery of the shoulder, may result in pulling on the nerves within the brachial plexus and is therefore a risk factor for obstetric brachial plexus palsy.

1.3 **B.** The Assisting Hand Assessment was developed for use with children 18 months to 12 years of age.

REFERENCES

1. Strombeck C, Krumlinde-Sundholm L, Forssberg H. Functional outcome at 5 years in children with obstetrical brachial plexus palsy with and without microsurgical reconstruction. *Dev Med Child Neurol.* 2000;42:148-157.

2. Eng GD, Koch B, Smokvina MD. Brachial plexus palsy in neonates and children. *Arch Phys Med Rehabil.* 1978;59:458-464.

3. Pondaag W, Malessy MJ, van Dijk JG, Thomeer RT. Natural history of obstetric brachial plexus palsy: a systematic review. *Dev Med Child Neurol.* 2004;46:138-144.

4. Thatte MR, Mehta R. Obstetric brachial plexus injury. *Indian J Plast Surg.* 2011;4:380-389.

5. Dunham EA. Obstetrical brachial plexus palsy. *Orthop Nurs.* 2003;22:106-116.

6. Michelow BJ, Clarke HM, Curtis CG, Zuker RM, Seifu Y, Andrews DF. The natural history of obstetrical brachial plexus palsy. *Plast Reconstr Surg.* 1994;93:675-680.

7. Clarke HM, Curtis CG. An approach to obstetrical brachial plexus injuries. *Hand Clin.* 1995;11:563-581.

8. Gordon M, Rich H, Deutschberger J, Green M. The immediate and long-term outcome of obstetric birth trauma. I. Brachial plexus paralysis. *Am J Obstet Gynecol.* 1973;117:51-56.

9. Hoeksma AF, ter Steeg AM, Nelissen RG, van Ouwerkerk WJ, Lankhorst G, de Jong BA. Neurological recovery in obstetric brachial plexus palsy: an historical cohort study. *Dev Med Child Neurol.* 2004;46:46-83.

10. Hoeksma AF, Wolf H, Oei SL. Obstetrical brachial plexus injuries: incidence, natural course and shoulder contracture. *Clin Rehabil.* 2000;14:523-526.

11. DiTaranto P, Campagna L, Price AE, Grossman JA. Outcome following nonoperative treatment of brachial plexus birth injuries. *J Child Neurol.* 2004;19:87-90.

12. Hoeksma AF, ter Steeg AM, Dijkstra P, Nelissen RG, Beelen A, de Jong BA. Shoulder contracture and osseous deformity in obstetrical brachial plexus injuries. *J Bone Joint Surg Am.* 2003;85:316-322.

13. Kon DS, Darakjian AB, Pearl ML, Kosco AE. Glenohumeral deformity in children with internal rotation contractures secondary to brachial plexus birth palsy: intraoperative arthrographic classification. *Radiology.* 2004;231:791-795.

14. Sibinski M, Woźniakowski B, Drobniewski M, Synder M. Secondary glenohumeral joint dysplasia in children with persistent obstetric brachial plexus palsy. *Int Orthop.* 2010;34:863-867.

15. Ibrahim AI, Hawamdeh ZM, Alsharif AA. Evaluation of bone mineral density in children with perinatal brachial plexus palsy: effectiveness of weight bearing and traditional exercises. *Bone.* 2011;49:499-505.

16. Narakas AO. Obstetric brachial plexus injuries. In: Lamb DW, ed. *The Paralyzed Hand.* Edinburgh: Churchill Livingstone; 1987:116-135.

17. McNeeley PD, Drake JM. A systematic review of brachial plexus surgery for birth-related brachial plexus injury. *Pediatr Neurosurg.* 2003;38:57-62.

18. Grossman JA, DiTaranto P, Yaylali I, Alfonso I, Ramos LE, Price AE. Shoulder function following late neurolysis and bypass grafting for upper brachial plexus birth injuries. *J Hand Surg Br.* 2004;29:356-358.

19. Gilbert A, Razaboni R, Amar-Khodja S. Indications and results of brachial plexus surgery in obstetrical palsy. *Orthop Clin North Am.* 1988;19:91-105.

20. Bain JR, Dematteo C, Gjertsen D, Hollenberg RD. Navigating the gray zone: a guide for surgical decision making in obstetrical brachial plexus injuries. *J Neurosurg Pediatr.* 2007;3:173-180.

21. Gilbert A, Pivato G, Kheiralla T. Long-term results of primary repair of brachial plexus lesions in children. *Microsurgery.* 2006;26:334-342.

22. Waters PM, Bae DS. The effect of derotational humeral osteotomy on global shoulder function in brachial plexus birth palsy. *J Bone Joint Surg Am.* 2006;88:1035-1042.

23. Kirkos JM, Papadopoulos IA. Late treatment of brachial plexus palsy secondary to birth injuries: rotational osteotomy of the proximal part of the humerus. *J Bone Joint Surg Am.* 1998;80:1477-1483.

24. Waters PM. Obstetric brachial plexus injuries: evaluation and management. *J Am Acad Orthop Surg.* 1997;5:205-214.

25. Waters PM, Peljovich AE. Shoulder reconstruction in patients with chronic brachial plexus birth palsy. A case control study. *Clin Orthop Relat Res.* 1999;364:144-152.

26. Waters PM, Bae DS. The early effects of tendon transfers and open capsulorrhaphy on glenohumeral deformity in brachial plexus birth palsy. *J Bone Joint Surg Am.* 2008;90:2171-2179.

27. Sundholm LK, Eliasson AC, Forssberg H. Obstetric brachial plexus injuries: assessment protocol and functional outcome at age 5 years. *Dev Med Child Neurol.* 1998;40:4-11.

28. Bellew M, Kay SP, Webb F, Ward A. Developmental and behavioural outcome in obstetric brachial plexus injury. *J Hand Surg Br.* 2000;25:49-51.

29. Spaargaren E, Ahmed J, van Ouwerkerk WJ, de Groot V, Beckerman H. Aspects of activities and participation of 7-8 year-old children with an obstetric brachial plexus injury. *Eur J Paediatr Neurol.* 2011;15:345-352.

30. Strombeck C, Krumlinde-Sundholm L, Remahl S, Sejersen T. Long-term follow-up of children with obstetric brachial plexus palsy. I. Functional aspects. *Dev Med Child Neurol.* 2007;49:198-203.

31. Partridge C, Edwards S. Obstetric brachial plexus palsy: increasing disability and exacerbation of symptoms with age. *Physiother Res Int.* 2004;9:157-163.

32. Bialocerkowski A, Galea M. Comparison of visual and objective quantification of elbow and shoulder movement in children with obstetric brachial plexus palsy. *J Brachial Plex Peripher Nerve Inj.* 2006;1:5.

33. Curtis C, Stephens D, Clarke HM, Andrews D. The active movement scale: an evaluative tool for infants with obstetrical brachial plexus palsy. *J Hand Surg Am.* 2002;27:470-478.

34. Mallet J. Paralysie obstétricale du plexus brachial. Traitement des séquelles. Primauté du traitement de l'épaule. — Méthode d'expression des résultats. [Obstetrical paralysis of the brachial plexus. II. Therapeutics. Treatment of sequelae. Priority for the treatment of the shoulder. Method for the expression of results.] *Rev Chir Orthop Reparatrice Appar Mot.* 1972;58(Suppl 1):166-168.

35. Phelps PE, Walker E. Comparison of the finger wrinkling test results to established sensory tests in peripheral nerve injury. *Am J Occup Ther.* 1977;31:565-572.

36. Tindall A, Dawood R, Povlsen B. Case of the month: The skin wrinkle test: a simple nerve injury test for paediatric and uncooperative patients. *Emerg Med J.* 2006;23:883-886.

37. Bialocerkowski A, O'shea K, Pin TW. Psychometric properties of outcome measures for children and adolescents with brachial plexus birth palsy: a systematic review. *Dev Med Child Neurol.* 2013;55:1075-1088.

38. Krumlinde-Sudholm L, Eliasson AC. Development of the assisting hand assessment: a Rasch-built measure intended for children with unilateral upper limb impairments. *Scand J Occup Ther.* 2003;10:16-26.

39. Haley SM, Coster WJ, Ludlow LH, Haltiwanger JT, Andrellos PA. *Pediatric Evaluation of Disability Inventory: Development, Standardization and Administration Manual.* Boston, MA: Trustees of Boston University; 1992.

40. Ho ES, Curtis CG, Clarke HM. Pediatric Evaluation of Disability Inventory: its application to children with obstetrical brachial plexus palsy. *J Hand Surg Am.* 2006;31:197-202.

41. Haley SM, Coster W. *PEDI-CAT: Development, Standardization and Administration Manual.* Boston, MA: CRECare LLC; 2010.

42. Daltroy LH, Liang MH, Fossel AH, Goldberg MJ. The POSNA Pediatric Musculoskeletal Functional Health Questionnaire: report on reliability, validity, and sensitivity to change. *J Pediatr Orthop.* 1998;18:561-571.

43. Huffman GR, Bagley AM, James MA, Lerman JA, Rab G. Assessment of children with brachial plexus birth palsy using the pediatric outcomes data collection instrument. *J Pediatr Orthop.* 2005;25:400-404.

44. Fewell RR, Folio MR. *Peabody Developmental Motor Scales.* 2nd ed. Austin, TX: Pro-Ed; 2000.

45. Murphy K, Rasmussen L, Hervey-Jumper S, Justice D, Nelson V, Yang L. An assessment of compliance utility of a home exercise DVD for caregivers of children and adolescents with brachial plexus palsy: a pilot study. *PM R.* 2012;4:190-197.

46. Ho ES, Roy T, Stephens D, Clarke HM. Serial casting and splinting of elbow contractures in children with obstetric brachial plexus palsy. *J Hand Surg Am.* 2010;35:84-91.

47. Basciani M, Intiso D. Botulinum toxin type-A and plaster cast treatment in children with upper brachial plexus palsy. *Pediatr Rehabil.* 2006;9:165-170.

48. DeMatteo C, Bain J, Galea V, Gjertsen D. Botulinum toxin as an adjunct to motor learning and therapy and surgery for obstetrical brachial plexus palsy. *Dev Med Child Neurol.* 2006;48:245-252.

49. Okafor U, Akinbo S, Sokunbi O, Okanlawon A, Woronha C. Comparison of electrical stimulation and conventional physiotherapy in functional rehabilitation in Erb's palsy. *Nig Q J Hosp Med.* 2008;18:202-205.

Spinal Cord Injury

Dana Robinson Johnson
Kimberly A. Scharff

CASE 2

A healthy and typically developing 14-year-old male was involved in a high-speed motor vehicle collision in which he was an unrestrained front-seat passenger. Upon assessment by first responders, he was unable to move any of his extremities. The patient was placed in a hard cervical collar and was immobilized on a backboard for transport to the trauma center. He was initially assessed in the emergency department. Radiographs revealed a fractured C6 vertebra. He was able to flex his elbows bilaterally against resistance and weakly extend his wrists. He demonstrated patchy sensation throughout his upper extremities and trunk. His initial International Standards for Neurological Classification of Spinal Cord Injury (ISNCSCI) score was C6 AIS B. He was placed on high-dose glucocorticoids and admitted to the intensive care unit for further management. Two days later, he underwent surgical fusion from C6 to T2 to stabilize his spine. Six days later, he was transferred to an acute rehabilitation hospital, where physical therapy evaluation and treatment started. A repeated ISNCSCI examination score of C7 AIS C showed that some neurologic recovery had occurred with fair muscle strength in bilateral triceps and finger flexors and trace contraction in bilateral hip flexors.

▶ Which outcome measure is used to determine the level and severity of a spinal cord injury (SCI)?
▶ What are the examination priorities?
▶ Describe a physical therapy plan of care based on the patient's age and level of injury.

KEY DEFINITIONS

AUTONOMIC DYSREFLEXIA: Potentially life-threatening condition that is triggered by a painful stimulus below the level of the SCI; typically characterized by headache, elevated blood pressure, bradycardia or tachycardia, and flushing above the level of the injury

HETEROTOPIC OSSIFICATION: Development of new, ectopic bone within soft tissues around peripheral joints in individuals with neurologic disorders

Objectives

1. Describe the unique mechanisms of injury associated with pediatric SCI.
2. Describe the purpose of the ISNCSCI examination and its reliability in the pediatric population.
3. Describe the common musculoskeletal impairments and complications associated with pediatric SCI.
4. Describe considerations for the short-term and long-term medical management of the adolescent with SCI.
5. Describe an appropriate physical therapy plan of care for an adolescent with SCI.
6. Identify the mobility-related durable medical equipment needs of a adolescent with SCI.

Physical Therapy Considerations

PT considerations during management of the adolescent with SCI:

▶ **General physical therapy plan of care/goals:** Promote independence with mobility and activities of daily living; promote quality of life; reduce/minimize risk of secondary complications and comorbidities

▶ **Physical therapy interventions:** Patient/family education regarding SCI and associated secondary complications; mobility training including balance and transfer training, wheelchair skills and upright mobility, when indicated; stretching and strengthening of intact/impaired muscles to maximize function; stretching of muscles below the level of injury to prevent contractures

▶ **Precautions during physical therapy interventions:** Monitor for signs/symptoms of autonomic dysreflexia (AD) in at-risk individuals; care when transferring/handling patients to prevent iatrogenic fractures due to decreased bone mineral density (BMD); orthostatic hypotension

▶ **Complications interfering with physical therapy:** AD, long bone fractures, scoliosis, hip subluxation/dislocation, skin breakdown, orthostatic hypotension, contractures, spasticity

Understanding the Health Condition

Pediatric SCI is a lifelong, low-incidence, high-cost disability that has a profound effect on both the child involved and his or her family. The National Spinal Cord Injury Association defines pediatric SCI as an acute traumatic lesion of the spinal cord and nerve roots in children from newborn to 15 years old.[1]

Spinal cord injuries can be divided into non-traumatic and traumatic. A non-traumatic SCI is any damage to the spinal cord that has not been caused by a major trauma. Common causes of non-traumatic SCI are myelopathies. These can be compressive, caused by some underlying structural abnormality combined with an antecedent trigger, like a fall, that leads to cord compression.[2] They also include neuroinflammatory disorders. Non-traumatic SCI can also be caused by a vascular insult, such as a spinal arteriovenous malformation or neoplasm. Individuals with non-traumatic SCIs do not necessarily enter major trauma or rehabilitation centers and thus are not easily tracked in SCI registries or databases, leading to variable epidemiologic data. A traumatic SCI is damage to the spinal cord that is due to a traumatic injury that results in a bruise or contusion, partial tear, or complete transection of the spinal cord. Common causes are motor vehicle collisions, falls, gunshot wounds, and sports-related injuries.

Every year 11,000 to 12,000 people in the United States sustain a SCI and an estimated 250,000 to 400,000 people are currently living with SCI.[1-3] SCIs in the pediatric population are relatively rare, with only 3.5% occurring in children younger than 15 years.[4] The overall incidence of pediatric SCI in the United States is 2 cases per 100,000 children, correlating with 1450 new pediatric SCI cases per year.[5] In the adult population, traumatic SCIs mainly affect males, accounting for more than 80% of all reported cases; during the adolescent years, the male-to-female ratio is similar. The higher incidence of males during the adolescent years can be attributed to increased risk-taking behaviors of adolescent boys.[6]

In general, the occurrence of pediatric SCI peaks between June and September, occurring most frequently in July and least frequently in February.[7,8] The most common etiology is motor vehicle collision, accounting for 40% to 50%. The second most common cause is accidental falls (14%), followed by acts of violence (gunshot wounds) and sports injuries.[9] Based on information gathered from the Kids' Inpatient Database and the National Trauma Database, there is a significantly higher incidence of SCI in African American children than in Native American and Hispanic children.

Other features of pediatric SCI include injuries without radiologic abnormalities, upper cervical injuries, birth trauma, child abuse, and lap-belt injuries. The interaction between growth and development is responsible for many of these unique features. In adults, traumatic SCIs result from various mechanisms of injury including flexion, hyperextension, flexion-rotation, axial loading, burst fractures, and compression fractures. However, a child's spine does not fully mature until 8 to 10 years of age and can subsequently lend itself to different mechanisms of injury.[10] Ligamentous laxity, disproportionately large head size relative to body size, inherent elasticity of the vertebral column, and horizontally oriented facet joints can create a fulcrum for sagittal force. These properties allow a large amount of translatory movement and render the pediatric spine exceedingly vulnerable to disruptive forces.[11] This explains why a significant number of pediatric patients present with signs and symptoms of SCI, but lack radiologic evidence of bony injury, also known as SCIWORA (spinal cord injury without radiographic abnormality). Mechanisms associated with SCIWORA are typically high-energy impacts with hinging forces that produce extreme stretching and whipping of the child's head and neck.[12] SCIWORA injuries occur nearly exclusively in children because of their immature anatomy and have been reported in 19% to 34% of all children who experience SCI.[13] A study by Pang and Wilberger[11] reported that 64% of children 5 years of age or younger at the time of injury will suffer a SCIWORA. However, the incidence of SCIWORA drops to 35% in ages 6 to 12 years and to 20% in children injured after the age of 12 years.[11] In children younger than 11 years, upper cervical injuries (C3 and above) are more common; over the age of 11, children have a greater propensity to sustain a lower cervical injury due to the slightly more mature upper cervical spine.[5]

The **ISNCSCI** were developed by the American Spinal Injury Association (ASIA) as a universal classification tool for the evaluation of neurologic impairment following SCI.[14] During this assessment, sensory (pinprick and light touch) and motor examinations are used to identify the level and severity of injury. At the end of the examination, a patient is assigned a neurologic level, a sensory level, a motor level, and a letter grade based on the ASIA Impairment Scale (AIS) to determine the degree of impairment and the level of completeness.[15,16] The neurologic level is the most caudal segment of the cord with intact motor and sensory function bilaterally. The motor level and the sensory level are the most caudal segments of the cord where there is intact bilateral motor and sensory function, respectively.[17] The AIS classification will designate whether an injury is complete (AIS A: no sensory or motor function is preserved in the sacral segments S4-S5) or incomplete and, if incomplete, designate the grade of incompleteness (AIS B, C, or D). AIS B is termed Sensory Complete in which sensory but not motor function is preserved below the neurologic level and includes the sacral segments S4-S5, *and* no motor function is preserved more than 3 levels below the motor level on either side of the body. AIS C, or Motor Incomplete, designates that motor function is preserved below the neurologic level, and more than half of key muscle functions below the single neurologic level of injury have a muscle grade less than 3. Last, AIS D is called Motor Incomplete. An AIS D level indicates that motor function is preserved below the neurologic level, and at least half of key muscle functions below the neurologic level have a muscle grade of 3 or greater. While the ASIA examination is a reliable tool for the neurologic assessment of an adult with SCI, it has been shown to have poor reliability for children younger than 4 years, secondary to an inability of the child to comprehend the instructions of the examination. Children younger than 10 years may have unreliable pinprick sensory examination secondary to anxiety, and the anal motor portion of the examination may be difficult to assess in children injured prior to achieving bowel continence. Based on research conducted at a model pediatric SCI rehabilitation hospital, formal testing should be delayed until the age of 4 years. Prior to this age, a modified examination consisting of observational motor activity and appreciation of sensation should be conducted. In the case of a modified examination, parents need to be informed that their child's young age will limit the reliability of classification and that only an estimated neurologic level can be provided.[18]

Based on the International Standards examination, SCIs are classified as either neurologically complete or incomplete, which is the most significant determinant of prognosis. A complete injury is described as the absence of sensory *and* motor function in the lowest sacral segments S4-S5 (i.e., AIS A). An incomplete injury is defined as preservation of sensory *or* motor function below the neurologic level that includes the lowest sacral segments S4-S5.[15] In individuals with complete SCIs, the extent of motor recovery is minimal to nonexistent. In contrast, there is frequently substantial recovery following incomplete SCI. A study by Burns et al.[19] reported that 20% to 75% of individuals with incomplete SCI regain the capacity to ambulate, to some degree, 1 year after injury. The majority of neurologic recovery occurs within the first 6 to 9 months, and the degree of improvement plateaus between 12 and 18 months after initial injury. Some studies have shown that 10% to 20% of complete injuries can change to incomplete during the first year, highlighting the importance of ongoing and reliable neurologic reassessment. The potential for a large amount of neurologic recovery in those with incomplete SCI can switch the focus of physical therapy from teaching compensatory techniques to recovering lost function.[10]

The location of spinal cord damage determines the extent of physical impairments. Injury to the cord in the cervical region results in tetraplegia, which is impairment or loss of motor and/or sensory function in all 4 extremities and the trunk, including the muscles of respiration. Injury to the cord in the thoracic, lumbar, or sacral regions results in paraplegia, which is an impairment or loss of motor and/or sensory function in all or part of the trunk and both lower extremities. Neurologic level and severity of injury vary as a function of age. In children aged 8 years and younger, 70% have paraplegia and approximately two-thirds have complete injuries. However, 50% of adolescents have paraplegia and 50% have complete lesions. Because of a proportionately larger head and underdeveloped neck musculature, younger children are more likely to have upper cervical injuries.[20]

Ultimately, the child with SCI is at risk for the same comorbidities and complications experienced by an adult with SCI. These comorbidities affect the neuromusculoskeletal, cardiovascular, and respiratory systems. However, the impact of such complications can be greater on the growing child and may persist into adulthood. The signs and symptoms of these conditions may vary in children, requiring more diligence on the part of the healthcare team.

The child with SCI is at risk for skeletal and joint deformity associated with bone growth in regions of the body where the muscles are paralyzed. In children with SCI, the incidence of hip subluxation (loss of containment of the femoral head within the acetabulum as seen on radiograph; Fig. 2-1) is between 29% and 82%. This typically occurs gradually over several years following SCI, but can be associated with trauma at the time of injury. The highest rate of hip dislocation occurs in children injured prior to age 10 years.[21] McCarthy and Betz[21] found that 93% of children injured prior to age 10 developed hip subluxation or dislocation, whereas only 9% of children injured after age 10 were affected. Aggressive prevention of hip dislocation is recommended for children injured prior to age 10. Prevention methods include soft tissue stretching, spasticity control, and prophylactic night bracing with a hip abduction orthosis. When prevention is ineffective, surgical treatment is

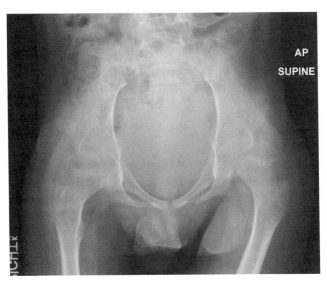

Figure 2-1. Anteroposterior (AP) radiograph of pelvis and hips showing poor containment of the femoral heads in the acetabula, indicating hip subluxation.

rarely indicated unless functional improvement is an anticipated surgical outcome. Although ambulation with bracing in children is typically unaffected by a dislocated hip, studies of adults with SCI have shown potential for future pain, skin breakdown, and sitting intolerance. Therefore, surgical correction of a dislocated hip in a child with SCI may be warranted (Fig. 2-2). Surgical treatment of hip

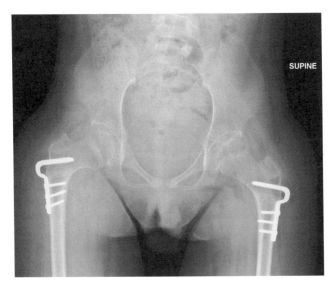

Figure 2-2. AP radiograph taken after proximal femoral derotational osteotomies to correct bilateral subluxed hips seen in Fig. 2-1.

dislocation may also include soft tissue releases, bony procedures (femoral and/ or acetabular osteotomies), and/or muscle transfers to ensure containment of the femoral head within the bony acetabulum. Surgery is typically followed by a period of immobilization in a hip spica cast or an abduction orthosis.[21]

Scoliosis affects 46% to 98% of children who sustain a SCI prior to their adolescent growth spurt.[22] Children with a scoliotic curve less than 20° may benefit from wearing a prophylactic brace, with the goal of preventing spinal surgery or reducing the extent of future surgery. For children with 20° to 40° curves, bracing may help delay the time until surgery. Bracing is not recommended when the child's curve has progressed beyond 40°, as bracing may cause skin breakdown.[22]

Children with SCI are at risk for development of severe contractures in paralyzed limbs. Commonly seen contractures include hip and knee flexion contractures and ankle plantar flexion or equinus contractures. Contractures can result in impaired sitting tolerance, inability to stand/ambulate, difficulty with skin hygiene, skin breakdown, joint damage, and impaired self-esteem. Prevention of joint contractures includes regular soft tissue stretching, splinting and bracing, and prone positioning to prevent flexion contractures at the hips and knees. When conservative management is ineffective, and contractures interfere with function such as upright mobility or sitting posture or result in discomfort, surgical intervention is warranted. Planning for surgical treatment of contractures requires commitment by the patient and family to intensive postoperative therapeutic interventions including stretching and bracing to prevent recurrence.[21]

As in the adult population with SCI, children with SCI are at risk for decreased BMD and osteoporosis. Following SCI, the trabecular bone of the pelvis and lower extremities is rapidly lost.[7] The pathogenesis of this process is complex and not fully understood. Immobilization and muscle atrophy result in decreased mechanical forces on the bones, which contribute to increased bone resorption and decreased bone formation.[23] Forty percent of BMD is lost via calcium secreted in the urine secondary to immobilization hypercalcemia. Treatment for immobilization hypercalcemia in the non-SCI population typically includes remobilization (*i.e.*, following a fracture). Because remobilization is typically not an option for the SCI population, treatment for immobilization hypercalcemia includes pharmacologically reducing calcium loss from bones and enhancing urinary excretion of calcium.[24] With or without intervention, a steady state between bone resorption and bone formation is typically reached approximately 2 years post-injury.[23]

Decreased BMD can result in pathologic fractures and heterotopic ossification (HO). Prevalence of fractures in children with SCI has been reported between 10% and 20%.[21] A child with SCI may not complain of pain associated with a fracture in an area of the body with impaired sensation; therefore, the caregiver as well as the physical therapist must be vigilant for signs of fracture that may include deformity, crepitus, swelling, erythema, and systemic fever. Treatment of long bone fractures typically consists of immobilization with a soft splint to decrease the risk of skin breakdown associated with casting an insensate limb.[21] Many studies have addressed pharmacologic management of osteoporosis in adults with SCI. Bisphosphonates are inhibitors of bone resorption and may have some effectiveness in reducing hypercalcemia and bone loss in the adult SCI population, particularly when administered during the first 12 months post-injury.[25] However, despite the use of bisphosphonates for more than 20 years in the adult SCI population, there is inadequate evidence to recommend use of bisphosphonates as routine prophylaxis for fractures in this population.[23] The research in the pediatric SCI population is even further limited. However, a recent case study reported that zoledronic acid (a common bisphosphonate) initiated approximately 1.5 years post-injury in a 12-year-old male with C3 incomplete SCI showed some benefit.[23] After 18 months of bisphosphonate therapy, the patient demonstrated improvements in bone mass, density, and strength that were not attributed to maturation and growth. The authors concluded that bisphosphonate therapy has the potential to prevent bone resorption and thus limit loss of trabecular bone in children. Management of decreased BMD may also be addressed through various physical therapy interventions, including standing and electrical stimulation. However, evidence for the effectiveness of these interventions in the SCI population is equivocal.

Related to the loss of BMD is the development of HO, which is the formation of new, ectopic bone in the soft tissues that surround peripheral joints. In individuals with SCI, HO forms only in joints below the level of the injury. Most commonly, HO occurs at the hip (70%-97%), followed by the knee, elbow, shoulder, and spine in descending order of incidence.[26] Development of HO is less common in children than in adults, with a reported incidence of 3% to 18% in children versus 20% to 50% in adults.[5] In the adult population, HO is most commonly diagnosed 1 to 6 months following injury. However, in pediatric patients with SCI, the onset of HO may be delayed by up to 14 months.[21] Signs and symptoms of HO include impaired joint range of motion (ROM), joint swelling, and a possible increase in spasticity. Pain may be present in those with preserved sensation below the level of injury. Clinical findings in children may be less obvious than those in adults, and spontaneous regression of HO is more likely to occur in children than in adults.[26] Pharmacologic treatment of HO may include sodium etidronate or nonsteroidal anti-inflammatory drugs. Irradiation may be used to prevent HO initially or following surgical treatment of HO to prevent recurrence. Surgical resection of HO is indicated when ROM restrictions interfere with movement or function, or when severe spasticity and pressure sores related to the presence of HO are a concern. However, surgical resection is associated with a high recurrence rate and complications.[26] Gentle passive ROM of the at-risk joints initiated early in the rehabilitation process may help prevent HO by maintaining the flexibility of the joint capsules and reducing the risk for contractures. This, in turn, will minimize the need for more aggressive intervention later, and thus reduce the risk for microtrauma to soft tissues, which may contribute to the formation of HO.[26]

Spasticity is an additional musculoskeletal complication that typically develops during the first 2 years following SCI. It is most often defined as an increase in muscle tone and deep tendon reflexes. About 65% to 78% of persons with SCI experience spasticity.[5] A study of spasticity in 403 individuals with SCI ranging in age from 15 to 82 years (mean age 31 years) at the time of injury with a range of 1 to 41 years (mean 14 years) post-injury was conducted.[27] Patients' self-reports of spasticity were correlated with impaired ROM and elicitable spasticity in the lower extremities; among those reporting spasticity, it could be manually elicited in 60% of patients. A significant correlation was found between elicitable spasticity and impaired hip abduction and extension and elbow flexion and extension ROM.[27] Half of pediatric patients with SCI experience spasticity. Spasticity may negatively impact quality of life, as it is associated with contractures and pressure ulcers. In addition, spasticity may interfere with performing activities of daily living such as dressing, bathing, and catheterizing, may result in a negative self-image, and may cause pain. In contrast, some individuals find spasticity functionally beneficial because it may provide increased trunk control or improve the ability to bear weight through the lower extremities.[5] Treatment of spasticity includes stretching, passive ROM exercises, and pharmacologic approaches. Management of localized spasticity may include injections of chemodenervation agents such as botulinum toxin. When global management of spasticity is indicated, skeletal muscle relaxant medications (*e.g.*, baclofen, diazepam, clonidine) may be used.

AD is a serious complication of SCI that affects both adults and children. It is characterized by a large increase in systolic and diastolic blood pressure and bradycardia, although tachycardia has also been reported. Symptoms include headache, goose flesh, paresthesias, shivering, nasal obstruction, flushing above the level of injury, malaise, nausea, feelings of anxiety, and blurry vision.[28] AD occurs in response to a noxious stimulus *below* the level of the injury, and typically in patients with SCI at or above T6. It occurs in persons with complete lesions as well as in those with incomplete lesions. Examples of noxious stimuli include distention of the bowel or the bladder, pain associated with urinary catheterization, disease of the upper gastrointestinal tract (such as a gastric ulcer or gastroesophageal reflux), skeletal fracture below the level of injury, sexual activity, and therapeutic electrical stimulation of the muscles.[28] In addition, tight clothing, excessive pressure on the skin (such as when sitting in a wheelchair for prolonged periods), and other injuries or wounds below the level of the SCI can result in AD.[5] Although the prevalence of AD is similar in children and adults with SCI, it is less often diagnosed in children because the signs and symptoms are more subtle.[29] If left untreated, hypertension can lead to stroke, seizure, and death.[24] Education about AD for caregivers of children with SCI is therefore critical to ensure that signs and symptoms of AD are recognized and immediate appropriate actions are taken to alleviate the causative noxious stimulus. They must also understand the importance of seeking emergency medical care when caregiver interventions are ineffective at resolving AD. Parents, other family members, teachers, coaches, and any other persons who will be caring for the child with SCI must be thoroughly educated regarding the signs and symptoms of AD, how to prevent it, how to manage it, and when to seek emergency medical intervention. Management of AD typically includes elevating the head of the bed (or sitting the child upright), loosening clothing, emptying the bowel and/or bladder,[5] or removing any other potential noxious stimulus that may be causing AD. The physical therapist, along with the nursing and medical staff, plays a critical role in providing this education to the child's caregivers.

Cardiovascular complications of SCI include dependent edema of the limbs, orthostatic hypotension, deep vein thrombosis (DVT), and cardiac disease. Individuals with pediatric-onset SCI are at even greater risk for later cardiovascular disease than are individuals with adult-onset SCI. Education on prevention strategies such as a regular home exercise program may help to minimize this risk.[24] DVT occurs less frequently in children with SCI than in adults with SCI.[30] Overall, there is a lower incidence of venous thromboembolism (which includes both DVT and pulmonary embolism) in children with SCI, with a rate of 1.1% in children younger than 14 years, 4.8% in children 14 to 19 years old, and 5.4% in adults.[5] Treatment for DVT may include prophylactic blood thinning agents and mechanical prophylaxis with graduated elastic stockings and sequential compression boots.[5]

Following the initial period of spinal shock when the bowel and bladder are usually hypotonic, the bowel and bladder develop spasticity as do the skeletal muscles below the level of the injury. This results in neurogenic bladder and neurogenic bowel. The spastic, or hyperactive, bladder muscle will contract against a closed sphincter, resulting in elevated bladder pressures. The inability to spontaneously void is therefore managed by clean intermittent catheterization of the bladder, typically every 3 to 4 hours. Pharmacologic intervention may be indicated when detrusor sphincter dyssynergy is present. Complications of neurogenic bladder can include AD, renal disease, and frequent urinary tract infections.[5] To manage a neurogenic bowel, a person with SCI must complete a regular bowel program to ensure continence of the bowel without constipation. This is typically completed at the same time every day or every other day. Oral stool softeners and/or laxatives may be used along with suppositories to stimulate evacuation of the bowel.

Skin care is critical to the care of the adolescent with SCI due to increased risk for pressure ulcers. Pressure ulcers are a common complication in children, adolescents, and adults with SCI alike[31] due to impaired or absent sensation, decreased mobility, impaired nutrition, and decreased lean body mass.[5] Pressure ulcers result from compression of soft tissues for a prolonged period of time; the tissue is thus deprived of nutrients and oxygen, resulting in ischemia, hypoxia, necrosis, and, ultimately, ulceration. Pressure ulcers occur most commonly over bony prominences, such as the sacrum, ischial tuberosities, and heels. Sequelae include sepsis, osteomyelitis, and malnutrition. In addition, pressure ulcers often result in significant financial costs to individuals with SCI and their families, as loss of time from work and school is common due to the need for prolonged bed rest to facilitate wound healing.[5,31] Prevention of pressure ulcers is therefore imperative to the health of a child with SCI. Preventive measures include: use of pressure-relieving surfaces such as an air mattress and an appropriate wheelchair cushion; frequent changes of position while in bed; performing weight-shifting while seated in the wheelchair; use of nighttime ankle-foot orthoses (AFOs) in bed to protect the heels; minimizing shear during transfers and repositioning; and ensuring adequate nutrition.[5] Caregivers must be instructed on positioning to reduce the risk of skin breakdown, especially for individuals with tetraplegia who are unable to reposition themselves independently. Skin inspection should be performed at least twice daily. Adolescents should be encouraged to assume independent responsibility for this task,[31] or for directing a caregiver to assist with skin inspection if they are physically unable to complete the task themselves. Persons with SCI are additionally at high risk for burn injuries to insensate areas due to contact with hot surfaces and spilled liquids.

Caregivers and patients must be instructed in the importance of avoiding potential sources of thermal injuries[5,31] such as seat warmers in vehicles, handling hot objects such as plates, cups, hair dryers, and curling irons, and placing hot objects in the lap (*e.g.*, laptop computers or pizza boxes).

While men with SCI often experience a loss of sexual response and decrease in fertility, the fertility of women with SCI is typically unaffected, although pregnancy is considered to be high risk with a higher rate of complications.[5] As a standard of practice, rehabilitation for adults with SCI typically addresses physical and psychologic issues related to sexuality after SCI.[31] Sexuality education must not be overlooked in the pediatric SCI rehabilitation setting. The approach to education of older adolescents regarding sexuality after SCI should typically be similar to that for adults. Adolescents should be offered sexual counseling without parents or caregivers present, and they may benefit from having a mentor with SCI to facilitate discussion and answer questions.[5] Whether parents initiate this discussion or not, the information should be included in the child's overall rehabilitation plan. The parents of a child with SCI must understand that the developmental process of sexuality will proceed in their child as it normally would; therefore, the child will need to be educated regarding sexuality in a developmentally appropriate manner.[31]

Children with complete injuries at C3 and above will be dependent upon long-term mechanical ventilation. Children with cervical injuries at C5 and below may acutely require ventilator support, but typically can be weaned from this support over time. However, these children remain at risk for pulmonary complications including recurrent aspiration, chronic atelectasis, dysphagia, mucous plugging, failure to thrive, impaired endurance, and sleep-disordered breathing.[31] In children with injuries at and above the C5 level, the potential for respiratory compromise is due not only to dysfunction of the phrenic nerves to the diaphragm, but also to dysfunction of the inspiratory and expiratory muscles of the chest and abdomen. Obvious signs and symptoms of respiratory insufficiency include recurrent pneumonias, fever, lethargy, and coughing. Chronic fatigue, irritability, and inattention are more subtle signs and symptoms of respiratory insufficiency that may occur in children with tetraplegia and are often overlooked.[32] The primary goals of pulmonary management of children with tetraplegia include maintaining respiratory health and preventing complications.[5,32] The physical therapist is often involved with providing many of these interventions to children with SCI.

Physical Therapy Patient/Client Management

The rehabilitation goals for the adolescent with SCI will be dictated by a combination of factors, including, but not limited to, patient/family goals, the patient and family's cultural and individual values, and the level and severity of the adolescent's injury. When assisting the patient and family to set and achieve goals, the physical therapist working with the adolescent with SCI must consider not only the age at the time of injury, but also the effects of the injury on his ongoing physical, cognitive, psychologic, and social development. However, it is important for parents and children to understand that "curing" the patient's SCI is *not* the goal of rehabilitation; rather, the goals are to maximize the patient's level of function and independence with the present impairments[5] and to ensure maintenance of his health and well-being. To ensure that the adolescent achieves his maximal functional potential, the physical therapist works closely with the rehabilitation team, including physiatrist, rehabilitation nurses, occupational therapist, speech-language pathologist, child-life specialist, social worker, psychologist, dietician, discharge planner, and the patient's family. Because adolescence is a time of transition between childhood and adulthood, rehabilitation for this age group aims to assist the adolescent with decreasing reliance on parents.[31] As with able-bodied peers, the adolescent with SCI may benefit from encouragement to obtain a part-time job or volunteer experience in anticipation of a future career. Encouraging the adolescent with SCI to participate in occupational activities such as housework/household maintenance, volunteer work, and recreational activities may assist with transitioning him to more successful outcomes in adulthood.[33] In addition, the rehabilitation team plays a role in providing SCI-related education regarding sexual health and reproduction. Peer discussion groups focusing on dating, self-esteem, and other issues important to this age group may also be beneficial.[5]

Discharge planning must begin when the patient is first admitted for rehabilitation. The rehabilitation team works closely with the family to ensure that the patient's needs will be adequately met upon discharge to the home. The physical or occupational therapist may perform an on-site evaluation of the home to make recommendations for accessibility (*e.g.*, installation of ramps or lifts, durable medical equipment such as bathing systems or grab bars). The team works with the family to ensure that transition to outpatient therapy services and medical care will be as seamless as possible. In addition, the rehabilitation team helps facilitate the adolescent's re-entry into school by working with school staff to ensure environmental access, educate staff and students about SCI, and facilitate the adolescent's transition to school-based therapies.[5]

Examination, Evaluation, and Diagnosis

A precise and thorough examination and evaluation is essential to establishing a plan of care and initiating rehabilitation of a patient with SCI. The history is a systematic gathering of information related to the injury and is obtained via chart review and patient and family interviews. It is imperative to gather information regarding the date and mechanism of injury and the acute medical treatments received. The physical therapist should be aware of any secondary injuries suffered. It is also imperative to determine if there was a loss of consciousness suffered during the initial injury to assess preliminary cognitive status and to give some insight into the possibility of a concurrent traumatic brain injury (TBI).[10] Because of the high velocity and trauma associated with traumatic SCI, the incidence of concomitant TBI is between 26% and 74%.[34,35] If the SCI is non-traumatic, information about the onset and progression of symptoms or when medical attention was sought is critical. This enables the therapist to determine the rate of deterioration resulting in paralysis.[36]

Past medical and surgical history highlights any premorbid deficits or limitations. In the pediatric population, developmental history, including prior level of function and age at major milestone attainment, is also pertinent to establish level of development prior to injury. The social history of the patient is crucial in determining discharge disposition, including primary caregiver information, anticipated discharge destination, living/home environment, and school set-up. The therapist must determine whether the patient had any premorbid learning issues or received any services (e.g., Individualized Education Program, IEP). In addition, any information on social interactions, support systems, leisure activities, sports, cultural beliefs, and future plans are helpful in maximizing the patient's outcomes.

Following a detailed history, the patient should be examined starting with a systems review. Appropriate monitoring of vital signs such as heart rate, blood pressure, and respiratory rate is a part of the cardiovascular assessment. The adolescent with SCI may suffer from orthostatic hypotension and may benefit from the use of an abdominal binder and/or thromboembolic devices (TEDs) for vascular support. Patients with injuries above the level of T6 are at risk for AD. In addition, an individual with a cervical injury such as the current patient is at risk for decreased respiratory efficiency and may require a detailed pulmonary assessment.

The integumentary assessment of an adolescent with SCI includes evaluation of color, integrity, current areas of skin breakdown, and areas of previous scarring. Neurovascular signs, including pulse, pain, temperature, and edema, are assessed.[10] The integumentary assessment can be the platform to initiate education of the patient and his family on the importance of adherence to pressure relief measures for the prevention of decubitus ulcers.

The musculoskeletal assessment consists of ROM, manual muscle testing (MMT), muscle tone and spasticity, posture, and sensation. In younger patients or those who have difficulty following directions, it may not be possible to conduct a standard MMT; therefore, the therapist may have to rely on functional observation, noting whether the patient has the ability to move against gravity. The modified Ashworth scale[37] is commonly used to measure the severity of spasticity because this tool grades increased muscle tone and tendon reflexes as elicited by passive movement.[27] Special attention is given to the assessment of clonus since these involuntary and rhythmic muscle contractions can considerably disrupt function, interfering with self-care and rehabilitation.[38,39] Ongoing postural assessment is critical as these patients are at high risk for developing pressure ulcers, joint deformities, and scoliosis related to postural imbalances. In patients with incomplete SCI, loss of strength and motor control is typically asymmetrical, resulting in imbalances in muscle strength around a specific joint. Weakness or inhibition of an agonist muscle causes shortening or over-facilitation of its antagonist. This 14-year-old adolescent with an incomplete cervical SCI will continue to experience physical growth in both height and weight and will therefore need frequent monitoring of his posture to assess for asymmetries. If asymmetries are present, appropriate interventions may include seating modifications or bracing to reduce the risk of progression of deformity and skin breakdown. Sensation is typically assessed during the ISNCSCI examination and needs to be reassessed frequently throughout the course of rehabilitation to determine the extent of neurologic recovery, if any. Pain should be assessed above, at, and below the level of injury.

In the neuromuscular assessment, functional movements are evaluated, including transfers, bed mobility, locomotion, balance and coordination, and wheelchair mobility. Function involves the way in which an individual carries out the physical demands of life. When evaluating function, the physical therapist must take into account the amount of physical assistance, verbal or visual cueing, and types of orthoses and/or assistive devices required to complete each task. The sitting balance assessment includes an evaluation of the patient's static and dynamic balance in long-sitting and short-sitting positions.

Following a thorough assessment of examination data, an appropriate physical therapy diagnosis can be established. Examples of physical therapy diagnoses for an adolescent with SCI include decreased strength, impaired balance, decreased ROM, decreased functional mobility, and limited activity tolerance. The physical therapy diagnosis guides the therapist toward prognosticating the optimal level of function the patient may achieve. Functional outcomes vary by individual, based on level and severity of injury, potential for neurologic recovery, presence of associated complications, and quality and quantity of rehabilitation training, as well as the patient's motivation and family support. Table 2-1 lists anticipated functional outcomes for each level of complete SCI, based on ideal circumstances.[10,40-42] Because individuals with incomplete injuries have significantly different motor and sensory function even at the same neurologic level of injury, it is impossible to predict functional outcomes based on level of SCI for incomplete injuries.[40]

Standardized outcome measures can measure the effectiveness and efficiency of rehabilitation in patients with SCI. The Functional Independence Measure (FIM), a widely used neurologic assessment tool, is an 18-item, 7-level scale that measures burden of care in the adult population.[43] Although reliable and valid, the FIM is not specific to the SCI population. The Functional Independence Measure for Children, or the WeeFIM, is a pediatric adaptation of the FIM, designed to assess and track functional abilities in children from 6 months to 7 years old[44] and can be used in children with developmental disabilities from 6 months to 21 years old. Because the WeeFIM has not been validated for 14-year-old adolescents with normal cognition, it would be inappropriate to use in this case.

The **Spinal Cord Independence Measure (SCIM)**, another well-known outcome measure, was designed specifically for patients with SCI, ages 13 and older, for the purpose of ability assessment, outcome assessment, and treatment goal determination. The SCIM is a valid and reliable comprehensive functional rating scale that measures functional achievements according to their value to the patient. It has been shown to demonstrate greater sensitivity to changes in function than the FIM.[45] The SCIM III includes 19 activities of daily living tasks, divided into 4 separate subgroups: self-care (scored from 0 to 20), respiration and sphincter management (scored from 0 to 40), mobility in room and toilet (scored from 0 to 10), and mobility indoors and outdoors (scored from 0 to 30). The final score ranges from 0 to 100,

Table 2-1   EXPECTED FUNCTIONAL OUTCOMES FOLLOWING COMPLETE SPINAL CORD INJURY

Level of Injury	Bed Mobility	Transfers	Wheelchair Mobility	Standing/ Ambulation
C1-C4 tetraplegia	Dependent	Dependent	**Manual:** Dependent **Power:** Independent with alternative drive controls, such as sip and puff, head array, or mini proportional joystick	**Standing:** Dependent **Ambulation:** Not indicated
C5 tetraplegia	Some assist	Some assist to dependent	**Manual:** Independent to some assist using grip enhancements or power-assist wheels on level, non-carpeted indoor surfaces; some assist to dependent outdoors **Power:** Independent using hand controls, such as joystick with or without adaptations	**Standing:** Dependent **Ambulation:** Not indicated
C6 tetraplegia	Independent to some assist	**Level:** Some assist to independent **Non-level:** Some assist to dependent	**Manual:** Independent indoors; some assist to dependent outdoors using grip enhancements **Power:** Independent using hand controls	**Standing:** Dependent **Ambulation:** Not indicated
C7-C8 tetraplegia	Independent	**Level:** Independent **Non-level:** Independent to some assist	**Manual:** Independent indoors and level outdoor terrain; some assist with uneven terrain	**Standing:** Independent to some assist with bracing or standing frame **Ambulation:** Not indicated
T1-T9 paraplegia	Independent	Independent	**Manual:** Independent indoors and outdoors on all terrain	**Standing:** Independent with bracing or standing frame **Ambulation:** Exercise ambulation with RGOs or HKAFOs and assistive device

(Continued)

			Wheelchair	Standing/
Level of Injury	**Bed Mobility**	**Transfers**	**Mobility**	**Ambulation**
T10-L1 paraplegia	Independent	Independent	**Manual:** Independent indoors and outdoors on all terrain	**Standing:** Independent with bracing **Ambulation:** Functional ambulation with KAFOs and assistive device
L2-S5 paraplegia	Independent	Independent	**Manual:** Independent indoors and outdoors on all terrain	**Standing:** Independent with or without bracing **Ambulation:** Functional ambulation with KAFOs or AFOs, with or without assistive device

Table 2-1   EXPECTED FUNCTIONAL OUTCOMES FOLLOWING COMPLETE SPINAL CORD INJURY (*CONTINUED*)

Abbreviations: AFO, ankle-foot orthosis; HKAFO, hip-knee-ankle-foot orthosis; KAFO, knee-ankle-foot orthosis; RGO, reciprocating gait orthosis.

where a score of 0 indicates total dependence and a score of 100 indicates complete independence.[46] The SCIM provides a good comprehensive start for establishing a baseline level of function during acute rehabilitation and for identifying weaknesses and focusing care.

The Walking Index for SCI (WISCI), the 6-minute walk test (6MWT), and the Spinal Cord Injury Functional Ambulation Inventory (SCI-FAI) are all valid and reliable functional outcome measures specific to ambulation. The WISCI II is a 20-item functional limitation scale used for the SCI population to categorize the level of physical assistance required for ambulation, as well as any requisite assistive devices and/or orthotics. Possible scores range from 0 (unable to walk despite any level of bracing, assistive device, or physical assistance) to 20 (ability to walk independently without braces or assistive device).[47] On initial assessment, the current patient's total WISCI score was 0; however, this assessment tool should be repeated in the rehabilitation setting to assess progress when standing and ambulation are initiated.

While the SCIM is the only comprehensive functional rating scale designed specifically for patients with SCI,[48] there are several standardized outcome measures that can be creatively modified for the SCI population, and may be useful to measure a patient's progress over the episode of care. It is the job of the physical therapist to be familiar with various standardized measures in order to choose the most appropriate one for each individual patient.

Plan of Care and Interventions

With an understanding of the functional deficits and potential complications of an adolescent with SCI, a comprehensive and individualized physical therapy plan of care is developed with the primary goal of maximizing function and independence in light of the deficits present. Pediatric interventions are similar to those for an adult, but with a different approach, as participation in an activity should be specific to the developmental stage of the child. For the current 14-year-old patient, the physical therapist noted the following impairments on initial evaluation: decreased strength in bilateral upper and lower extremities; impaired sensation, balance, and proprioception; and limited knowledge of his condition. Limitations in self-care and mobility included maximal assistance for bed mobility and dependence for static sitting balance and transfers. His initial total SCIM score was 26 out of 100. The patient's physical therapy plan of care will focus on functional mobility training (bed mobility, transfers, wheelchair mobility, gait), musculoskeletal interventions (skin management; exercises for balance, endurance, stretching, strengthening; standing), and education and equipment management.

Therapeutic exercise interventions should include ROM, strengthening, and balance training. ROM exercises begin as soon as possible after injury because loss of ROM in the extremities can decrease functional independence and increase the patient's energy demand during functional activities. ROM also helps prevent HO and decreases the risk for contractures by maintaining joint capsule flexibility.[26] To foster continued independence in the adolescent with an incomplete C7 SCI, self-ROM exercises can be taught with the assistance of adaptive equipment such as leg lifters or loops. For increased time efficiency, it is a good idea to teach the patient to do as much of his ROM as possible during regular daily activities such as dressing. Strength and endurance training are prerequisites for functional training.[49] An incomplete C7 SCI indicates that there is partial innervation of muscles below the level of injury. Therefore, it is imperative to perform an MMT to identify the muscles that can be trained, since this patient may require greater strength than normal in some muscle groups to compensate for those muscle groups that are no longer functioning.[10] Training can be accomplished via traditional progressive resistive exercises, circuit resistance training, functional electrical stimulation (FES), and body-weight-support treadmill training (BWSTT). Interventions to help reduce pulmonary complications related to cervical SCI may include respiratory muscle training, use of abdominal binders, noninvasive positive pressure ventilation and cough-assist devices, chest physical therapy, manually assisted or "quad" coughing, and use of positive expiratory pressure devices.[5,32] Balance training is an important component of SCI rehab. Tamburella et al.[50] postulated that balance is a significant factor for walking recovery. Balance training should occur in long-sitting, short-sitting, prone on elbows, standing (if appropriate), and during functional activities such as transfers and transitions. An adolescent with an incomplete SCI has more voluntary muscle function intact and thus more available balance strategies to employ. A study by Boswell-Ruys et al.[51] found that goal-oriented and task-specific balance training yields the most effective results. Unlike in the adult population, training needs to be accomplished while simultaneously engaging the young person (*e.g.*, incorporating video games into a sitting balance activity).

Functional mobility is the ability to move from one place or position to another and includes bed mobility, transfers, transitions, and wheelchair mobility.[5] The ability to perform bed mobility such as rolling or transitioning between supine and sitting depends on the individual's physical and developmental limitations. Devices such as an overhead trapeze bar or bed rails can assist the adolescent with SCI with sitting, scooting, and rolling in bed. With practice, this patient will be able to roll independently using either his elbow flexors to pull on the bed rails or his elbow extensors to push off the mattress. The ability to perform independent transfers also depends on his functional abilities and limitations. The option of a transfer board is useful to bridge the gap between transferring surfaces.[52] The physical therapist begins transfer training with teaching level transfer techniques using a transfer board and then progressing to level surfaces without a transfer board. The therapist then initiates non-level transfers with and without a transfer board. Transfer to and from level surfaces (*e.g.*, mat table to wheelchair) without a transfer board is a feasible independent goal for the individual with a C7 incomplete SCI (Table 2-1).

While therapeutic ambulation may be possible for an adolescent with an incomplete C7 SCI, *functional* ambulation is not. Therefore, it is the role of the physical therapist to facilitate alternate means of mobility because this is a critical component of an individual's life, fostering cognitive, social, and communication skills. For this patient, a wheelchair will be his primary means of mobility. The type of wheelchair (*i.e.*, power vs. manual) will depend on the adolescent's functional ability, balance, upper extremity strength, overall endurance and daily activity demand, and home environment/set-up. Based on his age, level of injury, prior independent level of function, and presentation on initial evaluation (ROM, MMT, static sitting balance), this patient should be able to propel a manual wheelchair over indoor and outdoor terrain.

Certain considerations should be taken into account when prescribing a wheelchair. The chair should be configured to promote decreased incidence of upper extremity strain and injury, because an adolescent with SCI needs to preserve upper extremity function for a lifetime of functional mobility using primarily his upper extremities. An adjustable axle allows the frame height and center of gravity to be adjusted, enabling placement of the rear axle as far forward as possible for optimal propulsion mechanics without compromising user stability. Since the patient may not have achieved his final adult height, the frame of the chair should accommodate adequate growth with respect to width and length. If necessary, the wheelchair will need to accommodate required orthoses. The seating assessment is a crucial part of the wheelchair evaluation. The wheelchair cushion should allow for proper positioning, dynamic stability, and adequate pressure relief.[5] Wheelchair cushions are available in various types and materials (*e.g.*, foam, gel, air, dynamic). While a solid back provides upright postural support, a solid seating surface facilitates neutral position of the pelvis and hips, reducing rotation and adduction.

Once optimal fit is achieved, wheelchair mobility training should be completed on multiple surface types, including indoor and outdoor surfaces, inclines, and curbs. Initial wheelchair mobility training must include proper propulsion techniques. The semicircular propulsion pattern (*i.e.*, the hands fall below the handrim during recovery phase or when the user is preparing for the next push) yields more efficient propulsion with decreased upper limb strain over time.[53] The patient should also be familiar with assisted stair management (*i.e.*, coaching others in appropriate method of ascending/descending stairs) and how to right the wheelchair in the event of a fall. Wheelchair mobility training should also be used as a time to continue education in weight shifting for the prevention of pressure ulcers over the buttocks, ischial tuberosities, and other bony prominences.[54] There are 4 basic types of weight shifts: anterior, lateral, vertical push-up, and posterior tilting. The most commonly taught pressure relief method for a patient with paraplegia is the vertical push-up method. It requires sufficient triceps strength for full elbow extension, in addition to adequate shoulder depression to assist with lifting the buttocks off the seating surface. However, in the interest of upper extremity preservation, an anterior weight shift followed by a left and right lateral weight shift is a more suitable option for the patient with a cervical level injury. There is significant variability in the literature regarding adequate duration of a weight shift. Documented durations range from 42 seconds to 3.5 minutes.[55] Using transcutaneous oxygen tension as an indicator of tissue viability, Coggrave and Rose[55] reported that the mean duration of various pressure relief positions required to raise tissue oxygen to unloaded levels was 1 minute 51 seconds. With respect to frequency, most rehabilitation programs recommend performing pressure reliefs every 15 to 30 minutes; however, research to support this practice is limited.

Up to 75% of individuals with an incomplete SCI will regain some ambulation.[19] In a study by Vogel and Lubicky[56] reviewing the ambulatory status of 207 individuals with SCI (ages 1-22 years), those with tetraplegia who ambulated were more likely to ambulate at the therapeutic level than at the community level. In general, an individual's potential as a therapeutic, household, or community ambulator depends on both the individual's physical presentation (Table 2-1) and the patient and family's level of motivation to pursue ambulation as a goal. An individual with incomplete SCI must be evaluated very carefully to determine if ambulation is a feasible goal, and if so, what type of orthoses and assistive devices will best meet his needs.

Limited evidence supports physiologic benefits of standing and walking programs for persons with SCI. A study of the effects of a **standing program** on adults within the first 2 years following SCI showed that those who stood for at least 1 hour per day, 5 days per week had significantly higher BMD in the lower extremities than those who did not participate in a standing program.[57] Importantly, this study showed that passive standing may help prevent *loss* of BMD in patients with *acute* SCI, as the patients initiated standing within 8 to 12 weeks of their SCI. However, a systematic review of the literature from 1960 to 2010 concluded that there was a lack of strong evidence to support the benefit of standing and walking on BMD, spasticity, or general health of persons with SCI.[58] Many of the studies reviewed were survey-based, thus offering a low level of evidence. Patient-reported problems with walking devices included difficulty with donning and doffing, poor cosmesis, fear of falling, and high energy expenditure. Thus, many studies reported a high rate of non-use within a short duration of receiving the orthosis.

Despite the lack of strong evidence to support the physiologic benefits of standing/walking on the health of young people with SCI, the psychologic benefits must be considered. Walking is often an important goal of persons with SCI and their families[56] and may offer psychologic benefits for children with SCI.[59,60] For these reasons, standing and upright mobility should be included in the rehabilitation program for this adolescent with SCI. The therapist must educate the patient and his family early on that ambulation with bracing is time- and energy-consuming and requires a long-term commitment to ensure success.

Static standing is often initiated in the acute phase of rehabilitation using a tilt table or standing frame. Children with sufficient upper body strength may progress to ambulating with braces supporting the lower extremities and using upper extremity support on an assistive device. The type of orthoses chosen depends on the child's level of injury, trunk control, amount of preserved lower extremity strength, and balance. A hip-knee-ankle-foot orthosis (HKAFO; Fig. 2-3) provides support for individuals with weak hip girdle and lower extremity muscles; a thoracic portion may be added when more proximal trunk support is needed.[5] HKAFOs

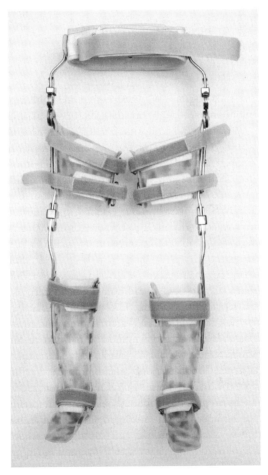

Figure 2-3. Hip-knee-ankle-foot orthosis (HKAFO) used to provide support for individuals with weak hip girdle and lower extremity muscles. Note drop locks at the knees and hips to maintain extension.

typically have drop locks at the knees and hips to maintain extension. A swing-to or swing-through gait pattern using bilateral upper extremity support on an assistive device is typical for those using HKAFOs. However, individuals with preserved active hip flexion and normal passive hip extension may prefer to ambulate with the hip joint unlocked in order to use a reciprocal gait pattern.

The metabolic cost for children who ambulate with locked HKAFOs is estimated to be up to 6 times higher than that for their typically developing peers.[60] The reciprocating gait orthosis (RGO) is an alternative to the HKAFO that reduces the metabolic cost of ambulation to only twice as much as that of typically developing peers. The RGO allows for a reciprocal gait pattern with an HKAFO (with or without the thoracic portion). While the knees remain locked in extension, the hips alternately flex and extend during the gait cycle. Sufficient upper body strength is required for use of either type of orthosis. For individuals with lower level injuries, or with incomplete injuries with significant preservation of strength in the lower extremities, less restrictive orthoses may be used. These include knee-ankle-foot orthoses (KAFOs) for those with insufficient quadriceps strength to maintain knee extension during stance[5] and AFOs for those with sufficient hip and knee strength to maintain extension in stance but impaired ankle strength.[61]

BWSTT (Fig. 2-4) provides opportunity for intensive step practice and training of lower extremity muscle strength and endurance. In recent years, the use of

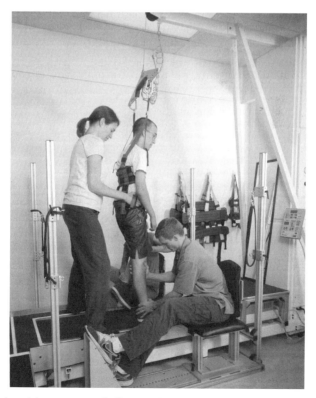

Figure 2-4. Body-weight-support treadmill training (BWSTT) with an adolescent with cervical level SCI.

BWSTT has become more widespread in the rehabilitation of adult and pediatric populations with neurologic conditions. A systematic review by Damiano and DeJong[62] investigated this intervention for pediatric populations through 21 years of age, including those with cervical level SCI. The reviewers found that a majority of the literature for use of **BWSTT in the pediatric SCI population** was generally of low quality, consisting of case reports and multiple case series. However, the authors concluded that because most of these studies showed positive effects, more rigorous studies are needed to explore the benefits of BWSTT in the pediatric population. The adolescent in this case with cervical incomplete SCI may benefit from BWSTT as a component of his rehabilitation program for a means of training the intact muscle groups in his lower extremities.

Cardiovascular disease and muscle atrophy are common sequelae of SCI,[63] with cardiovascular disease being a leading cause of death among adults with SCI.[64] Loss of muscle mass is additionally associated with insulin resistance, glucose intolerance, and type 2 diabetes.[63] Neuromuscular electrical stimulation (NMES) and FES may benefit individuals with SCI by reversing the loss of muscle mass and improving aerobic conditioning. A prospective cohort study of 14 sedentary adults with AIS A and AIS B SCI examined the efficacy of an 8-week subtetanic NMES training program on improving peak oxygen consumption.[64] NMES was applied to bilateral quadriceps and hamstring muscles 60 minutes per day, 5 days per week for 8 weeks, using frequencies of 2 to 4 Hz at intensities up to 200 mA. The participants were asked to increase the intensity as tolerated to a level of 13 to 15 on the Borg scale of perceived exertion. Exercise testing before and after training using wheelchair treadmill ergometry (*i.e.*, wheelchair propulsion exercise test performed on a treadmill at increasing speed and incline) demonstrated a mean increase in peak oxygen consumption of 22.65%.[64] In a second study, the same authors showed an increase in lean body mass and a decrease in regional body fat following a similar subtetanic training protocol in adults with SCI.[65] These studies demonstrated that a subtetanic NMES training program using a simple and convenient handheld device may have important health benefits in the adult population with SCI. However, more research is needed to study the benefits of such a program in the pediatric population.

The benefits of home-based FES cycling programs have been studied in adult and pediatric SCI populations. Adult males with C4 to T11 SCI (AIS A, B, and C) who cycled 40 to 60 minutes, 3 days per week for 8 weeks with home-based FES units experienced improved quality of life.[66] A study investigating the benefits of passive cycling, lower extremity FES cycling, and lower extremity NMES in children ages 5 to 13 years old with SCI levels ranging from C4 to T11 demonstrated benefits for both electrical stimulation groups.[63] All 3 groups exercised for 1 hour, 3 times per week for 6 months. Electrical stimulation was applied to the hamstrings, quadriceps, and gluteal muscles of the children in the stimulation groups. The **FES cycling group showed increases in both quadriceps muscle volume and stimulated muscle strength**, while the NMES group only showed increases in quadriceps muscle volume. Although increased muscle volume may be associated with decreased risk for cardiovascular disease, insulin resistance, glucose intolerance, and type 2 diabetes in this population, more research is needed.

Other studies have shown that FES may improve BMD in individuals with SCI. A randomized controlled trial comparing the benefits of FES cycling, passive cycling, and electrical stimulation without cycling was conducted with children with SCI ages 5 to 13 years with C4 to T11 SCI (AIS A, B, or C).[63] The children participated in either FES cycling, or passive cycling, or electrical stimulation to the hamstrings, quadriceps, and gluteal muscles for 1 hour per day, 3 times per week for 6 months. Although this study showed trends toward improved BMD at the proximal hips for both cycling groups, the differences were not statistically significant. The authors concluded that FES and passive cycling may be beneficial to bone health, but more research is needed. The current patient with C7 incomplete SCI may benefit from a home-based FES program to improve and maintain cardiovascular endurance and muscle mass.

Although many individuals with pediatric-onset SCI go on to achieve successful and stable adult lives, there is no cure for this life-altering condition. Therefore, public awareness and prevention of SCI are crucial to minimize the risk of sustaining an SCI and the lifelong disability associated with SCI. Prevention must include education on the use of age-appropriate vehicle restraint systems and proper safety equipment during sporting and recreational activities, water and diving safety, and gun safety. The physical therapist can play a key role in prevention education, helping to ensure that accidents and situations that may result in SCI can be avoided.

Evidence-Based Clinical Recommendations

SORT: Strength of Recommendation Taxonomy

A: Consistent, good-quality patient-oriented evidence
B: Inconsistent or limited-quality patient-oriented evidence
C: Consensus, disease-oriented evidence, usual practice, expert opinion, or case series

1. The International Standards for Neurological Classification of Spinal Cord Injury (ISNCSCI) examination is a reliable tool used to determine the severity of SCI injury in children older than 10 years. **Grade B**

2. The Spinal Cord Independence Measure (SCIM) is a reliable and valid tool to assess and track functional independence in individuals with SCI. **Grade A**

3. A standing program for 60 minutes per day, 5 days per week may help prevent loss of bone mineral density in individuals with acute SCI. **Grade B**

4. Body-weight-support treadmill training provides benefits for pediatric patients with SCI. **Grade C**

5. Cycling with lower extremity functional electrical stimulation (FES) and/or neuromuscular electrical stimulation (NMES) increases lower extremity muscle volume in children with SCI. **Grade B**

COMPREHENSION QUESTIONS

2.1 Which of the following does *not* contribute to the potential for SCIWORA?

A. Kyphoscoliosis in young child

B. Disproportionately large head relative to the child's body

C. Horizontally oriented facet joints in a child

D. Motor vehicle collision

2.2 Which of the following tests is used to determine the level and severity of SCI in the pediatric population?

A. WeeFIM

B. Spinal Cord Independence Measure (SCIM)

C. International Standards for Neurological Classification of Spinal Cord Injury (ISNCSCI)

D. Functional Independence Measure (FIM)

2.3 Which of the following is a true statement regarding autonomic dysreflexia?

A. It is always characterized by an increase in blood pressure and a decrease in heart rate.

B. It most commonly affects patients with SCI level at or above T12.

C. Distention of the bowel or bladder is a common cause.

D. Signs and symptoms are more obvious in younger children than in adolescents and adults.

ANSWERS

2.1 **D.** Motor vehicle collisions typically cause injuries that can be seen on MRI. Spinal cord injuries without radiologic abnormalities, or SCIWORA, are common in children due to the immaturity of the child's spine (option A). Characteristics of spinal immaturity include ligamentous laxity, horizontally oriented facet joints (option C), and inherent elasticity along with the disproportionately large head of a young child (option B). These features render the child's spine vulnerable to deforming forces and damage that may not be evident on imaging.

2.2 **C.** The ISNCSCI is the most common method for determining the level and severity of an SCI in the pediatric population. The WeeFIM, SCIM, and FIM are measures of function, not of level or severity of SCI.

2.3 **C.** Autonomic dysreflexia is commonly caused by distention of the bowel or bladder. It is most commonly experienced by patients with SCI *at or above* T6 (option B) and is characterized by an increase in blood pressure with *either* bradycardia or tachycardia (option A). Signs and symptoms are typically more *subtle* in infants and young children than in older children and adults (option D).

REFERENCES

1. National Spinal Cord Injury Association (NSCIA). Spinal cord injury statistics. http://www.spinalcord.org/. Accessed October 23, 2014.

2. McKinley WO, Seel RT, Hardman JT. Nontraumatic spinal cord injury: incidence, epidemiology, and functional outcome. *Arch Phys Med Rehabil.* 1999;80:619-623.

3. Whiteneck G, Gassaway J, Dijkers M, Jha A. New approach to study the contents and outcomes of spinal cord injury rehabilitation: the SCIRehab Project. *J Spinal Cord Med.* 2009;32:251-259.

4. National Spinal Cord Injury Statistical Center. Spinal cord injury facts and figures at a glance. Birmingham, AL: University of Alabama at Birmingham. March 2013. https://www.nscisc.uab.edu/PublicDocuments/fact_figures_docs/Facts%202013.pdf. Accessed October 23, 2014.

5. Greenberg JS, Ruutiainen AT, Kim H. Rehabilitation of pediatric spinal cord injury: from acute medical care to rehabilitation and beyond. *J Pediatr Rehabil Med.* 2009;2:13-27.

6. Ho CH, Wuermser LA, Priebe MM, Chiodo AE, Scelza WM, Kirshblum SC. Spinal cord injury medicine. 1. Epidemiology and classification. *Arch Phys Med Rehabil.* 2007;88:S49-S54.

7. Muzumdar D, Ventureyra EC. Spinal cord injuries in children. *J Pediatr Neurosci.* 2006;1:43-48.

8. Nobunaga AI, Go BK, Karunas RB. Recent demographic and injury trends in people served by the model spinal cord injury care systems. *Arch Phys Med Rehabil.* 1999;80:1372-1382.

9. Vitale MG, Goss JM, Matsumoto H, Roye DP Jr. Epidemiology of pediatric spinal cord injury in the United States: years 1997 and 2000. *J Pediatr Orthop.* 2006;26:745-749.

10. Atkinson H, Spearing EM. Traumatic and atraumatic spinal cord injury in pediatrics. In: Tecklin JS, ed. *Pediatric Physical Therapy.* Philadelphia, PA: Lippincott Williams & Wilkins; 2008:311-327.

11. Pang D, Wilberger JE. Spinal cord injury without radiographic abnormalities in children. *J Neurosurg.* 1982;57:114-129.

12. Collopy KT, Kivlehan SM, Snyder SR. Pediatric spinal cord injuries: anatomical differences bring different challenges with kids. *EMS World.* 2012;41:52-57.

13. Buldini B, Amigoni A, Faggin R, Laverda AM. Spinal cord injury without radiographic abnormalities. *Eur J Pediatr.* 2006;165:108-111.

14. Kirshblum SC, Biering-Sorensen F, Betz R, et al. International Standards for Neurological Classification of Spinal Cord Injury: cases with classification challenges. *J Spinal Cord Med.* 2014;37:120-127.

15. *American Spinal Injury Association: International Standards for Neurological Classification of Spinal Cord Injury.* Revised 2011; Atlanta, GA.

16. Kirshblum SC, Burns SP, Biering-Sorensen F, et al. International standards for neurological classification of spinal cord injury. *J Spinal Cord Med.* 2011;34:535-546.

17. Krisa L, Gaughan J, Vogel L, Betz RR, Mulcahey MJ. Agreement of repeated motor and sensory scores at individual myotomes and dermatomes in young persons with spinal cord injury. *Spinal Cord.* 2013;51:75-81.

18. Mulcahey MJ, Gaughan J, Betz RR, Johansen KJ. The International Standards for Neurological Classification of Spinal Cord Injury: reliability of data when applied to children and youth. *Spinal Cord.* 2007;45:452-459.

19. Burns AS, Marino RJ, Flanders AE, Flett H. Clinical diagnosis and prognosis following spinal cord injury. *Handb Clin Neurol.* 2012;109:47-62.

20. Vogel LC, DeVivo MJ. Pediatric spinal cord injury issues: etiology, demographics, and pathophysiology. *Top Spinal Cord Inj Rehabil.* 1997;3:1-8.

21. McCarthy JJ, Betz RR. Hip disorders in children who have spinal cord injury. *Orthop Clin North Am.* 2006;37:197-202.

22. Mehta S, Betz RR, Mulcahey MJ, McDonald C, Vogel LC, Anderson CJ. The effects of bracing on paralytic scoliosis secondary to spinal cord injury. *J Spinal Cord Med.* 2004;27:S88-S92.

23. Ooi HL, Briody J, McQuade M, Munnis CF. Zoledronic acid improves bone mineral density in pediatric spinal cord injury. *J Bone Miner Res.* 2012;27:1536-1540.

24. Shakhazizian KA, Massagli TL. Spinal cord injury. In: Campbell SK, vander Linden DW, Palisano RJ, eds. *Physical Therapy for Children*. St. Louis, MO: Saunders Elsevier; 2006:687-697.

25. Charmetant C, Phaner V, Condemine A, Calmels P. Diagnosis and treatment of osteoporosis in spinal cord injury patients: a literature review. *Ann Phys Rehabil Med*. 2010;53:655-668.

26. van Kuijk AA, Geurts AC, van Kuppevelt HJ. Neurogenic heterotopic ossification in spinal cord injury. *Spinal Cord*. 2002;40:313-326.

27. Skold C, Levi R, Seiger A. Spasticity after traumatic spinal cord injury: nature, severity, and location. *Arch Phys Med Rehabil*. 1999;80:1548-1557.

28. Karlsson AK. Autonomic dysreflexia. *Spinal Cord*. 1999;37:383-391.

29. Hickey KJ, Vogel LC, Wills KM, Anderson CJ. Prevalence and etiology of autonomic dysreflexia in children with spinal cord injury. *J Spinal Cord Med*. 2004;27:S54-S60.

30. Chen D, Apple DF, Hudson LM, Bode R. Medical complications during acute rehabilitation following SCI—current experiences of the Model Systems. *Arch Phys Med Rehabil*. 1999;80:1397-1401.

31. Vogel LC, Hickey KJ, Klass SJ, Anderson CJ. Unique issues in pediatric spinal cord injury. *Orthop Nurs*. 2004;23:300-308.

32. Porth SC. Recognition and management of respiratory dysfunction in children with tetraplegia. *J Spinal Cord Med*. 2004;27:S75-S79.

33. Anderson CJ, Vogel LC, Willis KM, Betz RR. Stability of transition to adulthood among individuals with pediatric-onset spinal cord injury. *J Spinal Cord Med*. 2006;29:46-56.

34. Macciocchi S, Seel RT, Thompson N, Byams R, Bowman B. Spinal cord injury and co-occurring traumatic brain injury: assessment and incidence. *Arch Phys Med Rehabil*. 2008;89:1350-1357.

35. Tolonen A, Turkka J, Salonen O, Ahoniemi E, Alaranta H. Traumatic brain injury is under-diagnosed in patients with spinal cord injury. *J Rehabil Med*. 2007;39:622-626.

36. Sisto SA, Ratner K. Evaluation. In: Sisto SA, Druin E, Sliwinski MM, eds. *Spinal Cord Injuries: Management and Rehabilitation*. St. Louis, MO: Mosby, Inc.; 2009:121-152.

37. Bohannon RW, Smith MB. Interrater reliability of a modified Ashworth scale of muscle spasticity. *Phys Ther*. 1987;67:206-207.

38. Yelnik AP, Simon O, Parratte B, Gracies JM. How to clinically assess and treat muscle overactivity in spastic paresis. *J Rehabil Med*. 2010;42:801-807.

39. Wallace DM, Ross TH, Thomas CK. Characteristics of lower extremity clonus after human cervical spinal cord injury. *J Neurotrauma*. 2012;29:915-924.

40. Sie I, Waters RL. Outcomes following spinal cord injury. In: Lin VW, ed. *Spinal Cord Medicine: Principles and Practice*. New York, NY: Demos Medical Publishing, Inc.; 2003:87-103.

41. McKinley W, Kulkarni U, Pai AB. Functional outcomes per level of spinal cord injury. Updated September 18, 2013: http://emedicine.medscape.com/article/322604-overview. Accessed October 23, 2014.

42. Burns AS, Ditunno JF. Establishing prognosis and maximizing functional outcomes after spinal cord injury: a review of current and future directions in rehabilitation management. *Spine*. 2001;26(24S):S137-S147.

43. Keith RA, Granger CV, Hamilton BB, Sherwin FS. The functional independence measure: a new tool for rehabilitation. *Adv Clin Rehabil*. 1987;1:6-18.

44. Wong V, Wong S, Chan K, Wong W. Functional independence measure (WeeFIM) for Chinese children: Hong Kong Cohort. *Pediatrics*. 2002;109:E36.

45. Catz A, Itzkovich M, Agranov E, Ring H, Tamir A. SCIM—spinal cord independence measure: a new disability scale for patients with spinal cord lesions. *Spinal Cord*. 1997;35:850-856.

46. Catz A, Itzkovich M. Spinal cord independence measure: comprehensive ability rating scale for the spinal cord lesion patient. *J Rehabil Res Dev*. 2007;44:65-68.

47. Dittuno PL, Dittuno JF Jr. Walking index for spinal cord injury (WISCI II): scale revision. *Spinal Cord*. 2001;39:654-656.

48. Furlan JC, Noonan V, Singh A, Fehlings MG. Assessment of disability in patients with acute traumatic spinal cord injury: a systematic review of the literature. *J Neurotrauma*. 2011;28:1413-1430.

49. Sliwinski MM, Druin E. Intervention principles and position changes. In: Sisto SA, Druin E, Sliwinski MM, eds. *Spinal Cord Injuries: Management and Rehabilitation*. St. Louis, MO: Mosby, Inc.; 2009:153-184.

50. Tamburella F, Scivoletto G, Molinari M. Balance training improves static stability and gait in chronic incomplete spinal cord injury subjects: a pilot study. *Eur J Phys Rehabil Med*. 2013;49:353-364.

51. Boswell-Ruys CL, Harvey LA, Barker JJ, Ben M, Middleton JW, Lord SR. Training unsupported sitting in people with chronic spinal cord injuries: a randomized controlled trial. *Spinal Cord*. 2010;48:138-143.

52. Mix CM, Specht DP. Achieving functional independence. In: Braddom RL, ed. *Physical Medicine and Rehabilitation*. Philadelphia, PA: Saunders; 1996:514-530.

53. Boninger ML, Souza AL, Cooper RA, Fitzgerald SG, Koontz AM, Fay BT. Propulsion patterns and pushrim biomechanics in manual wheelchair propulsion. *Arch PhysMed Rehabil*. 2002;83:718-723.

54. Beekman CE, Miller-Porter L, Schoneberger M. Energy cost of propulsion in standard and ultralight wheelchairs in people with spinal cord injuries. *Phys Ther*. 1999;79:146-158.

55. Coggrave MJ, Rose LS. A specialist seating assessment clinic: changing pressure relief practice. *Spinal Cord*. 2003;41:692-695.

56. Vogel LC, Lubicky JP. Ambulation in children and adolescents with spinal cord injuries. *J Pediatr Orthop*. 1995;15:510-516.

57. Alekna V, Tamulaitiene M, Sinevicius T, Juocevicius A. Effect of weight-bearing on bone mineral density in spinal cord injured patients during the period of the first two years. *Spinal Cord*. 2008;46:727-732.

58. Karimi MT. Evidence-based evaluation of physiological effects of standing and walking in individuals with spinal cord injury. *Iran J Med Sci*. 2011;36:242-253.

59. Kelly MA, Stokes KS. Standing and ambulation for the child with paraplegia or tetraplegia. In: Betz RR, Mulcahey MJ, eds. *The Child With a Spinal Cord Injury*. Rosemont, IL: The American Academy of Orthopaedic Surgeons; 1996:519, 528.

60. Katz DE, Haideri N, Song K, Wyrick P. Comparative study of conventional hip-knee-ankle-foot orthoses versus reciprocating-gait orthoses for children with high-level paraparesis. *J Pediatr Orthop*. 1997;7:377-386.

61. Calhoun CL, Schottler J, Vogel LC. Recommendations for mobility in children with spinal cord injury. *Top Spinal Cord Inj Rehabil*. 2013;19:142-151.

62. Damiano DL, DeJong SL. A systematic review of the effectiveness of treadmill training and body weight support in pediatric rehabilitation. *J Neurol Phys Ther*. 2009;33:27-44.

63. Johnston TE, Modlesky CM, Betz RR, Lauer RT. Muscle changes following cycling and/or electrical stimulation in pediatric spinal cord injury. *Arch Phys Med Rehabil*. 2011;92:1937-1943.

64. Carty A, McCormack K, Coughlan GF, Crowe L, Caulfield B. Increased aerobic fitness after neuromuscular electrical stimulation training in adults with spinal cord injury. *Arch Phys Med Rehabil*. 2012;93:790-795.

65. Carty A, McCormack K, Coughlan GF, Crowe L, Caulfield B. Alterations in body composition and spasticity following subtetanic neuromuscular electrical stimulation training in spinal cord injury. *J Rehabil Res Dev*. 2013;50:193-202.

66. Dolbow DR, Gorgey AS, Ketchum JM, Gater DR. Home-based functional electrical stimulation cycling enhances quality of life in individuals with spinal cord injury. *Ton Spinal Cord Inj Rehabil*. 2013;19:324-329.

Cerebral Hemispherectomy

Nisha Narula Pagan

A 5-month-old baby girl was admitted to the hospital due to infantile spasms. Seizures presented in clusters with a total of 30 to 40 seizures per day. Her medical history showed unresponsiveness to various antiepileptic drugs, which have been trialed since she was 2 months old. She has had multiple previous hospital admissions. Over time, her seizures have progressed to longer durations with forceful right arm and leg movements. Electroencephalography (EEG) confirmed epileptic activity arising from the left hemisphere. Magnetic resonance imaging (MRI) and positron emission tomography (PET) scans showed areas of cortical dysplasia in the left parietal occipital region with abnormalities extending toward the frontal region. Neurologic examination documented a right homonymous hemianopsia. A neurosurgeon recommended surgery for identification and removal of the epileptogenic region. She underwent a left hemicraniotomy and left cerebral functional hemispherectomy. The surgery was approximately 10 hours long and was performed without complications or excessive blood loss. Although the baby was awake and interactive the night after surgery, her interaction decreased slightly after 2 days. The parents were assured that this was expected due to postsurgical brain swelling. A complication after surgery was chemical meningitis; however, her fever subsided 2 weeks after surgery. At this time, the baby's intracranial pressure (ICP) was less than 16 mm Hg and the ventricular catheter was removed. Results of the head computed tomography (CT) scan confirmed that a ventriculoperitoneal (VP) shunt was not required. When the baby was able to adequately drink and eat (3 weeks after surgery), she was discharged from the hospital to home with her parents. Discharge instructions included scar management and precautions, as well as medical and rehabilitation follow-up. One month after surgery, early intervention was set up to include in-home physical and occupational therapy. A pediatric physical therapist assessed the infant in her home with her mother present.

► Discuss appropriate physical therapy interventions based on the child's expected clinical presentation.
► Describe a physical therapy plan of care across the child's lifespan: infant, toddler, and school age.
► Identify referrals to other medical team members.
► What is the child's rehabilitation prognosis based on etiology and age of surgery?

KEY DEFINITIONS

CHEMICAL MENINGITIS: Meningitis is an acute inflammation of the protective membranes (meninges) covering the brain and spinal cord; chemical meningitis (sometimes referred to as "aseptic" meningitis) may occur postsurgically and is associated with fever, stiff neck, and malaise.

CORTICAL DYSPLASIA: Congenital malformation of the cortex; a cause of seizures

HYDROCEPHALUS: Also known as "water on the brain"; swelling of the brain due to excessive accumulation of cerebrospinal fluid (CSF) that can occur when the normal flow or absorption of CSF around the brain is obstructed

INTRACRANIAL PRESSURE (ICP): Pressure measured inside the skull, and thus, the pressure exerted on the brain tissue and CSF (clear colorless fluid surrounding brain and spinal cord)

RIGHT HOMONYMOUS HEMIANOPSIA: Visual field defect involving the right halves of the visual field of both eyes

VENTRICULAR CATHETER: Plastic tube used in neurosurgery to drain fluid from the ventricles of the brain and thus keep them decompressed; used to monitor and relieve elevated ICP and hydrocephalus

VENTRICULOPERITONEAL (VP) SHUNT: Device used to treat hydrocephalus that allows fluid to move from a ventricle of the brain to the peritoneal cavity

Objectives

1. Define cerebral hemispherectomy.

2. Discuss the etiology leading to the necessity of a cerebral hemispherectomy.

3. Describe the clinical presentation of an individual status/post hemispherectomy.

4. Identify factors impacting physical recovery status/post hemispherectomy.

5. Describe rehabilitative needs and appropriate referrals for infants and children after hemispherectomy.

6. Describe related evidence available for physical therapy interventions that may be applied to children status/post cerebral hemispherectomy.

Physical Therapy Considerations

PT considerations during management of the individual status/post hemispherectomy in infancy and throughout the lifespan:

▶ **General physical therapy plan of care/goals:** Prevent/minimize loss of range of motion (ROM), strength, and aerobic functional capacity; maximize physical function and safety; minimize secondary impairments; optimize health-related quality of life

▶ **Physical therapy interventions:** Patient/family education; positioning and ROM exercises to prevent contractures at the neck, spine, and extremities (torticollis, elbow and hip flexion contractures, ankle plantar flexion contractures); equipment to increase mobility and/or to promote improved bone growth and equal weightbearing; graded exercises to optimize muscle strength with a focus on progression through developmental milestones; development and facilitation of home exercise program; therapeutic exercises to improve ROM, coordination, and strength; gait training (e.g., body-weight-support treadmill training); balance training; bilateral hand/arm exercises

▶ **Precautions during physical therapy interventions:** Delayed hydrocephalus that can develop at any time postsurgery; any gradual change, including a change in school performance, may indicate a need for a VP shunt or shunt revision; seizures may reoccur due to delayed hydrocephalus; seizures may indicate a need for additional surgery and/or change in medication management

▶ **Complications interfering with physical therapy:** Global delays in cognition, language, fine motor, gross motor, social, emotional, and adaptive development may interfere with physical therapy participation; functional skills may be impacted by visual and/or perceptual neglect; persistent hemiparesis with more distal extremity involvement; spasticity; sensory impairments with possible pain and sensory integration dysfunction

Understanding the Health Condition

Cerebral hemispherectomy is a complete surgical resection and/or disconnection of one hemisphere. It is a dramatic procedure typically performed to stop the detrimental effects of chronic and persistent drug-resistant seizures on a child's development.[1,2] Children who must undergo cerebral hemispherectomy often have medically intractable seizures arising from one hemisphere that has a structural abnormality. Patients with intractable seizures may be classified into 3 etiologic subgroups[3]: developmental (e.g., cortical dysplasia or hemimegalencephaly [one half of brain is abnormally larger than the other]); acquired (stable and nonprogressive brain lesions occurring perinatally or early in postnatal life, mostly consisting of ischemic or hemorrhagic pathology); and progressive (Rasmussen's encephalitis or Sturge-Weber syndrome). Patients with cortical dysplasia and hemimegalencephaly are typically younger at age of seizure onset and therefore younger at age of surgery compared with other etiologies.[4]

Cerebral hemispherectomy may offer the best possible opportunity to improve development.[5,6] It is often an option of last resort, in which the benefits outweigh the risks. The surgery may offer a viable option with improvements in quality of life[5] as compared to other nonsurgical treatments for pediatric intractable epilepsy.[7] In addition, it may provide better seizure control than other type of epileptic surgical procedures.[6] In a longitudinal study of 170 children, 112 (66%) were seizure-free after a mean follow-up period of 5.3 (± 3.3) years.[7] Other groups report seizure-free activity in up to 86% of patients at 5-year follow-up examinations. Patients usually take 3 antiepileptic drugs (AEDs) prior to surgery, whereas AED use declined to an average of one medication at 2 and 5 years after cerebral hemispherectomy and 17% required no AEDs after a 5-year follow-up.[8] Seizure etiology plays a large role in potential functional level, seizure-free rates, and need for use of medication after surgery.[3,4,9] For example, due to the integrity of residual brain tissue in a child with hemimegalencephaly or cortical dysplasia, cognitive and functional levels are limited and there is the possibility of seizure reoccurrence.[10]

According to a 2004 self-reported survey by the International League Against Epilepsy, hemispherectomy is a surgical procedure performed in approximately 36 pediatric epilepsy centers worldwide (including Asia, Australia, North America, and Latin America). One-third or more of the procedures are performed in children younger than 2 years. This procedure represents approximately 16% to 20% of all pediatric epilepsy surgeries.[8,11] The first reported hemispherectomy took place in 1928; it was performed to remove a malignant glioma of the nondominant hemisphere.[8] This was an "anatomical hemispherectomy" in which the hemisphere was completely removed. A decade later, this procedure was utilized to successfully obliterate intractable chronic seizure disorders. By 1966, Oppenheimer and Griffith[12] reported long-term complications following anatomical hemispherectomy. These long-term complications were later referred to as the syndrome "superficial cerebral hemosiderosis" (SCH). SCH manifested as neurological worsening and hydrocephalus after a mean interval of 8 years in about 25% of cases. Mortality rates were as high as 40%. With the increasing awareness of SCH, surgical procedures were modified. By decreasing the amount of brain removed, a lower incidence of complications occurred while still reducing seizures. In 1974, "functional" or "Rasmussen" hemispherectomies were introduced. In this procedure, only parts of a hemisphere are removed and the corpus callosum (fiber bundle connecting the two halves of the brain) is severed in order to disconnect the hemispheres.[13] Since the introduction of "functional" hemispherectomies, most hemispherectomies involve removal of brain tissue and a disconnection of the hemispheres.

Surgical approaches vary based on the surgeon's training and preference as well as patient characteristics such as age, size, and risk of blood loss. Since 1986, the University of California at Los Angeles (UCLA) Pediatric Epilepsy Program[8] has been one of the few programs offering the possibility of surgery to children with seizure disorders and is one of the few clinics to offer a hemispherectomy. Typically, children referred to UCLA for a cerebral hemispherectomy are younger than 3 years with severe cortical dysplasia and hemimegalencephaly. In 1998, the "modified UCLA functional cerebral hemispherectomy" was developed primarily to decrease blood loss and complications in infants and small children with small malformed ventricular systems from severe cortical dysplasia and other malformations of cortical development.[1] In a series of 96 patients who had a functional hemispherectomy at UCLA between 1998 and 2008, postsurgical complications included partial third nerve palsy, partial osteomyelitis of bone flap, CSF infections, and acquired hydrocephalus. Thirty-two percent of the patients eventually required cerebral shunts due to acquired hydrocephalus. The majority of the shunts were placed during the first 2 weeks after surgery; however, others were placed months and even years after surgery due to delayed hydrocephalus.

Shunt malfunctions or delayed hydrocephalus in children status/post hemispherectomy may produce atypical symptoms compared to other patient populations with shunts. It has been suggested that the increased space in the skull after hemispherectomy may not cause typical hydrocephalus signs and symptoms such as vomiting, lethargy, and headaches. Instead, the initial signs of shunt malfunctions may be seizures or subtle changes in behavior or performance in activities over weeks or months. Families and healthcare professionals are cautioned to monitor for the typical signs of increased ICP as well as reoccurrence of seizures and/or gradual behavioral changes.[8]

After cerebral hemispherectomy, children typically present with persistent motor and sensory deficits, including severe hemiparesis, spasticity, and impaired sensation on the contralateral side and a visual field cut. The clinical presentation of the resulting hemiplegia is similar to that of individuals with neurological disabilities such as stroke and cerebral palsy (CP).[14] Lower extremity return as it relates to ambulation can be expected in children who walked prior to surgery as well as infants learning for the first time after surgery.[15] Most often, the distal muscles of the upper extremity are more severely involved; however, upper extremity function varies and individuals demonstrate different degrees of hemiplegia.[14] **Functional recovery after a cerebral hemispherectomy** may be related to the etiology and/or the individual's age at the time of surgery.[9] Children with developmental etiology (cortical dysplasia and hemimegalencephaly) tend to have significantly diminished distal arm strength and hand function and show less improvement in gross motor function compared to those with acquired pathology (infarcts). Consistent with this finding, gross motor development had improved in a group of patients with acquired and progressive brain lesions, but not in children with the disorders of developmental etiology.[4]

The global impact and specific deficits associated with the complete removal or disconnection of one hemisphere continue to be investigated.[15,16] The functional recovery of a hemiparetic side in a child status/post hemispherectomy relies on neural reorganization or plasticity of the remaining tissues. Available remaining brain tissue includes the cortex of the remaining hemisphere (intact nonprimary motor and somatosensory areas), the ipsilateral corticospinal tract of the remaining hemisphere, and other subcortical tissue (corticoreticulospinal and spinocortical pathways).[2,17] Due to bilateral cortical input to proximal muscles, children status/post hemispherectomy will have more distal control impairments.[2] Studies on individuals who underwent hemispherectomy at an early age versus young adults who had later seizure onset and underwent hemispherectomy at a later age suggest that the timing of surgery also impacts the maturation and involvement of the intact structures. For example, during typical development, ipsilateral cortical pathways become inhibited by approximately 10 years of age. Therefore, an individual who had a hemispherectomy before 10 years of age may have more potential for recovery of the paretic side due to use of the remaining ipsilateral corticospinal tract. This use of the ipsilateral pathway has been shown to be independent of etiology and may be more impacted by timing of surgery.[2]

It has been suggested that there is a "critical maturational period" with respect to the timeframe for the greatest potential of sprouting new neurons and synapses.

Based on feline animal models, Villablanca and Hovda[18] have suggested that procedures such as hemispherectomies should be performed before the age of 3 years to maximize the ability of the brain to reorganize and recover after surgery. However, functional recovery with acute care rehabilitation has been demonstrated well beyond this suggested critical maturation period, as in a case study of a 28-year-old male who had a right hemispherectomy due to an increase in the frequency of seizures that he had first experienced at 5 years old.[17] Preoperatively, he was able to walk about 50 feet without an assistive device with gait deviations, compensational strategies, and frequent losses of balance due to left-sided weakness. Immediately after surgery, his affected (left) side was flaccid and he required complete assistance to perform transitions and transfers. By postoperative day 11 to 14, he was able to move his left arm and leg and walk up to 400 feet with physical assistance of one person.[17] It has been hypothesized that this individual's recovery was possible because his brain began reorganizing in response to an initial traumatic brain injury that occurred when he was 5 years old. In addition, this individual also had several smaller surgeries prior to a complete hemispherectomy. It is possible that the smaller surgeries over time may have been less stressful to the body and therefore aided in allowing neuroplasticity and reorganization. Therefore, it is possible that the right hemisphere functions gradually transferred to his left hemisphere in response to his initial injury and several surgeries.[17] The impact of rehabilitation and the neuroplasticity occurring years after surgery within this growing population of individuals post-cerebral hemispherectomy continue to be investigated.[19]

Physical Therapy Patient/Client Management

Follow-up throughout life from a multidisciplinary team is vital to the health and quality of life of children status/post cerebral hemispherectomy. The neurosurgery team typically plans follow-up visits 6 and 12 months after surgery and annually thereafter. Long-term follow-up is necessary due to the risk of late occurrence of seizures, hydrocephalus, possible shunt malfunctions, and persistent headaches.[8] To ensure optimal development of milestones, physical therapy, occupational therapy, and speech therapy are critical components of the healthcare team. In addition to the child's neurologist and neurosurgeon, other medical referrals may include: (1) orthopaedic specialist or surgeon for secondary impairments (e.g., contractures, leg length discrepancy, fractures); (2) neuropsychologist for cognitive deficits, behavioral difficulties, and mood disorders; (3) endocrinologist for postsurgical impact on hormones and growth, and (4) neuro-ophthalmologist for persistent visual field loss. Once the infant/child is medically stable, the physical therapist works with the patient and family to decrease the risk of contractures and other secondary impairments and increase functional mobility to enhance quality of life. The physical therapist may play a role in communicating with families and specialists about spasticity management options as well as possible orthopaedic surgical needs. Other providers that the physical therapist may communicate with include durable medical equipment vendors and orthotists.

Examination, Evaluation, and Diagnosis

Initially within the examination, a careful family interview and review of the medical history assists the therapist in formulating the plan of care and goals. If available, the physical therapist should obtain physical therapy and occupational therapy reports completed prior to the hemispherectomy because these can provide a clinical picture of the patient's previous level of motor functioning. Results and/or summaries of surgical reports, inpatient discharge recommendations, current medications, and any special tests such as imaging should be requested if they are not available in the medical record received at the time of the initial examination. From the subjective examination, the therapist must acquire an understanding of the impact of the underlying pathology or etiology and create a timeline of events. Specifically, the following should be noted: (1) when the seizures began and the determined etiology; (2) onset and frequency of seizures; (3) type, dosage, and frequency of AEDs; (4) the child's prior level of functioning, including achieved gross motor milestones prior to surgery; (5) type of surgeries and child's age; (6) any complications; and (7) potential medical treatments including shunt placements or medications. Due to the risk of delayed hydrocephalus, the therapist must consistently inquire about headaches, fatigue, and changes in behavior such as a decline in play or disruption of eating and feeding habits. If seizures reoccur, a neurologist will investigate potential delayed hydrocephalus, need for a shunt revision, and/or repeat surgery as neural connections may still exist with residual tissue.

The systems review for an infant or child status/post cerebral hemispherectomy is comprehensive and includes: sleep and feeding pattern; peripheral sensation and central processing of all sensations (vision, auditory, tactile, vestibular); observation of movement in all positions to inspect strength, symmetry, and strategies or preference of movements or positions; head and skull shape; visual deficits; ROM and flexibility of the neck, spine, and extremities; skin integrity; gait; upper extremity use; and safety and functional deficits. It is vital to collaborate with the child's occupational therapist to fully assess the child's adapted behavior (such as sleeping and eating) and organization of senses.

Functional mobility of children status/post hemispherectomy may be impacted by persistent spasticity in the upper and lower extremities. As a therapist applies a quick stretch, a muscle with spasticity may passively move freely for a short distance, followed by an abrupt catch, and then a rapidly increasing muscular resistance.[20] To assess for spasticity of the ankle plantar flexors in a 5-month-old baby, the therapist can examine the child at rest in supine while supporting the leg. After moving the joint passively throughout available range, the therapist quickly dorsiflexes the ankle to provide a quick stretch to the plantar flexors. Evaluating the joint at various speeds is helpful for planning and evaluating interventions.[21] Spasticity may be graded with the modified Tardieu scale (MTS). The original Tardieu scale dates back to the 1950s. It has been modified from the original scale to include use of the fastest velocity of passive movement possible (V3). The angle at which a clear "catch" in the passive movement has been felt is recorded. The MTS takes into account resistance to passive movement at both slow and fast speeds. Two joint positions are recorded: R1 and R2. The initial resistance to passive movement is recorded at the first catch (R1) and then the limb is moved slowly to the end range (R2). The MTS uses the same grading scale outlined in the original Tardieu scale; however, the modified version aimed to standardize the testing procedure by describing specific limb placement, alignment positions, and procedures. For children with CP, poor to adequate intra-rater/inter-rater reliability has been established and poor to excellent test-retest reliability has been observed in testing the gastrocnemius muscles.[22]

Impairment tests including those for strength, ROM, and sensation may be difficult to administer due to age or comprehension. However, careful observation of functional tasks can provide insight into the development of motor patterns as well as the interaction of impairment and activity in relation to participation.[21] Due to global delays, a developmental examination such as the **Bayley Scales of Infant and Toddler Development, Third Edition (Bayley-III)**[23] could be considered. The Bayley-III is a developmental instrument that assesses cognition, language, and motor skills for children ages 1 month to 42 months. The examination takes approximately 50 minutes to administer for children 12 months or younger and approximately 90 minutes for children 13 months or older. It assists in identifying developmental gross motor, fine motor, and cognitive delays and can be used to monitor progress. Bayley-III test scores correlate moderately or highly with scores on other instruments; internal consistency and test-retest reliability appear good.[23] An accommodated version of the test, known as Bayley-III Low Motor/Vision, was assessed and found to be useful in 19 children (ranging in age from 22 to 90 months). To enable assessment of children with motor and/or visual impairment, adaptations such as the removal of particular motor components in items designed to measure cognitive ability (e.g., removing pointing to connect similar pictures) were made to minimize impairment bias without altering what the test measures.[24]

To assess gross motor development, the physical therapist can use the Gross Motor Function Measure-66 (GMFM-66) or the GMFM-88 (which includes 22 more items). This well-known and standardized instrument is frequently used in children with CP and may also be applied to children with other disabilities from birth to 5 years of age. The GMFM is a clinical observational instrument and divides the dimensions of gross motor development into 5 categories. The GMFM-66 has good reliability and validity in assessing gross motor functions of children with CP who are younger than 3 years.[25]

The distal muscles of the upper extremity are often more severely involved in a child status/post hemispherectomy. In addition, mirrored movements in which the movement of one extremity is simultaneously "mirrored" by the opposite extremity may occur; this indicates that the undamaged hemisphere is controlling the movement of both hands.[26] The physical therapist should observe how the child or infant performs functional tasks with the paretic arm as well as the unaffected arm. In the case of an infant, hand-eye coordination and upper extremity strength and mobility should be observed in various positions. For example, in typical development, the 5-month-old infant's hands should actively reach to the knees, lower legs, and feet in supine. In prone, the 5-month-old can typically reach with both arms or weight shift and reach with one arm. In a supported position, such as in a caregiver's arms, the 5-month-old can hold a bottle when feeding, although the baby continues to need help to adequately sustain a proper position because of the bottle's weight and shape.[27] To further measure bimanual hand use, the therapist can use the Assisting Hand Assessment (AHA).[28] The AHA is a reliable and valid tool to measure bimanual activity in children (ages 18 months to 12 years old) who have a unilateral upper limb dysfunction, in particular children with hemiplegic CP or obstetric brachial plexus palsy (See Case 1). The AHA involves 2 steps. First, the assessor video records the child during a 10- to 15-minute play session utilizing bimanual toys from the AHA kit. Second, the assessor reviews the video and scores 22 items including general use, arm use, grasp and release, fine motor adjustments, coordination, and pace on a 4-point criterion-referenced rating scale. While not formally validated in this population, the AHA could be applied to children status/ post hemispherectomy since it has been designed for use with children who have unilateral upper limb dysfunction.[28]

Plan of Care and Interventions

Preliminary evidence suggests that rehabilitative techniques used for individuals with stroke and CP may be effective after cerebral hemispherectomy in children and young adults as young as 5 years old.[29,30] Many deficits in individuals with cerebral hemispherectomy may be irreversible due to the fact that the primary sensorimotor cortex has been unilaterally resected during hemispherectomy; however, partial recovery of motor functioning is possible as a result of major brain reorganization utilizing brain plasticity mechanisms.[17]

Many physical therapy interventions can be included in the plan of care. Due to global cognitive and motor delays, sensory/perceptual impairments,[31] and behavioral abnormalities (irritability, hyperactivity, aggressive and autistic behaviors),[32] a multisensory environment is recommended. Sensory input, such as swinging and rocking, may be used to modulate alertness and arousal levels of the infant or child for routine activities and participation in age-appropriate activities. Throughout therapy, a 5-month-old baby may require intermittent rocking or swinging to calm the nervous system to allow effective learning of new skills such as reaching, rolling, and coming up to sit.[33] In addition, play may be adequately stimulated with visual, tactile, and auditory stimulation. For example, with the visual stimulus of a toy, unilateral reaching across the body may occur when an object is presented to the side. This creates a weight shift, facilitating the baby to roll to her side. Careful consideration should be made of expected visual field cuts and sensory deficits.[31] Therapeutic activities should promote strength and flexibility in the spine and extremities while facilitating motor milestones with proper optimal alignment. This may be accomplished by utilizing handling techniques based on neurodevelopmental treatment (NDT) techniques. NDT is a common approach used in the treatment of children with CP and can serve as a form of therapeutic exercise for the pediatric population by grading assistance and progression through handling and positioning.[34,35] In addition to active rolling from supine to sidelying, the 5-month-old infant should have adequate head and trunk control to allow momentarily sitting while leaning forward on propped extended arms in a ring position of the lower extremities which is a wide, stable base of support. At the appropriate age, skills should be progressed to upright activities—from sitting to standing to gait training, as able. To facilitate bilateral upper extremity coordination, strength, and ROM, task-specific activities should be taught to the patient and encouraged and reinforced by family members. For the current patient, an example of a task-specific activity that challenges upper extremity coordination would be reaching for and grasping a toy using a palmar grasp and bringing it to the mouth in a supported sitting position. As the child enters school, the therapist must be involved to consult and train the patient, teachers, and caregivers to assure safety throughout transitions to new school environments and enhance physical fitness and integration into community activities.[36,37] As the child begins to stand, adaptive equipment such as a stander may be considered. One of the challenging and creative roles of the physical therapist is addressing equipment and positioning needs in the context of providing a stimulating environment to enhance mobility and exploration. Standing frames increase hamstring and hip flexor length, increase ankle dorsiflexion, and improve bone mineral density, which has been cited to be critical during onset of puberty.[38,39] Effective standing dosages range from 45 to 60 minutes daily.

To be effective, the therapist should design therapeutic interventions that incorporate active motor learning. The principles of motor learning pertain to how individuals acquire and perform motor activities. When motor learning principles are applied, such as facilitating repetitive, intense, and specific massed practice, permanent changes in functional motor abilities occur due to a cascade of neuroanatomical changes including the formation of new synapses, increase in astrocytic volume, dendritic sprouting, and angiogenesis.[40] In order to improve and successfully achieve a specific task, that *specific* task must be practiced. The capacity for the brain to reorganize has been investigated in a study of 12 children (11-19 years old) status/post cerebral hemispherectomy.[19] After 2 weeks of physical therapy focusing on locomotor training (overground and treadmill training; 30 hours guided by a physical therapist plus 40 hours walking with parents within the community), functional MRIs demonstrated increased volume and intensity of cortical activation in the sensorimotor and somatosensory cortices.

Further studies are required to determine the optimal dosage of physical therapy interventions (frequency, intensity, timing, type)[41] to achieve the best outcomes. Intensive mobility training (IMT) is a massed practiced format physical therapy treatment option designed to address specific gait, balance, and mobility deficits in individuals with chronic neurological deficits such as spinal cord injuries,[29,42] stroke,[29,43] Parkinson's disease,[29] and cerebral hemispherectomy.[29,30] IMT is a 10-day program with 3 hours of physical therapy per day (totaling 30 hours). Interventions include massed practice and repetitive task-specific training. The "dosage" is comparable to other effective rehabilitation studies that have used longer training periods over several weeks. IMT incorporates concepts from other successful therapies such as constraint-induced movement therapy (CIMT).[44] IMT focusing on mass practice of walking and active, voluntary gait-related activities may be a promising mode of intervention for individuals after hemispherectomy. In a study investigating the functional effects of IMT in 19 individuals (5-25 years old) post-hemispherectomy, improvements in balance and gait-related activities were greater in those who were 5 years or younger at the time of surgery compared with those who had surgery at an older age.[30] While there have been no published studies utilizing IMT on infants as young as 5 months of age, its principles, which share many principles of motor learning, could be used. For example, opportunities to practice specific motor skills such as reaching, rolling, or coming to sit may be set up in the home environment within a daily routine. The physical therapist could instruct a parent on specific handling and facilitation techniques to utilize during a frequent repetitive task such as rolling side to side and coming up to sit during routines such as diaper changes.

CIMT has mainly been used in the adult population status/post stroke. It has been used to increase functional use of the involved upper extremity through massed practice (increased repetitions with decreased rest periods) of hand and arm tasks while restraining the less affected upper extremity.[44] It should be noted that CIMT was developed to overcome learned "non-use" of an extremity and thus may not apply to an infant or young child who has never learned how to use her involved upper extremity. Therefore, modifications to CIMT continue to be suggested. In a study with 4 individuals aged 12 to 22 years with cerebral hemispherectomy, a modified CIMT program (3 hours/day of functional tasks with progressive complexity levels) was shown to improve quality of movement, spontaneous use of the upper extremity, and manual dexterity in outcome measures such as the Actual Amount of Use Test (AAUT) and Box and Block Test. In addition, post-training functional MRI changes occurred. For example, no signal was detected on one patient's paretic side before training; however, after training both hands were represented next to each other in the remaining hemisphere. During the CIMT intervention, subjects wore a resting splint 90% of waking hours for 10 days. This was considered a shortened version because more traditional programs include practice of functional tasks for 6 hours/day. Three hours was found to be more feasible due to low fitness level and cognition and emotional impairments present in the subjects.[14] A randomized, controlled, prospective parallel-group trial evaluating the adjustments to CIMT necessary to be appropriate and feasible for infants 3 to 8 months of age is currently in progress.[45] The study is described as a "baby-CIMT" protocol focusing on grasping and toy exploration. The need for a rich environment, selection of toys at the right ability level, optimal child positioning, and education and supervision of the parents as treatment providers are important components of the baby-CIMT intervention. It should be noted that caution must be taken when applying CIMT at a young age. Feline animal studies of CP suggest that maturation of the corticospinal tract may depend on early activity. Therefore, it is possible that intensive restraint at a young age may actually risk damage to the nonparetic upper extremity due to early decreased stimulation.[46]

Hand-arm bimanual intensive therapy (HABIT)[47] is another form of intense functional training (6 hours/day for 2 weeks); however, it focuses on improving coordination of the hands using structured task practice during bimanual play and functional activities. In a randomized clinical trial comparing 90 hours of CIMT to HABIT in 42 children ages 3.5 to 10 years, improvement on outcome measures of unimanual function (Jebsen-Taylor Test of Hand Function) and bimanual function (AHA) was similar in both CIMT and HABIT groups. However, since bimanual skills are of greater importance to caregivers, the HABIT group achieved greater perceived goal attainment. Due to potential advantages in each treatment approach (*e.g.*, CIMT may reduce specific impairments such as forearm supination, while HABIT assists in improving bilateral functional skills), combining both CIMT and HABIT in a "child-friendly" manner is suggested.[48]

Evidence-Based Clinical Recommendations

SORT: Strength of Recommendation Taxonomy

A: Consistent, good-quality patient-oriented evidence
B: Inconsistent or limited-quality patient-oriented evidence
C: Consensus, disease-oriented evidence, usual practice, expert opinion, or case series

1. Functional outcomes for children status/post cerebral hemispherectomy may be related to etiology and/or age at time of surgery; more functional improvements are noted in children with acquired etiologies and younger age at time of surgery. **Grade B**

2. The Bayley Scales of Infant and Toddler Development, Third Edition (Bayley-III) is a valid and reliable instrument to identify developmental gross motor, fine motor, and cognitive delays in children (ages 1 month to 42 months) and may be appropriate in assessing children with cerebral hemispherectomy. **Grade C**

3. Constraint-induced movement therapy (CIMT) improves motor function and increase use of the hemiparetic extremity in children with cerebral hemispherectomy. **Grade C**

COMPREHENSION QUESTIONS

3.1 The *most* common indication for a cerebral hemispherectomy is:
   A. Cortical tumor
   B. Medically intractable seizures
   C. Infarcts leading to hemiplegic cerebral palsy
   D. Seizures arising from several areas of the brain in both hemispheres

3.2 Typical clinical presentation of children status/post hemispherectomy includes:
   A. Increased spasticity with more involvement in the involved lower extremity as compared to the involved upper extremity
   B. Visual field cut without sensory deficits in the upper extremity
   C. Global delays in all areas with more involvement in the involved distal upper extremity
   D. Increased difficulty in walking recovery for children who walked previous to surgery

3.3 Physical therapy interventions for children status/post hemispherectomy:

  A. should be novel, task-specific, intense, and repetitive.

  B. are unlikely to change deficits due to complete disconnection of the involved cerebral hemisphere.

  C. are only necessary in the acute phase of recovery.

  D. have been shown to be ineffective when presented in massed blocked sessions.

ANSWERS

3.1 **B.** Cerebral hemispherectomy has been utilized as a treatment for cortical tumors (option A). However, it is a dramatic surgery most commonly used for intractable seizures resistant to medications. Unless infarcts lead to intractable seizures, infarcts alone are not indications for cerebral hemispherectomy (option C). Presurgical evaluation of children that are candidates for this surgery may show multifocal epileptic activity (seizures arising from several areas of the brain); however, the seizures are restricted to one hemisphere. This finding may be supported by neuroimaging scans showing abnormalities in one hemisphere. Although individuals with developmental etiologies such as hemimegalencephaly or cortical dysplasia may have abnormalities in both hemispheres, surgical candidates show seizures arising from only one hemisphere (option D).

3.2 **C.** A patient status/post hemispherectomy typically has spasticity with motor involvement in the lower extremity (option A); however, most involvement is in the distal upper extremity due to decreased subcortical innervation and/or etiology. Proximal muscles receive more bilateral cortical input than distal muscles, indicating that the unaffected hemisphere continues to provide input to those muscle groups after unilateral lesion or damage.[2] Functional recovery varies and patients may demonstrate minimal spontaneous movement, while others utilize their affected limb as a helper hand (the nondominant hand assists in bilateral tasks such as stabilizing a paper while cutting with the dominant, less involved hand). Others may be able to demonstrate crude grasp. Visual field cuts (option B) are present, but so are sensory deficits in the limbs. Although ambulation is difficult due to visual/perceptual, balance, strength, spasticity, sensory, and ROM limitations, partial recovery of motor functioning is possible as a result of major brain reorganization/neuroplasticity (option D).

3.3 **A.** Although more research is required regarding the effectiveness and dosage of physical therapy in clients status/post hemispherectomy, strategies implementing motor learning techniques (novel, massed practice) are feasible options for this population and positive changes may occur. Due to the younger ages of certain etiologies such as cortical dysplasia, children status/post cerebral hemispherectomy are aging with a chronic disability and would likely benefit from physical therapy throughout their lifespan.

REFERENCES

1. Cook SW, Nguyen ST, Hu B, et al. Cerebral hemispherectomy in pediatric patients with epilepsy: comparison of three techniques by pathologic substrate in 115 patients. *J Neurosurg.* 2004;100:125-141.

2. Samargia SA, Kimberley TJ. Motor and cognitive outcomes in children after functional hemispherectomy. *Pediatr Phys Ther.* 2009;21:356-361.

3. Devlin AM, Cross JH, Harkness W, et al. Clinical outcomes of hemispherectomy for epilepsy in childhood and adolescence. *Brain.* 2003;126:556-566.

4. van der Kolk NM, Boshuisen K, van Empelen R, et al. Etiology-specific differences in motor function after hemispherectomy. *Epilepsy Res.* 2013;103:221-230.

5. Griffiths SY, Sherman EM, Slick DJ, Eyrl K, Connolly MB, Steinbok P. Postsurgical health-related quality of life (HRQOL) in children following hemispherectomy for intractable epilepsy. *Epilepsia.* 2007;48:564-570.

6. Mani J, Gupta A, Mascha E, et al. Postoperative seizures after extratemporal resections and hemispherectomy in pediatric epilepsy. *Neurology.* 2006;66:1038-1043.

7. Moosa AN, Gupta A, Jehi L, et al. Longitudinal seizure outcome and prognostic predictors after hemispherectomy in 170 children. *Neurology.* 2013;80:253-260.

8. Lam S, Mathern GW. Functional hemispherectomy at UCLA. In: Cataltepe O, Jallo G, eds. *Pediatric Epilepsy Surgery: Preoperative Assessment and Surgical Treatment.* New York, NY: Thieme Medical Publishers, Inc.; 2010:230-240.

9. van Empelen R, Jennekens-Schinkel A, Buskens E, Helders PJ, van Nieuwenhuizen O; Dutch Collaborative Epilepsy Surgery Programme. Functional consequences of hemispherectomy. *Brain.* 2004;127:2071-2079.

10. Koh S, Nguyen S, Asarnow RF, et al. Five or more acute postoperative seizures predict hospital course and long-term seizure control after hemispherectomy. *Epilepsia.* 2004;45:527-533.

11. Harvey AS, Cross JH, Shinnar S, Mathern GW; ILAE Pediatric Epilepsy Surgery Survey Taskforce. Defining the spectrum of international practice in pediatric epilepsy surgery patients. *Epilepsia.* 2008;49:146-155.

12. Oppenheimer DR, Griffith HB. Persistent intracranial bleeding as a complication of hemispherectomy. *J Neurol Neurosurg Psychiatry.* 1966;29:229-240.

13. Daniel RT, Villemure JG. Hemispherectomy. *Epileptologie.* 2003;20:52-59.

14. de Bode S, Fritz SL, Weir-Haynes K, Mathern GW. Constraint-induced movement therapy for individuals after cerebral hemispherectomy: a case series. *Phys Ther.* 2009;89;361-369.

15. Choi JT, Vining EP, Reisman DS, Bastian AJ. Walking flexibility after hemispherectomy: split-belt treadmill adaptation and feedback control. *Brain.* 2009;132:722-733.

16. Choi JT, Vining EP, Mori S, Bastian AJ. Sensorimotor function and sensorimotor tracts after hemispherectomy. *Neuropsychologia.* 2010;48:1192-1199.

17. Bates AL, Zadai CC. Acute care physical therapist evaluation and intervention for an adult after right hemispherectomy. *Phys Ther.* 2003;83:567-580.

18. Villablanca JR, Hovda DA. Developmental neuroplasticity in a model of cerebral hemispherectomy and stroke. *Neuroscience.* 2000;95:625-637.

19. de Bode S, Mathern GW, Bookheimer S, Dobkin B. Locomotor training remodels fMRI sensorimotor cortical activations in children after cerebral hemispherectomy. *Neurorehabil Neural Repair.* 2007;21:497-508.

20. Scholtes VA, Becher JG, Beelen A, Lankhorst GJ. Clinical assessment of spasticity in children with cerebral palsy: a critical review of available instruments. *Dev Med Child Neurol.* 2006;48:64-73.

21. Wright M, Wallman L. Cerebral palsy. In: Campbell SK, Palisano RJ, Orlin MN, eds. *Physical Therapy for Children.* 4th ed. St. Louis, MO: Elsevier Saunders; 2012:577-627.

22. Fosang AL, Galea MP, McCoy AT, Reddihough DS, Story I. Measures of muscle and joint performance in the lower limb of children with cerebral palsy. *Dev Med Child Neurol.* 2003;45:664-670.

23. Bayley N. *Bayley Scales of Infant and Toddler Development.* 3rd ed. Technical Manual. Bloomington, MN: NCS Pearson, Inc.; 2006.

24. Visser L, Ruiter SA, van der Meulen B, Ruijssenaars W, Timmerman ME. Accommodating the Bayley-III for motor and/or visual impairment: a comparative pilot study. *Pediatr Phys Ther.* 2014;26:57-67.

25. Ko J, Kim M. Reliability and responsiveness of the Gross Motor Function Measure-88 in children with cerebral palsy. *Phys Ther.* 2013;93:393-400.

26. Kuhtz-Buschbeck JP, Sundholm LK, Eliasson AC, Forssberg H. Quantitative assessment of mirror movements in children and adolescents with hemiplegic cerebral palsy. *Dev Med Child Neurol.* 2000;42:728-736.

27. Bly L. *Motor Skills Acquisition in the First Year: An Illustrated Guide to Normal Development.* San Antonio, TX: Therapy Skills Builders; 1994.

28. Krumlinde-Sundholm L, Holmefur M, Kottorp A, Eliasson AC. The Assisting Hand Assessment: current evidence of validity, reliability, and responsiveness to change. *Dev Med Child Neurol.* 2007;49:259-264.

29. Fritz S, Merlo-Rains A, Rivers E, et al. Feasibility of intensive mobility training to improve gait, balance, and mobility in persons with chronic neurological conditions: a case series. *J Neurol Phys Ther.* 2011;35:141-147.

30. Fritz SL, Rivers ED, Merlo AM, Reed AD, Mathern GW, de Bode S. Intensive mobility training postcerebral hemispherectomy: early surgery shows best functional improvements. *Eur J Phys Rehabil Med.* 2011;47:569-577.

31. de Bode S, Fritz S, Mathern GW. Cerebral hemispherectomy: sensory scores before and after intensive mobility training. *Brain Dev.* 2012;34:625-631.

32. Lettoria D, Battaglia D, Saccoa A, et al. Early hemispherectomy in catastrophic epilepsy: a neuro-cognitive and epileptic long-term follow-up. *Seizure.* 2008;17:49-63.

33. Bhat AN, Landa RJ, Galloway JC. Current perspectives on motor functioning in infants, children, and adults with autism spectrum disorders. *Phys Ther.* 2011;91:1116-1129.

34. Fetters L, Kluzik J. The effects of neurodevelopmental treatment versus practice on the reaching of children with spastic cerebral palsy. *Phys Ther.* 1996;76:346-358.

35. Bly L. *Baby Treatment Based on NDT Principles.* San Antonio, TX: Therapy Skill Builders; 1999.

36. Damiano DL. Activity, activity, activity: rethinking our physical therapy approach to cerebral palsy. *Phys Ther.* 2006;86:1534-1540.

37. O'Neil ME, Fragala-Pinkham MA, Westcott SL, et al. Physical therapy clinical management recommendations for children with cerebral palsy-spastic diplegia: achieving functional mobility outcomes. *Pediatr Phys Ther.* 2006;18:49-72.

38. Gibson SK, Sprod JA, Maher CA. The use of standing frames for contracture management for nonmobile children with cerebral palsy. *Int J Rehabil Res.* 2009;32:316-323.

39. Glickman LB, Geigle PR, Paleg GS. A systematic review of supported standing programs. *J Pediatr Rehabil Med.* 2010;3:197-213.

40. Johnston MV. Plasticity in the developing brain: implications for rehabilitation. *Dev Disabil Res Rev.* 2009;15:94-101.

41. Kolobe TH, Christy JB, Gannotti ME, et al. Research summit III proceedings on dosing in children with an injured brain or cerebral palsy: executive summary. *Phys Ther.* 2014;94:907-920.

42. Fritz SL, Merlo-Rains AM, Rivers ED, et al. Intensive intervention for improving gait, balance, and mobility in individuals with chronic incomplete spinal cord injury: a pilot study of activity tolerance and benefits. *Arch Phys Med Rehabil.* 2011;92:1776-1784.

43. Fritz SL, Pittman AL, Robinson AC, Orton SC, Rivers ED. An intense intervention for improving gait, balance, and mobility for individuals with chronic stroke: a pilot study. *J Neurol Phys Ther.* 2007;31:71-76.

44. Gordon AM, Charles J, Wolf SL. Methods of constraint-induced movement therapy for children with hemiplegic cerebral palsy: development of a child-friendly intervention for improving upper-extremity function. *Arch Phys Med Rehabil.* 2005;86:837-844.

45. Eliasson AC, Sjöstrand L, Ek L, Krumlinde-Sundholm L, Tedroff K. Efficacy of baby-CIMT: study protocol for a randomised controlled trial on infants below age 12 months, with clinical signs of unilateral CP. *BMC Pediatr.* 2014;14:141-151.

46. Martin JH, Chakrabarty S, Friel KM. Harnessing activity-dependent plasticity to repair the damaged corticospinal tract in an animal model of cerebral palsy. *Dev Med Child Neurol.* 2011;53:9-13.

47. Gordon AM, Schneider JA, Chinnan A, Charles JR. Efficacy of a hand–arm bimanual intensive therapy (HABIT) in children with hemiplegic cerebral palsy: a randomized control trial. *Dev Med Child Neurol.* 2007;49:830-838.

48. Gordon AM. To constrain or not to constrain, and other stories of intensive upper extremity training for children with unilateral cerebral palsy. *DevMed Child Neurol.* 2011;53:56-61.

Hemipolymicrogyria: Bracing for Gait

Beth Ennis

A 14-month-old toddler diagnosed with right unilateral focal polymicrogyria, affecting her right frontal, temporal, and parietal cortices, is being seen for her weekly visit with the physical therapist through Part C Early Intervention. The patient has been seen regularly by the physical therapist since she was 9 months old. Occupational therapy visits were added at 1 year of age. Initially, she presented with left hemiparesis affecting her upper extremity more than lower extremity and she was not yet sitting, crawling, or bearing weight. Throughout six months of services, the child learned to sit, crawl, pull to stand, cruise, and take steps with a push toy. However, her therapist and her family have ongoing concerns about the impact of increased tone in her left arm and leg, and how this is impairing her function. Her team of therapists, in consultation with the orthopaedic surgeon, has initiated constraint-induced therapy for her arm. They are also considering the benefits of bracing for her left leg. While her skills are rapidly approaching age-appropriate levels, the physical therapist is concerned about the quality of her movement as well as the impact of increased tone on her bones, joints, and posture.

▶ What would be the most appropriate tools to evaluate gait in a child this young?
▶ What are the components of evaluation that need to be considered when determining if bracing is appropriate?
▶ What are the considerations in bracing a child at this early age?
▶ Identify team members that should be involved in the process of determining appropriate bracing.

KEY DEFINITIONS

DYNAMIC ANKLE-FOOT ORTHOSIS (DAFO): Category of ankle-foot brace that allows for anterior-posterior movement at the ankle (includes hinged and posterior leaf spring)

EQUINUS DEFORMITY: Limited ankle dorsiflexion

SOLID ANKLE-FOOT ORTHOSIS (AFO): Type of brace that keeps the foot in a neutral position, and does not allow movement at the ankle

SUPRAMALLEOLAR ORTHOSIS (SMO): Type of low-profile brace that limits ankle inversion and eversion, but generally allows dorsiflexion and plantar flexion

Objectives

1. Understand the role of muscle tone in the development of movement patterns.

2. Describe the common gait deviations expected in a child with hemiparesis.

3. Discuss musculoskeletal impairments that can be caused by altered muscle tone.

4. Relate the impairments caused by increased muscle tone to functional activity limitations.

5. Compare bracing options to determine the most appropriate for the given situation.

6. Discuss methods of monitoring appropriateness of bracing as a child grows and changes.

Physical Therapy Considerations

PT considerations for the young child with hemiparesis:

▶ **General physical therapy plan of care/goals:** Maintain range of motion (ROM) and activity in hemiparetic side to obtain typical or near-typical developmental milestones; address movement patterns to ensure that the child is using the most energy-efficient methods possible; prevention of musculoskeletal complications

▶ **Physical therapy interventions:** Weightbearing and activation of antagonist muscles to reduce tone; movement through typical progression and activation of hemiparetic side with activities that encourage participation in typical childhood activities; constraint-induced therapy; electrical stimulation; functional movement; dynamic bracing to allow functional movement without allowing movements into tonal patterns such as excessive plantar flexion

▶ **Precautions during physical therapy:** Significantly increased tone often requires pharmacologic management, such as oral medications for spasticity, botulinum toxin injections, or baclofen intrathecal pump to allow functional movement. Adverse drug reactions (ADRs) of these medications, such as decreased alertness and excessive weakness, must be monitored. Forcing movements against significantly increased tone can cause structural problems (*e.g.*, forcing dorsiflexion can cause a midfoot break)

▶ **Complications interfering with physical therapy:** Significantly increased speed or activity can increase tone in hemiparetic side; long-term use of constraint-induced therapy could interfere with bilateral limb use; significant tone reduction could negatively affect movement, especially if child was relying on the tone for stability.

Understanding the Health Condition

Polymicrogyria is defined as a condition related to the formation of gyri or folds in the brain before birth. This condition is diagnosed when there are too many gyri and the gyri are smaller than normal. The condition can be unilateral, which is a more mild form, or bilateral, with more significant sequelae. Polymicrogyria can exist on its own or with other brain abnormalities. Body structures and functions involved vary based on the area of the brain affected. Depending on the severity, the child may present with minimal signs and symptoms or severe developmental delay with hypertonicity/hypotonicity, seizures, and cognitive issues.[1] The cause and incidence of polymicrogyria is unknown. There is some evidence that an autosomal recessive form of inheritance is possible, but this is difficult to document because mild forms can often go undetected. It may also occur in families with no history of the disorder. Clinical management depends on the individual presentation and varies widely.

Since the current patient presented with hemiplegia secondary to unilateral focal polymicrogyria, decision making related to bracing and gait will be discussed. Gait deviations in children with hemiplegia vary based on severity. The Winters, Gage, and Hicks classification system from 1987 describes 4 distinct patterns of gait in children with spastic hemiplegia.[2] Group I is highlighted by foot drop during swing, flat foot or great toe strike at initial contact, excessive hip and knee flexion during swing, but adequate dorsiflexion during stance. As tone becomes more severe, there is more constant plantar flexion throughout the gait cycle (Group II), progressing to knee hyperextension and increased lumbar lordosis (Group III). The most severe pattern (Group IV) is characterized by limited hip movement and significantly increased lordosis. Studies evaluating the decreased efficiency and increased energy expenditure during gait in children with hemiplegia highlight compensations such as hip retraction in stance,[3] increased push-off on the unaffected side,[4] and early firing of the fibularis longus[5] as specific factors involved in increased effort and causes of deformity. Other studies discuss the influence of excessive plantar flexion on pelvic retraction and hip rotation.[6]

Failure to address atypical movement patterns and the compensations that occur with them can lead to increased energy expenditure, musculoskeletal deformities, and the need for surgical intervention. The goals for therapy and bracing are to normalize gait as much as possible and minimize the structural impact of atypical weightbearing that could require surgical corrections in the future.

Strengthening (to address weakness that often accompanies increased tone) is a major component of the necessary interventions. Strengthening is often integrated into daily activities to promote strengthening as a habit, since it is no longer thought of as just an intervention, but rather a lifestyle necessity for these children.[7] The impact of bracing on tone must be understood in order to choose the most appropriate brace type in children with hemiparesis. While the proper support from a brace could improve function, too much support can significantly impair the gait pattern, causing compensation further up the kinetic chain.

Physical Therapy Patient/Client Management

In the child with hemiplegia, multiple team members, including therapists, physicians, family, and/or other caregivers, are involved in managing the movement difficulties with the arm and the leg. Depending on the age of the child, the physical therapist encourages mobility and exploration, while monitoring the impact of altered tone on movement and development. Determining the need for bracing of the leg as well as other adaptive equipment is an ongoing process. Family education should focus on developing activities that are already a part of the family's life, so the family and child are not overwhelmed by extra work. Therapy could include active stretching, weightbearing activities, and other modalities such as aquatics or hippotherapy. Each intervention is designed to reduce the impact of increased muscle tone and improve movement patterns. Therapeutic interventions are also used following botulinum toxin injections or after surgical interventions to strengthen muscles while the tone in antagonistic muscles is decreased. When determining bracing, liaising with other healthcare professionals such as an orthotist, physician, or orthopaedic surgeon may be required by third party payors. Professionals with differing backgrounds and perspectives must work together for the best benefit of the child. Each professional needs to be aware of current literature and best practice related to the impact of bracing on gait.

Examination, Evaluation, and Diagnosis

Examination to determine appropriate bracing should include medical history, measurement of tone, gait assessment, and note of current developmental skill level. Collecting history information through parent interview gives the therapist an opportunity to develop rapport with the family and learn about their daily routine. This provides information to the therapist regarding the activities in which the child is involved and the skills the child needs to be able to achieve to fulfill her role.

Muscle tone is a difficult characteristic to quantify and therapists have struggled with this concept for decades. Two methods are classically used for measuring tone: the **Ashworth scale (and its modifications)** and the **Tardieu scale**. Table 4-1 presents the Ashworth scale and its modified version used to measure resistance to passive movement around a joint with varying amounts of speed. The bold numbers are used in the modified Ashworth scale, while those in parentheses are from the original Ashworth scale.

Score	Ashworth Scale (1964)	Modified Ashworth Scale (1987)
(0) **0**	No increase in tone	No increase in muscle tone
(1) **1**	Slight increase in tone giving a catch when the limb is moved in flexion or extension	Slight increase in muscle tone, manifested by a catch and release or by minimal resistance at the end of the ROM when the affected part(s) is moved in flexion or extension
(2) **1+**		Slight increase in muscle tone, manifested by a catch, followed by minimal resistance throughout the remainder (less than half) of the ROM (range of movement)
(3) **2**	More marked increase in tone but limb easily flexed	More marked increase in muscle tone through most of the ROM, but affected part(s) easily moved
(4) **3**	Considerable increase in tone, passive movement difficult	Considerable increase in muscle tone, passive movement difficult
(5) **4**	Limb rigid in flexion or extension	Affected part(s) rigid in flexion or extension

Table 4-1   ASHWORTH SCALE[8] AND MODIFIED ASHWORTH SCALE[9]

In both the original and modified Ashworth scales, test-retest reliability in children with cerebral palsy (CP) varies from poor to adequate depending on the joint tested. Intra-rater reliability tends to be higher than inter-rater reliability.[10] The Tardieu scale measures resistance to passive movement at 3 velocities: (1) as slow as possible; (2) limb falling against gravity; and (3) as fast as possible and includes two range calculations at each velocity: the first at the feel of a catch and the second at full ROM. In use with children with CP, test-retest reliability varies from adequate to excellent in the lower extremity, and inter-rater reliability is adequate.[11] Although no studies have assessed the reliability and validity of these scales in children with polymicrogyria, the use of these methods to measure tone appears to have at least face validity for use with children that present with hemiparesis and increased tone.

Gait pattern must be evaluated to establish which components are atypical and may be addressed by bracing. While multi-plane video analysis has become the gold standard for evaluating gait, it is not readily available in many clinical settings. There are several other tools available, but many still require video or a system similar to the GAITRite (portable gait analysis tool). In 2013, Sagawa et al.[12] evaluated the impairments identified in 3-dimensional (3D) video kinematic analysis using clinical gait assessments such as the Gait Deviation Index (GDI). The GDI provides a way to score multidimensional gait analysis and compare it to typical gait, with a score of 100 or greater indicating an absence of pathology.[13] Sagawa et al.[12] found that hip extensor weakness, adductor spasticity, knee hyperextension, and ankle spasticity and weakness correlated with low GDI.

The classic clinical method of assessing gait in children with hemiparetic CP is the Winter classification,[2] but recent studies have found that children with minimally affected body structures and functions may not be able to be classified under this system. It has been suggested that a Group 0 be added to the Winter classification for children who are unable to be classified in Group 1.[12,14] Given that the toddler in this case has very mild impairments, using the entire Winter classification may not be appropriate. However, the Winter system provides parameters for physical therapists to use when evaluating gait, such as foot position during swing and initial contact, knee position in stance, and hip position throughout the cycle, which could be helpful with this child.

New observational assessment tools such as the Salford Gait Tool (SF-GT) and the Visual Gait Assessment Scale have recently emerged. SF-GT was developed to visually assess the hip, knee, and ankle during 6 points of gait, and was found to have good criterion validity[15] as well as good intra- and inter-observer reliability.[16] The Visual Gait Assessment Scale also notes positions of the hip, knee, and ankle at several points along the gait cycle. This scale also has good validity (compared to 3D gait analysis) and good reliability in experienced observers.[17] Interestingly, a systematic review on classification of gait in children with CP found that while many analytic methods are used for diagnosis, they have limited clinical value because they tend to place participants in categories that are not clinically relevant.[18]

Regardless of which tool the physical therapist uses to assess gait, it is advantageous to consistently use the chosen tool to demonstrate how using a brace changes the angles of specific joints during the gait cycle. A functional outcome measure such as the Gross Motor Function Measure (GMFM) can be used to show functional progress with use of bracing. The GMFM measures the child's function in a variety of dimensions (A: lying and rolling; B: sitting; C: crawling and kneeling; D: standing; and E: walking, running, and jumping). The GMFM is valid and reliable when used with children with CP and meaningful clinically important differences (MCIDs) for dimensions D and E were established in a study of 381 children with CP in 2008.[19] The Gross Motor Functional Classification System (GMFCS) describes functional abilities for children with CP across age bands and provides classification based on functional ability, with Level I being highly functional and Level V being dependent.[20] Table 4-2 shows the MCIDs for 3 GMFCS levels for a large effect size. For example, a highly functional child with CP would need a change of 6.5 points in the walking, running, and jumping dimension (E) to show a clinically significant change from pretest to post-test.

The toddler in this case was evaluated to determine the need for an appropriate type of brace. On the modified Ashworth scale, her tone was 1+ in her left plantar flexors and 1 in her left hamstrings. No atypical tone was noted at her hip. During gait observation, the therapist thought she fell in the range of a Group 1 on the Winter scale: plantar flexion through the swing phase, initial contact with her first metatarsal, then moving quickly to foot flat. On initial assessment, no knee hyperextension was noted in midstance. During terminal stance, the child had active dorsiflexion and good tibial translation. Given these parameters, the physical

Table 4-2 MINIMALLY CLINICALLY IMPORTANT DIFFERENCE FOR LARGE EFFECT SIZE[19]			
Dimension	GMFCS Level I	GMFCS Level II	GMFCS Level III
Dimension D	3.8	5.3	2.4
Dimension E	6.5	4.5	3.0

therapist recommended a dynamic AFO. One of the physicians did not agree with this recommendation because he was concerned about the risk of a midfoot break if the ankle were allowed to move into dorsiflexion. Although the clinicians' observations and examinations resulted in the same findings, their recommendations differed based on experience and perceived knowledge of the literature. The team decision was made to provide the child with a solid AFO to wear only at night to prevent loss of dorsiflexion ROM. Within a few months, the left knee hyperextension became apparent in the stance phase of gait, so she began to wear the solid AFO during gait to prevent damage to her knee. However, the solid AFO did not allow forward tibial translation during terminal stance, making her gait unstable. Therefore, the therapist initiated another discussion with the physician to request that the child use a dynamic AFO.

Plan of Care and Interventions

As the physical therapist begins to address gait in the child with hemiplegia, limitations in body structures and functions that are noted in the examination need to be considered. Limitations in joint ROM that prevent optimal gait mechanics should be addressed using therapeutic techniques, medical management, and adaptive equipment, as appropriate. Even if the child has one or more AFOs, therapy is often conducted without braces. While braces can reduce atypical gait parameters and assist in developing more typical walking patterns, activities outside of the braces are necessary to develop isolated strength and control. There is some evidence that weightbearing activities are beneficial in reducing tone. Strengthening may be appropriate as muscles with increased tone can be weak, and research has shown that strengthening activities do not increase spasticity.[21] According to Damiano,[7] strengthening should not be uniquely a therapy activity, but rather a lifestyle choice. Physical therapy is often seen as a chore; if strengthening activities are integrated into everyday life, they shift from "homework" to a part of life.

Because the goals for this patient included independent ambulation on level and unlevel surfaces, stair climbing, and jumping in place, the treatment plan included a variety of activities to promote weightbearing, reduce the mild to moderate increased tone in the gastrocsoleus complex, and encourage upright activities with equal use of both legs. Manual guidance was provided through her pelvis or through her knee down into her foot to encourage a foot flat position. This strategy was successful since her tone was mild to moderate in intensity. Increased speed can often promote increased stiffness. Therefore, the therapist encouraged her to move slowly until more control was gained.

Typically, a combination of strategies is used to manage increased tone in the young child. Nonsurgical interventions, which are recommended if the child is younger than 8 to 9 years, include botulinum toxin injections, electrical stimulation, bracing, and physical therapy. **Botulinum toxin injections** temporarily reduce spasticity so that antagonist muscles can be strengthened and new motor plans can be learned.[22] Other studies have shown that factors correlated with botulinum toxin injections being successful in reducing spasticity and improving motor planning and gait include younger age, fewer number of injections, child motivation, and higher parental stress.[23,24] These studies also emphasize the importance of physical therapy after the botulinum toxin injections for the successful acquisition of new motor plans. In children with hemiparesis, activity in the anterior tibialis needs to be assessed to determine whether there is adequate muscle strength to counter the antagonist muscles with increased tone. If the anterior tibialis muscle is able to actively contract, reducing the tone of the antagonist gastrocsoleus complex—even temporarily—can provide the therapist with time to strengthen dorsiflexion and counter the pull of the plantar flexor tone. This tone reduction could be in the form of medical intervention (e.g., botulinum toxin injections) and/or external support (e.g., bracing). Because children are growing, muscles with increased tone can restrict growth if they are not stretched and used. Therefore, reduction of tone is a constant consideration. Modified constraint-induced therapy[25] and functional electrical stimulation for motor retraining following botulinum toxin injections[26] have shown promise in modifying gait parameters, although generally in children rated GMFCS Levels I-III.

Because there is evidence to support specific types of bracing for children with differing abilities, thorough clinical evaluation is necessary to determine the appropriate brace for the child at each point in her life. In children with more significant impairments, a solid AFO continues to be the most recommended device.[27] In contrast, there is growing recognition that **children with less significant tone** show more functional improvement and better gait characteristics, such as heel strike, stride length, and cadence, in dynamic AFOs.[28-31] One study of 11 children with hemiplegia, GMFCS Levels I-II, reinforced the fact that a hinged AFO not only reduced energy expenditure, but also controlled equinus deformity.[31] Clinical interpretation suggests that a child with more significant involvement might need more support to prevent deformity, whereas the child with less involvement could be provided slightly less support to allow more typical movement during gait.

The current child was re-examined to assess the effect of the dynamic AFO on her gait performance. The therapist noted that she had a neutral ankle position in swing with a gradual decrease in excessive hip flexion over time, heel strike on initial contact with slow transition through loading, and forward tibial translation in terminal stance. The physical therapist instructed the parent in donning the dynamic AFO and applying the straps so that the child's heel was seated well in the brace to ensure that dorsiflexion was generated at the ankle and not at the midfoot.

Evidence-Based Clinical Recommendations

SORT: Strength of Recommendation Taxonomy

A: Consistent, good-quality patient-oriented evidence
B: Inconsistent or limited-quality patient-oriented evidence
C: Consensus, disease-oriented evidence, usual practice, expert opinion, or case series

1. The modified Ashworth scale and Tardieu scales appear to have face validity for use with children with polymicrogyria that present with hemiparesis and increased tone. **Grade C**

2. In children with cerebral palsy (GMFCS Levels I-III), botulinum toxin injections followed by physical therapy temporarily reduce spasticity so that antagonist muscles can be strengthened and new motor plans can be learned. **Grade A**

3. Bracing to reduce tone and normalize gait parameters is an effective intervention in children with lower extremity spasticity, but the specific bracing type needs to be individualized to the child. **Grade A**

COMPREHENSION QUESTIONS

4.1 All of the following are true regarding children with hemiplegia, except:
   A. They have an asymmetrical gait pattern.
   B. They sometimes present with equinus deformity.
   C. They always need bracing to normalize gait.
   D. They have involvement of the arm and leg on the same side.

4.2 Children who present with increased tone may benefit from all of the following, except:
   A. Medical management of tone
   B. Strengthening programs
   C. Bracing during movement
   D. Increasing tone for stability

4.3 A valid and reliable tool for measuring tone is:
   A. GMFM
   B. Modified Ashworth scale
   C. Manual muscle testing
   D. Palpation of the muscle

ANSWERS

4.1 **C.** Bracing may not always be needed, depending on the amount of tone present. Generally, some amount of asymmetry in gait is present, even if it is mild (option A).

4.2 **D.** Increasing tone in children with spasticity can lead to even more inefficient movements and increased energy expenditure.

4.3 **B.** The modified Ashworth scale is the only tool listed that measures tone.

REFERENCES

1. Genetics Home Reference. Polymicrogyria. 2009. http://ghr.nlm.nih.gov/condition/polymicrogyria. Accessed September 30, 2014.

2. Winters TF, Gage JR, Hicks R. Gait patterns in spastic hemiplegia in children and young adults. *J Bone Joint Surg Am.* 1987;69:437-441.

3. Böhm H, Döderlein L. Gait asymmetries in children with cerebral palsy: do they deteriorate with running? *Gait Posture.* 2012;35:322-327.

4. Böhm H, Stief F, Dussa CU, Döderlein L. Predictors of pelvic retraction in children with cerebral palsy derived from gait parameters and clinical testing. *Gait Posture.* 2012;35:250-254.

5. Boulay C, Pomero V, Viehweger E, et al. Dynamic equinus with hindfoot valgus in children with hemiplegia. *Gait Posture.* 2012;36:108-112.

6. Brunner R, Dreher T, Romkes J, Frigo C. Effects of plantarflexion on pelvis and lower limb kinematics. *Gait Posture.* 2008;28:150-156.

7. Damiano DL. Muscle size matters. *Dev Med Child Neurol.* 2009;51:416-417.

8. Ashworth B. Preliminary trial of carisoprodal in multiple sclerosis. *Practitioner.* 1964;192:540-542.

9. Bohannon RW, Smith MB. Interrater reliability of a modified Ashworth scale of muscle spasticity. *Phys Ther.* 1987;67:206-207.

10. Ashworth scale/modified Ashworth scale. *Rehab Measures* 2012. http://www.rehabmeasures.org/Lists/RehabMeasures/PrintView.aspx?ID=902. Accessed September 30, 2014.

11. Tardieu scale/Modified tardieu scale. *Rehab Measures* 2012. http://www.rehabmeasures.org/Lists/RehabMeasures/PrintView.aspx?ID=1038. Accessed September 30, 2014.

12. Sagawa Y Jr, Watelain E, De Coulon G, Kaelin A, Gorce P, Armand S. Are clinical measurements linked to the Gait Deviation Index in cerebral palsy patients? *Gait Posture.* 2013;38:276-280.

13. Schwartz MH, Rozumalski A. The gait deviation index: a new comprehensive index of gait pathology. *Gait Posture.* 2008;28:351-357.

14. Riad J, Haglund-Akerlind Y, Miller F. Classification of spastic hemiplegic cerebral palsy in children. *J Pediatr Orthop.* 2007;27:758-764.

15. Toro B, Nester CJ, Farren PC. The development and validity of the Salford Gait Tool: an observation-based clinical gait assessment tool. *Arch Phys Med Rehabil.* 2007;88:321-327.

16. Toro B, Nester CJ, Farren PC. Inter- and intraobserver repeatability of the Salford Gait Tool: an observation-based clinical gait assessment tool. *Arch Phys Med Rehabil.* 2007;88:328-332.

17. Brown CR, Hillman SJ, Richardson AM, Herman JL, Robb JE. Reliability and validity of the Visual Gait Assessment Scale for children with hemiplegic cerebral palsy when used by experienced and inexperienced observers. *Gait Posture.* 2008;27:648-652.

18. Dobson F, Morris ME, Baker R, Graham HK. Gait classification in children with cerebral palsy: a systematic review. *Gait Posture.* 2007;25:140-152.

19. Oeffinger D, Bagley A, Rogers S, et al. Outcome tools used for ambulatory children with cerebral palsy: responsiveness and minimum clinically important differences. *Dev Med Child Neurol.* 2008;50:918-925.

20. Palisano R, Rosenbaum P, Walter S, Russell D, Wood E, Galuppi B. Development and relaiblity of a system to classify gross motor function in children with cerebral palsy. *Dev Med Child Neurol.* 1997;39:214-223.

21. Finlay H, Ainscough J, Craig J, et al. Current clinical practice in the use of muscle strengthening in children and young people with cerebral palsy: a regional survey of paediatric physiotherapists. *J Assoc of Paediatric Chartered Physiotherapists.* 2012;3:27-41.

22. Degelaen M, de Borre L, Kerckhofs E, et al. Influence of botulinum toxin therapy on postural control and lower limb intersegmental coordination in children with spastic cerebral palsy. *Toxins.* 2013;5:93-105.

23. Yap R, Majnemer A, Benaroch T, Cantin MA. Determinants of responsiveness to botulinum toxin, casting, and bracing in the treatment of spastic equinus in children with cerebral palsy. *Dev Med Child Neurol.* 2010;52:186-193.

24. de Souza ME, Duarte NAC, Franco RC, Secco MFM, Politti F, Oliveira CS. Effect of botulinum toxin A on spasticity and function in children with cerebral palsy: a systematic review. *Med Sci Technol.* 2014;55:11-15.

25. Coker P, Karakostas T, Dodds C, Hsiang S. Gait characteristics of children with hemiplegic cerebral palsy before and after modified constraint-induced movement therapy. *Disabil Rehabil.* 2010;32:402-408.

26. Seifart A, Unger M, Burger M. Functional electrical stimulation to lower limb muscles after botox in children with cerebral palsy. *Pediatr Phys Ther.* 2010;22:199-206.

27. Cobeljic G, Bumbasirevic M, Lesic A, Bajin Z. The management of spastic equinus in cerebral palsy. *Orthopaed Trauma.* 2009;23:201-209.

28. Radtka SA, Skinner SR, Johanson ME. A comparison of gait with solid and hinged ankle-foot orthoses in children with spastic diplegic cerebral palsy. *Gait Posture.* 2005;21:303-310.

29. Desloovere K, Molenaers G, Van Gestel L, et al. How can push-off be preserved during use of an ankle foot orthosis in children with hemiplegia? A prospective controlled study. *Gait Posture.* 2006;24:142-151.

30. Van Gestel L, Molenaers G, Huenaerts C, Seyler J, Desloovere K. Effect of dynamic orthoses on gait: a retrospective control study in children with hemiplegia. *Dev Med Child Neurol.* 2008;50:63-67.

31. Balaban B, Yasar E, Dal U, Yazicioglu K, Mohur H, Kalyon TA. The effect of hinged ankle-foot orthosis on gait and energy expenditure in spastic hemiplegic cerebral palsy. *Disabil Rehabil.* 2007;29:139-144.

Extreme Prematurity and the Neonatal Intensive Care Unit

Anastasiya Ruiz

CASE 5

A 32-year-old pregnant female presented to the emergency department with severe preeclampsia. Male infant was born by emergency cesarean section at 25 weeks 2 days, weighing 550 g. Apgar scores were 1 at 1 minute, 4 at 5 minutes, and 7 at 10 minutes. The infant was intubated in the delivery room due to poor respiratory effort and transferred to a Level IV neonatal intensive care unit (NICU). Of note, the mother's past medical history is significant for chronic hypertension. The prenatal medical screening, including Group B streptococcus, was negative. Perinatal course was significant for preeclampsia superimposed on chronic hypertension and administration of antenatal steroids. The infant's pertinent history of present illness is as follows: apnea of prematurity (AOP), neonatal respiratory distress syndrome (RDS), bronchopulmonary dysplasia (BPD), intrauterine growth restriction (IUGR), and patent ductus arteriosus (PDA). The infant is now 34 weeks 3 days (post-conceptual age) and weighs 1040 g. The physical therapist receives a consult to evaluate and treat. At the bedside, the therapist notes that the infant is in left sidelying in an incubator on 5 L/min high-flow nasal cannula and a nasogastric tube for feeding is present. From the cardiorespiratory monitor, the vital signs are: heart rate, 155 to 160 beats/min; respiratory rate, 65 to 75 breaths/min; oxygen saturation, 94% to 95%. The baby's mother is at the bedside.

▶ What are the examination priorities?
▶ What are the possible complications interfering with physical therapy?
▶ What precautions should be taken during physical therapy examination and interventions?
▶ Describe a physical therapy plan of care based on each stage of the health condition.

KEY DEFINITIONS

APGAR: Test performed by the delivering medical team at 1, 5, and 10 minutes after birth; each of the 5 sections (respiratory effort, heart rate, muscle tone, reflexes, skin color) is scored on a scale of 0 to 2; the higher the score, the better the health of the infant

GROUP B STREPTOCOCCAL INFECTION: Bacterial infection present in the woman's vagina, rectum, or urinary bladder that can be passed to the infant during delivery; although rare, infants who become infected are at risk for pneumonia, sepsis, and meningitis.

HIGH-FLOW NASAL CANNULA: Oxygen delivery device that delivers heated and humidified air at higher fractions of inspired oxygen than room air

INCUBATOR: Apparatus used to control environmental factors for infants who are ill or born preterm; primary purpose is to provide a thermal environment that helps the infant maintain appropriate body temperature

LEVEL IV NEONATAL INTENSIVE CARE UNIT: Neonatal unit that provides the highest level of comprehensive care for critically ill infants, including advanced respiratory support, 24-hour on-site neonatology team, advanced imaging, and urgent on-site access to pediatric medical and surgical subspecialists

POST-CONCEPTUAL AGE: Gestational age plus weeks since birth (chronological age)

PREECLAMPSIA: One of the most common complications of pregnancy, marked by hypertension and proteinuria; places the mother at increased risk for brain injury, blood clotting issues, and kidney and liver injury; it also decreases blood flow to the placenta, leading to IUGR or prematurely born infants

Objectives

1. Identify common medical sequelae of prematurity.

2. Identify possible developmental consequences of prematurity.

3. Describe how the infant's history of present illness (prematurity, AOP, RDS, BPD, IUGR) may impact development.

4. Describe the neonatal physical therapist's role in the NICU.

5. Identify precautions associated with treating the premature infant.

6. Identify appropriate interventions for the premature infant.

Physical Therapy Considerations

PT considerations during management of the premature infant:

▶ **General physical therapy plan of care/goals:** Facilitate typical development and achievement of developmental milestones from birth age to discharge; prevent or minimize secondary impairments; promote appropriate muscle tone and movement pattern development; encourage development of self-regulatory skills and state of arousal; promote infant role (procuring, social interaction, exploratory play, feeding); educate caregivers on proper handling techniques, positioning, and developmental activities; promote parental role

▶ **Physical therapy interventions:** Determine and facilitate infant's movement patterns, tone, posture, behavioral organization (including stress signs), and physiologic stability; facilitate quiet alert state and state transitions; minimize stress; promote age-appropriate postural and movement activities; facilitate proper handling techniques and positioning; provide environmental modifications; nursing and caregiver education

▶ **Precautions during physical therapy interventions:** Continuous monitoring of vital signs and behavioral cues throughout sessions; monitor medical lines and tubes; determine whether physiologic cost of the examination/intervention outweighs anticipated benefits

▶ **Complications interfering with physical therapy:** Pain and stress; decline in physiologic stability (apnea, bradycardia); fractures

Understanding the Health Condition

Development is a complex and dynamic process fostered by the intrauterine environment, which is rhythmic, rich in diverse stimuli, and gravity-free. Prematurity (birth before 37 weeks of gestation), and especially extreme prematurity (birth before 28 weeks of gestation), occurs at a critical point in neurobehavioral and physiologic maturation.[1] The immature infant is forced to adapt to the NICU environment and experience stress, pain, effects of various medical conditions associated with premature birth, overstimulation from the environment (lights, sounds, medical interventions), and multisensory understimulation due to the absence of the intrauterine environment.[1,2] Put simply, prematurity is the complicated interaction between the environment and the immature organ systems of the infant.[3] As a result, prematurity alters the trajectory of optimal development and has a negative impact on all systems including cognitive, behavioral, and motor.[1]

Premature birth can occur for various genetic, toxic, metabolic, and infectious reasons leading to preterm labor, premature rupture of membranes, and/or fetal or maternal illness.[3] The majority of infant morbidity and mortality is related to compromised development due to preterm birth in addition to the illnesses that precipitated preterm birth, any delivery complications, and medical interventions after birth.[1,3] With advances in medicine, including antenatal steroids, surfactant therapy, and ventilation therapy, survival for premature infants has improved in the last several decades. As of 2009, an infant born at 25 weeks gestational age and below 1500 g has a survival rate of 67% and 90%, respectively.[4-6] However, morbidity in this population continues to persist. In the preterm population, gestational age and weight are strong predictors of outcome, with gestational age being more significant than birth weight.[1,3,4,6-10] Other factors that negatively impact survival and health status in extremely premature infants include male sex, multiple births, and lack of antenatal steroids.[6,9]

It is important to recognize that prematurity is not a single disease; deficits can overlap and impact on one another not only at birth, but also into adolescence and adulthood.[3] Infants born preterm are at risk for many conditions such as AOP, RDS, BPD, visual impairments (e.g., retinopathy of prematurity), brain injury (e.g., intraventricular hemorrhage [IVH], periventricular leukomalacia), PDA, feeding intolerance, osteopenia of prematurity, gastroesophageal reflux, and necrotizing enterocolitis. AOP is the absence of respiration for 20 seconds or more, usually accompanied by bradycardia and/or oxygen desaturation.[11] AOP is related to respiratory control immaturity. In infants born weighing less than 1000 g, the incidence of AOP is 90%.[11] Medical management usually includes supplemental oxygen and medications such as caffeine.[11] RDS is caused by insufficient surfactant in the underdeveloped lung.[11] Other contributing factors include an overly compliant chest wall, decreased intrathoracic pressure, and cardiovascular shunting. Risk factors include prematurity, male sex, maternal diabetes, and chorioamnionitis.[11] Medical management requires surfactant and supplemental oxygenation, including mechanical ventilation. BPD is the most common cause of chronic lung disease (CLD) in infants, increasing the risk of rehospitalization in the first year.[12-14] The hallmarks of BPD are oversimplified alveoli (larger and fewer in number) and abnormal pulmonary vasculature.[12,14] Pathogenesis is related to antenatal and postnatal factors such as mechanical ventilation and supplemental oxygen, which promote the release of inflammatory cytokines that causes subsequent damage to the lungs.[12,14] BPD is defined as requiring supplemental oxygen for at least 28 days of life.[12,13] The severity of the condition is based on oxygen requirement at 36 weeks post-conceptual age.[12,13] Factors contributing to the susceptibility of acquiring BPD include lower gestational age, lower weight, intubation, fluid overload, PDA in the first week of life, and high peak inspiratory pressure during mechanical ventilation.[12,14,15] The use of nasal continuous positive airway pressure and nasal intermittent positive pressure ventilation decreases the risk of developing BPD.[11] BPD is a major cause of neonatal illness and poorer outcomes in psychomotor, language, and cognitive domains, as well as decreased exercise capacity when compared to full-term infants.[13,14,16] Symptoms of BPD can persist into early adulthood.[12-14] PDA is the failure of the ductus arteriosus to close, causing heart failure (right and left), redistribution of systemic blood flow, and reduction of renal, mesenteric, and cerebral blood flow. The risk of PDA increases with decreasing gestational age. The larger the PDA, the higher the risk for IVH, BPD, and increased mortality and morbidity.[17] IUGR is a condition characterized by poor growth, wherein the infant's weight is below the 10th percentile for its gestational age.[18] It can be classified as symmetric or asymmetric (head-sparing). Infants with IUGR are at higher risk for mortality and neurodevelopmental morbidity, and are at higher risk to be born preterm.[19] Infants with IUGR have poor memory performance, learning disabilities, and deficits in visual-motor function and attention span.[19] IUGR is associated with maternal comorbidities including hypertension, preeclampsia, HELLP syndrome, and gestational diabetes.[19] The most significant factor in neurodevelopmental and cognitive performance at 9 to 10 years old is the amount of head-sparing, with better outcomes in those with greater head-sparing.[18]

The developing infant brain is especially susceptible to injury. Premature birth alone—with no other associated conditions—predisposes the infant to neurodevelopmental deficits.[2] It was previously thought that the developing brain had the advantage of plasticity to recover from an injury.[2] However, it is clear that the lower the gestational age and birth weight, the poorer the motor outcomes.[1,20] Brain development may be affected by inflammation, hypoxia, excitotoxicity, or ischemic events associated with severe illness and stress from necessary procedures crucial to sustain the infant's life.[21,22] Studies comparing premature infants at 40 weeks of gestation to full-term infants consistently show white matter abnormalities, as well as decreased total cerebral volumes, smaller cortical surface areas, grey matter injury, and altered neural pathways.[1,2,4,20,21] These differences even persist into school age.[1] White matter abnormalities are strongly associated with cognitive and motor delays and cerebral palsy (CP) at 2 years of age.[4]

Medical management in the extremely premature, very low-birth-weight (<1500 g) infant most often includes surfactant administration, respiratory support, parenteral and enteral nutrition, and early caffeine initiation.[11,23,24] Prior to the infant's birth, the mother may be given antenatal steroids because they have been shown to reduce neonatal death, RDS, IVH, necrotizing enterocolitis, system infections, and the need for respiratory support in the first 48 hours of life.[11]

Survivors of preterm birth demonstrate a variety of disabilities, each having an effect on one another in a complex and interweaving way.[3] Impaired cognitive, motor, and behavioral development can occur in the presence of significant, mild, or no apparent brain injury.[2] For instance, mild motor impairments, called minor neuromotor dysfunction, may present as reflex, postural, or tonal abnormalities, ataxia, or asymmetries even in the absence of CP.[20] While differences in motor performance between preterm and term infants may not initially be evident, the disparity becomes obvious at preschool age and into adolescence, even in children with no obvious neurologic damage.[1] This may be related to the increased complexity of motor task demands, such as balance skills and manual dexterity. Other common developmental deficits include behavioral and emotional issues (*e.g.*, attention deficit/hyperactivity disorder), problems forming social relationships, difficulties in school, lower cognitive scores, impaired processing speed, deficits in executive function, and inattention.[1,3,8,10,25,26] These behavioral, academic, and cognitive issues tend to persist into adulthood.[8,10] In addition, several studies have demonstrated that lower socioeconomic status negatively impacts outcomes of preterm infants.[4,8,16,23,25]

Premature birth not only impacts the infant, but also creates a traumatic and stressful experience to the parents by interrupting antenatal bonding and causing parental fears of infant survival and the possibility of developmental disabilities.[27] The mother-infant attachment and relationship is crucial because it sets the stage for future social interactions and behavioral and cognitive development.[1,27,28] Preterm birth negatively impacts the quality of the mother-infant relationship as well as the mother's perception of her relationship with her infant.[27] Low socioeconomic status and education level are risk factors for problems in the mother-infant relationship.[1,4,27]

Physical Therapy Patient/Client Management

The NICU team includes a neonatologist, medical resident, nurse practitioner and/ or physician assistant, registered neonatal nurse (the infant is usually assigned a primary nurse for consistency), respiratory therapist, social worker, lactation specialist, developmental specialist, and therapist (physical, occupational, and/or speech). Care is provided in a goal-directed, developmentally supportive way. The family is a vital and active part of the NICU team that is involved in decisions and encouraged to provide input into their baby's care. The infant is at the center of all decisions regarding timing and degree of interventions and evaluations provided.[29] The NICU is a highly specialized environment and an advanced practice area for physical therapists.[30] All direct care in the NICU requires constant reassessment of safety and necessity to ensure that the benefits of care outweigh the possible harm, since even routine evaluation and examination techniques may harm the infant.[29] For this reason, students, physical therapy assistants, and physical therapists without specialized training are not appropriate providers of care in the NICU.[29] Physical therapists who provide services in this environment must complete a mentoring and competency process that includes extensive knowledge of neonatal care, the critical care environment, common neonatal conditions, typical and atypical neonatal development, and family education and interaction in the NICU.[31] The primary role of the physical therapist in the NICU is to promote typical development, prevent secondary sequelae, and support and educate caregivers.[32] There are several theoretical frameworks guiding physical therapy in the NICU. In the dynamic systems model, multiple components (infant, environment, and task of the infant) interact simultaneously to influence functional movement and postural control.[33] One component may constrain another in an infant who is medically fragile and physiologically immature. The infant's attempts to perform a task or complete a goal, such as self-soothing or transitioning to an awake state, is the optimal time for the physical therapist or caregiver to provide support so that the infant is successful because this is the time that the system is most responsive to change.[33] While the dynamic system theory focuses on movement, the synactive theory describes behavioral organization. Behavioral organization and maintenance is influenced by the interaction between the immature system of the infant, the caregiver, and the environment.[31] The autonomic system is the foundation on which motor ability, state transitions, attention/interaction, and self-regulation components are built upon. While these components are hierarchical, each component also influences the other and instability in one system influences the rest. In the preterm infant, the systems are immature and behavior is characterized by behavioral disorganization and stress.[31] Behavioral organization is one of the most important capacities underlying the infant's ability to perform his expected occupation.[31]

Examination, Evaluation, and Diagnosis

The physical therapy evaluation begins with a thorough chart review. Relevant information includes: infant's age and weight at birth and at evaluation, mother's history (past medical history, education level, number of previous pregnancies, medications taken during pregnancy), pregnancy course and complications (*e.g.,* cause of premature birth, substance abuse, extent of prenatal care), perinatal history (*e.g.,* Apgar scores, complications during delivery), infant's medical history, and family's social history (*e.g.,* involvement in social services, supports available).[31] A comprehensive chart review provides the therapist a strong foundation for the evaluation. Prior to the evaluation, the therapist should also consult the chart and the nurse to learn if there were any significant medical events over the last few days, such as changes in medical stability or increased irritability. Laboratory values and imaging should be reviewed, as well as evaluations from services consulted thus far (*e.g.,* neurology, genetics, orthopaedics). The therapist should always speak with the nurse to determine whether the time chosen for the evaluation is suitable. To allow the infant to sleep and conserve energy for neurodevelopment and growth, the therapist must consider clustering care and timing the evaluation prior to feeding or around nursing care.

Once at the bedside, the therapist notes the infant's vital signs at rest, respiratory support (*e.g.,* high-flow nasal cannula), and all lines and tubes attached to the infant, since these will need to be carefully monitored during the hands-on evaluation. The observational portion of the assessment begins by noting the infant's position and posture in the incubator, presence of developmental positioning equipment, and state of arousal. It should be noted if the infant appears supported and comfortable. It is also valuable to observe nursing care as this can provide information about the infant's stability, movement patterns, and tolerance to handling. The observational assessment provides information about the infant's baseline status and readiness for intervention.[33,34]

The hands-on portion of the evaluation should be initiated by providing contained touch, performed by placing the weight of the therapist's hand on the infant's trunk, buttocks, or head for several minutes. This is a way to grade tactile input and allow the infant to accommodate to touch. In an effort to maintain homeostasis while processing the clinician's input, the infant may initially demonstrate stress signs. These may include arching of the spine, extension of the upper and lower extremities, and irritability.[35] During stressful experiences, the infant tries to regain and maintain neurophysiologic balance through self-regulatory behaviors, which may include suck search, hand clasping, attempts to achieve a flexed posture, searching for boundaries, and bracing of the legs. Observe whether the infant is able to recover from stress without support. If the infant is unable to calm, the therapist should provide external support. This may include providing hand grasp, promoting hands together and to the mouth, facilitating flexed posture, providing boundaries, and offering non-nutritive sucking. It is important for neurobehavioral development that the therapist responds to the infant while allowing the infant the opportunity to recruit self-regulatory skills and calm on his own.[31] This is a delicate balance and may take experience for the therapist to develop. Once the infant regains behavioral organization, either through external support or internal strategies, the therapist should note which strategy was most effective, the amount of stimulation required to calm the infant, the amount of time it took for the infant to calm, and the degree of physiologic cost to the infant. These variables are essential to the physical therapy evaluation because they factor into the assessment of tolerance to handling and degree of behavioral organization.[31]

Pain in the premature infant is also an important aspect of the evaluation. It is well established that preterm infants feel the pain of invasive procedures, such as a heel stick, and have the peripheral and central nervous system structures necessary for processing and sensing pain.[36] In fact, preterm infants have lower pain thresholds than their term counterparts due to the immaturity of their nervous system.[36] Preterm infants may also feel the noxious stimuli long after it has ended, which may contribute to sensitization to repeated painful input. Lucas-Thompson et al.[36] determined that the lower the gestational age at birth, the more vulnerable infants are to a painful procedure and less able they are to recover from this noxious input. In the preterm infant, pain can be measured by changes in vital signs and facial expressions such as increased heart rate, nasolabial furrowing, eyebrow bulging, and eye squeezing.[34,36] Preterm infants may have difficulty enlisting self-regulatory behaviors or even signaling when they have pain.[34,36] The physical therapist can help alleviate pain through provision of non-pharmacologic interventions such as facilitated tucking or non-nutritive sucking as well as educating caregivers or other clinicians on the importance of providing such interventions during noxious procedures.[37]

The benefits of continuing with a hands-on assessment must always be weighed against the potential risks and physiologic cost to the infant. The therapist should use changes in vital signs and signs of stress and pain as a guide for when an evaluation needs to be paused or terminated. These indications should not be taken lightly as they are the infant's only way of communicating that the environment is supportive or appropriate. Infants who are premature may not be able to cope with the degree of stimulation and handling due to neurologic immaturity, impaired musculoskeletal tone, and environmental factors (e.g., gravity, light, sound). The infant may only be able to organize behaviorally with the external support from the caregiver. Therefore, providing appropriately timed and graded support is vital in strengthening neural connections and teaching self-soothing behaviors. Ignoring important distress cues may cause the infant to progress into significant medical instability manifested by bradycardia, apnea, and severe oxygen desaturation requiring medical intervention. Other signs of instability that require immediate intervention include pallor, cyanosis, limpness, stiffness, and unresponsiveness.[31] The therapist should also be careful of fractures in these medically fragile infants. Elevated alkaline phosphatase levels (>800 IU/L) and osteopenia of prematurity increase fracture risk.[34]

Once the infant is able to achieve and maintain behavioral organization after the initial tactile touch, the therapist can continue with the assessment. Active muscle function with and without tactile input can be assessed next. When the infant is moving without boundaries, the quality (i.e., fluidity, midline orientation, organization, symmetry) and frequency of movements should be noted. It is important for the therapist to be aware of typical and atypical development since it is expected that preterm infants demonstrate less coordinated movements with a poorer repertoire.[31] For infants with respiratory issues such as BPD, neck extension and scapular retraction may occur during active movements as a strategy to optimize respiratory status.[34] Another way to assess the degree of infant movements is through the quality of general movements (GMs). GMs are part of the infant's spontaneous movement repertoire and "involve the whole body in a variable sequence of arm, leg, neck and trunk movements."[38] They are complex and demonstrate considerable variability in speed, intensity, and force. GMs have a gradual beginning and end and appear fluent and elegant.[39,40] In the preterm period, GMs are normally variable, possibly having large amplitudes and fast speed.[38] Movements that lack complexity and variability may indicate abnormalities in the central nervous system.[38] An asymmetry in active movement is an atypical finding. Observing GMs has value in predicting neurodevelopmental issues.[39] In a systematic review, Noble and Boyd[41] found that **GMs are valid and reliable in predicting the incidence of CP when compared to other neonatal assessments** (*e.g.*, Assessment of Preterm Infants' Behavior, Neonatal Intensive Care Unit Network Neurobehavioral Scale, Test of Infant Motor Performance, Neurobehavioral Assessment of the Preterm Infant).

Another way to assess the maturing central nervous system is to test for the presence of primitive reflexes. Reflexes are the foundation for development of movement; abnormalities may impede movement acquisition.[22,42] Reflexes develop in a caudocephalad (lower extremities to upper extremities) and centripetal (distal to proximal) pattern.[43] The palmar grasp and plantar grasp are established by 32 weeks of age and it is important to assess their presence during the examination.[31,34,42] Based on the infant's tolerance, the asymmetric tonic neck reflex, which appears at 35 weeks of gestation, can also be performed.[42]

Tone also develops in a caudocephalad and centripetal pattern.[43] In the lower extremities, tone begins to emerge between 33 and 35 weeks; in the upper extremities, tone begins between 35 and 37 weeks.[31,43,44] It is expected that preterm infants have lower flexor tone. Even when compared to their term counterparts at term equivalent age, premature infants have lower tone and movement patterns that are different.[45] Assessment of tone should include the scarf sign, upper and lower extremity recoil, and the popliteal angle.[34,42]

The infant's state of arousal has a significant impact on the evaluation and further interventions. Responses, including active movements, tone, and reflexes, are dampened in a drowsy and sleeping state and exaggerated in an active alert or crying state.[31] Ideally, the evaluation should be performed in a variety of states. However, assessment of GMs is most accurate in the active alert state.[40] For preterm infants, transitioning to and maintaining an awake state are physiologically costly. As such, preterm infants tend to sleep longer.[31] By 36 weeks, the infant should be able to achieve brief periods of arousal, but will likely not be able to stay awake for long periods of time.[31] The ability of the infant to achieve and maintain a state of arousal while preserving homeostasis indicates his level of behavioral organization.[35] The quiet alert state that is optimal for feeding, interaction, and exploration appears in only a few preterm infants and only closer to term.[31]

Assessment of head shape deformities and head preference is important in premature infants. Since the initiation of sudden infant death syndrome (SIDS) guidelines by the American Association of Pediatrics in 1992 that advocated infants sleep on their backs, the incidence of head shape deformities has increased, especially in the preterm population.[46,47] Nuysink et al.[47] observed that 44.8% of infants younger than 32 weeks gestational age had a head rotation preference (referred to as a "head preference"), wherein the infant's head was mainly turned to one side and there was impaired active movement to the opposite side. By comparison, the incidence of this type of posturing preference was only 13% to 20% in infants born full term. In their sample, in those infants who had a head preference, 91% had a head preference to the right. In those born preterm, a head preference can be attributed to various factors, including the infant's position in utero, musculoskeletal and neuromuscular immaturity, and the effects of gravity on the immature system.[47] Caregiver practices in the NICU also contribute to a head preference. By approaching the infant from the right or positioning equipment on the infant's right side, caregivers often stimulate the infant largely to the right due to their own handedness or preference.[47]

A head preference can lead to persistent pressure on one side of the skull that results in a positional head deformity such as positional plagiocephaly (PP). PP is an obliquity in head shape accompanied by displacement of the ear anteriorly on the same side. Risk factors include preterm birth, supine sleeping, male sex, decreased awake time (less time to perform "tummy time"), and congenital torticollis.[46] Nuysink et al.[47] also found that at term equivalent age, for infants born at less than 32 weeks, CLD was the only factor associated with an increased risk of PP.[47] However, one predictor of PP at 6 months of age was a positional preference at term equivalent age, with the frequency of PP being highest in males and multiples. Recent research confirms that there may be a correlation between PP and persistent asymmetric performance, as well as abnormalities in visual, auditory, and motor system development.[46,48] Knowing that multiples, males, and infants with CLD are at highest risk for development of PP, the therapist can focus on these infants to provide timely education and prevention strategies to caregivers. While assessing head shape can be challenging due to constraints of the incubator, observing for a head-turn preference at rest and with active movements should be completed during the evaluation.

Throughout the examination, the therapist should observe for any musculoskeletal abnormalities (e.g., joint contractures) and edema, especially if presentation is asymmetrical. For instance, edema in the entire left lower extremity may alert the clinician to internal damage, such as a fracture. Last, there are many factors affecting the examination. Abnormal findings may be transient and may not always correlate to abnormal outcomes. The evaluation may be influenced by various factors, such as the infant's state or procedures endured in the preceding days (e.g., immunization shots, PDA repair). However, persistent abnormalities observed over several examinations are significant.

Plan of Care and Interventions

Developmental interventions have a positive effect on infant development, oxygenation, weaning from mechanical ventilation, feeding, growth, and length of hospital stay.[28,35] Therefore, physical therapy is an important intervention in the NICU. The physical therapy plan of care should be geared toward findings from the last session and maximizing the infant's roles of procuring, exploration, interaction, and feeding.[31] For each session, interventions should be task-specific and goal-oriented to take advantage of the infant's emerging skills and to facilitate his development. This is also important to ensure the session is focused, given the infant's immaturity and impaired tolerance to handling. As always, the therapist should monitor the infant's stress and vital signs to guide the interventions. Progression of interventions from simple (*e.g.*, contained touch, contained movements) to complex (*e.g.*, exploratory movements, movements against gravity) should solely be based on the aforementioned behavioral and physiologic cues. Another consideration in treating an infant in an incubator is whether to remove the infant from the incubator for the session (Fig. 5-1A). The incubator can restrict which interventions can be performed, but the transition out of the incubator may disrupt temperature regulation and produce stress leading to physiologic instability and weight loss. Factors that should be considered include: the infant's weight gain over the last several days, ability to maintain temperature (*i.e.*, is the infant close to being transitioned to an open crib), and the benefits of providing interventions out of the incubator.

Promoting behavioral organization and preventing stress are important physical therapy goals because early experiences affect brain development and neural organization.[31,35,44] The dilemma is that the NICU environment is inherently not conducive to the premature infant's development and physiologic stability, but it is necessary to sustain extrauterine life. Environmental modifications that are in line with developmental care consist of: turning unnecessary overhead lights off or cycling of light, limiting sound (*e.g.*, opening incubator doors softly, avoiding loud conversations directly over the infant), and decreasing unnecessary handling by clustering care to allow for periods of deep sleep. Note that the environment can and should be modified to facilitate developmental activities and skills. Since multimodal sensory input can compromise the infant's autonomic stability, especially in those with BPD and low activity tolerance, sensory input should be introduced one modality at a time, allowing the infant to accommodate to the

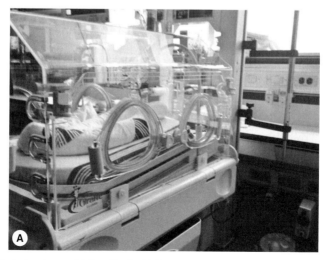

Figure 5-1. **A.** An incubator with "nest" in the NICU.

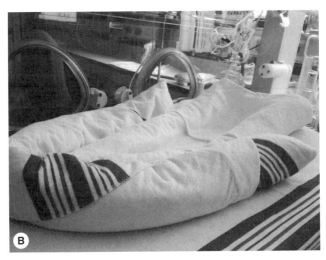

Figure 5-1. (*Continued*) **B.** Close-up view of oval nest made of blankets. A deep nest is created to surround the infant on all sides to promote midline orientation while still allowing some active movement.

introduction of a new input. For example, to facilitate state transition the therapist should be mindful of speaking over the infant and may consider shielding of light to facilitate eye opening.

Once the environment is optimal, the therapist can enlist other strategies during the session to decrease stressors and pain, which can facilitate motor organization and development. Containment is one way to accomplish this. Containment is a principle that caregivers follow that has been shown to promote behavioral organization by decreasing stressors.[44] Containment is a way of providing the boundaries that an infant lacks. For example, one way the therapist can accomplish containment is through contained touch. This involves placing a firm hand over the infant's trunk, head, or buttocks and keeping the body part still for several minutes. One reason containment is effective may be its ability to mimic the boundaries of the intrauterine environment, which do not restrict movement but rather guide movements and provide sensory feedback. Containment also grades tactile input and allows the premature infant to accommodate to touch and subsequent interventions by giving him time to recruit self-regulatory behaviors.

Another way to mimic the intrauterine environment to promote behavioral organization or self-regulatory behaviors is through positioning. For infants born premature, lack of the intrauterine environment has a significant effect on musculoskeletal alignment, postures, and movement acquisition. The lack of the antigravity environment in which the infant can move freely, absence of the mother's organs to provide boundaries that are crucial for motor pattern development and behavioral organization, and musculoskeletal immaturity impair the infant's ability to move and reposition. In addition, experiences in the NICU cause stress and pain, and may reinforce extension patterns as the infant attempts to self-regulate. Common sequelae of poor positioning include neck hyperextension, trunk extension, scapular retraction, and anterior pelvic tilt. Therefore, the goal of positioning is to mimic the intrauterine environment. Positioning that promotes postures similar to that in utero can facilitate appropriate musculoskeletal alignment, typical movement patterns, development of flexor tone, self-regulation, and restful sleep. For positioning to be consistent and supportive, it is crucial for the therapist to collaborate with nursing, since they are the primary caregivers in the NICU.

Guidelines of proper positioning focus on regular repositioning of the trunk and cervical spine, neutral neck alignment, midline positioning, facilitation of flexion (*e.g.*, extremities flexed and close to body, trunk flexed, hands together and close to mouth), and firm 3-dimensional boundaries. It is important to reiterate that there is a fine line between containing an infant and limiting all his movements with boundaries. The boundaries should assist, but not eliminate movement because the infant's ability to move within the boundaries allows for sensory and proprioceptive feedback that is crucial for sensory and motor development. While in an incubator, the infant may be positioned in a "nest," which is a deep oval made of blankets and/ or positioning aids (Fig. 5-1B), surrounding the infant on all sides while allowing some movement. This type of "nest" assists in maintaining flexed posture and promotes more midline orientation with active movement.[44]

Promoting varied positions within the infant's tolerance is also important for development, head shape and rotation preference, skin integrity, and decreasing the risk of contractures.[44] There are specific benefits of each position. The prone position is best for oxygenation, decreasing episodes of apnea, improving sleep, reducing reflux, and stabilizing vital signs.[35,44] The sidelying position can assist with bringing hands together and to the mouth for self-regulation and exploratory play.[35,44] Both the sidelying and prone positions can provide containment and facilitate recovery from stress.[44] In infants requiring supplemental oxygen, the **prone and left lateral positions** improve lung function and breathing efficiency.[49] Gouna et al.[49] also found that apneic and hypoxemic events decreased when these infants were placed in these positions. Providing developmental positioning in supine is most challenging because gravity promotes extension in this position. However, one of its benefits is that it allows for unrestricted access for procedures.

Each position can be augmented to ensure that the premature infant is flexed, contained, aligned, and comfortable. Monterosso et al.[50] found that in the prone position, a **postural support nappy and a support roll** encouraged flexed posture, midline orientation, and neuromotor function in the lower extremities. In this study, a postural support roll was placed around the pelvis to provide hip elevation leading to improved alignment at the hips and ability of the infant to move the lower extremities. A support roll positioned the infant in a quarter turn from prone, enabling flexion and alignment of the upper and lower extremities. Together, these supports resulted in better musculoskeletal alignment and lower incidence of scapular retraction, abduction of the hips, and anterior pelvic tilt. In sidelying, a roll placed along the anterior trunk can promote alignment at the shoulder and hip joints. The therapist can also use a rolled cloth to assist in scapular protraction and hands together in sidelying and supine.

In addition to contained touch and positioning, the therapist can use other strategies to decrease stress during the session, such as palmar grasp, non-nutritive sucking, promoting hands together and to the mouth, and avoiding abrupt positional changes and handling since these may overstimulate the fragile infant and disrupt homeostasis.[35] If external support (e.g., contained touch, repositioning, palmar grasp) is unsuccessful in decreasing stress, the therapist should withdraw touch and observe the infant. If the infant calms, the session should be stopped, as this may be the limit of his tolerance to handling. Appropriately responding to the infant's stress signs reinforces future behavior in similar situations.[31]

As with positioning, facilitation of infant movement should also be done in a variety of positions to allow for diverse experiences in order to achieve optimal outcomes. All infants learn to move by pushing through and against a supportive surface. Premature infants are at a disadvantage due to their immaturity, gravity, and environment stressors. This can be provided through contained movement. During contained movement, the caregiver or therapist provides boundaries while the infant participates in active movement.[44] When the infant is at rest, the infant should be in a flexed position. If the premature infant can tolerate contained movement, a more challenging activity is exploratory movements. Exploratory movements are active movements without boundaries and should also be performed in the supine, sidelying, and prone positions. Initially, the infant may need support proximally at the trunk and neck, gravity eliminated, and/or support at the extremities, allowing active movement of one extremity at a time. One important consideration is respiratory status, which is less optimal and more demanding in supine and sidelying as compared to prone, especially in infants with CLD.[44] Elevation of the head and upper trunk to 30° to 45° may reduce the strain on the respiratory system.[44] With all movements and in all positions, the therapist should aim to encourage symmetrical movement patterns.

Other interventions may include guided flexion and extension of the lower extremities. This is similar to the infant's alternating, rhythmic movements in utero and may help with strengthening the lower extremities and facilitation of typical motor patterns. The therapist should be careful not to apply traction or produce forceful movements due to risk of fractures in this population. Also, caution should be taken as the infant may require external support for self-regulation during this activity (e.g., hands to mouth, contained touch). For infants experiencing significant stress, the therapist can grade the activity by performing the intervention on one extremity at a time and allowing rest and external support between repetitions. Promotion of scapular protraction is also important because premature infants tend to have restrictions in scapular retractors due to extension patterns related to stress, pain, and immaturity in the neuromusculoskeletal system. This may compromise achievement of future milestones, such as reaching for objects in midline or crawling. Scapular retraction is even more evident in infants with CLD who tend to use postural muscles as accessory respiratory muscles.[44] A gentle stretch of the scapular retractors can be applied in supine, sidelying, or prone to achieve appropriate muscle length.

Family education and training is one of the most important physical therapy interventions in the NICU. Infant development is affected by the parent-infant relationship, which can be reinforced through parent education and involvement in their infant's care.[1,27,28,31,51] Incorporating the parents as an active and vital part of the NICU team is a component of developmentally supportive care called family-centered care (FCC). FCC decreases hospital length of stay, improves the infant-parent relationship, and improves long-term outcomes.[51,52] The therapist can facilitate FCC by encouraging skin-to-skin care, breastfeeding, and hand swaddling, which can improve bonding and empower parents in their roles.[44,51,53] In the NICU, the parent can be taught the importance of providing external support and how to do so during stressful or painful events, such as nursing care or skin-breaking procedures.

Given the importance of the parent-infant relationship and its role in development, it is important that the therapist supports this interaction and provides opportunities for parents to participate.[27] Consultation with the social worker prior to the family education session is useful to learn pertinent information regarding the family dynamic.[53] In interacting with the infant's family, the physical therapist must understand the grief process the family is likely undergoing. Parents in the NICU often experience a loss of control, a loss of their parental role, and fear of their child's survival and developmental outcome.[28,53] Caregivers may experience uncertainty in being able to provide competent and developmentally appropriate care for their infant, deeming medical professionals more skilled.[28,53] Many express fear of "hurting" their child during repositioning or with diaper changes due to how fragile they appear. Physical therapy can empower parents by providing techniques on how to care for their infants in a developmentally appropriate and medically safe way. **Caregiver training and education** should be provided using diverse teaching strategies, including observation of therapy sessions, verbal instruction, and written material.[28] Hands-on practice can also increase competence and confidence during the transition from the NICU to the home environment.[53]

All through the NICU stay, parent education should include: infant's current and expected development, consequences of prematurity, importance of flexor tone and flexed posture, interpretation of stress signs and ways to promote behavioral organization, head preference and prevention of head shape deformities, appropriate handling techniques and positions, play activities aimed at facilitating achievement of milestones, "Back to Sleep" education with emphasis on "Tummy to Play," and follow-up programs and early intervention.[28,53] Parents should be encouraged to talk to their infant because this has been linked to intellectual achievements. This is especially true when parents increase "extra talk" (conversational talk, positive reinforcement, complex ideas, and varied vocabulary) in addition to "business talk" (essential commands for parents and children).[25]

Parents should also be educated in varying infant positions (for sleep, play, and feeding) and the orientation of the infant's head to outside activity to facilitate development and prevent plagiocephaly and head preference. For instance, during skin-to-skin care, if the infant's head is turned to the right, the parent should turn the infant's head to the left during the next skin-to-skin care session. Parental awareness and education is key in decreasing persistence of head preference and plagiocephaly.[46,48] Factors having a negative impact on PP include low socioeconomic status and the mother's educational level, as these caregivers are less likely to place infants in tummy time and more likely to bottle feed infants from the same side.[46] These practices may be related to inadequate education from clinicians regarding positioning guidelines, resulting in parental confusion.[46] Prevention of positional skull deformities, such as PP, includes: tummy time when awake and supervised;

alternating the infant's supine head position to the right and left occiputs during the day and at night through stimulation to outside activity, manually turning the infant's head, or by changing the infant's supine position in the crib (e.g., if the crib is against a wall, alternating the side to which the infant will turn to outside activity); and avoiding prolonged placement in car seats (when not a passenger in a car) and infant seats or swings.[54]

It is crucial for the therapist to emphasize the importance of Tummy to Play when educating on SIDS guidelines because tummy time is related not only to decreasing the incidence of head shape and head preference, but also to earlier achievement of supine, prone, and sitting milestones.[46] The American Association of Pediatrics guidelines recommend performing tummy time at least 30 minutes per day, on a firm surface such as a play mat, when the infant is awake and supervised, gradually increasing frequency and duration based on the infant's tolerance.[46]

Evidence-Based Clinical Recommendations

SORT: Strength of Recommendation Taxonomy

A: Consistent, good-quality patient-oriented evidence
B: Inconsistent or limited-quality patient-oriented evidence
C: Consensus, disease-oriented evidence, usual practice, expert opinion, or case series

1. Assessment of general movements (GMs) is valid and reliable in identifying infants at risk for developmental delay and cerebral palsy. **Grade A**

2. In infants requiring supplemental oxygen, the left lateral and prone positions improve lung function and breathing strategies and result in fewer events of apnea and hypoxia compared to the supine position. **Grade C**

3. In the prone position, a postural support nappy and support roll promote flexed posture, midline orientation, musculoskeletal alignment, and neuromotor function in the lower extremities of very low-birth-weight infants. **Grade B**

4. Education provided to parents is most effective when multiple methods are utilized, including observation of therapy, verbal instruction, and written handouts. **Grade C**

COMPREHENSION QUESTIONS

5.1 Which of the following increases the risk of positional plagiocephaly in preterm infants?

A. Spending at least 30 minutes per day in supervised, awake tummy time

B. Diagnosis of chronic lung disease

C. Female sex

D. Reducing time spent in swings and infant seats

5.2 Which of the following strategies promotes behavioral organization in the preterm infant during the physical therapy session?

A. Providing multimodal sensory input when the infant is stressed

B. Positioning the infant in sidelying without 3-dimensional boundaries or a nest

C. Grading tactile input and allowing rest between positional changes

D. Timing the session between feeding times, when the infant is in a deep sleep state

5.3 The therapist is at the bedside for the initial evaluation. List the following in the order that would promote optimal neurobehavioral organization during the physical therapy session:

1. Observe the infant's state, position, and movement patterns

2. Open the incubator doors softly

3. Provide contained touch

4. Take note of the vital signs at rest and all lines and tubes attached to the infant

A. 2, 3, 1, 4

B. 1, 2, 3, 4

C. 2, 3, 4, 1

D. 4, 1, 2, 3

ANSWERS

5.1 **B.** Male sex and chronic lung disease are factors that increase the risk of positional plagiocephaly. Options A and D are recommended ways to *decrease* the risk of positional skull deformities.

5.2 **C.** Factors that increase stress in the premature infant are multimodal input (option A) and lack of appropriate boundaries or support (option B). Deep sleep is difficult for preterm infants to achieve in the NICU due to environmental factors and neurobehavioral immaturity, which limits the infant's ability to self-regulate. Deep sleep is vital to development and growth and therefore timing a therapy session during this time is not appropriate (option D).

5.3 **D.** Providing developmental interventions while limiting stress and pain to the premature infant is crucial to achieve optimal outcomes. The therapist must remember that even routine interventions and evaluations can be stressful to the infant. Noting the environment (*e.g.*, lines and tubes) as well as the infant's baseline status can guide the therapist to a more organized and focused session prior to a hands-on evaluation. Opening and closing of incubator doors can be noisy, and contribute to the infant's stress. Last, providing contained touch is a good way to grade tactile input and begin the hands-on portion of the evaluation or treatment.

REFERENCES

1. Sansavini A, Guarini A, Caselli MC. Preterm birth: neuropsychological profiles and atypical developmental pathways. *Dev Disabil Res Rev.* 2011;17:102-113.

2. Bennet L, Van Den Heuij L, Dean JM, Drury P, Wassink G, Gun AJ. Neural plasticity and the Kennard principle: does it work for the preterm brain? *Clin Exp Pharmacol Physiol.* 2013;40:774-784.

3. Leppert M, Allen MC. Neurodevelopmental consequences of preterm birth: causes, assessment, and management. In: Coleman CC, Feldman E, eds. *Developmental-Behavioral Pediatrics.* Philadelphia, PA: Saunders Elsevier; 2009:259-268.

4. Raz S, Debastos AK, Newman JB, Batton D. Extreme prematurity and neuropsychological outcome in preschool years. *J Int Neuropsychol Soc.* 2010;16:169-179.

5. Hintz SR, Kendrick DE, Vohr BR, Poole WK, Higgins RD; National Institute of Child Health and Human Development Neonatal Research Network. Community supports after surviving extremely low-birth-weight, extremely preterm birth: special outpatient services in early childhood. *Arch Pediatr Adolsc Med.* 2008;162:748-755.

6. Arnold C, Tyson JE. Outcomes following periviable birth. *Semin Perinatol.* 2014;38:2-11.

7. Hintz SR, Kendrick DE, Wilson-Costello DE, et al. Early-childhood neurodevelopmental outcomes are not improving for infants born at <25 weeks' gestational age. *Pediatrics.* 2011;127:62-70.

8. Watts JL, Saigal S. Outcome of extreme prematurity: as information increases so do the dilemmas. *Arch Dis Child Fetal Neonatal Ed.* 2006;91:F221-F225.

9. Tyson JE, Parikh NA, Langer J, Green C, Higgins RD; National Institute of Child Health and Human Development Neonatal Research Network. Intensive care for extreme prematurity—moving beyond gestational age. *N Engl J Med.* 2008;358:1672-1681.

10. Aarnoudse-Moens CS, Weisglas-Kuperus N, van Goudoever JB, Oosterlaan J. Meta-analysis of neurobehavioral outcomes in very preterm and/or very low birth weight children. *Pediatrics.* 2009;124:717-728.

11. Gomella TL, Cunningham MD, Eyal FG, Tuttle D, eds. *Neonatology: Management, Procedures, On-Call Problems, Diseases, and Drugs.* New York: McGraw-Hill Co; 2009.

12. Bhandari A, Bhandari V. Pitfalls, problems, and progress in bronchopulmonary dysplasia. *Pediatrics.* 2009;123:1562-1573.

13. Short EJ, Kirchner HL, Asaad GR, et al. Developmental sequelae in preterm infants having a diagnosis of bronchopulmonary dysplasia: analysis using a severity-based classification system. *Arch Pediatr Adolesc Med.* 2007;161:1082-1087.

14. O'Reilly M, Sozo F, Harding R. Impact of preterm birth and bronchopulmonary dysplasia on the developing lung: long-term consequences for respiratory health. *Clin Exp Pharmacol Physiol.* 2013;40:765-773.

15. Cuhna GS, Mezzacappa-Filho F, Ribeiro JD. Risk factors for bronchopulmonary dysplasia in very low birth weight newborns treated with mechanical ventilation in the first week of life. *J Trop Pediatr.* 2005;51:334-340.

16. Sullivan MC, Msall ME, Miller RJ. 17-year outcome of preterm infants with diverse neonatal morbidities: part 1—impact on physical, neurological, and psychological health status. *J Spec Pediatr Nurs.* 2012;17:226-241.

17. Sellmer A, Bjerre JV, Schimdt MR, et al. Morbidity and mortality in preterm neonates with patent ductus arteriosus on day 3. *Arch Dis Child Fetal Neonatal Ed.* 2013;98:F505-F510.

18. Leitner Y, Fattal-Valevski A, Geva R, et al. Neurodevelopmental outcomes of children with intrauterine growth retardation: a longitudinal 10-year prospective study. *J Child Neurol.* 2007;22:580-587.

19. von Beckerath A, Kollmann M, Rotky-Fast C, Karpf E, Lang U, Klaritsch P. Perinatal complications and long-term neurodevelopmental outcome of infants with intrauterine growth retardation. *Am J Obstetr Gynecol.* 2013;208:130-136.

20. Allen MC, Cristofalo EA, Kim C. Preterm birth: transition to adulthood. *Dev Disabil Res Rev.* 2010;16:323-335.

21. de Kieviet JF, Zoetebier L, van Elburg RM, Vermeulen RJ, Oosterlaan J. Brain development of very preterm and very low-birthweight children in childhood and adolescence: a meta-analysis. *Dev Med Child Neurol.* 2012;54:313-323.

22. Smith GC, Gutovich J, Smyser C, et al. Neonatal intensive unit stress is associated with brain development in preterm infants. *Ann Neurol.* 2011;70:541-549.

23. Barrington KJ. Management during the first 72 h of age of the periviable infant: an evidence-based review. *Semin Perinatol.* 2014;38:17-24.

24. Dobson NR, Patel RM, Smith PB, et al. Trends in caffeine use and association between clinical outcomes and timing of therapy in very low birth weight infants. *J Pediatr.* 2014;164:992-998.

25. Msall ME, Park JJ. The spectrum of behavioral outcomes after extreme prematurity: regulatory, attention, social, and adaptive dimensions. *Semin Perinatol.* 2007;32:42-50.

26. Doyle LW, Anderson PJ. Adult outcome of extremely premature infants. *Pediatrics.* 2010;126:342-351.

27. Korja R, Latva R, Lehtonen L. The effects of preterm birth on mother-infant interaction and attachment during the infant's first two years. *Acta Obstet Gynecol Scand.* 2012;91:164-173.

28. Dusing SC, Murray T, Stern M. Parent preferences for motor development education in the neonatal intensive care unit. *Pediatr Phys Ther.* 2008; 20:363-368.

29. Sweeney JK, Heriza CB, Blanchard Y; American Physical Therapy Association. Neonatal physical therapy. Part I: clinical competencies and neonatal intensive care unit clinical training models. *Pediatr Phys Ther.* 2009;21:296-307.

30. Ludwig S. Poll question: do you know why infants in the neonatal intensive care unit need neonatal therapy services? *Newborn Infant Nurs Rev.* 2013;13:2-4.

31. Vergara ER, Bigsby R. *Developmental and Therapeutic Interventions in the NICU.* Baltimore, MD: Brookes Publishing Co; 2007.

32. Sturdivant C. A collaborative approach to defining neonatal therapy. *Newborn Infant Nurs Rev.* 2013;13:23-26.

33. Sweeney JK, Heriza CB, Blanchard Y, Dusing SC. Neonatal physical therapy. Part II: practice frameworks and evidence-based practice guidelines. *Pediatr Phys Ther.* 2010;22:2-16.

34. Byrne E, Campbell SK. Physical therapy observation and assessment in the neonatal intensive care unit. *Phys Occup Ther Pediatr.* 2013;33:39-74.

35. Mahoney MC, Cohen MI. Effectiveness of developmental interventions in the neonatal intensive care unit: implications for neonatal physical therapy. *Pediatr Phys Ther.* 2005;17:194-208.

36. Lucas-Thompson R, Townsend EL, Gunnar MR, et al. Developmental changes in the responses of preterm infants to a painful stressor. *Infant Behav Dev.* 2008;31:614-623.

37. Liaw J, Yang L, Wang KK, Chen C, Chang Y, Yin T. Non-nutritive sucking and facilitated tucking relieve preterm infant pain during heel-stick procedures: a prospective, randomized, controlled crossover trial. *Int J Nurs Stud.* 2012;49:300-309.

38. Einspieler C, Prechtl HFR. Prechtl's assessment of general movements: a diagnostic tool for the functional assessment of the young nervous system. *Ment Retard Dev Disabil Res Rev.* 2005;11:61-67.

39. Zuk L. Fetal and infant spontaneous general movements as predictors of developmental disabilities. *Dev Disabil Res Rev.* 2011;17:93-101.

40. Nakajima Y, Einspieler C, Marschik PB, Bos AF, Prechtl HFR. Does a detailed assessment of poor repertoire general movements help to identify those infants who will develop normally? *Early Hum Dev.* 2006;82:53-59.

41. Noble Y, Boyd R. Neonatal assessments for the preterm infant up to 4 months corrected age: a systematic review. *Dev Med Child Neurol.* 2012;54:129-139.

42. Kotagal S. Neurological examination of the newborn. *Up To Date*. 2013. http://www.uptodate.com/contents/neurological-examination-of-the-newborn?source=search_result&search=infant+neuro+exam&selectedTitle=2%7E150. Accessed November 4, 2014.

43. Sweeney JK, Gutierrez T. Musculoskeletal implications of preterm infant positioning in the NICU. *J Perinat Neonat Nurs*. 2002;16:58-70.

44. Byrne E, Garber J. Physical therapy interventions in the neonatal intensive care unit. *Phys Occup Ther Pediatr*. 2013;33:75-110.

45. Mercuri E, Guzzetta A, Laroche S, et al. Neurologic examination of preterm infants at term age: comparison with term infants. *J Pediatr*. 2003;142:647-655.

46. Shweikeh F, Nuno M, Danielpour M, Krieger MD, Drazin D. Positional plagiocephaly: an analysis of the literature on the effectiveness of current guidelines. *Neurosurg Focus*. 2013;35:1-9.

47. Nuysink J, van Haastert IC, Eijsermans MJ, et al. Prevalence and predictors of idiopathic asymmetry in infants born preterm. *Early Hum Dev*. 2012;86:387-392.

48. Nuysink J, Eijsermans MJ, van Haastert IC, et al. Clinical course of asymmetric motor performance and deformational plagiocephaly in very preterm infants. *J Pediatr*. 2013;163:658-665.

49. Gouna G, Rakza T, Kuissi E, Pennaforte T, Mur S, Storme L. Positioning effect on lung function and breathing pattern in premature newborns. *J Pediatr*. 2013;162:1133-1137.

50. Monterosso L, Kristjanson LJ, Cole J, Evans SF. Effect of postural supports on neuromotor function in very preterm infants to term equivalent age. *J Paediatr Child Health*. 2003;39:197-205.

51. Gooding JS, Cooper LG, Blaine AI, Franck LS, Howse JL, Berns SD. Family support and family-centered care in the neonatal intensive care unit: origins, advances, impact. *Semin Perinatol*. 2011;35:20-28.

52. Cockroft S. How can family centered care be improved to meet the needs of parents with a premature baby in the neonatal intensive care unit? *J Neonatal Nurs*. 2011;18:105-110.

53. Goldstein LA. Family support and education. *Phys Occup Ther Pediatr*. 2013;33:139-161.

54. Laughlin J, Luerssen TG, Dias MS; Committee on Practice and Ambulatory Medicine, Section on Neurological Surgery. Prevention and management of positional skull deformities in infants. *Pediatrics*. 2011;128:1236-1241.

Cerebral Palsy—Early Intervention

Kimberly D. Ward
Barb Kellar

A 26-month-old female is currently receiving early intervention services. She was born prematurely at 28 weeks of gestational age via cesarean section due to maternal preeclampsia and subsequent fetal distress. She had an initial Apgar score of 4 at 1 minute and 6 at 5 minutes, requiring supplemental oxygen. The child remained in the neonatal intensive care unit (NICU) for 9 weeks due to prematurity, poor feeding, and difficulty with lung development. She was referred for physical therapy following discharge from the NICU, but the child's mother did not follow through with medical recommendations. Subsequently, the child, her mother, and her mother's live-in boyfriend moved to a neighboring community. The hospital medical staff lost contact with the family following this move. At 7 months of age, the child was referred for early intervention services under the Individuals with Disabilities Education Improvement Act Part C (IDEA Part C) due to failure to progress with gross motor skills and spasticity in her upper and lower extremities, as well as difficulties with feeding. The child qualified for an Individualized Family Service Plan (IFSP) with teacher support, and occupational, physical, and speech therapies at home. A social worker assisted the family in obtaining medical services and helped facilitate consistent follow-up with services for the child. The mother was given support for transportation to the hospital where the child was followed by a pediatrician, orthopaedist, neurologist, and a team of professionals including physical, occupational, and speech therapists. The mother works part-time at a local pizza restaurant and has more consistently attended her daughter's medical appointments and therapy sessions. The mother has difficulty understanding many of the medical terms and concerns regarding her daughter's health and diagnosis. The mother's boyfriend has not been involved with the family since a drug conviction just after the move. The child has received physical therapy services from age 8 months until her current age of 26 months. At 20 months of age, she was diagnosed with spastic diplegic cerebral palsy (CP). Since initiation of physical and occupational therapy, her gross motor skills have improved. She independently rolls from supine to prone and can maintain sitting on the floor, though she needs assistance to be placed in sitting. She was initially fitted with bilateral ankle-foot orthoses (AFOs) to support the posture of her feet during stance and ambulation, as well as bilateral knee immobilizers and resting night orthoses due to hamstring and Achilles tendon tightness, respectively. She was also provided with a supine stander. Currently, she has bilateral hip and knee contractures and demonstrates lower extremity hypertonicity, especially during movement for transfers, walking, and all static and dynamic balance activities. She can walk short distances indoors with a posterior wheeled walker and adult support to help her with turning and managing the walker. When she is not using her AFOs, she toe walks and demonstrates hyperlordosis. The outpatient physical therapy evaluation reveals that her mobility skills are consistent with Gross Motor Function Classification System (GMFCS) Level III. She requires moderate assistance with self-care activities, transfers, and all mobility. She seeks opportunities to be as independent as she can and she is often impulsive. The child attends day care 5 days per week.

▶ Based on the child's diagnosis and family support, what do you anticipate will be contributing factors to activity limitations?
▶ What educational needs should be addressed for the child at this time?
▶ What are the implications regarding the mother's understanding and participation that might affect the child's progress?

KEY DEFINITIONS

ANKLE-FOOT ORTHOSIS (AFO): Custom or prefabricated brace worn on the foot and/or lower extremity to maintain appropriate positioning of the ankle and/or to provide support during weightbearing activities

APGAR SCORES: Quick assessment performed on a neonate at 1 minute and 5 minutes after birth. The 1-minute score indicates how well the baby tolerated the birthing process, while the 5-minute score indicates how well the baby is doing outside the mother's womb. The examiner looks at: breathing effort, heart rate, muscle tone, reflexes, and skin color. Each category is scored with 0, 1, or 2, depending on the observed condition, with a maximum score of 10. Scores of ≥ 7 are considered normal; scores <7 indicate that medical attention is needed. Low Apgar scores at 1 and 5 minutes are significantly associated with CP.[1]

EARLY INTERVENTION: Federally funded program of support and services designed to meet the developmental needs of children with a disability and their families. Needs may be related to physical, cognitive, communication, social/emotional, and/or adaptive development.

GROSS MOTOR FUNCTION CLASSIFICATION SYSTEM (GMFCS): 5-level classification system based on self-initiated mobility of children with CP; sitting, walking, and wheeled mobility are the primary forms of mobility used in the GMFCS.[2]

INDIVIDUALIZED FAMILY SERVICE PLAN (IFSP): For infants and toddlers with disabilities who receive services through IDEA Part C; multidisciplinary assessment of the family resources, priorities and concerns, the strengths and needs of the child with the disability, needed services, and an individualized service plan to meet these needs. This plan is evaluated at least once per year and reviewed at least every 6 months.

INDIVIDUALS WITH DISABILITIES EDUCATION IMPROVEMENT ACT:[3]

PART B: (IDEA Part B): Federal legislation that establishes school-aged services for students (3-21 years of age) with disabilities

PART C: (IDEA Part C): Federal legislation that establishes early intervention services for infants and toddlers (birth to 3 years of age) with disabilities and their families

KNEE IMMOBILIZER: External support worn on lower extremity that provides support during stance and/or to provide prolonged stretch of the hamstrings

POSTERIOR WHEELED WALKER: Wheeled walker that provides upper extremity support for increased balance during ambulation; designed to promote upright posture and decrease forward leaning during ambulation by wrapping behind the user and being open in front of the user

PREECLAMPSIA: Pregnancy complication (usually after 20 weeks of gestation) in which the mother experiences hypertension that may lead to significant complications including morbidity or mortality of the mother or unborn child[4]

SUPINE STANDER: Positioning device that enables supported standing in a supine position for individuals that are unable to maintain independent standing

Objectives

1. Describe typical characteristics of children with CP.
2. Understand and define the classification of types of CP.
3. List appropriate testing used for children with CP with respect to the IFSP.
4. List the potential benefits and complications of physical therapy intervention as per the Early Intervention and day care programming, including involvement of family and other professionals involved in the child's care.

Physical Therapy Considerations

PT considerations for the young child with CP in the early intervention setting:

▶ **General physical therapy plan of care/goals:** Initiation of early intervention services; maximize independent mobility (wheelchair, walker) and physical function, activity, and participation; minimize secondary impairments

▶ **Physical therapy interventions:** Coordination and communication with parent, IFSP team, and medical team; patient-related instruction (targeted toward parent and other caregivers) regarding topics such as handling, positioning, caregiving, biomechanical safety for lifting-related tasks, and equipment usage; procedural interventions including procuring appropriate equipment for positioning, mobility, and caregiving; gait training, strengthening activities, orthoses and bracing, maintenance of range of motion (ROM); play and child engagement

▶ **Precautions during physical therapy:** Close monitoring of skin integrity with use of AFOs; close positioning of physical therapist to the child during gait training and transfers; safety monitoring during all movement due to potential impulsivity of the child

▶ **Complications interfering with physical therapy:** Parental need to learn about diagnosis and its implications and how best to help her daughter learn, play, and gain independence; parent with limited financial means that requires assistance from social worker at hospital for obtaining equipment and transportation to and from clinic appointments

Understanding the Health Condition

Cerebral palsy (CP) is a term used to describe a group of permanent disorders of movement and posture attributed to non-progressive disturbances that occurred in the developing fetal or infant brain.[5] While the brain lesion is static, musculoskeletal impairments that may result from the brain lesion are progressive. Worldwide, it is estimated that the prevalence of CP is roughly 2 cases per 1000 live births.[6] For babies born *before* 28 weeks of gestation, the prevalence of CP is significantly higher at approximately 112 per 1000 live births.[6]

There are various systems used to classify CP. Classification may be based on functional ability, distribution of motor involvement, or impairments of muscle tone that affect movement.[5,7]

Three systems classify individuals with CP based on their functional abilities: the GMFCS, the Manual Ability Classification System (MACS), and the Communication Function Classification System (CFCS). The GMFCS classifies individuals based on their functional mobility including ambulation or wheeled mobility. The GMFCS uses specific age bands including those for children younger than 2 years, 2 to 4 years of age, 4 to 6 years of age, 6 to 12 years of age, and 12 to 18 years of age.[2] The MACS classifies individuals with CP based on their ability to use their hands to manipulate objects and on their need for assistance in daily activities during play, eating, and dressing. This classification is designed to reflect the child's *typical* manual performance, not the child's maximal capabilities.[8] The MACS was developed for children 4 to 18 years of age. Last, the CFCS classifies individuals based on their communication abilities.[9] The CFCS has been developed for children 2 years of age and older. Each of the three systems (GMFCS, MACS, CFCS) consists of five levels of ability, with level 1 representing the highest level of ability and level 5 representing the most limited level of ability.

Classification of CP by distribution of motor involvement[7] is based on an individual's clinical presentation. Individuals are typically classified into one of four categories: hemiplegia, diplegia, triplegia, or quadriplegia (tetraplegia). Hemiplegia describes primary motor involvement of one side of the body, including one upper and one lower extremity. Individuals with diplegia present with primary motor involvement of the lower extremities, and may have some minor involvement of the upper extremities. Triplegia describes motor involvement of three extremities, usually both lower extremities and one upper extremity. Persons with quadriplegia or tetraplegia have motor involvement of all four extremities.

Finally, classification of CP may be based on impairments of muscle tone that affect movement, and includes spastic, dyskinetic, ataxic, and mixed.[10] In spastic CP, spasticity is defined as hypertonia in which passive resistance to movement of a joint increases with increasing speed of movement. Individuals with spasticity experience abnormal movement patterns that can lead to joint contractures and difficulty with positioning and mobility. Dyskinetic CP (includes athetoid, choreoathetoid, and dystonic) is characterized by variable muscle tone and "atypical patterns of posture and involuntary, uncontrolled, recurring, and occasionally stereotyped movement of affected body parts."[10, p. 577] Athetoid CP is characterized by "slow, continuous, writhing movements that prevent maintenance of a stable posture."[10, p. 577] Dystonic CP is characterized by "involuntary sustained or intermittent muscle contraction with repetitive movements and abnormal postures."[10, p. 577] In ataxic CP, the individual demonstrates movement that is uncoordinated, abnormal, and unstable. This movement pattern is not due to weakness or involuntary muscle activity. Individuals with mixed CP may demonstrate varying types, though the most common type is spastic-dyskinetic CP.

For children with CP ages 1 to 15 years, gross motor developmental curves have been developed.[11] The primary impairments may include spasticity, reduced postural control, reduced selective voluntary motor control, and impaired sensory processing.[5]

These primary impairments may lead to secondary impairments such as contractures, skeletal deformities, decreased strength, and limited endurance.[5] Over time, skeletal abnormalities such as torsional deformities (femoral anteversion and tibial torsion), acetabular malformations, hip subluxation and dislocation, ankle and foot deformities, and differing rates of skeletal maturation may arise.[12] Individuals with CP are also at risk for low bone mineral density that may result in osteopenia and osteoporosis.[13]

Primary and secondary impairments associated with CP may contribute to activity limitations and participation restrictions. Individuals with CP may ambulate independently with few gait deviations, utilize hand-held assistive devices for ambulation, or utilize manual or power wheelchairs for mobility.

Individuals with CP may also have a variety of other associated impairments (behavioral, speech, hearing, vision), cognitive delays, seizure disorders, urinary incontinence, or constipation.[14] It is important to note that while these impairments are more prevalent in individuals with CP, they are not inherent to *all* individuals with CP.

Physical Therapy Patient/Client Management

In order to provide family-centered services,[15] it is important that the physical therapist supports goals that have been identified by the family and that are addressed through shared planning and implementation of interventions.[16-19] The early intervention physical therapist should consider not only the child's abilities and participation in her home environment, but also her abilities and participation in the community and child care environments. The physical therapist should communicate with and provide consultation to the child's family, educational team (teachers and other early intervention providers), medical team (primary care physician, developmental pediatrician, neurologist, orthopaedic physician, orthotist, occupational therapist, and speech-language pathologist), and other physical therapists providing services to the child.[16,20]

Physical therapy services for children with CP during the preschool years should focus on maximizing independent mobility (which may include wheelchair mobility and/or use of a walker) and physical function, activity, and participation while also minimizing secondary impairments. Children with CP who are not able to independently walk or crawl may benefit from assistive devices (*e.g.*, walkers) or wheeled mobility to increase their ability to access their environment. Independent mobility is especially important during the preschool years, as children develop cognitive skills from exploring their environment.[21] Children with CP who are not able to stand independently may also benefit from **supported standing programs** in which the child stands in a supine or prone stander to allow for upright positioning and lower extremity weightbearing. Lower extremity weightbearing through supported standing programs provides a variety of physiologic benefits including improved bone density, hip stability, lower extremity ROM, and reduced spasticity.[22] Sustained standing helps promote more typical weightbearing forces through the developing lower extremity bones, allowing for more typical remodeling of the head of the femur and acetabulum.[22] Upright positioning may also be important for psychosocial benefits, including improved social interaction and alertness.[22] Physical therapists should help minimize the development of contractures that may occur with hypertonicity and atypical positioning over time. Children with CP may benefit from AFOs to provide for more typical ankle-foot positioning and support when standing and ambulating.[23,24] Positioning should include using a variety of postures throughout the day to promote participation and to encourage development of motor skills.[24] Positioning also provides low-load, prolonged stretches to musculature that is at risk for developing contractures.[24]

Examination, Evaluation, and Diagnosis

The examination and evaluation of a young child with CP should be comprehensive and address the child's impairments of body structures and functions, activity limitations, participation restrictions, and environmental and personal factors that impact the child. The needs and priorities of the child's family should also be taken into consideration.[17,18]

The physical therapist should begin with interviews of the parent and other key caregivers (e.g., teachers) to gather information about the child's developmental history, previous interventions including all therapies, medical and surgical interventions, and family or caregiver goals, concerns, and priorities.[18,20, 24] The examination should also include observation of the child in settings that are typical for the child's same-aged peers (e.g., home, day care, playground)[20,24] and observation of the child and caregiver/family interactions.[24]

Examination of primary impairments of body structures and functions includes assessment of spasticity, balance and postural control, selective voluntary motor control, and sensory processing.[24] Examination of secondary impairments of body structures and functions includes assessment of postural alignment, trunk and extremity ROM (including muscular flexibility), muscular strength, and endurance. Additional impairments that should be assessed include pain, cardiopulmonary status (e.g., heart rate, respiratory rate), and skin integrity.[24] Additional considerations include nutrition, feeding, seizures, vision, hearing, and bowel/bladder function. Examination of activity limitations and participation restrictions includes assessment of mobility, gross motor performance, fine motor performance, self-care performance, and play.

Muscle tone, including hypertonicity, hypotonicity, or dystonia, may be assessed through clinical observation and/or through use of the modified Ashworth scale (MAS).[24-26] The MAS is a measurement scale used to assess muscle tone on a 0 to 4 scale, with 0 indicating no increase in muscle tone, and 4 indicating rigidity in flexion or extension.[27] Spasticity may be assessed through use of the modified Tardieu scale.[25,26] The modified Tardieu scale (see Case 3) assesses spasticity through measurement of joint ROM at both slow and fast velocities. Measurements are taken at the point of first catch when the joint is moved at a fast velocity (Tardieu's R1) and at the point of full passive ROM when the muscle is at rest after the joint has been moved at a slow velocity (Tardieu's R2).[25,26]

Balance and postural control in young children with CP may be assessed using a wide variety of balance tools[28] including the Movement Assessment of Infants (MAI),[29] the Pediatric Balance Scale (PBS),[30] or the Early Clinical Assessment of Balance (ECAB).[31] Balance may also be assessed through functional observation of reaching and playing in sitting, standing, and walking, and during transitions between positions.[24] Postural alignment and ROM may be measured via goniometry or through the use of the Spinal Alignment and Range of Motion Measure (SAROMM).[32] Special attention should be given to hip abduction with knee flexion and extension, hip extension with knee flexion and extension, knee extension with hip flexion, and ankle dorsiflexion with knee flexion and extension because these muscle groups are particularly prone to contractures.[24] It is also important to assess postural symmetry, hip joint integrity, lower extremity alignment, leg length discrepancies, and scoliosis. Muscular strength may be assessed through functional testing, especially in young children.[24] Endurance may be assessed using the Early Activity Scale for Endurance (EASE) for children with CP, 2 to 6 years of age.[33]

Child engagement, self-care, and participation may be assessed through the Pediatric Evaluation of Disability Inventory (PEDI)[34] or the **Child Engagement in Daily Life (CEDL)**.[35] The CEDL is a reliable and valid assessment of a child's participation (17-59 months of age) in and enjoyment of family and community life and recreational activities, as well as participation in self-care.[35] To help determine the parents' needs related to caregiving for the current child, the therapist could use the **Ease of Caregiving for Children**, a reliable and valid parent-completed measure of how difficult it is for them to safely help their child participate in activities of daily living.[36] In a study with 429 parents of children with CP and 100 children without CP (18-60 months of age), Ward et al.[36] found that the ease of caregiving for parents of children without motor difficulties varied by the children's ages. In contrast, for parents of children with CP, there was no significant difference based on the child's age, but parents of children with less gross motor ability reported more difficulties in caregiving than parents of children with higher gross motor abilities.[36]

Standardized tests that measure gross motor performance in children with CP include the Gross Motor Function Measure (GMFM) and the Quality Function Measure (QFM). The **GMFM** is a clinical measure of gross motor mobility, including: lying and rolling; sitting, crawling, and kneeling; standing; and walking, running, and jumping.[37] It includes motor skills that are typical of normal developmental milestones up to 5 years of age. The GMFM may be used to assess motor skills, to evaluate change over time, and to guide treatment for children with CP. The GMFM is a well-recognized and reliable tool that has been validated for use with individuals with CP and for children with Down syndrome.[37-40] The QFM is an observational tool to assess the *quality* of movement in individuals with CP (GMFCS I, II, or III; ages 4 and older).[41]

The physical therapist assesses the child's physical environment and the social/cultural environment of the family and child. Considerations of the physical environment include the setting (home, school, community), available equipment, and transportation. Considerations of the social/cultural environment include caregiver-child interaction, support and resources, caregiver learning styles and needs, language, and cultural beliefs. Assessment of the child's personal charac-teristics includes consideration of cognition, play, communication, language, social/emotional skills, behavior, and motivation.[24]

Plan of Care and Interventions

Physical therapy interventions for young children with CP who receive services through early intervention should include communication and collaboration, patient-related education, and procedural interventions[16,20] to meet established goals as developed in the IFSP.[24] When working with a family and their young child with CP, the physical therapist should help the family understand CP and the implications for their child.[14] This may include helping the family be hopeful, but realistic, about the child's prognosis.[11,42] The therapist should recognize that the family may need support to adapt to having a child diagnosed with CP and the therapist should be able to refer to other service providers if specialized assistance is identified for these needs.[43] The physical therapist can help parents maximize their ability to care for and interact with their child.[20,36] Families may benefit from strategies to help increase ease in caregiving tasks, especially related to positioning, feeding, dressing, and transporting the child out in the community.[36] The physical therapist may be a key facilitator to help the family identify and utilize community and recreational resources that may help their child participate in their community for leisure, play, and fitness.[20]

Recommended interventions should be structured so that they fit within a family's daily routine, thereby allowing for increased practice and adherence, while mini-mizing extra burden on the family.[19,43-45] For the 26-month-old child in this case, the physical therapist determined that one of the goals was to facilitate ambula-tion to increase the child's ability to move within her current educational environ-ment. One intervention that the therapist practiced twice per week in day care was gait training with a posterior wheeled walker while the child wore her AFOs. The therapist progressively decreased the amount of assistance required to man-age the forward movement of the walker and facilitate the child's upright stance. The therapist also provided intermittent verbal cueing for hip flexion to help the child move her lower extremities forward in order to take a forward step. To enable increased practice and adherence for gait training in the child's natural environment (day care, home), the therapist made recommendations and trained both the preschool staff and the mother in gait training with the child.

Many play-based, activity-focused, or function-focused interventions help children achieve goals, especially related to mobility, endurance, and motor devel-opment.[24,46] Interventions may also address changing or adapting environmen-tal factors to help increase the child's participation and improve performance of activities.[47] As the treating early intervention physical therapist working with this 26-month-old child, various age-appropriate activities at home and within the class-room could be recommended. At home, a prone-propped position while watching television can facilitate trunk extensor strength. In the classroom, the child should be encouraged to transfer from her seated position to stand with her peers and practice gait training during activity times to improve gross motor activity. During movement from the class to the outside playground, ambulation with the child's posterior walker should be encouraged to facilitate transfers and ambulation.

Interventions may help improve the child's postural stability and independent mobility[21] to promote participation.[48] The therapist should encourage and educate the mother to position her daughter in a variety of positions throughout the day to help prevent secondary impairments[49] and encourage motor development, exploration, and play. Positions such as prone lying and supported standing programs that provide a gentle, prolonged stretch are also beneficial to children with CP.[24] The physical therapist should assist with obtaining and managing the equipment and assistive technology necessary for positioning, mobility, and participation (e.g., orthoses, standers, walkers).[47,50,51]

Evidence-Based Clinical Recommendations

SORT: Strength of Recommendation Taxonomy

A: Consistent, good-quality patient-oriented evidence
B: Inconsistent or limited-quality patient-oriented evidence
C: Consensus, disease-oriented evidence, usual practice, expert opinion, or case series

1. For children with cerebral palsy who are non-ambulatory, supported standing programs reduce spasticity and improve bone density, hip stability, social interaction, and alertness. **Grade B**

2. The Child Engagement in Daily Life (CEDL) and the Ease of Caregiving for Children measures are valid and reliable tools to assess participation for young children with CP (17-59 months of age for the CEDL) and the difficulty of caregiving for young children (18-60 months of age for the Ease of Caregiving for Children) with CP. **Grade B**

3. The Gross Motor Function Measure (GMFM) is a valid and reliable tool to measure gross motor function and evaluate change over time in children with CP. **Grade A**

4. Physical therapy interventions structured within the family's daily routine facilitate increased adherence and practice while minimizing the burden on the family. **Grade B**

COMPREHENSION QUESTIONS

An early intervention physical therapist is working with a 26-month-old child diagnosed with CP at age 20 months. The child is able to sit independently, but does not pull to stand independently. She plays with toys and blocks like her 2-year-old cousin, but she log rolls on the floor to get to different toys. When held in standing, she tends to keep her legs very stiff and crosses them like a pair of scissors with her hips adducted and internally rotated. Her legs are significantly more involved than her arms, and she uses her arms for functional tasks with greater ease than her legs.

6.1 The child's mother tells the physical therapist that she heard that children with CP have brain damage, and asks if this brain damage will get worse over time. The most appropriate response to the mother's concern would be:

    A. CP is an inherited genetic disorder that directly affects muscle.

    B. CP results from brain damage that does not change over time and the signs that the child demonstrates now will thus also not change over time.

    C. Children with CP have non-progressive damage or disturbance to the brain, although secondary changes in the musculoskeletal system may progress over time.

    D. Children with CP have progressive brain damage that worsens over time and results in increased musculoskeletal changes over time.

6.2 Based on extent and location of limb involvement, what type of CP does this child most likely demonstrate?

    A. Diplegia

    B. Hemiplegia

    C. Monoplegia

    D. Quadriplegia

6.3 Based on the child's lower extremity posture and motor skills, what intervention is most important to initiate first?

    A. Daily passive ROM for 20 minutes in the morning and 20 minutes in the evening

    B. Passive standing in a prone stander daily

    C. Body-weight-supported treadmill training

    D. Patterning done 6 hours per day

ANSWERS

6.1 **C.** The brain lesions that occur in the fetal or developing brain are static and do not progress. However, there may be further progressions of musculoskeletal impairments due to the child's hyper/hypotonicity and/or atypical positioning.

6.2 **A.** The child demonstrates primary motor involvement of the lower extremities, as noted by spasticity in the lower extremities in scissoring (legs crossing midline) with standing and gait, and extensor tone noted as "stiffness" in standing and walking. She has some minor involvement in the upper extremities with more involvement in the lower extremities.

6.3 **B.** There are many forms of treatment that will benefit this child. However, lower extremity weightbearing through supported standing programs is important to initiate to promote the physiologic and psychosocial benefits.

REFERENCES

1. O'Callaghan ME, MacLennan AH, Gibson CS, et al. Epidemiologic associations with cerebral palsy. *Obstet Gynecol*. 2011;118:576-582.

2. Palisano RJ, Rosenbaum P, Bartlett D, Livingston MH. Content validity of the expanded and revised Gross Motor Function Classification System. *Dev Med Child Neurol*. 2008; 50:744-750.

3. Individuals with Disabilities Education Improvement Act of 2004. Pub L No. 108-446, 118 Stat 2647.

4. Backes CH, Markham K, Moorehead P, Cordero L, Nankervis CA, Giannone PJ. Maternal preeclampsia and neonatal outcomes. *J Pregnancy*. 2011;2011:214365. Epub Apr 4, 2011.

5. Rosenbaum P, Paneth N, Leviton A, et al. A report: the definition and classification of cerebral palsy April 2006. *Dev Med Child Neurol Suppl*. 2007;109:8-14.

6. Oskoui M, Coutinho F, Dykeman J, Jette N, Pringsheim T. An update on the prevalence of cerebral palsy: a systematic review and meta-analysis. *Dev Med Child Neurol*. 2013;55:509-519.

7. Rethlefsen SA, Ryan DD, Kay RM. Classification systems in cerebral palsy. *Orthop Clin North Am*. 2010;41:457-467.

8. Eliasson AC, Krumlinde-Sundholm L, Rösblad B, et al. The Manual Ability Classification System (MACS) for children with cerebral palsy: scale development and evidence of validity and reliability. *Dev Med Child Neurol*. 2006;48:549-554.

9. Hidecker MJ, Paneth N, Rosenbaum PL, et al. Developing and validating the Communication Function Classification System for individuals with cerebral palsy. *Dev Med Child Neurol*. 2011;53:704-710.

10. Wright M, Wallman L. Cerebral palsy. In: Campbell SK, Palisano RJ, Orlin MN, eds. *Physical Therapy for Children*. 4th ed. St. Louis, MO: Elsevier; 2012:577-627.

11. Beckung E, Carlsson G, Carlsdotter S, Uvebrant P. The natural history of gross motor development in children with cerebral palsy aged 1 to 15 years. *Dev Med Child Neurol*. 2007;49:751-756.

12. Carter DR, Tse B. The pathogenesis of osteoarthritis in cerebral palsy. *Dev Med Child Neurol*. 2009;51:79-83.

13. Fehlings D, Switzer L, Agarwal P, et al. Informing evidence-based clinical practice guidelines for children with cerebral palsy at risk of osteoporosis: a systematic review. *Dev Med Child Neurol*. 2012;54:106-116.

14. Wong C, Bartlett DJ, Chiarello LA, Chang HJ, Stoskopf B. Comparison of the prevalence and impact of health problems of pre-school children with and without cerebral palsy. *Child Care Health Dev*. 2012;38:128-138.

15. Dunst CJ, Trivette CM, Hamby DW. Meta-analysis of family-centered helpgiving practices research. *Ment Retard Dev Disabil Res Rev*. 2007;13:370-378.

16. An M, Palisano RJ. Family-professional collaboration in pediatric rehabilitation: a practice model. *Disabil Rehabil*. 2014;36:434-440.

17. Brewer K, Pollock N, Wright FV. Addressing the challenges of collaborative goal setting with children and their families. *Phys Occup Ther Pediatr*. 2014;34:138-152.

18. Chiarello LA, Palisano RJ, Maggs JM, et al. Family priorities for activity and participation of children and youth with cerebral palsy. *Phys Ther*. 2010;90:1254-1264.

19. Wiart L, Ray L, Darrah J, Magill-Evans J. Parents' perspectives on occupational therapy and physical therapy goals for children with cerebral palsy. *Disabil Rehabil*. 2010;32:248-258.

20. Chiarello LA, O'Niel M, Dichter CG, et al. Exploring physical therapy clinical decision making for children with spastic diplegia: survey of pediatric practice. *Pediatr Phys Ther*. 2005;17:46-54.

21. Lobo MA, Harbourne RT, Dusing SC, McCoy SW. Grounding early intervention: physical therapy cannot just be about motor skills anymore. *Phys Ther*. 2013;93:94-103.

22. Paleg GS, Smith BA, Glickman LB. Systematic review and evidence-based clinical recommendations for dosing of pediatric supported standing programs. *Pediatr Phys Ther*. 2013;25:232-247.

23. Dalvand H, Dehghan L, Feizi A, Hosseini SA, Amirsalari S. The impacts of hinged and solid ankle-foot orthoses on standing and walking in children with spastic diplegia. *Iran J Child Neurol.* 2013;7:12-19.

24. O'Neil ME, Fragala-Pinkham MA, Westcott SL, et al. Physical therapy clinical management recommendations for children with cerebral palsy-spastic diplegia: achieving functional mobility outcomes. *Pediatr Phys Ther.* 2006;18:49-72.

25. Numanoglu A, Gunel MK. Intraobserver reliability of modified Ashworth scale and modified Tardieu scale in the assessment of spasticity in children with cerebral palsy. *Acta Orthop Traumatol Turc.* 2012;46:196-200.

26. Yam WK, Leung MS. Interrater reliability of Modified Ashworth Scale and Modified Tardieu Scale in children with spastic cerebral palsy. *J Child Neurol.* 2006;21:1031-1035.

27. Bohannon RW, Smith MB. Interrater reliability of a modified Ashworth scale of muscle spasticity. *Phys Ther.* 1987;67:206-207.

28. Saether R, Helbostad JL, Riphagen II, Vik T. Clinical tools to assess balance in children and adults with cerebral palsy: a systematic review. *Dev Med Child Neurol.* 2013;55:988-999.

29. Chandler LS, Andrews MS, Swanson MW. *Movement Assessment of Infants: A Manual.* Rolling Bay, WA: Chandler, Andrews, and Swanson; 1980.

30. Franjoine MR, Gunther JS, Taylor MJ. Pediatric balance scale: modified version of the berg balance scale for the school-age child with mild to moderate motor impairment. *Pediatr Phys Ther.* 2003;15:114-128.

31. McCoy SW, Bartlett DJ, Yocum A, et al. Development and validity of the early clinical assessment of balance for young children with cerebral palsy. *Dev Neurorehabil.* 2014;17:375-383.

32. Bartlett D, Purdie B. Testing of the spinal alignment and range of motion measure: a discriminative measure of posture and flexibility for children with cerebral palsy. *Dev Med Child Neurol.* 2005;47:739-743.

33. Westcott McCoy SW, Yocum A, Bartlett DJ, et al. Development of the Early Activity Scale for Endurance for children with cerebral palsy. *Pediatr Phys Ther.* 2012;24:232-240.

34. Haley SM, Coster WJ, Ludlow LH, Haltiwanger JT, Andrellos PJ. *Pediatric Evaluation of Disability Inventory (PEDI): Development, Standardization and Administration Manual.* Boston, MA: PEDI Research Group; 1992.

35. Chiarello LA, Palisano RJ, McCoy SW, et al. Child Engagement in Daily Life: a measure of participation for young children with cerebral palsy. *Disabil Rehabil.* 2014;36:1804-1816.

36. Ward KD, Chiarello LA, Bartlett DJ, Palisano RJ, McCoy SW, Avery L. Ease of Caregiving for Children: a measure of parent perceptions of the physical demands of caregiving for young children with cerebral palsy. *Res Dev Disabil.* 2014;35:3403-3415.

37. Russell DJ, Rosenbaum PL, Avery LM, Lane M. *Gross Motor Function Measure (GMFM-66 & GMFM-88) User's Manual.* London: Mac Keith Press; 2002.

38. Russel DJ, Avery LM, Rosenbaum PL, et al. Improved scaling of the gross motor function measure for children with cerebral palsy: evidence of reliability and validity. *Phys Ther.* 2000;80:873-885.

39. Russell DJ, Avery LM, Walter SD, et al. Development and validation of item sets to improve efficiency of administration of the 66-item Gross Motor Measure in children with cerebral palsy. *Dev Med Child Neurol.* 2010;52:e48-e54.

40. Brunton LK, Bartlett DJ. Validity and reliability of two abbreviated versions of the Gross Motor Function Measure. *Phys Ther.* 2011;91:577-588.

41. Wright FV, Rosenbaum P, Fehlings D, Mesterman R, Breuer U, Kim M. The Quality Function Measure: reliability and discriminant validity of a new measure of quality of gross motor movement in ambulatory children with cerebral palsy. *Dev Med Child Neurol.* 2014;56:770-778.

42. Bartlett DJ, Palisano RJ. Physical therapists' perceptions of factors influencing the acquisition of motor abilities of children with cerebral palsy: implications for clinical reasoning. *Phys Ther.* 2002;82:237-248.

43. Rone-Adams SA, Stern DF, Walker V. Stress and compliance with a home exercise program among caregivers of children with disabilities. *Pediatr Phys Ther*. 2004;16:140-148.

44. Myrhaug HT, Ostensjo S. Motor training and physical activity among preschoolers with cerebral palsy: a survey of parents' experiences. *Phys Occup Ther Pediatr*. 2014;34:153-167.

45. An M, Palisano RJ. Family-professional collaboration in pediatric rehabilitation: a practice model. *Disabil Rehabil*. 2014;36:434-440.

46. Ketelaar M, Vermeer A, Hart H, van Petegem-van Beek E, Helders PJ. Effects of a functional therapy program on motor abilities of children with cerebral palsy. *Phys Ther*. 2001;81:1534-1545.

47. Ostensjo S, Carlberg EB, Vollestad NK. The use and impact of assistive devices and other environmental modifications on everyday activities and care in young children with cerebral palsy. *Disabil Rehabil*. 2005;27:849-861.

48. Carey H, Long T. The pediatric physical therapist's role in promoting and measuring participation in children with disabilities. *Pediatr Phys Ther*. 2012;24:163-170.

49. Porter D, Michael S, Kirkwood C. Is there a relationship between preferred posture and positioning in early life and the direction of subsequent asymmetrical postural deformity in non-ambulant people with cerebral palsy? *Child Care Health Dev*. 2008;34:635-641.

50. Ryan SE, Campbell KA, Rigby PJ. Reliability of the family impact of assistive technology scale for families of young children with cerebral palsy. *Arch Phys Med Rehabil*. 2007;88:1436-1440.

51. Ryan SE, Campbell KA, Rigby PJ, Fishbein-Germon B, Hubley D, Chan B. The impact of adaptive seating devices on the lives of young children with cerebral palsy and their families. *Arch Phys Med Rehabil*. 2009;90:27-33.

Cerebral Palsy— Elementary School

Kimberly D. Ward
Barb Kellar

The child from Case 6 is now 5 ½ years old. She is attending half-day preschool at her local child care center 5 days per week and will begin attending full-day kindergarten at her local public elementary school in 3 months. The physical therapy services she receives are transitioning from Early Intervention (services provided under the Individuals with Disabilities Education Improvement Act—IDEA, Part C) to school-aged programming (services provided under IDEA, Part B). As part of this process, she has been referred for a full educational evaluation that will be completed by the elementary school's educational team. The evaluation consists of the typical testing performed on every child entering kindergarten, in addition to evaluations completed by the school district's educational psychologist, occupational therapist, speech-language pathologist, and physical therapist. At her current preschool, the child is in a classroom with one teacher, a classroom assistant, and 14 additional preschoolers. In addition, she is assigned a classroom assistant whose primary role is to assist her throughout the day. At the preschool, she receives physical therapy services 45 minutes twice per week and occupational therapy services 30 minutes twice per week. Although the educational team has tried to include her in the majority of preschool activities, her participation in outdoor playground activities continues to be a challenge and she prefers to play inside with her friends. As part of the transition evaluation, the school-based physical therapist from the kindergarten will conduct interviews with the child, her mother, and her preschool educational team to identify the child's strengths and needs associated with accessing and participating in her preschool environment and their related concerns regarding her upcoming transition to kindergarten. Using the Gross Motor Function Measure (GMFM) and results from a full evaluation, the physical therapist determined that the child's gross motor skills were consistent with Gross Motor Function Classification System (GMFCS) level III. The therapist recommended physical therapy services as a part of school-based programming to help her access her educational environment and to provide training and consultation with her kindergarten educational team. Currently, the child sits in a classroom chair with a high back, pelvic positioning belt, and arm rests.

Since she has not demonstrated the endurance and sitting balance to safely maintain sitting for a 30-minute lunch period, the physical therapist is concerned that the child will require adaptive seating in the public school lunchroom because the bench seats do not provide back support. Although the child can walk up and down a short flight of stairs using two handrails and moderate assistance from an adult, the school team anticipates having her use the elevator to access the second floor where her kindergarten classroom and library are located. In addition, the child will require an evacuation plan in the event of an emergency (*e.g.*, fire) and appropriate staff must be trained in safe emergency evacuation procedures. Although the kindergarten offers an adapted physical education class that includes children with various gross motor challenges, the child's mother requested that her daughter not attend this adapted programming, but rather be included in the regular physical education class with appropriate modifications. The child's kindergarten physical education team has explained to the school-based physical therapist that they are willing to incorporate the child to the best of their abilities, but they are anxious due to the large class size and their limited experience working with students with similar physical challenges. The child's mother asked about obtaining a power wheelchair to enable her daughter to have more independent and efficient mobility for increased distances in the elementary school. The preschool physical therapist had recommended to the child's mother that they attend a seating clinic at the local children's hospital to obtain this equipment and the child's mother made this appointment. The child's mother has also been in contact with a local support agency and received financial assistance to support her daughter's medical equipment needs and physical therapy services through a local outpatient physical therapy clinic.

► Based on the child's strengths and needs, what do you anticipate will be contributing factors to activity limitations and participation restrictions when she begins kindergarten?
► What are the educational needs that should be addressed for the child at this time?
► What equipment might be required in her educational programming starting in the fall, including all aspects of her day (*e.g.*, lunchroom, classroom, evacuation, playground, physical education, transportation)?
► What training needs to be completed with the school staff prior to the child's transition to kindergarten?
► What is the best way to address the upcoming needs for her participation in the regular physical education programming?

KEY DEFINITIONS

EVALUATIVE REPORT (ER): Multidisciplinary report containing at least two student evaluations completed by the school district; if a student is found to qualify for special education, the educational team has 30 calendar days to complete an IEP.

INDIVIDUALIZED EDUCATION PROGRAM (IEP)[1]: Legally binding document developed annually for students who require specially designed instruction; identifies the special education and related services the student will receive for one calendar year

NOTICE OF RECOMMENDED EDUCATIONAL PLACEMENT (NOREP): Document that classifies type of classroom and programming that a child will receive for the duration of the IEP

PERMISSION TO EVALUATE (PTE): Document that parents/guardians are required to sign before a school system may evaluate a student for special education services

SECTION 504 OF THE REHABILITATION ACT OF 1973: Federal legislation that makes discrimination against individuals with disabilities illegal; Section 504 provides that students who do not require specially designed instruction may receive accommodations and services including physical therapy if they are considered to have a disability that impacts a major life function.

Objectives

1. Describe typical characteristics of school-aged children with cerebral palsy (CP).
2. List appropriate components of a school-based physical therapy evaluation for a child with CP.
3. Identify opportunities for consultation, collaboration, and patient/client-related instruction within school-based physical therapy practice.

Physical Therapy Considerations

PT considerations for management of the child with CP who is transitioning from early intervention to school-based services:

▶ **General physical therapy plan of care/goals:** Coordinate transition to kindergarten with related services needed to support the child in her educational program; provide efficient means to access the school environment including classroom, general school building, cafeteria, and playground; create meaningful adaptations to promote participation in school activities (*e.g.,* classroom, recess, field trips)

▶ **Physical therapy interventions:** Coordination and communication with all members of the educational team; education to school staff including strategies to promote increased student self-efficacy and safe strategies for assistance with transfers and mobility; procedural interventions for specific goals (*e.g.*, mobility, balance, and strength related to participation in the school environment and school activities); development of an emergency evacuation plan; varied positioning during school day to meet the child's needs; accommodation of school activities (*e.g.*, physical education class, extracurricular activities) and environments (*e.g.*, student areas of the classroom, playground) to enhance participation

▶ **Precautions during physical therapy:** Fatigue, especially throughout the school day

▶ **Complications interfering with physical therapy:** Increased time required for educational activities and related services; increased energy/time demands of activity throughout the school day; increased energy/time demands of mobility with assistive devices

Understanding the Health Condition

Please refer to this section in Case 6 (Cerebral Palsy—Early Intervention).

Physical Therapy Patient/Client Management

Federal legislation provides for physical therapy services in educational settings for students with disabilities if those services are necessary for the students to participate in and benefit from their education. The IDEA mandates that these physical therapy services support the participation of students with disabilities.[1] Similarly, Section 504 of the Rehabilitation Act of 1973 provides that students with disabilities may receive physical therapy services if those services are required to "allow the student with a disability to receive a free and appropriate education as adequately as a non-disabled student."[2] Service requirements and the role of the collaborative educational team differ from a more traditional medical model.[3,4] The goal of physical therapy services provided within the educational setting is to ensure that a student is able to access and participate effectively in school activities and benefit from available learning opportunities.[5] School-based physical therapists utilize their knowledge and a wide variety of skills and professional competencies[6] to provide evidence-based[7] assessments and interventions including procedural interventions, student-related instruction, and collaboration and consultation with students, families, educational teams, and medical teams.

In educational environments, physical therapists are members of the educational team[1] and physical therapy is a related service, considered part of a student's comprehensive educational program. The educational team also includes the student and individuals who interact with the student, including: parents/guardians, regular and special education teachers, individual aide, school nurse, occupational therapist, special area teachers (*e.g.*, physical education teacher), and transportation personnel.

In the school setting, student-centered services[5] support goals that have been identified by the educational team. This type of collaborative goal setting is an important part of student-centered care and is associated with positive outcomes.[8]

As children get older, they should gradually take a more active role in this decision-making process.[5,9,10] Goals that are included in a student's IEP should be meaningful and educationally relevant,[5] measurable and observable, and should identify quantitative criteria and relate to school function in the curriculum or in a general school activity (e.g., participation in or access to the cafeteria, gym, or classroom).[11]

Beyond the traditional physical school environments (school buildings and grounds and outdoor recreational facilities), there are a variety of settings that are also considered school settings. These non-traditional school settings include individual or group homes and skilled nursing facilities for medically fragile students, individual homes for students who are home-schooled, community environments for educational activities that take place off of school grounds (educational/field trips, community-based instruction, and pre-vocational training), and school-related transportation.

The physical therapist in an educational setting often serves as a liaison between the student's medical team and the educational team.[6] The school-based physical therapist should communicate and provide consultation to the student's family, educational team, and medical team. Consultation with the student's family and educational team should address services, accommodations, and adaptations required to meet the student's needs within the educational setting.[6,12] Consultation with the student's medical team should address the student's strengths and needs within the community and school settings and their relationship to medical interventions. For example, if the student undergoes medical or surgical procedures, the physical therapist should address the child's particular needs upon return to school.

Examination, Evaluation, and Diagnosis

The school-based examination and evaluation of a student with CP should identify the goals of the student, family, and educational team, identify the student's strengths and needs related to body structures and functions, activity, and participation, and identify and assess environmental and personal factors that impact the student. Based on this information, the school-based therapist and the educational team then determine if the student requires physical therapy services to benefit from her educational program.[1]

The physical therapist begins by interviewing the parent, student, and members of the educational team[4] to gather information about her developmental history, concerns, and priorities, particularly as they relate to her educational program.[9,12] This is especially important as the student's, parents', and educational team members' perceptions of the student's strengths and needs may differ.[13]

The examination includes observation and assessment of the student's function in the natural contexts of her school environment and activities.[5,9,12] The physical location of classrooms, as well as the time required to travel within the greater school campus, should be assessed. To assess function within the school setting for elementary school students, the physical therapist can use the **School Function Assessment (SFA)**.[14] The SFA is a criterion-referenced tool that measures participation in the school setting and activity in physical and cognitive/behavioral tasks for students in kindergarten through

6th grade.[14] Participation is assessed in the regular or special education classroom and in five non-classroom settings, namely: playground/recess, transportation, bathroom/toileting, transitions, and mealtime/snack time. Activity categories include travel, maintaining and changing positions, recreational movement, manipulation with movement, hygiene, eating and drinking, clothing management, up/down stairs, and others. Any educational professional familiar with the child's function in the school environment may complete the SFA. Raw scores can be converted to criterion scores for each individual section of the SFA. The student's scores can then be compared to criterion cut-off scores. The SFA includes two separate criterion cut-off score scales, one for kindergarten through 3rd grade and one for 4th through 6th grade.

For the child presented in this case, the physical therapist observed that she ambulates with a posterior rolling walker on level surfaces within her preschool. She needs intermittent assistance or verbal cues for attention because she occasionally bumps her walker into peers or environmental barriers. She requires increased time to ambulate and transition between student activity areas in her classroom, and benefits from being able to move from place to place when it is less crowded. For all transfers, she requires moderate assistance from her one-on-one aide. She propels herself in her manual wheelchair to all indoor and outdoor recess activities. For longer distances such as class field trips, she has someone else propel her. She is unable to ambulate with her walker on uneven surfaces such as the grass or wood chips on the playground, so an adult's assistance is required to help her move in these areas. She also has insufficient muscle strength, coordination, and motor planning necessary to access the playground equipment. With assistance from her aide, she can ascend the ramped playground equipment to access a small slide. She enjoys being pushed on the adapted swing, though she needs maximal assistance to get into and out of the swing.

Examination of primary impairments of body structures and functions should include assessment of spasticity, balance and postural control, selective voluntary motor control, and sensory processing.[9] Examination of secondary impairments should include assessment of postural alignment, trunk and extremity range of motion (ROM), muscular strength, and endurance. Additional impairments that should be assessed include pain, cardiopulmonary status (heart rate, respiratory rate), and skin integrity. Muscle tone may be assessed through clinical observation or through the modified Ashworth scale (MAS)[9] and spasticity may also be assessed using the modified Tardieu scale. For the current student, the therapist noted that she demonstrates a toe-walking pattern when ambulating. She uses a pronounced lateral weight shift and a shortened step length, and demonstrates increased tone and spasticity (MAS score of 3 in bilateral lower extremities). The student has an upcoming appointment with a physician to evaluate the need for possible medical intervention (e.g., botulinum toxin injections) to decrease tightness in lower extremity muscles. On the Wong-Baker FACES pain scale, the child rated her lower extremity pain during ambulation as "2—hurts a little bit."

Balance and postural control in young children with CP may be assessed using a wide variety of balance tools. For the student in this case, appropriate measures include the Pediatric Balance Scale,[15] Pediatric Reach Test,[16] and the Early Clinical Assessment of Balance.[17] The therapist noted that the student's balance and righting reactions were limited and that she had difficulty protecting herself when she lost her balance. In static standing, she uses a wide base of support. She was able to walk four steps when given hand-held assistance, but fell when attempting to independently weight shift. Though she can transition to standing from her classroom chair, she needed close supervision and a stable surface such as a chair or classroom desk to help her push up or pull to standing. She required contact guard assistance and verbal cues to transition to use her posterior rolling walker. She can independently move from a prone position on the floor to a quadruped position, but requires moderate assistance to transition to standing due to decreased balance.

There are a variety of valid and clinically feasible functional mobility and endurance assessments for use with students with CP.[18] For students who are ambulatory, mobility may be assessed using the 30-second walk test,[19] 6-minute walk test (6MWT),[20,21] Timed Up and Go (TUG) test,[22] and the Timed Up and Down Stairs.[23] For students 4 to 13 years of age with CP who are able to walk (GMFCS levels I-III), mobility may also be assessed through parent report using the MobQues28.[24] The MobQues28 is a mobility questionnaire that asks parents to rate their child's level of difficulty completing a variety of mobility tasks including level surface mobility, mobility on uneven surfaces or over changes in elevation, transitioning between positions (*e.g.*, transitioning from sitting on the floor or on a chair; transitioning out of a shower or car), and recreational activities (*e.g.*, kicking a ball, running on various terrains). Each task is rated on a 5-point scale from "impossible without help" to "not difficult at all."[24] Endurance may be assessed by parent report using the Early Activity Scale for Endurance (EASE)[25] or the 6MWT (for ambulatory students).[20,21] For students 6 years and older, cardiorespiratory fitness may be assessed with the Energy Expenditure Index (EEI).[26] For students classified at GMFCS level I or II, aerobic fitness may be assessed using the Shuttle Run Test I (SRT-I) and Shuttle Run Test II (SRT-II).[27] During performance of these tests, appropriate self-report measures of exertion include the Pictorial Children's Effort Rating Table (PCERT) or the Children's OMNI Walk/Run Scale of Perceived Exertion.[28] Because of this student's age and ambulatory ability, the therapist chose the 6MWT and the TUG test (using her posterior wheeled walker) as the best initial assessments. The student was able to walk 190 m during the 6MWT, though she rated her exertion as "6—tired" on the Children's OMNI Walk/Run Scale of Perceived Exertion, indicating increased energy expenditure. On a daily basis, the student walks with her posterior rolling walker within and between classrooms, but at a pace that is slower than her peers. She can also climb up and down a short flight of three stairs to access the school stage, using both handrails and moderate assistance from an adult.

Engagement and participation in school-aged children may be assessed via the Children's Assessment of Participation and Enjoyment (CAPE)[29] and the Preference for Activity of Children (PAC). Health-related quality of life may be assessed through the Cerebral Palsy Quality of Life Questionnaire for Children (CP QOL-Child),[30] the Pediatric Quality of Life Inventory (PedsQL),[31] or the Caregiver Priorities and Child Health Index of Life with Disabilities (CPCHILD).[32] The use and impact of assistive technology (*e.g.*, mobility devices, adaptive devices for self-care, technology for communication and education) should also be assessed.[33]

Two common standardized tests that measure gross motor performance in students with CP are the GMFM[34] and the Quality Function Measure (QFM).[35] Gross motor function is often classified by using the GMFCS. For the current student, the therapist determined that her gross motor skills were consistent with GMFCS level III, meaning that she ambulates using a walker, uses a wheelchair for traveling longer distances or outdoors, and can sit in a regular chair with pelvic or trunk support.

Plan of Care and Interventions

Physical therapy interventions for the student with CP who is transitioning from early intervention to school-aged services should focus on educational-based services intended to ensure that the student is able to access and participate in her educational programming. In addition, prevention or minimization of secondary conditions that may impact health, wellness, and quality of life both in the short term and long term should be considered.[36]

When working with a student with CP within the school setting, the physical therapist should help the student, family, and educational team members understand CP, implications for the student,[6] and strategies and interventions to address the student's needs to improve access to and participation in her education.[1] Table 7-1 highlights specific physical therapy areas of instruction. As students with CP age, instruction should be directed toward fostering their independence, self-advocacy, positive self-concept, self-management of their disability, and participation in medical and educational decision making.[9,10,36,37] Physical therapists can assist families in understanding **transition planning** when children begin school-based services.[38] In a study using semi-structured interviews of program managers, therapists, and parents of children with CP, parents expressed that they felt unprepared for changes in service delivery models, that they did not fully understand the factors (including legislation) that impact services in school-based practice, and that they needed more general information regarding community-based services and supports.[38] Families and educational staff may also benefit from strategies to ease caregiving tasks, especially related to positioning, feeding, dressing, and transporting the student out in the community. Strategies and recommendations to help families and educational staff utilize community and recreational resources and supports may help families and students with CP participate in their community for leisure, play, and fitness.[5,6,12]

Physical therapists may also serve as a resource for community-based disability support and socialization networks.[37] School teachers often feel that they do not have the training or support needed to work with students with physical disabilities. Therefore, physical therapists working in educational environments should provide training and support to create a more successful experience for the teachers and the students with whom they work.[6,39]

Recommended interventions must address how to best include the student in the educational setting with the focus on inclusion into the least restrictive environment.[1] Physical therapy services should promote the student's independence and self-advocacy, particularly as she gets older.[5] These services may directly address

Table 7-1 PHYSICAL THERAPY AREAS OF INSTRUCTION TO STUDENT, FAMILY, AND SCHOOL PERSONNEL		
Student[37]	Family[37]	School Personnel[6,39,40]
Increase understanding of the individual's disability and precautions	Increase understanding of student's disability and precautions	Increase understanding of student's disability, disease progression, and medical precautions
Increase independence	Provide strategies to help increase student's independence	Provide strategies to help increase student's independence
Increase self-management of disability	Provide strategies to help foster student's self-management of disability	Increase disability awareness (individual, classroom, school)
Improve problem solving regarding disability	Instruct in techniques or strategies for daily care	Provide information regarding daily care and handling during the school day (personal care needs)
Develop or improve coping strategies	Instruct in home exercise programs	Instruct in proper transfer and assistance techniques
Increase self-advocacy	Assist in understanding and navigating special education and school district policies and procedures	Instruct in emergency evacuation procedures
Assist in learning how to instruct others in their care or assistance	Provide wellness training on proper body mechanics and injury prevention	Provide wellness training on proper body mechanics and injury prevention
Increase general disability awareness	Consult regarding equipment needs and proper use	Consult regarding equipment needs and proper use
Identify community resources	Provide resources for disability support	Consult regarding field trip planning
Prepare for transitions during school and post-secondary transition	Identify community resources	Identify and implement task and environmental adaptations
	Coordinate with other healthcare providers	Identify signs and symptoms of fatigue

impairments or activity limitations, but should also address adapting the environment to help increase the student's participation and improve performance of activities.[41,42] Important considerations for direct services include maximizing independent mobility, physical function, activity, and participation. Aspects of the environment that may be adapted include physical, relationships, attitudes, and assistive technology, as well as systems or policies. Accommodations including allowing the student to use school elevators or to leave classes a few minutes early and/or arrive a few minutes late may be appropriate to enable her to travel within the school building. Within classrooms, students may require adapted chairs and desks for proper positioning, or may require room set-ups that allow ease of access into and out of the classroom. In this case, the student's mother requested that her daughter be included in the regular physical education class with appropriate modifications, but the kindergarten physical education team was anxious to include her due to the large class size and their limited experience working with students with similar physical challenges. The physical therapist could provide activity accommodations to help ensure that the student can safely participate and could provide staff training to help the staff feel comfortable carrying out these strategies. Many play-based, function-focused, or participation-based interventions help achieve goals, especially related to independence, mobility, endurance, and motor development.[9,43] Both student- or context-focused therapy interventions result in equivalent and significant improvements in self-care, mobility, and participation outcomes.[41]

Students with CP who are not able to ambulate independently may benefit from assistive devices (e.g., walkers, crutches) or wheeled mobility to increase their ability to access their environment. Physical therapists should assist with obtaining and managing equipment necessary for positioning, mobility, and participation.[42,44] In school settings, physical therapists need to take into consideration the energy expenditure and time required for mobility,[45] specifically ensuring that the energy and time required for independent mobility do not negatively impact the student's ability to benefit from her educational program.[46] The student in this case ambulates with a posterior rolling walker on level surfaces, though she requires intermittent assistance to negotiate environmental barriers and increased time to ambulate longer distances. She propels herself in her manual wheelchair indoors and is pushed by an adult for longer distances and outdoor activities. Prior to this evaluation, the mother had begun the process of obtaining a power wheelchair. The evaluating therapist agreed with the mother's request for a power wheelchair because use of power mobility would increase her daughter's access to the school environment, decrease energy expenditure, and help facilitate participation in more activities. **Independent mobility** is especially important during the school years to enable children to interact with peers and to learn from exploring their environment.[47]

To help prevent secondary impairments and to encourage motor development, exploration, and play, the therapist should educate and encourage families and daily caregivers to place the student that is unable to independently ambulate in a variety of positions throughout the day.[9] Factors that facilitate the use of postural management programs within schools include availability of equipment, staff knowledge regarding the benefits of postural management, communication between school staff and therapists, scheduling postural management programs around activities throughout the school day, and school staff motivation. Factors that hinder use of postural management programs in schools include complicated equipment, poorly maintained equipment, insufficient time, and insufficient school staff skills.[40]

Students with CP who are not able to stand independently may also benefit from supported standing programs in which the student stands in a supine or prone stander. Weightbearing via supported standing programs improves bone density, hip stability, lower extremity ROM, and spasticity.[48] Sustained standing provides more typical weightbearing forces to the developing lower extremity bones. This helps remodel the head of the femur and acetabulum in a manner that mimics typical weightbearing during development.[48] Upright positioning may also be important for psychosocial benefits, including improved social interactions and improved alertness.[48]

Interventions to address ROM, pain, and nutrition are particularly important in older students with CP with more motor involvement (GMFCS levels III to V), particularly as studies have found declines in gross motor capacity of adolescents with CP.[49] Decreased gross motor capacity is associated with decreased ROM, pain, and suboptimal anthropometric measurements.[50] Physical therapists should consider methods to prevent muscular contractures that may occur with hypertonicity and atypical positioning over time. Low-load, prolonged stretching of muscles that are at risk for tightness is more effective than manual stretching.[51] Students with CP may benefit from orthoses for more typical ankle-foot positioning and support when standing and ambulating.[9,52]

Last, physical therapists should incorporate interventions to improve strength and cardiorespiratory fitness for students with CP.[53] Progressive resistance exercise programs have been found to increase strength of select muscle groups and improve independent mobility without adverse effects on spasticity in individuals with CP.[46,54] Aerobic exercise in students with CP improves cardiorespiratory fitness.[46] For students with CP who are independently ambulatory (GMFCS levels I and II), functional physical training programs improve aerobic endurance, anaerobic capacity, walking distance, agility, muscle strength, and functional ambulation. In this case, the therapist noted that the student lacked sufficient muscle strength, coordination, motor planning, and cardiorespiratory fitness to efficiently access playground equipment and her school environment. The physical therapist worked with the school's physical education teacher to incorporate activities to improve strength and fitness within her physical education classes. The therapist also worked with the student and her mother to develop a home program that incorporated strengthening and aerobic activities in their daily home routine and identified physical activity–based recreational opportunities that the student was interested in trying. The student and her mother decided that one particular activity they would like to try is bicycling, particularly since they live close to a bike path. They contacted a local bicycle vendor to trial an adaptive bike. Incorporation of such activities and exercise programs might improve this student's muscle strength, mobility, and aerobic endurance to enable her to improve her mobility, physical activity, and endurance throughout her day.

Evidence-Based Clinical Recommendations

SORT: Strength of Recommendation Taxonomy

A: Consistent, good-quality patient-oriented evidence
B: Inconsistent or limited-quality patient-oriented evidence
C: Consensus, disease-oriented evidence, usual practice, expert opinion, or case series

1. The School Function Assessment is a reliable and valid tool for assessment of participation and activity in elementary school students. **Grade A**
2. Physical therapists can help families understand the transition planning when children begin school-based services. **Grade C**

3. Independent mobility is especially important during the school years to enable children with disabilities to interact with peers and to learn from exploring their environment. **Grade B**

COMPREHENSION QUESTIONS

A school-based physical therapist is working with a kindergarten student diagnosed with CP, GMFCS level III. The student is able to ambulate with use of a rolling walker. She enjoys being with her classmates, but becomes frustrated when she has difficulty keeping up with classmates during physical education class or while outside on the playground and school sports fields. The student is on grade level for all academic areas.

7.1 Which of the following tools would be *most* appropriate to measure this student's participation in the school setting and activity in school-related tasks?

A. Children's Assessment of Participation and Enjoyment (CAPE)

B. Gross Motor Function Measure (GMFM)

C. Quality Function Measure (QFM)

D. School Function Assessment (SFA)

7.2 Which of the following objective measures would be *most* appropriate to measure this student's mobility and endurance?

A. 6-minute walk test (6MWT)

B. 30-second walk test

C. Early Activity Scale for Endurance

D. MobQues28

7.3 To address the student's frustration with keeping up with her classmates during physical education and recess, which intervention is *most* important for the physical therapist to initiate?

A. Convene a meeting with the student's physical education teacher to provide the student with a separate physical education class.

B. Help the student problem solve and identify strategies to increase her participation in physical education and recess.

C. Increase lower extremity strength and balance.

D. Request that the student's teacher allow the student to play inside during recess.

ANSWERS

7.1 **D.** The School Function Assessment (SFA) is a criterion-referenced tool for children in kindergarten through 6th grade. The SFA measures participation in the school setting and activity in physical and cognitive/behavioral tasks. The CAPE (option A) measures children's engagement and participation in recreation and leisure activities while not in the school environment. The GMFM (option B) and the QFM (option C) are two common standardized tests that measure gross motor performance in students with CP.

7.2 **A.** The 6MWT is an objective measure used to assess both mobility and endurance. While the 30-second walk test (option B) and MobQues28 (option D) both measure mobility, they do not measure endurance. The Early Activity Scale for Endurance (option C) measures endurance, but does not specifically measure mobility in children.

7.3 **B.** It is important to include the student in addressing such issues, in order to help increase her independence, self-advocacy, and problem-solving ability regarding her disability. Options A and D would isolate the student and not allow her to integrate with her peers. Increasing her lower extremity strength and balance (option C) may help her keep up with her classmates, but it neither directly addresses the student's current frustration, nor allows her the opportunity to problem-solve.

REFERENCES

1. Individuals with Disabilities Education Act (IDEA), Pub. L. No. 108-446 (2004).

2. Birmingham G, Coultes K, Geddes R, et al. *Pennsylvania Physical Therapy Association Guidelines for the Practice of Physical Therapy in Educational Settings*. Harrisburg, PA: Pennsylvania Physical Therapy Association; 2009.

3. McEwen IR, ed. *Providing Physical Therapy Services Under Parts B & C of the Individuals With Disabilities Education act (IDEA)*. 2nd ed. Section on Pediatrics, American Physical Therapy Association; 2009.

4. McEwen IR, Shelden ML. Pediatric therapy in the 1990s: the demise of the educational versus medical dichotomy. *Occup Phys Ther Educat Environ*. 1995;15:33-45.

5. Laverdure PA, Rose DS. Providing educationally relevant occupational and physical therapy services. *Phys Occup Ther Pediatr*. 2012;32:347-354.

6. Effgen SK, Chiarello L, Milbourne SA. Updated competencies for physical therapists working in schools. *Pediatr Phys Ther*. 2007;19:266-274.

7. Schreiber J, Stern P, Marchetti G, Provident I, Turocy PS. School-based pediatric physical therapists' perspectives on evidence-based practice. *Pediatr Phys Ther*. 2008;20:292-302.

8. Brewer K, Pollock N, Wright FV. Addressing the challenges of collaborative goal setting with children and their families. *Phys Occup Ther Pediatr*. 2014;34:138-152.

9. O'Neil ME, Fragala-Pinkham MA, Westcott SL, et al. Physical therapy clinical management recommendations for children with cerebral palsy-spastic diplegia: achieving functional mobility outcomes. *Pediatr Phys Ther*. 2006;18:49-72.

10. Andersen CS, Dolva A. Children's perspective on their right to participate in decision-making according to the United Nations Convention on the Right of the Child article 12. *Phys Occup Ther Pediatr*. May 27, 2014. [Epub ahead of print]

11. Dole RL, Arvidson K, Byrne E, Robbins J, Schasberger B. Consensus among experts in pediatric occupational and physical therapy on elements of individualized education programs. *Pediatr Phys Ther*. 2003;15:159-166.

12. Chiarello LA, O'Niel M, Dichter CG, et al. Exploring physical therapy clinical decision making for children with spastic diplegia: survey of pediatric practice. *Pediatr Phys Ther*. 2005;17:46-54.

13. Dunn N, Shields N, Taylor NF, Dodd KJ. A systematic review of the self-concept of children with cerebral palsy and perceptions of parents and teachers. *Phys Occup Ther Pediatr*. 2007;27:55-71.

14. Coster W, Deeney T, Haltiwanger J, Haley S. *School Function Assessment*. San Antonio, TX: Psychological Corporation; 1998.

15. Franjoine MR, Gunther JS, Taylor MJ. Pediatric balance scale: a modified version of the Berg Balance Scale for the school-age child with mild to moderate motor impairment. *Pediatr Phys Ther*. 2003;15:114-128.

16. Bartlett D, Birmingham T. Validity and reliability of a pediatric reach test. *Pediatr Phys Ther*. 2003;15:84-92.

17. McCoy SW, Bartlett DJ, Yocum A, et al. Development and validity of the Early Clinical Assessment of Balance for young children with cerebral palsy. *Dev Neurorehabil*. 2014;17:375-383.

18. Chrysagis N, Skordilis EK, Koutsouki D. Validity and clinical utility of functional assessments in children with cerebral palsy. *Arch Phys Med Rehabil*. 2014;95:369-374.

19. Knutson LM, Bushman B, Young JC, Ward G. Age expansion of the thirty-second walk test norms for children. *Pediatr Phys Ther*. 2009;21:235-243.

20. Geiger R, Strasak A, Treml B, et al. Six-minute walk test in children and adolescents. *J Pediatr*. 2007;150:395-399.

21. Klepper SE, Muir N. Reference values on the 6-Minute Walk Test for children living in the United States. *Pediatr Phys Ther*. 2011;23:32-40.

22. Williams EN, Carroll SG, Reddihough DS, Phillips BA, Galea MP. Investigation of the timed 'Up & Go' test in children. *Dev Med Child Neurol*. 2005;47:518-524.

23. Zaino CA, Marchese VG, Westcott SL. Timed up and down stairs test: preliminary reliability and validity of a new measure of functional mobility. *Pediatr Phys Ther*. 2004;16:90-98.

24. Dallmeijer AJ, Scholtes VA, Becher J, Roorda LD. Measuring mobility limitations in children with cerebral palsy: Rasch model fit of a mobility questionnaire, MobQues28. *Arch Phys Med Rehabil*. 2011;92:640-645.

25. McCoy SW, Yocum A, Bartlett DJ, et al. Development of the Early Activity Scale for Endurance for children with cerebral palsy. *Pediatr Phys Ther*. 2012;24:232-240.

26. Rose J, Gamble JG, Lee J, Lee R, Haskell WL. The Energy Expenditure Index: a method to quantitate and compare walking energy expenditure for children and adolescents. *J Pediatr Ortho*. 1991;11:571-578.

27. Verschuren O, Blowmen M, Kruitwagen C, Takken T. Reference values for aerobic fitness in children, adolescents, and young adults who have cerebral palsy and are ambulatory. *Phys Ther*. 2010;90:1148-1156.

28. Roemmich JN, Barkley JE, Epstein LH, Lobarinas CL, Whit TM, Foster JH. Validity of PCERT and OMNI walk/run ratings of perceived exertion. *Med Sci Sports Exerc*. 2006;38:1014-1019.

29. Imms C. Review of the children's assessment of participation and enjoyment and the preferences for activity of children. *Phys Occup Ther Pediatr*. 2008;28:389-404.

30. Waters E, Davis E, Boyd R, et al. *Cerebral Palsy Quality of Life Questionnaire for Children (CP QOL-Child) Manual*. Melbourne: Deakin University; 2006.

31. Varni JW, Seid M, Kurtin PS. PedsQL 4.0: reliability and validity of the Pediatric Quality of Life Inventory Version 4.0 generic core scales in healthy and patient populations. *Med Care*. 2001;39:800-812.

32. Narayanan UG, Fehlings D, Weir S, Knights S, Kiran S, Campbell K. Initial development and validation of the Caregiver Priorities and Child Health Index of Life with Disabilities (CPCHILD). *Dev Med Child Neurol*. 2006;48:804-812.

33. Henderson S, Skelton H, Rosenbaum P. Assistive devices for children with functional impairments: impact on child and caregiver function. *Dev Med Child Neurol*. 2008;50:89-98.

34. Russell DJ, Rosenbaum PL, Avery LM, Lane M. *Gross Motor Function Measure (GMFM-66 & GMFM-88) User's Manual*. London: Mac Keith Press; 2002.

35. Wright FV, Rosenbaum P, Fehlings D, Mesterman R, Breuer U, Kim M. The Quality Function Measure: reliability and discriminant validity of a new measure of quality of gross motor movement in ambulatory children with cerebral palsy. *Dev Med Child Neurol.* 2014;56:770-778.

36. Campbell SK. Therapy programs for children that last a lifetime. *Phys Occup Ther Pediatr.* 1997;17:1-15.

37. Shields N. Self-concept is a concept worth considering. *Phys Occup Ther Pediatr.* 2009;29:23-26.

38. Darrah J, Wiart L, Magill-Evans J, Ray L, Andersen J. Are family-centered principles, functional goal setting and transition planning evident in therapy services for children with cerebral palsy? *Child Care Health Dev.* 2010;38:41-47.

39. O'Keeffe MJ, McDowell M. Bridging the gap between health and education: words are not enough. *J Paediatr Child Health.* 2004;40:252-257.

40. Maher CA, Evans KA, Sprod JA, Bostock SM. Factors influencing postural management for children with cerebral palsy in the special school setting. *Disabil Rehabil.* 2011;33:146-158.

41. Ostensjo S, Carlberg EB, Vollestad K. The use and impact of assistive devices and other environmental modifications on everyday activities and care in young children with cerebral palsy. *Disabil Rehabil.* 2005;27:849-861.

42. Palisano RJ, Chiarello LA, King GA, Novak I, Stoner T, Fiss A. Participation-based therapy for children with physical disabilities. *Disabil Rehabil.* 2012;34:1041-1052.

43. Ryan SE, Campbell KA, Rigby PJ. Reliability of the Family Impact of Assistive Technology Scale for families of young children with cerebral palsy. *Arch Phys Med Rehabil.* 2007;88:1436-1440.

44. Lephart K, Utsey C, Wild DL, Fisher SR. Estimating energy expenditure for different assistive devices in the school setting. *Pediatr Phys Ther.* 2014;26:354-359.

45. Fowler EG, Kolobe TH, Damiano DL, et al. Promotion of physical fitness and prevention of secondary conditions for children with cerebral palsy: section on pediatrics research summit proceedings. *Phys Ther.* 2007;87:1495-1510.

46. Livingstone R, Field D. Systematic review of power mobility outcomes for infants, children, and adolescents with mobility limitations. *Clin Rehabil.* 2014;28:954-964.

47. Paleg GS, Smith BA, Glickman LB. Evidence-based clinical recommendations for dosing of pediatric supported standing programs. *Pediatr Phys Ther.* 2013;25:232-247.

48. Bartlett DJ, Hanna SE, Avery L, Stevenson RD, Galuppi B. Correlates of decline in gross motor capacity in adolescents with cerebral palsy in Gross Motor Function Classification System levels III to V: an exploratory study. *Dev Med Child Neurol.* 2010;52:e155-e160.

49. Pin T, Dyke P, Chan M. The effectiveness of passive stretching in children with cerebral palsy. *Dev Med Child Neurol.* 2006;48:855-862.

50. Abd El-Kafy EM. The clinical impact of orthotic correction of lower limb rotational deformities in children with cerebral palsy: a randomized controlled trial. *Clin Rehabil.* 2014;28:1004-1014.

51. Johnson CC. The benefits of physical activity for youth with developmental disabilities: a systematic review. *Am J Health Promotion.* 2009;23:157-167.

52. Martin L, Baker R, Harvey A. A systematic review of common physiotherapy interventions in school-aged children with cerebral palsy. *Phys Occup Ther Pediatr.* 2010;30:294-312.

53. Gorter H, Holty L, Rameckers EE, Elvers HJ, Oostendorp RA. Changes in endurance and walking ability through functional physical training in children with cerebral palsy. *Pediatr Phys Ther.* 2009;21:31-37.

54. Verschuren O, Ketelaar M, Gorter JW, Helders PJ, Utterwaal CS, Takken T. Exercise training program in children and adolescents with cerebral palsy: a randomized controlled trial. *Arch Pediatr Adoles Med.* 2007;161:1075-1081.

Cerebral Palsy— Postsecondary Education and Transition to Adulthood

Kimberly D. Ward
Barb Kellar

CASE 8

The youth from Cases 6 and 7 with spastic diplegic cerebral palsy (CP) did well in high school and completed a college-preparatory track for computer science. When she was re-evaluated for a transitional Individualized Education Program (IEP) at age 16, the team determined that she no longer required specially designed instruction to access her educational programming. She continued to receive consultative physical therapy services, guidance services, and orientation and mobility training via a service agreement plan through Section 504 of the Rehabilitation Act of 1973. She was accepted to a public four-year university accessible from her home by regional rail lines. In high school, she worked with her guidance counselor and school-based physical therapist to help her develop self-advocacy skills and learn what resources and accommodations were available and how to request needed accommodations. She learned about her rights and protections as an individual with a disability under the Rehabilitation Act of 1973 and under the Americans with Disabilities Act of 1990. She also worked with a mobility and orientation specialist to learn how to take the city subways and regional rail lines in preparation for attending college. She is currently a senior in college, with a major in computer design and a minor in marketing. She has worked closely with the University's Office of Accommodations and receives accommodated on-campus dormitory housing and academic accommodations, including extended time on assignments and examinations and the option to use a note taker for courses. She ambulates with bilateral forearm crutches in her dormitory and college classrooms. She uses her power wheelchair for longer distances such as between her room and the cafeteria and between classes. In high school, she preferred not to use her power wheelchair. However, she has realized that the power wheelchair is the fastest and most energy-efficient means of long-distance mobility. The dormitory has a push-button-activated automatic door to access the building. She is independent with self-care tasks and her room has an adjacent privately accessible bathroom with grab bars near the toilet and shower and a zero-threshold enlarged shower stall that accommodates a shower bench. She wears bilateral molded ankle-foot orthoses and is independently donning and doffing them. Her friends help her with tasks such as taking her laundry to the basement laundry room. While the transition from high school to the university setting was relatively smooth, her transition to adult healthcare services has been challenging. She has had difficulty finding an adult-oriented primary care physician that she feels has a thorough understanding of CP. During her freshman year, she tried to maintain her ambulation skills and keep up with her home exercise and stretching program, but academic and social time demands made this difficult. During her sophomore year, it was more difficult for her to ambulate and she also began experiencing hip and low back pain. She found a pediatric physical therapist experienced in working with teenagers and young adults with CP and received physical therapy services twice per week for 6 weeks to address her pain. She is not attending physical therapy at this time and wants to find an adult-oriented primary care physician and physical therapist with a good understanding of the long-term effects of CP on adults. She is also interested in receiving botulinum toxin A (BTX-A) injections in her hamstrings again because her spasticity continues to limit her hamstring range of motion (ROM) and transfer ability. Through social media and online research, she learned that some adults with CP have had positive outcomes from selective dorsal rhizotomy surgery and wants to know if this is an option for her. She has started applying and interviewing for jobs at local marketing firms. While potential employers have expressed interest in her resume and portfolio, she feels that some seem hesitant due to her physical disability. The University's Career Center has been working with the Office of Vocational Rehabilitation in her state to help potential employers understand her physical disability and her ability to meet the expectations of the positions to which she is applying.

► Based on her strengths and needs, what activity limitations and participation restrictions do you anticipate will impact her ability to begin a job?
► What work accommodations may she benefit from?
► What strategies or accommodations will be helpful as she graduates from college and prepares to live on her own?

KEY DEFINITIONS

AMERICANS WITH DISABILITIES ACT OF 1990 (ADA): Federal civil rights legislation that prohibits discrimination against individuals with disabilities in employment, transportation, public accommodations, communications, and governmental activities[1]

BOTULINUM TOXIN A (BTX-A): One of seven neurotoxins (labeled A-G) produced by the bacterium *Clostridium botulinum*; therapeutic uses for botulinum toxin injection include focal dystonia and spasticity; injected muscles are temporarily weakened or paralyzed for several months.

SECTION 504 OF THE REHABILITATION ACT OF 1973: Federal legislation that provides protections such that individuals with a disability that impacts one or more major life activities shall not be discriminated against or denied benefits or services from any employer or agency that receives federal financial assistance.[2] Section 504 ensures access and accommodations for students in public primary and secondary schools who do not require special education, for students in colleges and universities, for adults employed by governmental agencies or other employers that receive federal financial assistance, and for individuals seeking the services of governmental agencies or other agencies that receive federal financial assistance.

Objectives

1. List areas to be addressed to help ensure the health and wellness of young adults with CP.

2. Describe interventions to prevent or minimize common secondary conditions in adults with CP.

3. Identify strategies that may be used to help young adults with CP transition from pediatric healthcare services into adult healthcare services.

4. Identify strategies that may be used to help young adults with CP transition from high school to postsecondary opportunities.

Physical Therapy Considerations

PT considerations for management of the young adult with CP who is transitioning from high school to postsecondary opportunities such as attending college or joining the work force:

▶ **General physical therapy plan of care/goals:** Coordinate transition and support into the work environment; assistance to facilitate workplace acceptance and accommodations for employment; provide adaptations needed to support participation in a full-time working environment; successful transition into adult-oriented healthcare systems

▶ **Physical therapy interventions:** Coordination and communication with the high school educational team, University Accommodations office, orientation and mobility specialist, public transportation accessibility office, and adult-oriented healthcare providers (e.g., physicians, therapists); instruction on health promotion and energy conservation; assistance in transitioning to adult-oriented healthcare providers who are familiar with adults with CP and its long-term sequelae

▶ **Precautions during physical therapy interventions:** Fatigue, pain, postural asymmetries, decreased balance

▶ **Complications interfering with physical therapy:** Medical insurance plan restrictions; increased time and energy demands for daily tasks, employment, and exercise; decline of mobility and increases in secondary impairments from CP; transition to adult-oriented healthcare providers; lack of public transportation accessibility

Understanding the Health Condition

As individuals with CP age, impairments and activity limitations occur at a higher prevalence and progress faster than in individuals without CP. These impairments and activity limitations include increased pain and fatigue, postural asymmetries, decreased balance, decreased gross motor capacity, reduced physical activity and physical fitness, decreased ambulation, and decreased function.[3-11] Youth and adults with CP are also at a greater risk for having a lower self-concept and have a higher prevalence of depressive symptoms compared to those without CP.[8,12]

For adults with CP, pain is most frequently reported in the lower back, hips, legs, and feet.[13] Associated musculoskeletal disorders that may progress during adulthood include osteoarthritis, patella alta, hip dysplasia, spondylolysis, and cervical stenosis.[14] Patella alta is most frequently seen in individuals with spastic diplegic CP who use a crouch-type gait pattern. Patella alta may result in anterior knee pain, decreased functional ambulation, patellar stress fractures, or subluxation and dislocation of the patella.[14] Spondylolysis is estimated to be present in up to 30% of adults with CP, particularly in those who have undergone selective dorsal rhizotomy or who have increased anterior pelvic tilt.[14] Adults with CP demonstrate a much higher prevalence of early cervical disc degeneration and mid-cervical instability with a narrowed spinal canal, which may lead to loss of function and progressive neurologic deficits.[14]

Physical Therapy Patient/Client Management

The transition to adulthood is a critical time for individuals with pediatric-onset disabilities such as CP.[15] Transition is defined as "a period of biologic, social and emotional change, in which the adolescent has four major developmental tasks: to consolidate their identity; to achieve independence from their parents; to establish adult relationships outside the family; to find a vocation."[16, p. 111] Thus, the transition to adulthood for a youth with CP should address health, psychosocial, and educational/vocational needs. Physical therapists in educational and in medical settings may be integral players in helping young adults transition to postsecondary education, employment, and adult-oriented medical services.[15,17]

Self-awareness, self-efficacy, persistence, and resilience are important personal characteristics for individuals with CP[3,10] and they may benefit from specific attention to help develop these skills.[15] Young adults with CP may benefit from learning about their rights as individuals with disabilities and from learning about available resources, services, and accommodations.[15] For example, young adults with CP have reported dissatisfaction with public transportation and report that they need to be able to plan ahead before traveling in the community.[10] Young adults who want or need to utilize public transportation may benefit from learning how to access such services and from learning strategies to manage these services.

Young adults with CP are transitioning from child/family-oriented services to adult-oriented healthcare services. This transition is often challenging because adult-oriented services are frequently more centered on the individual rather than the family-centered model more typical of pediatric healthcare.[4] This transition is also challenging because many adult-oriented medical professionals have limited experience with individuals with pediatric-onset disabilities. In addition, adults with CP require healthcare services that address not only impairments associated with CP, but that also address adult-onset conditions and promote health and wellness.[16,17]

During the transition into adulthood, patient/client-related instruction should help foster independence, self-concept, self-advocacy, self-management of disability, and participation in medical and educational decision making.[3,12,18,19] When needed, physical therapists should refer young adults and their families to other practitioners such as psychologists, social workers, or guidance counselors to help address significant psychosocial-related needs. Physical therapists may be instrumental in helping young adults develop the means to cope with their disability and may serve as a resource for community-based disability support and socialization networks.[12,15] Last, physical therapists may consult with medical teams regarding episodic care needs, health promotion and wellness, or with medical or surgical procedures for skeletal alignment, muscle function, contracture management, or spasticity management.[17,20-22]

Examination, Evaluation, and Diagnosis

The examination and evaluation of a young adult with CP should be comprehensive and address impairments of body structures and functions, activity limitations, participation restrictions, and environmental and personal factors, including her strengths and needs.[23] The physical therapist should start the examination with an interview of the young adult to gather information about her medical history, concerns, needs, and priorities.[19,23] As appropriate, other caregivers, family members, educational team members, or healthcare team members may also be interviewed.

Examination of primary impairments of body structures and functions should include assessment of spasticity, balance and postural control, selective voluntary motor control, and sensory processing.[19] Examination of secondary impairments includes assessment of postural alignment, trunk and extremity ROM (including muscular flexibility), muscular strength, and endurance. ROM can be assessed via goniometry and muscular strength can be assessed through functional testing and hand-held dynamometry. Other impairments that should be assessed include pain, cardiopulmonary status, and skin integrity. Additional considerations include nutrition, feeding, seizures, vision, hearing, and bowel/bladder function. Special attention should be paid to examination of signs and symptoms of patella alta, hip dysplasia, spondylolysis, and cervical stenosis because these conditions progress in adulthood.[14] Concerns regarding patella alta, hip dysplasia, spondylolysis, and cervical stenosis may necessitate a referral for further medical examination and imaging.

Examination of activity limitations and participation restrictions should include assessment of mobility, gross and fine motor performance, self-care performance, leisure activities, environmental access, and participation in natural environments.[19] Assessment should include the physical and social/cultural environments relevant to the young adult. Considerations include physical settings (*e.g.*, home, dorm room, school, potential job location, community settings), equipment, and transportation. The physical location layout of the environment, as well as the time required to travel within the environment, should be assessed. Considerations of the social/cultural environment include caregiver-young adult interaction, support, and resources. Assessment of the young adult's personal characteristics should include consideration of cognition, communication, language, social/emotional skills, behavior, culture, and motivation.

Few assessment tools have been validated on young adults with CP. Although developed for individuals up to 18 years of age, the Gross Motor Function Classification System (GMFCS; see Case 6) has been found to be a reliable tool to classify and describe gross motor function in adults with CP.[24] In the literature, balance, postural control, ambulation, endurance, cardiorespiratory fitness, physical activity, and quality of life in young adults with CP have been assessed using a wide variety of tools. Posture and postural ability in young adults with CP may be assessed via the Posture and Postural Ability Scale (PPAS).[25] The PPAS uses a 7-point ordinal scale to assess mobility into and out of prone, supine, sitting, and standing postures, and assesses the quality of posture in these static positions in the frontal and sagittal planes.[25] It is also important to assess postural symmetry, hip joint integrity, lower extremity alignment, leg length discrepancies, and scoliosis. Although the Gross Motor Function Measure (GMFM; see Case 6) was designed to assess typical developmental milestones up to 5 years of age,[26] it has also been used in studies with adults with CP.[22] It was determined that this young woman's gross motor function was consistent with GMFCS level III.

For the young adult in this case, balance was assessed using several standardized tests (Balance Evaluation Systems Test [BESTest],[27] Observational Gait Scale,[28] Tinetti Performance Oriented Mobility Assessment[29]) and through observation of reaching in sitting, standing and walking, and during transitions between positions.[19] Ambulation and endurance was assessed using the 6-minute walk test,[30-32] sit-to-stand test,[33] and the Timed Up and Go.[31,33] Cardiorespiratory fitness was assessed through a progressive protocol using a cycle ergometer.[34] Fatigue was assessed using the fatigue severity scale[7] and physical activity was assessed using the Physical Activity Scale for Individuals with Physical Disabilities.[7] Quality of life was assessed using the health-related quality of life instrument, Short Form 36 Version 2.0 (SF-36v2).[35] The SF-36v2 is a self-report assessment of physical functioning, performance in physical roles, bodily pain, general health perceptions, vitality, social functioning, performance in emotional roles, and mental health over a 4-week or 1-week recall period.[35]

Plan of Care and Interventions

Physical therapy interventions for young adults with CP who are transitioning from high school and into adult roles should focus on their ability to access and participate in postsecondary education, employment, and adult roles, management of primary impairments, prevention of secondary impairments, and promotion of health and wellness.[18,20,36-38] Interventions may also directly address environmental barriers in home, school, work, or community settings.[39-41] Many activity-focused, function-focused, or participation-based interventions help achieve goals, especially related to mobility, endurance, and motor development.[19,38,42] In this case, the young woman benefited from accommodations including allowing increased travel time and use of elevators in her high school and college buildings. She also used adapted chairs in lecture halls and classrooms to allow for proper positioning and used accessible desks and work spaces to accommodate use of her forearm crutches and power wheelchair. She was instrumental at working with school personnel to identify and implement strategies for improved environmental organization to increase ease of access.

The physical therapist should help the young adult become aware of the effects of her activity on pain and endurance and identify strategies for energy conservation and fatigue management.[3] The key point is that the energy and time required for independent mobility should not significantly negatively impact participation.[43] The young woman in this case used a variety of adaptive equipment, depending on the particular setting and activity circumstances. For example, she used her bilateral forearm crutches in her dorm and college classrooms, but used her power wheelchair for longer distances and times when she needed to conserve energy or needed to maintain pace with peers.

Interventions to address mobility, ROM, strength, positioning, weightbearing, and pain are particularly important in young adults with CP. Decline in gross motor capacity in adults with CP is associated with pain, decreased ROM, and suboptimal anthropometric measurements.[44] Physical therapy including mobility, ROM exercises, and strengthening programs have been used to reduce pain in adults with CP.[13] Contractures may occur with hypertonicity and atypical positioning over time. Interventions such as low-load prolonged stretching, orthoses, and positioning can be used to maintain ROM. Young adults with CP with severe spasticity may benefit from **botulinum toxin type A (BTX-A)** to reduce spasticity and pain, increase passive ROM, and improve positioning.[17,20,21,45] Functional weightbearing and maintenance of mobility and transfer skills are important, particularly for young adults with reduced or limited independent mobility.[20] Supported standing programs for individuals who are not able to stand independently provide a variety of physiologic and psychosocial benefits.[46]

Health promotion and wellness is important for young adults with CP,[47] especially because young adults with CP have lower levels of physical activity and physical fitness than peers without CP.[10,11,48] For young adults with CP, progressive resistance exercise (PRE) programs significantly increase strength of targeted muscle groups[43,49] and aerobic exercise programs improve cardiorespiratory fitness and body composition.[43,50] The young adult in this case worked with her physical therapist to develop an exercise program that she could complete at her local gym 2 to 3 days per week.[51] This program included PRE and use of a stationary bike and recumbent cross-training for aerobic exercise.[43,50,52]

Adults with CP who undergo surgery may have specific preoperative or postoperative needs for physical therapy intervention. Initial studies on adults with spastic diplegic CP who have undergone selective dorsal rhizotomy in adulthood demonstrate significant improvement in hamstring and gastrocnemius passive ROM, improved gross motor function for crawling and kneeling, and decreased lower extremity spasticity, along with subjective reports of improvement in function.[22]

Evidence-Based Clinical Recommendations

SORT: Strength of Recommendation Taxonomy

A: Consistent, good-quality patient-oriented evidence
B: Inconsistent or limited-quality patient-oriented evidence
C: Consensus, disease-oriented evidence, usual practice, expert opinion, or case series

1. Interventions for youth and young adults with CP can facilitate a positive transition to postsecondary education, employment, and adult-oriented medical services, address health, psychosocial, and educational/vocational needs, and promote independence, decision making, and self-advocacy. **Grade C**

2. Botulinum toxin type A (BTX-A) injected into muscles with severe spasticity can reduce spasticity and pain, increase passive ROM, and improve positioning in young adults with CP. **Grade B**

3. Progressive resistance exercise increases strength in youth and young adults with CP. **Grade B**

COMPREHENSION QUESTIONS

An outpatient physical therapist is working with a 22-year-old young adult diagnosed with diplegic CP, GMFCS level III. She reports that she has been experiencing increased pain with ambulation, anterior knee pain, and decreased endurance, all of which have become more pronounced over the past year.

8.1 Which of the following tools would be *most* appropriate to measure this young woman's cardiorespiratory fitness?

A. Gross Motor Function Measure (GMFM)
B. Progressive protocol test with a cycle ergometer
C. Short Form 36 Version 2.0 (SF-36v2)
D. Tinetti Performance Oriented Mobility Assessment

8.2 Anterior knee pain in an adult with spastic diplegic CP is *most* likely to be the result of which of the following?

   A. Hip dysplasia

   B. Osgood-Schlatter disease

   C. Patella alta

   D. Spondylolysis

8.3 This young woman is interested in starting an exercise program for health promotion and wellness. Which of the following is the *most* appropriate recommendation for her?

   A. Progressive resistance exercise and aerobic exercise using a stationary bike or recumbent cross-trainer

   B. Exercise for health promotion is not recommended for this young woman, as secondary impairments will continue to progress with age.

   C. Passive stretching 20 minutes per day

   D. Walking 20 minutes per day in the community

ANSWERS

8.1 **B.** A progressive protocol test using a cycle ergometer has been found to be an appropriate means to test cardiorespiratory fitness in adults with CP. The GMFM (option A) assesses typical developmental milestones. The SF-36v2 (option C) assesses physical functioning, pain, general health perceptions, vitality, social functioning, performance in emotional roles, and mental health. The Tinetti Performance Oriented Mobility Assessment (option D) is a balance assessment.

8.2 **C.** Patella alta in adults with spastic diplegic CP presents as anterior knee pain and occurs most frequently in individuals who use a crouch-type gait pattern. While hip dysplasia (option A) and spondylolysis (option D) are common in adults with CP, these conditions do not present as anterior knee pain. While anterior knee pain can be the result of Osgood-Schlatter disease (option B), it is not the most likely cause of this young woman's knee pain.

8.3 **A.** Progressive resistance exercise and aerobic exercise programs have been found to create significant improvements in strength and cardiorespiratory fitness in young adults with CP. Passive stretching (option C) will not improve health and wellness. Walking 20 minutes per day (option D) is not ideal for increasing or maintaining her aerobic fitness, given her ambulation status.

REFERENCES

1. Americans with Disabilities Act of 1990 (including ADA Amendments Act of 2008 [P.L. 110-325]). http://www.ada.gov/pubs/adastatute08.pdf. Accessed March 20, 2015.

2. Section 504, Rehabilitation Act of 1973, 29 U.S.C. § 701. http://www.dol.gov/oasam/regs/statutes/sec504.htm. Accessed March 20, 2015.

3. Brunton LK, Bartlett DJ. The bodily experience of cerebral palsy: a journey to self-awareness. *Disabil Rehabil*. 2013;35:1981-1990.

4. Camfield P, Camfield C. Transition to adult care for children with chronic neurological disorders. *Ann Neurol*. 2011;69:437-444.

5. Hanna SE, Rosenbaum PL, Bartlett DJ, et al. Stability and decline in gross motor function among youth with cerebral palsy aged 2 to 21 years. *Dev Med Child Neurol*. 2009;51:295-302.

6. Opheim A, Jahnsen R, Olsson E, Stanghelle JK. Walking function, pain, and fatigue in adults with cerebral palsy: a 7-year follow-up study. *Dev Med Child Neurol*. 2009;51:381-388.

7. Russchen HA, Slaman J, Stam HJ, et al. Focus on fatigue amongst young adults with spastic cerebral palsy. *J Neuroeng Rehabil*. 2014;11:161.

8. Van der Slot WM, Nieuwenhuijsen C, Van den Berg-Emons RJ, et al. Chronic pain, fatigue, and depressive symptoms in adults with spastic bilateral cerebral palsy. *Dev Med Child Neurol*. 2012;54:836-842.

9. Rodby-Bousquet E, Czuba T, Hagglund G, Westbom L. Postural asymmetries in young adults with cerebral palsy. *Dev Med Child Neurol*. 2013;55:1009-1015.

10. Palisano RJ, Shimmell LJ, Stewart D, Lawless JJ, Rosenbaum PL, Russell DJ. Mobility experiences of adolescents with cerebral palsy. *Phys Occup Ther Pediatr*. 2009;29:133-153.

11. Nooijen C, Slaman J, van der Slot W, et al. Health-related physical fitness of ambulatory adolescents and young adults with spastic cerebral palsy. *J Rehabil Med*. 2014;46:642-647.

12. Shields N. Self-concept is a concept worth considering. *Phys Occup Ther Pediatr*. 2009;29:23-26.

13. Hirsh AT, Kratz AL, Engel JM, Jensen MP. Survey results of pain treatments in adults with cerebral palsy. *Am J Phys Med Rehabil*. 2011;90:207-216.

14. Murphy KP. Cerebral palsy lifetime care: four musculoskeletal conditions. *Dev Med Child Neurol*. 2009;51(Suppl. 4):30-37.

15. Stewart DA, Law MC, Rosenbaum P, Willms DG. A qualitative study of the transition to adulthood for youth with physical disabilities. *Phys Occup Ther Pediatr*. 2001;21:3-21.

16. Chamberlain MA, Kent RM. The needs of young people with disabilities in transition from paediatric to adult services. *Eur Medicophys*. 2005;41:111-123.

17. Murphy KP, Sobus K, Bliss PM. The adult with cerebral palsy: a provider-consumer perspective. *Phys Med Rehabil Clin N Am*. 2009;20:509-522.

18. Campbell SK. Therapy programs for children that last a lifetime. *Phys Occup Ther Pediatr*. 1997;17:1-15.

19. O'Neil ME, Fragala-Pinkham MA, Westcott SL, et al. Physical therapy clinical management recommendations for children with cerebral palsy - spastic diplegia: achieving functional mobility outcomes. *Pediatr Phys Ther*. 2006;18:49-72.

20. Murphy KP. The adult with cerebral palsy. *Orthop Clin N Am*. 2010;41:595-605.

21. Olver J, Esquenazi A, Fung VS, Singer BJ, Ward AB. Botulinum toxin assessment, intervention and aftercare for lower limb disorders of movement and muscle tone in adults: international consensus statement. *Eur J Neurol*. 2010;17:57-73.

22. Reynolds MR, Ray WZ, Strom RG, Blackburn SL, Lee A, Park TS. Clinical outcomes after selective dorsal rhizotomy in an adult population. *World Neurosurg*. 2011;75:138-144.

23. Effgen SK. *Meeting the Physical Therapy Needs of Children*. 2nd ed. Philadelphia, PA: F.A. Davis; 2013.

24. Jahnsen R, Aamodt G, Rosenbaum P. Gross Motor Function Classification System used in adults with cerebral palsy: agreement of self-reported versus professional rating. *Dev Med Child Neurol*. 2006;48:734-738.

25. Rodby-Bousquet E, Agustsson A, Jonsdottir G, Czuba T, Johansson A, Hagglund G. Interrater reliability and construct validity of the Posture and Postural Ability Scale in adults with cerebral palsy in supine, prone, sitting and standing positions. *Clin Rehabil*. 2014;28:82-90.

26. Russell DJ, Rosenbaum PL, Avery LM, Lane M. *Gross Motor Function Measure (GMFM-66 & GMFM-88) User's Manual.* London: Mac Keith Press; 2002.

27. Opheim A, Jahnsen R, Olsson E, Stanghelle JK. Balance in relation to walking deterioration in adults with spastic bilateral cerebral palsy. *Phys Ther.* 2012;92:279-288.

28. Mackey AH, Lobb GL, Walt SE, Stott NS. Reliability and validity of the Observational Gait Scale in children with spastic diplegia. *Dev Med Child Neurol.* 2003;45:4-11.

29. Tinetti ME, Williams TF, Mayewski R. Fall risk index for elderly patients based on number of chronic disabilities. *Am J Med.* 1986;80:429-434.

30. Geiger R, Strasak A, Treml B, et al. Six-minute walk test in children and adolescents. *J Pediatr.* 2007;150:395-399.

31. Maanum G, Jahnsen R, Froslie KF, Larsen KL, Keller A. Walking ability and predictors of performance on the 6-minute walk test in adults with spastic cerebral palsy. *Dev Med Child Neurol.* 2010;6:e126-e132.

32. Andersson C, Asztalos L, Mattsson E. Six-minute walk test in adults with cerebral palsy. A study of reliability. *Clin Rehabil.* 2006;20:488-495.

33. Chrysagis N, Skordilis EK, Koutsouki D. Validity and clinical utility of functional assessments in children with cerebral palsy. *Arch Phys Med Rehabil.* 2014;95:369-374.

34. De Groot S, Janssen TW, Evers M, Van Der Luijt P, Nienhuys KN, Dallmeiher AJ. Feasibility and reliability of measuring strength, sprint power, and aerobic capacity in athletes and non-athletes with cerebral palsy. *Dev Med Child Neurol.* 2012;54:647-653.

35. Ware JE, Kosinski M, Bjorner JB, et al. *User's Manual for the SF-36v2TM Health Survey.* 2nd ed. Lincoln, RI: QualityMetric Incorporated; 2007.

36. Carey H, Long T. The pediatric physical therapist's role in promoting and measuring participation in children with disabilities. *Pediatr Phys Ther.* 2012;24:163-170.

37. Laverdure PA, Rose DS. Providing educationally relevant occupational and physical therapy services. *Phys Occup Ther Pediatr.* 2012;32:347-354.

38. Palisano RJ, Chiarello LA, King GA, Novak I, Stoner T, Fiss A. Participation-based therapy for children with physical disabilities. *Disabil Rehabil.* 2011;34:1041-1052.

39. Hemmingson H, Borell L. Environmental barriers in mainstream schools. *Child Care Health Dev.* 2002;28:57-63.

40. Hemmingson H, Borrell L. Accommodation needs and student-environment fit in upper secondary schools for students with severe physical disabilities. *Can J Occup Ther.* 2010;67:162-172.

41. Roy L, Rousseau J, Allard H, Feldman D, Majnemer A. Parental experience of home adaptation for children with motor disabilities. *Phys Occup Ther Pediatr.* 2008;28:353-368.

42. Valvano J. Activity-focused motor interventions for children with neurological conditions. *Phys Occup Ther Pediatr.* 2004;24:79-107.

43. Fowler EG, Kolobe THA, Damiano DL, et al. Promotion of physical fitness and prevention of secondary conditions for children with cerebral palsy: section on pediatrics research summit proceedings. *Phys Ther.* 2007;87:1495-1510.

44. Bartlett DJ, Hanna SE, Avery L, Stevenson RD, Galuppi B. Correlates of decline in gross motor capacity in adolescents with cerebral palsy in Gross Motor Function Classification System levels III to V: an exploratory study. *Dev Med Child Neurol.* 2010;52:e155-e160.

45. Intiso D, Simone V, Di Rienzo F, et al. High doses of a new botulinum toxin type A (NT-201) in adult patients with severe spasticity following brain injury and cerebral palsy. *Neurorehabilitation.* 2014;34:515-522.

46. Paleg GS, Smith BA, Glickman LB. Systematic review and evidence-based clinical recommendations for dosing of pediatric supported standing programs. *Pediatr Phys Ther.* 2013;25:232-247.

47. Thorpe D. The role of fitness in health and disease: status of adults with cerebral palsy. *Dev Med Child Neurol.* 2009;51:52-58.

48. Slaman J, Bussman J, van der Slot WM, et al. Physical strain of walking relates to activity level in adults with cerebral palsy. *Arch Phys Med Rehabil.* 2013;94:896-901.

49. Jeglinsky I, Surakka J, Carlberg EB, Autti-Ramo I. Evidence on physiotherapeutic interventions for adults with cerebral palsy is sparse. A systematic review. *Clin Rehabil.* 2010;24:771-788.

50. Slaman J, Roebroeck M, van der Slot W, et al. Can a lifestyle intervention improve physical fitness in adolescents and young adults with spastic cerebral palsy? A randomized controlled trial. *Arch Phys Med Rehabil.* 2014;95:1646-1655.

51. Taylor NF, Dodd KJ, Baker RJ, Willoughby K, Thomason P, Graham HK. Progressive resistance training and mobility-related function in young people with cerebral palsy: a randomized controlled trial. *Dev Med Child Neurol.* 2013;55:806-812.

52. Peterson MD, Lukasik L, Muth T, et al. Recumbent cross-training is a feasible and safe mode of physical activity for significantly motor-impaired adults with cerebral palsy. *Arch Phys Med Rehabil.* 2013;94:401-407.

Fitness in Cerebral Palsy

Lisa K. Kenyon

CASE 9

A 12-year-old boy with spastic quadriplegic cerebral palsy (CP), Gross Motor Function Classification System (GMFCS) level II is undergoing a physical therapy examination. When asked about his desired goals and outcomes for physical therapy, the child reports that he would like to participate in sports activities with his friends. Further questioning reveals that he rarely participates in play activities that involve physical activity and that his preference is to partake in sedentary activities such as watching television and playing video games. The boy's parents support his goals and state that they have been concerned about their son's physical fitness. However, they are also concerned about their son's safety and specifically that playing sports might not be good for him. They are especially concerned that participation in sports activities might increase his spasticity and deteriorate his quality of movement.

- ▶ Are exercise programs targeted at improving fitness safe and appropriate for adolescents with CP?
- ▶ What tests and measures should be used to determine the physical fitness levels in this adolescent?
- ▶ Are there any tests and measures that can be used in those who use assistive devices to ambulate?

KEY DEFINITIONS

AEROBIC CAPACITY: Maximal amount of work a person can perform (*i.e.*, production of adenosine triphosphate) using oxygen-based energy production systems

AGILITY: Ability to move quickly and rapidly change directions in an effective and efficient manner

ANAEROBIC CAPACITY: Maximal amount of work a person can perform using non-oxygen-based energy production systems (*e.g.*, creatine phosphate and lactate production) during short duration exhaustive exercise

GROSS MOTOR FUNCTION CLASSIFICATION SYSTEM (GMFCS): 5-level classification system used to describe the gross motor function of children 18 years or younger with CP.[1] GMFCS focuses on a child's typical performance in the areas of sitting, walking, and wheeled mobility; level I represents the highest level of gross motor function and level V represents the lowest level of gross motor function.

Objectives

1. Discuss the role of the physical therapist in promoting wellness and fitness in children with CP.

2. Identify valid and reliable tests and measures related to physical fitness for use with children and adolescents with CP.

3. Administer and interpret select tests and measures related to physical fitness for use with children and adolescents with CP.

4. Integrate evidence-based concepts related to physical fitness into the physical therapy plan of care for children and adolescents with CP.

5. Identify when exercise is contraindicated in an individual with CP.

6. Develop intervention strategies to target improvement of physical fitness and function in children and adolescents with CP.

Physical Therapy Considerations

PT considerations during management of the pre-teen with CP who presents with physical fitness concerns:

▶ **General physical therapy plan of care/goals:** Promote health and wellness by improving fitness parameters such as aerobic and anaerobic capacity, agility, strength, and flexibility

▶ **Physical therapy interventions:** Customized exercise programs to meet the individual physical demands of desired outcome activities

▶ **Precautions during physical therapy:** Appropriate warm-up and cool-down activities to decrease risk of injury; monitor biomechanical alignment issues and adverse effects such as musculoskeletal-related pain

▶ **Complications interfering with physical therapy:** Overuse injuries

Understanding the Health Condition

Cerebral palsy (CP) is a term used to describe a group of non-progressive neurologic disorders that materialize during infancy or early childhood and permanently impact a person's ability to move and coordinate muscle activity.[2] The Centers for Disease Control and Prevention (CDC) estimates that 1 in every 303 children in the United States has CP.[3] **Children with CP exhibit decreased levels of physical activity and physical fitness** as compared to their typically developing peers.[3-10] Measures of fitness such as aerobic capacity,[6] anaerobic capacity,[9] and muscle strength[4] are frequently decreased in children and adolescents with CP. Deficits in aerobic capacity may result from factors such as compromised circulation, ineffective ventilation, and increased fatigue in spastic musculature.[6] The submaximal anaerobic endurance and lower peak muscle power often exhibited by children with spastic CP may be related to quantitative and qualitative differences in spastic musculature.[9] As a result of decreased activity levels, disuse atrophy may also contribute to decreased anaerobic capacity in individuals with spastic CP.[9] Strength deficits have been ascribed to decreased central activation,[4,10-12] altered muscle physiology,[10] and secondary myopathy.[13-15]

Exercise programs for children and adolescents with CP are often avoided due to concerns that the demands of maximal exercise programs could negatively impact movement quality or increase spasticity.[7] However, such concerns have yet to be validated. In fact, multiple studies in children with CP have concluded that exercise programs are safe, feasible, and beneficial.[7,16-20] In a study by Verschuren et al.,[17] children with CP classified at GMFCS levels I to II who were randomly assigned to a circuit training program demonstrated significant positive training effects in anaerobic capacity, aerobic capacity, agility, and quality of life compared to children with CP in a control group. Unnithan et al.[19] found that a strength and aerobic interval training program resulted in significant improvements in aerobic capacity and gross motor function in 7 children and adolescents with spastic diplegic CP. A randomized clinical trial found that a strength training program for 21 children with CP who were ambulatory (with or without an assistive device) resulted in a trend toward improved gross motor function and improvements in muscle strength.[21] Qualitatively, McBurney et al.[22] reported that young people with CP who participated in a home-based strength training program for 6 weeks experienced an increased sense of well-being and improved participation in school and leisure activities. Last, exercise may be beneficial for cognitive development in children with and without disabilities.[17,23]

Similar to the typically developing population, those with developmental disabilities are impacted by the health consequences of a sedentary lifestyle.[24-27] Conditions such as CP can result in a vicious cycle of deconditioning in which a sedentary lifestyle leads to difficulties performing physical activities that contribute to greater deconditioning and a further decline in function and physical fitness.[25,28] As individuals with CP age, many experience a loss of functional mobility and an increased reliance on others to perform activities of daily living.[29,30] Subsequent to this loss of physical function is decreased quality of life[31,32] and increased mortality rates.[24,25,27] Perhaps most striking is the report that adults with CP exhibit a 2 to 3 fold greater death rate from coronary artery disease than the general population.[24,27]

Despite evidence supporting the many benefits of improving the physical fitness of children and adolescents with CP, pediatric physical therapists may feel they lack the time, resources, or knowledge to develop and implement fitness programs to meet the goals and needs of this patient population.[33] According to the *Guide to Physical Therapist Practice (Guide)*,[34] physical therapists provide preventative services to promote wellness, fitness, and quality of life. The *Guide* further asserts that promoting health, wellness, and fitness is an integral aspect of physical therapist practice. The American Physical Therapy Association's Section on Pediatrics task force on fitness also states that promoting activity, fitness, health, and wellness is the responsibility of all physical therapists and that physical therapists should "routinely apply research relevant to health-related fitness when treating children and adolescents."[35, p.208]

Physical Therapy Patient/Client Management

Contraindications to exercise programs for children with CP include uncontrolled seizure activity and severe osteoporosis.[36,37] The primary goal for a child with CP who presents with decreased physical fitness includes promoting health and wellness by improving aerobic and anaerobic capacity, agility, strength, and other fitness parameters.

Examination, Evaluation, and Diagnosis

The physical therapy examination begins with an interview with the child and parents/caregivers to obtain a complete history and to identify risk factors, goals, and resources. Formal pre-participation screening using tools such as the Physical Activity Readiness Questionnaire (PAR-Q) may be helpful to determine if there are any medical or other concerns related to increasing the child's level of physical activity.[38] The PAR-Q is a screening tool designed to determine the potential risk of exercising for an individual based on his answers to seven specific health history questions. To help identify activities that a child enjoys performing and to help set activity-related goals and outcomes, tools such as the Children's Assessment of Participation and Enjoyment (CAPE) and Preference for Activity of Children (PAC) can be used.[39] The CAPE examines how children participate in everyday activities outside of mandatory school activities and provides information related to the five dimensions of participation including diversity, intensity, and enjoyment of activities. The PAC is a companion tool that further evaluates participation by tapping into children's preferences for involvement in various activities. The CAPE and the PAC were developed for children ages 6 to 21 years with disabilities (including CP) and without disabilities. They consist of 55 activities related to children's day-to-day participation in activities outside of the school curriculum. Each of these tools can be completed in a self-administered version or through an interviewer-assisted option.

Anthropometric measurements such as weight, height, and body mass index (BMI) may be particularly helpful in the examination of health and wellness.

For *all* children 2 years or older, the CDC recommends use of BMI-for-age growth charts to monitor a child's weight in relation to stature.[40] Because BMI in children and adolescents is both age- and sex-specific, the BMI-for-age percentile is best to use when determining whether a child is underweight, healthy weight, overweight, or obese.[40]

In addition to the traditional components of the examination (*e.g.*, muscle tone, range of motion, gross motor skills, balance), tests and measures related to fitness should include assessment of aerobic and anaerobic capacity, agility, and muscle strength. Much of the research involving fitness tests in children with CP has focused on children in GMFCS levels I and II who have higher gross motor function and who can walk without the use of hand-held assistive devices.[41,42] Use of classic treadmill protocols such as the Bruce or the Balke to assess aerobic capacity is not recommended due to the inherent difficulties that children with CP may experience related to the demands of these protocols (*i.e.*, increasing gait speed and incline of the treadmill).[41] However, the 6-minute walk test is a reproducible and valid submaximal test of aerobic capacity in children with CP who function at GMFCS level I or II.[41] Two valid and reliable 10-m shuttle run tests have been developed to measure aerobic capacity in children who have CP and who function at either GMFCS level I or II: the **GMFCS level I–specific shuttle run test (SRT-I) and the GMFCS level II–specific shuttle run test (SRT-II)**.[42] Reference values for these two shuttle run tests are available for children with CP ages 6 to 12 years who are classified in GMFCS level I or II.[43] For children with CP who are classified in GMFCS level III, the 10-m GMFCS level III–specific shuttle run test (SRT-III) has been found to have good test-retest reliability.[44] For children in GMFCS levels III and IV who are able to propel themselves in a wheelchair, the 1-stroke push test and the 6-minute push test are promising tests that show good preliminary reliability.[45]

Despite the attention given to aerobic capacity, most activities in daily life are performed in short bursts of activity that require anaerobic capacity and agility skills.[46] Because of the functional need for quick bursts of energy, anaerobic capacity has even been suggested as a better indicator of functional ability in children with neuromuscular conditions.[47] The **Muscle Power Sprint Test (MPST)** is a valid and reliable tool for assessing anaerobic power in children and adolescents with CP who function at a GMFCS level I or II.[48] Reference values for the MPST are available for typically developing children ages 6 to 12 years of age.[48] Children with CP may also have difficulties with activities such as making sudden changes of direction. The **10 × 5-m sprint test** is a valid and reliable tool to measure agility in children and adolescents with CP who function at a GMFCS level of I or II.[49]

Muscle strength testing is often considered an essential component of a routine physical therapy examination.[34] Although many therapists rely on manual muscle testing (MMT) to document muscle strength and changes in strength over the course of treatment, the reliability of MMT has been questioned.[50] Hand-held dynamometry offers an additional method to assess strength in children with CP, but may be difficult to accurately use in clinical settings. Functional strength tests are an alternative means of testing muscle strength in task-specific activities. Verschuren et al.[50] developed three such functional lower extremity strength tests that are reliable in children with CP who function at GMFCS level I or II: a lateral step-up test, a sit-to-stand test, and a half-kneel-to-stand test. In each of these functional strength tests, the number of qualified repetitions completed during a 30-second timeframe is counted and scored.

Plan of Care and Interventions

Exercise programs to improve fitness in children with CP are safe, feasible, and effective.[7,16-21] Intervention to improve fitness parameters in children and adolescents with CP should follow the basic principles of training: specificity, overload, and reversibility.[28] *Specificity* refers to the need to individualize intervention programs to meet the specific needs of each child. Programs should also be customized to meet the specific demands of the anticipated outcome activities. For example, if improving the ability to perform rapid changes in body position during short bursts of walking and running is desired, the training program should target improvements in anaerobic capacity and agility. For fitness to improve, the body must also experience *overload* such that the demands placed on the targeted system are greater than those typically placed on the system. Simply put, interventions to improve fitness must demand more from the body than typical daily activities. *Reversibility* refers to the well-known concept that inactivity leads to a return to baseline fitness levels in as little as 4 to 8 weeks.

Customizing programs to meet the interests and needs of a particular individual may promote program compliance and encourage continued activity. The Personalized Exercise and Nutrition Program for Youth (PEP-for-Youth) Model[51] begins with a needs assessment that helps therapists ensure that fitness programs are designed based on the specific needs of each individual. The PEP-for-Youth Model employs an ecologic framework to identify and address potential barriers to physical activity in adolescents with disabilities. After the needs assessment, the therapist collaborates with the child to develop a personalized physical activity and nutrition plan. The resulting intervention plan is created to be flexible to adapt to the changing needs and unanticipated barriers encountered as the plan is carried out. This flexibility allows the intervention plan to be easily adapted to accommodate not only changes in growth and development, but also changes in the child's activity preferences.

Several studies indicate that children with CP may benefit from interval training programs that combine short bursts of high-intensity exercise activity interchanged with periods of active rest.[17,19] In a study by Verschuren et al.,[17] 86 children ages 7 to 20 years with spastic CP were assigned to either an intervention group or a control group (usual rehabilitation care). The intervention group participated in a circuit-style training program that included a 5-minute warm-up, 25 to 35 minutes of functional aerobic, anaerobic, and muscle-strengthening exercises in circuit setup, and a 5-minute cool-down. The intervention group trained 2 days per week for 8 months. Functional activities included task-specific exercises such as running and abruptly changing direction, step-ups, and ascending/descending stairs. Aerobic capacity, anaerobic capacity, strength, athletic competence, gross motor function, and participation significantly improved in the intervention group compared to the control group.

Some fitness programs have emphasized the use of various exercise equipment to target quality of life and physical fitness parameters in individuals with CP.[24,52,53] The Pediatric Endurance and Limb Strengthening (PEDALS)[53] program was a randomized controlled trial utilizing a stationary bicycling program in community-based physical therapy clinics for 62 ambulatory children with spastic diplegic CP (GMFCS levels I-III). Features of the stationary bicycle included a semi-recumbent design with a wide padded seat, trunk support, and foot straps. More recently, Peterson et al.[24] employed a NuStep Recumbent Cross Trainer to explore the feasibility and safety of an exercise program for adults with CP. These studies have demonstrated that minor adaptations can be made to address the fitness needs of individuals with CP who are non-ambulatory or who ambulate with assistive devices.[24,52,53]

Monitoring exercise intensity during exercise is important to ensure that a training effect is achieved. Although heart rate is not an accurate indicator of exercise intensity in young children, it becomes a more appropriate indicator in the mid- to late teen years.[54] Pictorial scales such as the OMNI scale of perceived exertion have been found to be more valid and reliable than the Borg scale when establishing a perceived rate of exertion in children and adolescents.[55,56]

Based on a critical review of the existing evidence, recommendations for strength training have been developed for children and adolescents with spastic CP.[37] These recommendations include a focus on simple, single-joint resistance training conducted under the direction of a physical therapist to stabilize and control movement. Children and adolescents with CP require increased rest between sets of strengthening exercises and may benefit from up to 3 minutes of rest between sets.[37] Intervention periods of more than 12 weeks are often needed for improvements in strength in children with CP.[37] Strengthening programs should also be customized to meet the specific demands of the anticipated outcome activities. For example, if the desired functional improvements relate to activities that are performed in a weightbearing position, then the strengthening program should consist of closed chain activities. Children with CP often have difficulties with selective motor control and may have difficulties isolating specific joint movements. In such instances, strengthening programs based on functional movement tasks may better promote the desired training effect.[37] In addition to these recommendations, a systematic review by Mockford and Caulton[57] concluded that isotonic strengthening exercises were more beneficial for children with CP than isokinetic strengthening exercises.

Evidence-Based Clinical Recommendations

SORT: Strength of Recommendation Taxonomy

A: Consistent, good-quality patient-oriented evidence
B: Inconsistent or limited-quality patient-oriented evidence
C: Consensus, disease-oriented evidence, usual practice, expert opinion, or case series

1. Children with cerebral palsy demonstrate lower levels of physical activity and physical fitness compared to their typically developing peers. **Grade A**

2. In children with CP in GMFCS levels I and II, tools such as the 10-m shuttle run test, the Muscle Power Sprint Test, and the 10 × 5-m sprint test are reliable and valid measures of aerobic capacity, anaerobic power, and agility, respectively. **Grade B**

3. Exercise programs aimed at improving fitness in children with CP are safe and effective. **Grade A**

COMPREHENSION QUESTIONS

9.1 Which of the following statements *best* describes the training principle of overload?

A. The exact demands of the activity and individual needs of the child must be met to achieve carry-over.

B. The demands placed on the system must be greater than those typically placed on the system.

C. Inactivity following training will lead to a return to baseline function in a period of 4 to 8 weeks.

D. Fitness activities must be fun and motivating to ensure compliance and participation.

9.2 Which of the following tests is *best* to use when assessing agility in children with CP who function at GMFCS level I or II?

A. 10-m shuttle run test

B. Muscle Power Sprint Test

C. 10 × 5-m sprint test

D. Functional lower extremity strength tests

9.3 Which of the following tests is *best* to use when assessing aerobic capacity in children with CP who function at GMFCS level I or II?

A. 10-m shuttle run test

B. Muscle Power Sprint Test

C. 10 × 5-m sprint test

D. 6-minute walk test

ANSWERS

9.1 **B.** The principle of overload relates to placing demands on the system that are greater than the demands typically placed on the system.

9.2 **C.** The 10 × 5-m sprint test is used to test agility in children with CP in GMFCS levels I and II. The 10-m shuttle run test is a test of aerobic capacity (option A), the Muscle Power Sprint Test is a test of anaerobic capacity (option B), and functional lower extremity strength tests assess strength (option D).

9.3 **A.** The 10-m shuttle run test is the best test to use when seeking information concerning maximal aerobic capacity in children with CP who function at GMFCS level I or II. The 6-minute walk test is a submaximal test of aerobic capacity (option D). The Muscle Power Sprint Test is a test of anaerobic capacity (option B) and the 10×5-m sprint test is used to test agility (option C).

REFERENCES

1. Palisano R, Rosenbaum P, Bartlett D, Livingston M. The Gross Motor Function Classification System—expanded and revised. 2007. Canchild Centre for Childhood Disability Research. http://motorgrowth.canchild.ca/en/GMFCS/resources/GMFCS-ER.pdf. Accessed October 31, 2014.

2. National Institutes of Health. National Institute of Neurological Disorders and Stroke. Cerebral palsy information page. http://www.ninds.nih.gov/disorders/cerebral_palsy/cerebral_palsy.htm. Accessed October 13, 2014.

3. Centers for Disease Control and Prevention. Cerebral palsy. http://www.cdc.gov/ncbddd/cp/index.html. Accessed October 13, 2014.

4. Wiley ME, Damiano DL. Lower-extremity strength profiles in spastic cerebral palsy. *Dev Med Child Neurol*. 1998;40:100-107.

5. van den Berg-Emons HJ, Saris WH, de Barbanson DC, Westerterp KR, Huson A, van Baak MA. Daily physical activity of school children with spastic diplegia and of healthy control subjects. *J Pediatr*. 1995;127:578-584.

6. Hoofwijk M, Unnithan V, Bar-Or O. Maximal treadmill performance of children with cerebral palsy. *Pediatr Exerc Sci*. 1995;7:305-313.

7. Verschuren O, Ketelaar M, Takken T, Helders PJ, Gorter JW. Exercise programs for children with cerebral palsy: a systematic review of the literature. *Am J Phys Med Rehabil*. 2008;87:404-417.

8. van Eck M, Dallmeijer AJ, Beckerman H, van den Hoven PA, Voorman JM, Becher JG. Physical activity level and related factors in adolescents with cerebral palsy. *Pediatr Exerc Sci*. 2008;20:95-106.

9. Parker DF, Carriere L, Hebestreit H, Bar-Or O. Anaerobic endurance and peak muscle power in children with spastic cerebral palsy. *Am J Dis Child*. 1992;146:1069-1073.

10. Stackhouse SK, Binder-Macleod SA, Lee SC. Voluntary muscle activation, contractile properties, and fatigability in children with and without cerebral palsy. *Muscle Nerve*. 2005;31:594-601.

11. Rose J, McGill KC. Neuromuscular activation and motor-unit firing characteristics in cerebral palsy. *Dev Med Child Neurol*. 2005;47:329-336.

12. Elder GC, Kirk J, Stewart G, et al. Contributing factors to muscle weakness in children with cerebral palsy. *Dev Med Child Neurol*. 2003;45:542-550.

13. Friden J, Lieber RL. Spastic muscle cells are shorter and stiffer than normal muscle cells. *Muscle Nerve*. 2003;27:157-164.

14. Foran JR, Steinman S, Barash I, Chambers HG, Lieber RL. Structural and mechanical alterations in spastic skeletal muscle. *Dev Med Child Neurol*. 2005;47:713-717.

15. Lieber RL, Steinman S, Barash IA, Chambers HG. Structural and functional changes in spastic muscle. *Muscle Nerve*. 2004;29:615-627.

16. Fragala-Pinkham MA, Haley SM, Goodgold S. Evaluation of a community-based group fitness program for children with disabilities. *Pediatr Phys Ther*. 2006;18:159-167.

17. Verschuren O, Ketelaar M, Gorter JW, Helders PJ, Uiterwaal CS, Takken T. Exercise training program in children and adolescents with cerebral palsy: a randomized controlled trial. *Arch Pediatr Adolesc Med*. 2007;161:1075-1081.

18. Schlough K, Nawoczenski D, Case LE, Nolan K, Wigglesworth JK. The effects of aerobic exercise on endurance, strength, function and self-perception in adolescents with spastic cerebral palsy: a report of three case studies. *Pediatr Phys Ther*. 2005;17:234-250.

19. Unnithan VB, Katsimanis G, Evangelinou C, Kosmas C, Kandrali I, Kellis E. Effect of strength and aerobic training in children with cerebral palsy. *Med Sci Sports Exerc.* 2007;39:1902-1909.

20. Fowler EG, Ho TW, Nwigwe AI, Dorey FJ. The effect of quadriceps femoris muscle strengthening exercises on spasticity in children with cerebral palsy. *Phys Ther.* 2001;81:1215-1223.

21. Dodd KJ, Taylor NF, Graham HK. A randomized clinical trial of strength training in young people with cerebral palsy. *Dev Med Child Neurol.* 2003;45:652-657.

22. McBurney H, Taylor NF, Dodd KJ, Graham HK. A qualitative analysis of the benefits of strength training for young people with cerebral palsy. *Dev Med Child Neurol.* 2003;45:658-663.

23. Ploughman M. Exercise is brain food: the effects of physical activity on cognitive function. *Dev Neurorehabil.* 2008;11:236-240.

24. Peterson MD, Lukasik L, Muth T, et al. Recumbent cross-training is a feasible and safe mode of physical activity for significantly motor-impaired adults with cerebral palsy. *Arch Phys Med Rehabil.* 2013;94:401-407.

25. Thorpe D. The role of fitness in health and disease: status of adults with cerebral palsy. *Dev Med Child Neurol.* 2009;51:52-58.

26. Rimmer JH. Exercise and physical activity in persons aging with a physical disability. *Phys Med Rehabil Clin N Am.* 2005;16:41-56.

27. Rimmer JH, Chen MD, McCubbin JA, Drum C, Peterson J. Exercise intervention research on persons with disabilities: what we know and where we need to go. *Am J Phys Med Rehabil.* 2010;89:249-263.

28. Verschuren O. Physical fitness in children and adolescents with cerebral palsy. [Dissertation] Utrecht the Netherlands: Utrecht University, 2007.

29. Bottos M, Feliciangeli A, Sciuto L, Gericke C, Vianello A. Functional status of adults with cerebral palsy and implications for treatment of children. *Dev Med Child Neurol.* 2001;43:516-528.

30. Dunstan DW, Owen N. New exercise prescription: don't just sit there: stand up and move more, more often: comment on "Sitting time and all-cause mortality risk in 222 497 Australian adults." *Arch Intern Med.* 2012;72:500-501.

31. Turk MA, Geremski CA, Rosenbaum PF, Weber RJ. The health status of women with cerebral palsy. *Arch Phys Med Rehabil.* 1997;78:10-17.

32. Turk MA, Scandale J, Rosenbaum PF, Weber RJ. The health of women with cerebral palsy. *Phys Med Rehabil Clin N Am.* 2001;12:153-168.

33. Goodgold S. Wellness promotion beliefs and practices of pediatric physical therapists. *Pediatr Phys Ther.* 2005;17:148 -157.

34. Guide to Physical Therapist Practice-Second Edition. *Phys Ther.* 2001;81:9-746.

35. Ganely KJ, Paterno MV, Miles C, Stout J, Brawner L, Girolami G, Warren M. Health-related fitness in children and adolescents. *Pediatr Phys Ther.* 2011;23:208-220.

36. Fowler EG, Kolobe TH, Damiano DL, Thorpe DE, Morgan DW, Brunstrom JE, et al. Promotion of physical fitness and prevention of secondary conditions for children with cerebral palsy: Section on Pediatrics Research Summit Proceedings. *Phys Ther.* 2007;87:1495-1510.

37. Verschuren O, Ada L, Maltais DB, Gorter JW, Scianni A, Ketelaar M. Muscle strengthening in children and adolescents with spastic cerebral palsy: considerations for future resistance training protocols. *Phys Ther.* 2011;9:1130-1139.

38. Physical Activity Readiness Questionnaire (PAR-Q). The Canadian Society for Exercise Physiology. Available at:http://www.csep.ca/cmfiles/publications/parq/par-q.pdf. Accessed October 13, 2014.

39. King GA, Law M, King S, Hurley P, Hanna S, Kertoy M, Rosenbaum P. Measuring children's participation in recreation and leisure activities: construct validation of the CAPE and PAC.*Child Care Health Dev.* 2007;33:28-39.

40. Centers for Disease Control and Prevention. Growth Charts. http://www.cdc.gov/growthcharts/growthchart_faq.htm. Accessed October 14, 2014.

41. Nsenga Leunkeu A, Shephard RJ, Ahmaidi S. Six-minute walk test in children with cerebral palsy Gross Motor Function Classification System Levels I and II: reproducibility, validity, and training effects. *Arch Phys Med Rehabil.* 2012;93:2233-2339.

42. Verschuren O, Takken T, Ketelaar M, Gorter JW, Helders PJ. Reliability and validity of data for 2 newly developed shuttle run tests in children with cerebral palsy. *Phys Ther.* 2006;86:1107-1117.

43. Verschuren O, Bloemen M, Kruitwagen C, Takken T. Reference values for aerobic fitness in children, adolescents, and young adults who have cerebral palsy and are ambulatory. *Phys Ther.* 2010;90:1148-1156.

44. Verschuren O, Bosma L, Takken T. Reliability of a shuttle run test for children with cerebral palsy who are classified at Gross Motor Function Classification System level III. *Dev Med Child Neurol.* 2011;53:470-472.

45. Vershuren O, Ketelaar M, De Groot J, Nova FV, Takken T. Reproducibility of two functional field exercise tests for children with cerebral palsy who self-propel a manual wheelchair. *Dev Med Child Neurol.* 2013;55:185-190.

46. Bailey RC, Olsen J, Pepper SL, Porszasz J, Barstow TJ, Cooper DM. The level and tempo of children's physical activities: an observational study. *Med Sci Sports Exerc.* 1995;27:1033-1041.

47. Bar-Or O. Role of exercise in the assessment and management of neuromuscular disease in children. *Med Sci Sports Exerc.* 1996;28:421-427.

48. Verschuren O, Takken T, Ketelaar M, Gorter JW, Helders PJ. Reliability for running tests for measuring agility and anaerobic muscle power in children and adolescents with cerebral palsy. *Pediatr Phys Ther.* 2007;19:108-115.

49. Douma-van Riet D, Verschuren O, Jelsma D, Kruitwagen C, Smits-Engelsman B, Takken T. Reference values for the muscle power sprint test in 6- to 12-year-old children. *Pediatr Phys Ther.* 2012;24:327-232.

50. Verschuren O, Ketelaar M, Takken T, van Brussel M, Helders PJ, Gorter JW. Reliability of hand-held dynamometry and functional strength tests for the lower extremity in children with cerebral palsy. *Dis Rehabil.* 2008;30:1358-1366.

51. Rimmer JA, Rowland JL. Physical activity for youth with disabilities: a critical need in an underserved population. *Dev Neurorehabil.* 2008;11:141-148.

52. Demuth SK, Knutson LM, Fowler EG. The PEDALS stationary cycling intervention and health-related quality of life in children with cerebral palsy: a randomized controlled trial. *Dev Med Child Neurol.* 2012;54:654-661.

53. Fowler EG, Knutson LM, DeMuth SK, et al.; Physical Therapy Clinical Research Network. Pediatric endurance and limb strengthening (PEDALS) for children with cerebral palsy using stationary cycling: a randomized controlled trial. *Phys Ther.* 2010;90:367-381.

54. Plowman SA. Children aren't miniature adults: similarities and differences in physiological responses to exercise. Parts 1 and 2. *ACSM's Health Fitness J.* 2001;5:11-18.

55. Pfeiffer KA, Pivarnik JM, Womack CJ, Reeves MJ, Malina RM. Reliability and validity of the Borg and OMNI rating of perceived exertion scales in adolescent girls. *Med Sci Sports Exerc.* 2002;34:2057-2061.

56. Robertson RJ. *Perceived Exertion for Practitioners: Rating Effort With the OMNI Picture System.* Champaign, IL: Human Kinetics; 2004.

57. Mockford M, Caulton JM. Systematic review of progressive strength training in children and adolescents with cerebral palsy. *Pediatr Phys Ther.* 2008;20:318-333.

Down Syndrome

Kathy Martin

CASE 10

A family has recently moved into the area and has scheduled an appointment to initiate outpatient physical therapy services for a 15-month-old girl with Down syndrome (DS). The child has received Individuals with Disabilities Education Improvement Act (IDEA) Part C early intervention services in the past, and will continue those services in their new community. However, the family also wants to obtain additional physical therapy services at this time. The child began to roll over at 6 months, sit independently at 10 months, and belly crawl at 12 months. Currently, she is able to stand at a support if placed there, but she is not yet pulling to stand. Her past medical history includes a moderate ventricular septal defect (VSD) that was repaired through open heart surgery (median sternotomy) at 4 months of age. She required supplemental oxygen by nasal cannula prior to the surgery, but has not required it since then. She has hypothyroidism and her current medications include thyroxine and ranitidine. She is the youngest child in a family with two older children (boy age 5 years and girl age 7 years). Her parents have recently divorced and her mother has full custody of all three children. Her father sees her one day per week and has her overnight every other weekend.

▶ What examination signs may be associated with her diagnosis?
▶ How would this individual's contextual factors influence or change your patient/client management?
▶ What are the most appropriate physical therapy outcome measures to assess this child's overall sensorimotor development?
▶ What are the most appropriate physical therapy interventions?

KEY DEFINITIONS

HYPOTHYROIDISM: Condition in which the thyroid gland does not produce enough thyroid hormone

INDIVIDUALS WITH DISABILITIES EDUCATION IMPROVEMENT ACT (2004), PART C: Federal law that provides financial assistance to states to implement an early intervention program that is comprehensive, coordinated, and multidisciplinary to enhance the family's capacity to meet the developmental needs of their child with a disability

RANITIDINE: Histamine H2-receptor antagonist that inhibits stomach acid production and is commonly used to treat gastroesophageal reflux

STERNOTOMY: Surgical approach that involves cutting the sternum lengthways (from top to bottom) in order to expose the thoracic cavity

THYROXINE: Synthetic thyroid hormone replacement used to treat hypothyroidism

VENTRICULAR SEPTAL DEFECT: Hole in the wall (septum) that separates the lower chambers of the heart (*i.e.*, the ventricles)

Objectives

1. Identify signs and symptoms of complications from inadequate medical management of a VSD and hypothyroidism.

2. Identify red flag signs and symptoms that would trigger a referral to evaluate possible atlantoaxial instability.

3. Identify an appropriate developmental assessment tool to record the current status and motor development progress of a child with DS.

4. Describe the expected prognosis for gross motor skill acquisition for the young child with DS in the next 12 to 36 months.

5. Design an appropriate physical therapy program for a young child with DS.

Physical Therapy Considerations

PT considerations during management of the young child with DS:

▶ **General physical therapy plan of care/goals:** Improve quality of motor control for achievement of motor milestones; initial focus on pulling to stand, standing, and independent ambulation; caregiver education regarding how to facilitate motor development at home; monitor lower extremity alignment and need for orthoses

▶ **Physical therapy interventions:** Caregiver education regarding how to create an environment conducive to independent exploration and gross motor play; strengthening in the form of play activities to encourage pull to stand, standing, and core control/balance such as reaching outside of base of support; assisted ambulation; evaluation for orthoses

▶ **Precautions during physical therapy:** Protect joints from extreme range of motion (ROM) secondary to hypotonia and ligamentous laxity; observe for signs and symptoms of atlantoaxial instability; observe for signs of inadequate management of thyroid and cardiopulmonary comorbidities

▶ **Complications during physical therapy:** Behavioral challenges secondary to young age and intellectual disability; atlanto-occipital instability, though uncommon, is potentially devastating if not identified and treated; rare medical complications

Understanding the Health Condition

Down syndrome (DS), or trisomy 21, is the most common chromosomal abnormality and is characterized by three copies (trisomy) of the 21st chromosome. It is also the most common cause of intellectual disability (cognitive delay) in the United States. The incidence of DS increases with increasing maternal age. For women at age 20 years, the incidence is 1 in 2000, but rises to 1 in 100 when the mother is 40 years old.[1] Approximately 6000 babies per year are born in the United States with DS.[1,2]

The medical diagnosis of DS can be made prenatally during the first trimester with a rate of detection of 82% to 87% with screening that involves maternal age, nuchal translucency (using ultrasound to measure the size of the clear space in the posterior tissues of the neck of the fetus), and maternal blood tests.[3] Second trimester quad screening (measurement of four substances in maternal serum) has a detection rate of 80%. However, integrated first and second semester screening improves the detection rate to 95%.[3]

At birth, physical appearance leads to the suspected diagnosis of DS. The most reliable characteristics include small ears, a wide space between the first and second toes, small internipple distance, Brushfield's spots (colored speckles in the iris of the eye), and an increased nuchal (neck) skinfold thickness.[4] Other reliable and discriminative signs include hypotonia, a flat face with upward slant of the eye slit, and brachycephaly (flattened posterior aspect of the skull).[4] Chromosome analysis (karyotyping) is needed to confirm the suspected diagnosis. Karyotyping is the gold standard for diagnosis but it takes several days for results to be available.[4]

DS is characterized by reduced brain volume and an increased risk of abnormality in nearly every organ system.[3] Children with DS are globally delayed in meeting developmental milestones and all have some degree of intellectual disability. The gross motor delays are the result of hypotonia, ligamentous laxity, and reduced brain volume, especially in the cerebellum.[3] They are most delayed in achieving gross motor milestones that require postural control and coordination such as walking, running, and jumping. Ultimately, the factors that most limit participation for persons with DS are their cognitive impairment and deficits in expressive language and verbal short-term memory.[3,5,6]

Musculoskeletal and neurologic abnormalities are present to some degree in every child with DS and these pathoanatomical features are most important in describing the clinical presentation relevant to physical therapy. Key musculoskeletal system impairments include hypotonia (reduced resting muscle tone and decreased resistance to passive stretch) and ligamentous laxity that results in joint hypermobility.[3] Important neurologic impairments include reduced brain volume, smaller frontal and temporal areas, smaller cerebellum (critical for postural control and balance), and a smaller hippocampus (critical for long-term memory).[3,6]

The involvement of other systems varies in individuals with DS. Thyroid disorders, particularly hypothyroidism, are much more frequent (28 to 54 times higher) in individuals with DS than the general population.[7] Thyroid hormone replacement is the current standard of care for hypothyroidism.[8] The most frequent problems with this medication are either underdosing so that symptoms are not fully resolved, or excessive drug plasma levels that can produce signs of hyperthyroidism.[9] Hypothyroidism may present as fatigue and poor endurance, muscle and joint aching, increased sensitivity to cold, decreased motivation, weight gain, dry skin, and constipation.[3,10] Hyperthyroidism may be characterized by nervousness, weight loss, tachycardia, insomnia, increased appetite, heat intolerance, and goiter.[9]

Congenital heart defects such as septal defects are present in 44% to 58% of persons with DS.[4] Common medications used in the management of these defects include diuretics, angiotensin-converting enzyme (ACE) inhibitors, and digoxin (digitalis). Diuretics are used to decrease blood pressure by increasing the kidneys' ability to excrete water, thus decreasing the fluid load on the heart.[9] The most serious adverse effects of diuretics include dehydration and electrolyte imbalances. Orthostatic hypotension, weakness, and fatigue may also occur and be problematic for physical therapy interventions. ACE inhibitors also decrease blood pressure and are generally tolerated well.[9] Adverse reactions may include gastrointestinal discomfort, dizziness, chest pain, or a persistent dry cough.[9] Digoxin is used to increase the force of the heart muscle contractions, thus improving the heart's effectiveness. Adverse effects include cardiac arrhythmias, gastrointestinal distress, drowsiness, fatigue, confusion, and visual disturbances.[9] Surgery to correct anatomical heart defects is often performed via a median sternotomy approach at 2 to 4 months of age.

Additional features are present in some persons with DS. Gastrointestinal tract abnormalities are present in up to 10% of children with DS and may include celiac disease (5%-7%), duodenal stenosis/atresia (1%-5%), imperforate anus (1%-4%), Hirschsprung's disease (1%-3%), and tracheoesophageal fistula or esophageal atresia (0.4%-0.8%).[4] Medical management of these conditions may include a combination of special diet, medication, and surgery. Although the overall incidence of leukemia in children with DS is less than 1%, this rate is 20 times higher than that of the general population.[11] Skin disorders such as eczema, palmoplantar hyperkeratosis, xerosis, seborrheic dermatitis, folliculitis, and cutis marmorata are present in up to 87% of persons with DS.[12] Medical management is condition-specific, but may involve topical or oral medication. Seizures occur in 6% to 8% of children with DS and are managed by antiepileptic medications.[3,4,12] Obstructive sleep apnea is another significant issue with 57% of 3-year-olds with DS having an abnormal sleep study.[3] Continuous positive airway pressure (CPAP) therapy during sleep is a common intervention for this condition. Behavioral or mental health disorders affect 18% to 38% of those younger than 20 years old.[4] Common disorders include attention-deficit/hyperactivity disorder (ADHD), autism, conduct/oppositional disorder, or aggressive behavior. Interventions include behavioral therapy and medication.

Finally, up to 78% of persons with DS will have a hearing impairment[12] and up to 80% will have a visual impairment[4] requiring corrective lenses or surgery. For thorough discussion of the medical and surgical management of disorders and anomalies associated with DS, several resources are available.[3,4,9]

Guidelines for monitoring the health of persons with DS have been developed for children,[13] adolescents,[14] and adults.[15] While these guidelines are directed toward physicians, some of these recommendations are relevant for physical therapists.

Physical Therapy Patient/Client Management

Management of the young child with DS requires a team approach. Because of the multiple comorbidities and global delays, this team often includes a physical therapist, occupational therapist, speech therapist, special education teacher, and several physician specialties, including a developmental pediatrician. The physical therapist objectively documents the child's gross motor development, including body structure and function impairments, activity limitations, and participation concerns not only for the child, but also for the entire family unit. The overall goal of physical therapy is to promote functional independence and gross motor skill acquisition in addition to preventing secondary complications resulting from motor delays, hypotonia, and ligamentous laxity. The physical therapist in an outpatient setting focuses not only on direct interventions with the child with DS, but also on family and caregiver education regarding how to structure the child's environment and experiences to promote development. Typical physical therapy interventions address strengthening and postural control through appropriate play activities. Prescribing an appropriate orthosis to improve lower extremity biomechanics and efficiency is common. The outpatient physical therapist should also be aware of the services provided to the family under Part C of the IDEA law and coordinate efforts with the early intervention team as appropriate. Although relatively uncommon, persons with DS are at risk for atlanto-occipital , or atlanto-axial, instability (AAI) due to ligamentous laxity. Up to 15% of persons with DS have this problem, but only 2% are symptomatic.[3,7] The signs and symptoms include easy fatigability; difficulty walking; abnormal gait or a change in gait; neck pain or torticollis; limited neck mobility; change in hand function; new onset of urinary retention or incontinence; increase in incoordination or clumsiness; sensory impairments; and spasticity, hyperreflexia, or a Babinski's sign.[7] Screening for AAI by physicians is controversial; different opinions on how and when screening should occur can be found in the literature. The American Academy of Pediatrics[13] published guidelines stating that if the child is symptomatic, plain cervical radiographs should be obtained in neutral position. If abnormalities are noted, immediate referral to a neurosurgeon is indicated; if no radiologic abnormalities are noted, the radiographs should be repeated in flexion and extension.[13]

Examination, Evaluation, and Diagnosis

Beyond the diagnosis of DS and the age of the child, the outpatient physical therapist is probably not going to have access to information about the child prior to meeting her and her parents. Getting a detailed birth, developmental, and medical history is a priority for the first appointment. During the interview of the parent, the physical therapist should also be observing the child's preferred movement patterns and interests. Setting up a safe area with developmentally appropriate toys and allowing the child to play while the physical therapist gathers information can facilitate this.

The history should include questions regarding any complications during the mother's pregnancy, age at which motor milestones were achieved, and medical management of comorbidities, including surgeries and medications. Because every system of the body can potentially be affected, the history should include a thorough review of systems with emphasis on asking about signs and symptoms that might suggest dysfunction. For example, hearing and vision can by screened by asking, "Does your daughter startle at loud noises, or turn to look at visually interesting toys?" Behavior management issues can be discovered by asking the parents what upsets their child, how readily she calms when upset, and what activities or toys help the child to calm.

The objective part of the examination focuses on both the quantity and quality of gross motor skills the child has. The quantity of skills should be documented using a standardized developmental assessment tool, while the quality is more descriptive of the movement patterns observed. Although the focus should be on functional gross motor skills, body structure/function impairments, activity limitations, and participation restrictions should be documented. During the initial examination, anthropomorphic measures such as height, weight, and body mass index (BMI) should be screened and then tracked periodically. Measurement of waist circumference may also be helpful in monitoring obesity. Vital signs such as heart rate, respiratory rate, and blood pressure should be taken at each session, especially in a child with a history of congenital heart defect. Standard goniometric measurements should be taken at joints where ROM (either limited or excessive) is a concern. For children with DS who can follow simple directions, strength can be formally assessed through manual muscle testing (MMT). One study found that testing children with DS between the ages of 7 and 15 years was successful with hand-held dynamometry with "practice, encouragement and feedback."[16] These authors used the mean of the best three trials and found that reliability was better with eight trials, but still acceptable with four trials.[16] For children unable to follow directions for MMT such as the 15-month-old in this case, careful observation of functional movements against gravity can provide a gross assessment of strength. To assess postural control and balance, individualized tests can be used. This could be as simple as measuring time in single-leg stance, or could be more formal using a test such as the Berg Balance Scale or the Pediatric Balance Scale (for older children).[17] Observational gait analysis remains the most common method of gait analysis in the clinical setting. Martin et al.[18] have designed a gait analysis tool specifically for children with DS based on the most common gait deviations observed. This scale uses a 0 to 3 scoring system (0 = within normal range, 1 = inconsistently normal, 2 = mild to moderate deviation, and 3 = marked deviation) for six aspects of gait: upper extremities, trunk, hip position in terminal stance, knee position in midstance, foot position at initial contact, and base of support. Scores for each body segment were operationally defined and the inclusion of "inconsistently normal" was intended to help identify emerging skill. Although this tool is quick and easy to use, has acceptable intra- and inter-rater reliability, and provides an objective description of gait, its validity and clinically meaningful change in score has not been investigated.

There are many standardized developmental assessment tools available. In children with DS, the test with the strongest research supporting its use is the **Gross Motor Function Measure (GMFM)**. The GMFM is a criterion-referenced test that has been specifically validated for children with DS.[19] It has become a standard in research and is the basis for some of the best prognostic data available. This test is divided into five subscales: lying and rolling; sitting; crawling and kneeling; standing; and walking, running, and jumping. While a specific age range for use with the GMFM has not been identified, the gross motor skills included are ones that a typically developing 5-year-old would pass. Based on the expected motor delays seen with DS, this test could likely be used through middle childhood years without reaching a ceiling effect. The GMFM uses a 4-point scoring system and has been shown to be sensitive to small but meaningful changes. Perhaps the greatest value of the GMFM is that motor growth curves for children with DS have been developed, making it possible to help identify if a child is advanced, age-appropriate, or delayed compared to expectations for a child with DS.[20] Palisano et al.[20] have also published data predicting the probability of a child with DS mastering a gross motor skill at a particular age. (Table 10-1).

Gémus et al.[21] found that the GMFM was relatively more responsive to change than *Bayley Scales of Infant Development* (2nd edition) in infants with DS, which has long been the gold standard in research. Gémus et al.[21] also made several recommendations to improve the ease and accuracy of testing children with DS with the GMFM, including: (1) use of parent report when a child is not cooperative with testing; (2) use of modeling or imitation in place of verbal cues and keeping verbal

Table 10-1   PREDICTED PROBABILITY (%) OF ACHIEVING GROSS MOTOR FUNCTIONS ACROSS AGES FOR CHILDREN WITH DS BASED ON LOGISTIC REGRESSION[20]

Milestone	Age in Months								
	6	12	18	24	30	36	48	60	72
Rolling	51	64	74	83	89	93	97	99	100
Sitting	8	78	99	100	100	100	100	100	100
Crawling	10	19	34	53	71	84	96	99	100
Standing	4	14	40	73	91	98	100	100	100
Walking	1	4	14	40	74	92	99	100	100
Running	1	2	3	5	8	12	25	45	67
Climbing steps	0	0	1	1	3	5	18	46	77
Jumping forward	0	0	0	1	2	5	18	52	84

"Reproduced with permission from Palisano RJ, Walter SD, Russell DJ, Rosenbaum PL, Gémus M, Galuppi BE, Cunningham L. Gross motor function of children with Down syndrome: creation of motor growth curves. *Arch Phys Med Rehabil.* 2001;82:494-500."

communication limited, simple, and direct; (3) tag team with another person so that one person interacts and models skills, while the other observes and scores; (4) structure the environment to limit distractions; (5) avoid open-ended questions; and (6) start with items that reflect the child's preferred postures and movements. In addition, performance of a more difficult skill can lead to automatic scoring of precursor skills, and for children older than 3 years, testing only Dimensions D (standing) and E (walking, running, and jumping) is acceptable.

A few other standardized tests are appropriate for this population. The Peabody Developmental Motor Scales, 2nd edition (PDMS-2) is a norm-referenced test for children from birth to 72 months that provides age-equivalent scores, percentile ranks, and scaled scores for gross motor and fine motor skills.[22] Scaled scores allow for comparing a child's performance over time to assess progress from one testing date to the next. Next, the Bayley Scales of Infant Development, which is appropriate for children aged 1 to 42 months, is the gold standard to which many other developmental assessment tools are compared.[23] This tool evaluates global development, including cognitive, language, motor, adaptive behavior, and social-emotional areas. Last, a relatively new tool developed in the Netherlands has been specifically designed for children with DS younger than 3 years. The Test of Basic Motor Skills of Children with Down Syndrome has 15 items developed within a postural control framework, and reportedly has similar sensitivity to change as the GMFM.[24]

Participation has been the least researched area for all children with disabilities, but this is especially true for children and adults with DS. As a result, few tools and little data are available on this topic. One tool currently available that covers very young children with DS is the Social Function section of the Pediatric Evaluation of Disability Inventory (PEDI).[25] The two other sections of the PEDI (Self-Care, Mobility and Transfers) assess activity limitations. The PEDI is designed for children (6 months-7.5 years) and allows for consideration of environmental changes and caregiver support necessary for a child to participate. Newer tools that have recently been developed for children aged 6 to 21 years include the Children's Assessment of Participation and Enjoyment (CAPE) and its companion measure, the Preferences for Activities for Children (PAC).[26]

Plan of Care and Interventions

In general, the goals of physical therapy interventions are to enhance the acquisition rate of motor skills, prevent occurrence of secondary problems resulting from compensatory strategies to overcome hypotonia and joint instability,[27] and improve the child's participation in life activities. Palisano et al.[20] suggested that for children with mild motor impairments whose motor function is age-appropriate or advanced relative to expectations for children with DS, motor goals could be met through structured play and recreation activities (vs. physical therapy). However, children who have moderate to severe motor impairments and whose motor function is delayed relative to expectations for children with DS are less likely to achieve their goals without physical therapy intervention.[20]

Key goals for an infant or toddler with DS include acquisition of postural control, righting, balance reactions, and motor milestones—especially independent ambulation. General strengthening to help accomplish these goals may be achieved by repetitive transitions, such as squat-to-stand or sit-to-stand to strengthen the leg extensors. Activities requiring the child to reach across midline help encourage trunk rotation and thus improve abdominal control. Any position or activity on a moveable surface (therapy ball, rocker board, bolster, etc.) can contribute to improved core strength and postural control.

Table 10-2 provides a summary of current evidence and dosage recommendations for common interventions utilized in persons with DS from infancy to approximately 8 years. Of note, while some research has been done on the efficacy of various interventions for persons with DS, many studies have small sample sizes

Table 10-2   COMMON INTERVENTIONS FOR PERSONS WITH DOWN SYNDROME

Intervention	Age Range	Summary of Evidence	Dosage Guidelines
Early intervention	Birth to 3 years	Neurodevelopmental treatment (NDT) focus[28] and training of the person providing the intervention[27,29] are *not* significant factors in obtaining best results. Intensity of intervention and parent investment are likely keys to progress.[27] Parents prefer **home-based programs** that empower them to provide low-tech strengthening programs for their child.[29]	No conclusive data, but intensity does seem to matter. Parental involvement and ability to implement daily activities to promote development are likely more important than number of therapy visits per week.[27]
Treadmill training	Appropriate when infant able to sit alone for 30 sec[30,31] or take 6 steps on treadmill in 1 min[31,32] (≈10 months) OR Able to take 3 to 6 independent steps[33]	Teaching parents to suspend child over a **motorized treadmill** to stimulate stepping led to significantly earlier onset of independent walking (mean improvement of 101 days).[30] Kinematics and maturity/stability of gait pattern improved.[32,33] Achievement of other motor milestones positively affected.[34] Best to begin when stepping pattern is still quite variable, inconsistent, and unstable.[31]	8 min/day, 5 days/wk enough to produce significant results.[30] Adding ankle weights and increasing belt speed improve results, but asking parents to track and manipulate too many variables at once can be overwhelming.[31,34]

(Continued)

Table 10-2 COMMON INTERVENTIONS FOR PERSONS WITH DOWN SYNDROME *(CONTINUED)*			
Intervention	Age Range	Summary of Evidence	Dosage Guidelines
Postural control	15 to 31 months and 4 to 6 years[35]	Focus on development and refinement of postural synergies. Include specific practice and changing task conditions to improve motor coordination.[35,36]	No conclusive data to provide guidelines.
Orthoses	3.5 to 8 years[37] Mean age of 28 months[37] 3 to 6 years[38] 19 to 24 months[38] When able to pull to stand[39] 4 to 7 years[40]	**Shoe inserts/foot orthoses and supramalleolar orthoses** improve gait, balance, and gross motor skills.[37,38,41,42] Standard of care has been to provide orthoses when child begins to stand with support. Small study suggested that introducing orthoses too soon (*i.e.,* before independent walking) may be detrimental because they limit exploration and variability of movement.[39] Current debate is which of these two orthoses is more effective and when to introduce it. Height, weight, BMI, and degree of hypermobility may be key factors in decision of which orthosis to use.[40]	No conclusive data. Standard of care is to wear orthoses during waking hours, especially during periods of increased activity.

or poor internal validity. Thus, there are many gaps in our knowledge of the most appropriate interventions for this population and the standard of care is still dictated mostly by therapist experience and preference.

Given the intellectual disability and language impairments that are universal for persons with DS, intervention strategies to improve gross motor skills must accommodate for this population's unique learning needs. Regarding communication, sign language and augmentative communication devices should be used to improve effectiveness, regardless of age.[43] As noted previously, Gémus et al.[21] recommend limiting verbal cues and instead using more modeling or imitation of desired movements to improve effectiveness.

In addition to the communication issues, Wishart[44] has described the learning style of children with DS as overly dependent on social skills in that they will pretend to be interested in something else or "turn on the charm" when faced with a difficult task. She also describes a tendency of children with DS to just opt out and refuse to engage when their avoidance strategies are not successful. This means that effective intervention for persons with DS must include appropriate behavioral as well as communication strategies and collaborative planning with the parent or caregiver to find activities that are motivating and engaging enough to circumvent the typical pattern of avoidance of difficult tasks. Depending on the age and cognitive development of the child, distraction and redirection, offering age-appropriate choices, and earning rewards for appropriate behavior may be effective strategies.

Evidence-Based Clinical Recommendations

SORT: Strength of Recommendation Taxonomy

A: Consistent, good-quality patient-oriented evidence
B: Inconsistent or limited-quality patient-oriented evidence
C: Consensus, disease-oriented evidence, usual practice, expert opinion or case series

1. The Gross Motor Function Measure is appropriate for children with Down syndrome (DS) and especially useful because motor growth curves for children with DS have been developed, making it possible to help identify if a child is advanced, age-appropriate, or delayed compared to expectations for a child with DS. **Grade B**

2. Caregiver education to provide low-tech strengthening opportunities in the home environment is preferred by parents and helps to achieve the necessary intensity of intervention to produce change in skill level. **Grade C**

3. Body-weight-support treadmill training for pre-ambulatory infants at 8 minutes per day, 5 days per week can help an infant with DS learn to walk on average 3 months earlier. **Grade B**

4. Providing either foot orthoses or supramalleolar orthoses to ambulatory children with DS can improve functional gross motor skills (**Grade A**) and improve balance and stability in those who are pulling to stand or willing to stand when placed on their feet, possibly leading to earlier onset of independent ambulation (**Grade C**).

COMPREHENSION QUESTIONS

10.1 Children with Down syndrome show delayed development of postural control that is *most* affected by:

   A. Hydrocephalus

   B. Smaller than normal cerebellum

   C. Visual impairment

   D. Tendency toward obesity

10.2 Which of the following has been shown to help a young child with DS learn to walk independently earlier?

A. Supramalleolar orthoses

B. Early intervention programming

C. Treadmill training

D. Aquatic therapy

10.3 Poor activity tolerance, as evidenced by the child's refusal to participate in active play for more than a few minutes, could be a symptom of inadequate management of:

A. Hypothyroidism

B. Visual deficits

C. Gastroesophageal reflux

D. Postural control deficits

ANSWERS

10.1 **B.** The cerebellum is a critical part of the brain that controls balance and postural control. The smaller cerebellum seen in children with DS is considered to be one explanation for why persons with DS have diminished postural control at all ages. Hydrocephalus (option A) is not a common comorbidity and visual impairment (option C) is rarely severe enough to affect postural control. Although obesity (option D) may adversely affect postural control, all persons with DS, regardless of their weight, have deficits in postural control.

10.2 **C.** Treadmill training has been shown to help infants with DS learn to walk independently an average of 101 days earlier than the control group.[60] Although orthoses (option A) are the current standard of care, the timing of when to introduce them (before or after acquisition of independent walking) remains controversial. No research to date has specifically looked at the effect of early intervention (option B) or aquatic therapy (option D) on the acquisition of independent walking.

10.3 **A.** Common symptoms of hypothyroidism include poor endurance and fatigue, decreased motivation, and muscle and joint aches. None of the other choices are likely to cause poor activity tolerance.

REFERENCES

1. National Down Syndrome Society. Down syndrome facts. http://www.ndss.org/Down-Syndrome/Down-Syndrome-Facts/. Accessed March 11, 2014.

2. Centers for Disease Control and Prevention. Facts about Down syndrome. http://www.cdc.gov/ncbddd/birthdefects/DownSyndrome.html. Accessed March 11, 2014.

3. Roizen NJ. Down syndrome. In: Batshaw ML, Roizen NJ, Lotrecchiano GR, eds. *Children With Disabilities*. 7th ed. Baltimore, MD: Paul H. Brookes Publishing Co; 2013:307-318.

4. Weijerman ME, de Winter JP. Clinical practice: the care of children with Down syndrome. *Eur J Pediatr*. 2010;169:1445-1452.

5. Chapman RS, Hesketh LJ. Behavioral phenotype of individuals with Down syndrome. *Ment Retard Dev Disabil Res Rev*. 2000;6:84-95.

6. Pennington BF, Moon J, Edgin J, Stedron J, Nadel L. The neuropsychology of Down syndrome: evidence for hippocampal dysfunction. *Child Dev*. 2003;74:75-93.

7. Cohen WI. Current dilemmas in Down syndrome clinical care: celiac disease, thyroid disorders, and atlanto-axial instability. *Am J Med Genet C Semin Med Genet*. 2006;142C:141-148.

8. Hawli Y, Nasrallah M, El-Hajj Fuleihan G. Endocrine and musculoskeletal abnormalities in patients with Down syndrome. *Nat Rev Endocrinol*. 2009;5:327-334.

9. Ciccone CD. *Pharmacology in Rehabilitation*. 4th ed. Philadelphia, PA: FA Davis Co; 2007.

10. Pitetti KH, Fernhall B. Comparing run performance of adolescents with mental retardation, with and without Down syndrome. *Adapt Phys Act Q*. 2004;21:219-228.

11. Ravindranath Y. Down syndrome and leukemia: new insights into the epidemiology, pathogenesis, and treatment. *Pediatr Blood Cancer*. 2005;44:1-7.

12. Roizen NJ, Patterson D. Down's syndrome. *Lancet*. 2003;361:1281-1289.

13. Bull MJ; Committee on Genetics. Health supervision for children with Down syndrome. *Pediatrics*. 2011;128:393-406.

14. Roizen NJ. Medical care and monitoring for the adolescent with Down syndrome. *Adolesc Med*. 2002;13:345-358.

15. Smith DS. Health care management of adults with Down syndrome. *Am Fam Physician*. 2001;64:1031-1038.

16. Mercer V, Lewis CL. Hip abductor and knee extensor muscle strength of children with and without Down syndrome. *Pediatr Phys Ther*. 2001;13:18-26.

17. Franjoine MR, Gunter JS, Taylor MJ. Pediatric balance scale: a modified version of the Berg balance scale for the school-aged child with mild to moderate motor impairment. *Pediatr Phys Ther*. 2003;15:114-128.

18. Martin K, Hoover D, Wagoner E, et al. Development and reliability of an observational gait analysis tool for children with Down syndrome. *Pediatr Phys Ther*. 2009;21:261-268.

19. Russell DJ, Rosenbaum PL, Avery LM, Lane M. *Gross Motor Function Measure (GMFM-66 & GMFM-88) User's Manual*. Ontario, CA: Wiley-Blackwell Publishing, Inc.; 2007.

20. Palisano RJ, Walter SD, Russell DJ, et al. Gross motor function of children with Down syndrome: creation of motor growth curves. *Arch Phys Med Rehabil*. 2001;82:494-500.

21. Gémus M, Palisano R, Russell D, et al. Using the Gross Motor Function Measure to evaluate motor development in children with Down syndrome. *Phys Occup Ther Pediatr*. 2001;21:69-79.

22. Folio MR, Fewell RR. *Peabody Developmental Motor Scales Examiner's Manual*. 2nd ed. Austin, TX: PRO-ED, Inc.; 2000.

23. Bayley N. *Bayley Scales of Infant and Toddler Development Administration Manual*. 3rd ed. San Antonio, TX: Harcourt Assessment, Inc.; 2006.

24. van den Heuvel ME, de Jong I, Lauteslager PE, Voman MJ. Responsiveness of the Test of Basic Motor Skills of children with Down syndrome. *Phys Occup Ther Pediatr*. 2009;29:71-85.

25. Haley SM, Coster WJ, Ludlow LH, Haltiwanger JT, Andrellos PJ. *Pediatric Evaluation of Disability Inventory*. Boston, MA: New England Medical Centre; 1992.

26. King G, Law M, King S, et al. *Children's Assessment of Participation and Enjoyment (CAPE) and Preferences for Activities of Children (PAC)*. San Antonio, TX: Harcourt Assessment; 2004.

27. Mahoney G, Robinson C, Fewell RR. The effects of early motor intervention on children with Down syndrome or cerebral palsy: a field-based intervention. *J Dev Behav Pediatr*. 2001;22:153-162.

28. Harris SR. Effects of neurodevelopmental therapy on motor performance of infants with Down's syndrome. *Dev Med Child Neurol.* 1981;23:477-483.

29. Sayers LK, Cowden JE, Sherrill C. Parents' perceptions of motor interventions for infants and toddlers with Down syndrome. *Adapt Phys Act Q.* 2002;19:199-219.

30. Ulrich DA, Ulrich BD, Angulo-Kinzler RM, Yun J. Treadmill training of infants with Down syndrome: evidence-based developmental outcomes. *Pediatrics.* 2001;108:84-91.

31. Wu J, Looper J, Ulrich BD, Ulrich DA, Angulo-Barroso RM. Exploring effects of different treadmill interventions on walking onset and gait patterns in infants with Down syndrome. *Dev Med Child Neurol.* 2007;49:839-845.

32. Wu J, Looper J, Ulrich DA, Angulo-Barroso RM. Effects of various treadmill interventions on the development of joint kinematics in infants with Down syndrome. *Phys Ther.* 2010;90:1265-1276.

33. Looper J, Wu J, Angulo-Barroso R, Ulrich D, Ulrich BD. Changes in step variability of new walkers with typical development and with Down syndrome. *J Motor Behav.* 2006;38:367-372.

34. Ulrich DA, Lloyd MC, Tiernan CW, Looper JE, Angulo-Barroso RM. Effects of intensity of treadmill training on developmental outcomes and stepping in infants with Down syndrome: a randomized controlled trial. *Phys Ther.* 2008;88:114-122.

35. Shumway-Cook A, Woollacott MH. Dynamics of postural control in the child with Down syndrome. *Phys Ther.* 1985;65:1315-1322.

36. Galli M, Rigoldi C, Mainardi L, Tenore N, Onorati P, Albertini G. Postural control in patients with Down syndrome. *Disabil Rehabil.* 2008;30:1274-1278.

37. Martin K. Effect of supramalleolar orthoses on postural stability in children with Down syndrome. *Dev Med Child Neurol.* 2004;46:406-411.

38. Tamminga JS, Martin KS, Miller EW. Single-subject design study of 2 types of supramalleolar orthoses for young children with Down syndrome. *Pediatr Phys Ther.* 2012;24:278-284.

39. Looper J, Ulrich DA. Effect of treadmill training and supramalleolar orthosis use on motor skill development in infants with Down syndrome: a randomized clinical trial. *Phys Ther.* 2010;90:382-390.

40. Looper J, Benjamin D, Nolan M, Schumm L. What to measure when determining orthotic needs in children with Down syndrome: a pilot study. *Pediatr Phys Ther.* 2012;24:313-319.

41. Pitetti KH, Wondra VC. Dynamic foot orthosis and motor skills of delayed children. *J Prosthet Orthot.* 2005;17:21-24.

42. Selby-Silverstein L, Hillstrom HJ, Palisano RJ. The effect of foot orthoses on standing foot posture and gait of young children with Down syndrome. *Neuro Rehabilitation.* 2001;16:183-193.

43. Chapman RS. Language development in children and adolescents with Down syndrome. *Ment Retard Dev Disabil Res Rev.* 1997;3:307-312.

44. Wishart J. Motivation and learning styles in young children with Down syndrome. *Down Syndr Res Pract.* 2001;7:47-51.

Duchenne Muscular Dystrophy

Christine A. Cronin

A 12-year-old male with Duchenne muscular dystrophy (DMD) lives with his parents and sister in a split-level style home in a suburban town. He attends the local middle school and, when the weather is amenable, drives home from school in his power wheelchair. He is a good student and is able to write his own class notes. He has an aide to help him at school, as needed. American history stirs his interest and he enjoys politics. He is a sports enthusiast. He and his parents make a great effort to allow him to participate in typical activities. He enjoys the benefit of swimming with an adapted flotation device one to two evenings per week at the local YMCA and he is an active member of the Boy Scouts. This young male is approximately 5 feet 9 inches tall and weighs 190 lbs. His bedroom is on the lower floor of the house that is accessible from the garage. There is a small bathroom/shower on this floor and the doorframe has been widened to accommodate his wheelchair. He has a hospital bed and the family's van is wheelchair accessible. He recently stopped ambulating following a femoral fracture and is becoming proficient in using a power wheelchair. He requires maximal assistance of one to roll, to sit up, and to perform a pivot transfer. He is able to sit at the edge of his bed with close supervision. Maximal assistance is required for dressing and toileting care. He is independent in use of utensils during meals, but requires assistance to lift a cup with liquid. There is a hydraulic sling lift in the house, but it is usually in storage due to its size and appearance. He wears bilateral hand splints for a short time each day to prevent further contractures of his wrists, hands, and fingers. He also has bilateral fixed ankle-foot orthoses (AFOs). Impairments include decreased vital capacity with a weak cough, limitations in range of motion (ROM) of extremity joints, global decreased strength, hypotonia, developing scoliosis, and pain in his lumbar spine and both hips. He is unable to shift his weight front to back and side-to-side while seated in his wheelchair. His multidisciplinary team consists of a pediatrician, physiatrist, orthopaedic surgeon, school physical therapist, and home physical therapist. His physical therapists fabricated his orthoses, assisted in the selection of his power chair, and have provided appropriate advice for home adaptations. His frequent colds often develop into bronchitis. Significant medical history includes two femoral fractures. Most recently, he fractured the left mid-femur during a transfer in a makeshift lift from his wheelchair to the above-ground pool in his backyard. Medications include calcium and a stool softener. He is not taking any glucocorticoids due to his parents' concerns of further weight gain and bone density loss. His mother does not work and is able to care for his needs. When he does not drive his wheelchair home, she picks him up from school and helps him complete his homework. This appears to be a close-knit family, but he frequently expresses concern about the burden he presents to his parents and other family members and is worried about his own longevity. The home physical therapist currently sees him twice weekly for 45-minute sessions emphasizing community and home mobility and assisted technology access.

▶ What distinctive examination sign may be associated with this diagnosis?
▶ Which three tests are most appropriate to assess function and participation?
▶ What do you anticipate may be the contributing factors to his condition?
▶ What are the most critical physical therapy interventions for this individual?

KEY DEFINITIONS

CREATINE KINASE (also known as creatine phosphokinase): Enzyme that catalyzes the conversion of adenosine diphosphate (ADP) and phosphocreatine into adenosine triphosphate (ATP) and creatine; expressed in many tissues, but in higher concentrations in the brain, striated muscle, and other tissues that rapidly regenerate ATP

GOWERS' SIGN: When an individual rises from the floor using a 4-point stance placing hands on the knees and then hyperextending the knees while pushing on the thighs to compensate for hip extension weakness

HYPERCAPNIA: Excess carbon dioxide (CO_2) in the blood; usually results from lung disease, hypoventilation, or impaired consciousness

PSEUDOHYPERTROPHY: Increase in the size of a muscle that is not due to an increase in the size of individual skeletal muscle fibers; in DMD, muscles are replaced by fibrous tissue and fat.

TRANSAMINASE: Enzyme that catalyzes the transfer of an amino group from one molecular group to another, which is an important process in forming amino acids in the metabolism of proteins; elevated transaminase levels in the blood may indicate liver dysfunction

Objectives

1. Describe the medical treatment plan for an individual with DMD.

2. Examine the benefits and disadvantages (*i.e.*, adverse drug reactions, ADRs) of glucocorticoids prescribed to prolong functional ambulation.

3. Understand the importance of the provision of physical therapy services that incorporate the individual's personal goals, promote self-advocacy, and emphasize participation.

4. Identify precautions and when to refer to other healthcare professionals.

Physical Therapy Considerations

PT considerations during management of the pre-teen with DMD:

▶ **General physical therapy plan of care/goals:** Maximize safe participation and function at home and in the community; optimize positioning throughout the day and night to minimize contractures; improve/maintain lower extremity strength, ROM, and endurance; maintain respiratory status; optimize transfers to and from wheelchair, bathing area, and toilet; progress standing tolerance and ambulation with and without an assistive device; maximize safe and functional independence; promote self-advocacy

▶ **Physical therapy interventions:** Practice negotiating wheelchair through tight spaces, over ramps, into and out of home, van, and bus; practice safe and effective transfers into and out of family pool; review strengthening, ROM, and respiratory program taught during therapy and integrate into a home program; weight shifting in wheelchair and sitting balance at the edge of bed; promote self-advocacy in daily tasks and activities and instructing family members and caregivers in activities such as ROM, transfers, and proper transportation techniques

▶ **Precautions during physical therapy:** No resisted or forceful ROM to the extremities or trunk due to high fracture risk and damage to muscles; pain, weakness, fatigue; assistance with weightbearing activities required during transfers to decrease risk of fall or injury; close monitoring of skin when wearing orthoses

▶ **Complications interfering with physical therapy:** Patient discomfort with AFOs and prolonged positioning; patient and parent anxiety regarding potential fractures

Understanding the Health Condition

Muscular dystrophy is a progressive neuromuscular disorder characterized by a predictable pattern of muscle group deterioration that leads to atrophy, progressive weakness, deformity, contracture, and progressive disability. DMD is caused by a genetic mutation (locus Xp21.2) that encodes for a muscle protein called dystrophin. Individuals with DMD lack dystrophin, which causes the muscle cells to be easily damaged. DMD is the most common X-linked disease occurring in about 1 out of 3,500 to 6,000 male births.[1] Weakness is the primary impairment due to progressive loss of myofibrils. The presence of a Gowers' sign and pseudohypertrophy in males may suggest a diagnosis of DMD and justify further diagnostic testing. Although symptoms typically are present at 2.5 years, the average age of a definitive diagnosis is 4.9 years.[2]

Early signs and symptoms reported by families and caregivers of children with DMD include delayed motor development, abnormal walking and running, decreased ability to climb stairs and get up from the floor, and frequent falling. Gait characteristics include an anteriorly tilted pelvis with increased lumbar lordosis, a waddling gait pattern, and foot pronation and eversion. Toe walking with plantar flexion at the ankle may be present to stabilize the knee.[2] Weakness in the neck flexors, shoulder girdle, anterior abdominals, and hip muscles occurs early. More than 40% to 50% of muscle power is lost by 6 years of age.[3] In untreated males, ambulation typically ceases at 10 to 12 years of age; 80% of these children develop scoliosis after they stop walking.[4] In the normal course of the disease, contractures frequently affect wrist flexors, elbow flexors, iliotibial bands, knee flexors, and plantar flexors by 13 years of age. Behavioral studies have identified that boys with DMD have speech delays, cognitive impairment, and a lower IQ (average 85).[5] DMD should be suspected if a young child (almost always male due to X-linked inheritance pattern) presents with abnormal muscle function, elevated serum creatine kinase (indicating increased muscle breakdown), and elevated serum transaminases.[6]

A 2010 review of four trials completed between 2005 and 2007 investigated the effects of prolonged use (5.5-8 years) of **systemic glucocorticoids** (prednisone and deflazacort) on the course of the DMD disease process.[7] The authors concluded that the earlier the glucocorticoid was initiated, the more sustained the neuromuscular function.[7] Participants were able to ambulate two to five years longer than those not taking glucocorticoids. Other benefits of long-term use included a decreased need for spinal stabilization, decreased rate of pulmonary dysfunction, and postponement of the need for nasal intermittent positive pressure ventilation (NIPPV). In two of the trials, left ventricular ejection fraction was maintained when compared to those not on the medication regimen. Moxley et al.[7] identified decreased height and increased weight as the most common ADRs of long-term use of deflazacort or prednisone in the DMD population. Vertebral and limb fractures also occurred more frequently. In 2013, a longitudinal study reported on the effects of long-term use of deflazacort on the development of scoliosis in 54 males with DMD.[8] Prior to becoming non-ambulatory, 30 boys took the drug and 24 did not. At the 15-year follow-up, 78% of survivors taking the glucocorticoid were able to avoid spinal surgery (because spinal curves were not ≥ 20°) compared to only 8.3% of those not treated. After 10 years of this drug treatment, none of the boys in the glucocorticoid group developed scoliosis. However, 70% of those taking deflazacort developed cataracts, had decreased longitudinal growth (mean height 17 cm shorter than those not taking deflazacort), and had an increased mean weight (55 kg vs. 51 kg in the non-medication group). Notably, there was no significant difference in long bone fractures between groups.

Death in persons with DMD usually results from respiratory insufficiency and typically occurs between 20 and 25 years of age.[9] Once daytime hypercapnia is present, mean survival is 9.7 months without ventilator support.[10] In a recent study of 43 patients with DMD, the probability of survival to 30 years of age was 85% with a median survival of 35 years.[11] The authors hypothesized that increasing survival rates may be due to increased use of assisted mechanical ventilation and therapeutic options such as cardiomyopathy treatment and spinal fusion surgery.

Physical Therapy Patient/Client Management

Taking into account several factors such as insurance status, location of residence, and stage of the disease, the multidisciplinary treatment team for an individual with DMD may consist of a pediatrician, pediatric orthopaedic surgeon, pediatric neurologist, pulmonologist, cardiologist, physiatrist, gastroenterologist, psychologist, physical therapist, occupational therapist, respiratory therapist, dietician, social worker, and orthotist. Members of the team should inform the patient and the family about the natural progression of the disease, expected function decline, and optimal therapy interventions. For the latter, these interventions include glucocorticoids and assisted technology options including powered mobility. In the more advanced stages of the disease, respiratory support such as NIPPV with manually and mechanically assisted cough protocols is important. Education on home and community accessibility and transportation information should be provided. The physical therapist's charge is to develop and implement a treatment plan to optimize the patient's function and participation. Physical therapy is aimed at maximizing function and minimizing secondary impairments (e.g., joint contractures, muscle imbalance, joint asymmetry, orthosis management).[12] The therapist teaches: strategies to maintain balance, strength, and ROM; teaches and monitors glossopharyngeal breathing; and promotes self-advocacy. The therapist teaches the parents, adult caretakers, and the patient in each tailored strategy. The implementation of these strategies should be reviewed periodically and adjusted as needed.

Examination, Evaluation, and Diagnosis

Optimally, the physical therapist should obtain pertinent information prior to performing the initial examination. This includes the patient's current team of multidisciplinary providers, medical history (including past surgeries and x-ray reports), medications, and allergies. It is important for the therapist to be familiar with current literature supporting that glucocorticoid treatment prolongs functional ambulation and stair climbing, prevents scoliosis, and helps maintain pulmonary function.

After reviewing the medical history, the physical therapist may request that the patient (in collaboration with his parents) complete self-reports of participation levels and quality of life. Examples include the Children's Assessment of Participation and Enjoyment (CAPE), a tool that examines how children interact in everyday routines, and the Pediatric Quality of Life Inventory (PedsQL) that measures health-related quality of life for both healthy children and those with chronic health conditions. In a study comparing 50 boys with DMD to 25 unaffected age-matched boys, self-reports from the CAPE and PedsQL indicated that boys with DMD had significantly lower physical activity participation and lower perceived quality of life compared to age-matched norms, except in emotional measures.[13] While the frequency of activity participation and social activities decreased with age in those with DMD, it did not decline in older, healthy boys.[13] Responses on these self-reports can provide the therapist with insight as to the patient's current level of participation.

The patient interview will provide the physical therapist valuable information to assist the child with DMD and his family. Mental status and communication are noted and demographic information is reviewed. The medication list and allergies should be updated. The therapist should ask the patient why he is present for the evaluation and what he hopes to achieve. Family members' contributions to the interview may be helpful. Results from the patient's self-assessments may be discussed at this time in order to assist in providing meaningful goals.

Baseline measurements should include examination of the musculoskeletal system, measurements of body structure and function, activity limitations, and participation restrictions. Appropriate measurement instruments must take into consideration the age of the child, functional status, his requested outcomes, pharmacologic management, home/work/school environment, and available support.

For the initial assessment of the pre-teen with DMD in the home setting, the physical therapist should assess strength,[14-16] ROM,[17] balance (e.g., Functional Reach Test[18]), and posture. A wheelchair assessment[19] should also be performed. Given that there is no respiratory therapist involved in this case, it is also critical to assess respiratory pattern and capacity.

In the area of activity limitations, the therapist should evaluate the pre-teen's self-care and physical activities at home, in school (as able), and/or in the community. Multiple tests can be converted into timed testing.[14] While the 6-minute walk test is an outcome measure recently performed in the DMD population,[20,21] a more appropriate test to administer in this case is the Gait, Stair, Gower and Chair Assessment (GSGC) due to his non-ambulatory status. Further examination should include assessment of upper extremity function with tools such as the Brooke Scale[14] and/or the Jebsen Hand Function Test.[22] To assess motor function of the lower limbs, a scale specific to individuals with muscular dystrophy is the Modified Vignos Lower- Extremity Scale.[23,24] The Motor Function Measure (MFM) assesses changes in motor function, which can be useful to show improvement resulting from therapeutic interventions or to predict loss of ambulation.[25-27] The MFM consists of 32 tasks scored on a 4-point Likert scale. An ideal outcome tool for the current child would be the **Egen Klassification Scale (EK scale)**. The EK scale takes about 10 minutes to administer and measures the functional ability for non-ambulatory individuals with DMD to perform daily activities.[28] The scale predicts ongoing loss of physical ability in individuals with DMD. It has ten categories, namely: the ability to use a wheelchair, transfer from a wheelchair, balance in the wheelchair, stand, move arms, use hands and arms for eating, turn in bed, cough, speak, and physical well-being. Performance on the EK scale, in combination with forced vital capacity (FVC%), has been found to predict the need for assisted ventilation.[29]

In the home setting, ideal assessments for general function and/or participation for this patient could include the Functional Independence Measure (FIM),[30] the Pediatric Evaluation of Disability Inventory (measures functional skills for children between 6 months and 7 years of age and individuals who are functioning under the developmental age of 7 years),[31] or the Enderle-Severson Transitional Rating Scale. The latter scale is designed to assess an individual with mild disabilities in the areas of jobs/job training, leisure, and recreation, who is living at home and negotiating the community.[32]

Based on the evaluation so far, the therapist may choose to formally assess the pre-teen's difficulties in interacting in life experiences. These may be measured using the Pediatric Quality of Life Inventory and Neuromuscular Module (PedsQL 3.0 NMM)[33] or the CAPE.[13]

Plan of Care and Interventions

Using the information gathered from the patient, the family, and the assessments, the therapist develops a plan of care and implements appropriate interventions. In 2010, the DMD Care and Considerations Working Group (DMDCCWG) recommended a comprehensive multidisciplinary approach based on stages of the disease.[12] The five stages (1-5) identified are: presymptomatic, early ambulatory, late ambulatory, early non-ambulatory, and late non-ambulatory. The patient in this case would be classified as Stage 4 (early non-ambulatory). While the physician in this case may have recommended the use of glucocorticoids to prolong his ambulation, the child was not taking them due to his parents' concerns of further weight gain and bone density loss. Physical therapy interventions include stretching to manage joint flexibility and contractures, exercise prescription and progression, and recommendations for and provisions of assistive devices. Since the disease progresses in a predictable fashion, therapy goals should anticipate future impairments and address their mitigation or prevention. Therapists should monitor for scoliosis (and its progression), provide basic respiratory management, share positioning recommendations, and participate in team decisions regarding standers, seating systems, and home modifications. The patient and supportive family members and educators should be involved in goal setting and plan of care development to facilitate the integration of recommended strategies and interventions into identified routines.

Joint contractures occur due to muscle imbalance, lack of mobility, and changes in muscle tissue.[14] Maintaining joint extensibility is important for optimal function and alignment and requires a team effort. Stretching should include passive, active assisted, and active stretching for the ambulatory and non-ambulatory phases. The DMDC-CWG recommended stretching 4 to 6 days per week during the patient's daily routines, at home, school, or in the clinic. Prolonged stretching using orthoses, splinting, and standing programs (e.g., standing frames) should be implemented to preserve flexibility and mobility. The patient may be more accepting of night orthoses to preserve ankle dorsiflexion. Knee-ankle-foot orthoses (KAFOs) may permit short-distance ambulation in the late ambulatory stage of DMD and permit stand pivot transfers and standing in the early non-ambulatory stage.[14] However, in a review of 35 studies, the authors concluded that although the use of KAFOs prolongs assisted walking and standing, it is questionable whether they prolong *functional* walking for patients with DMD.[34] Hyde et al.[35] performed a prospective, randomized study comparing two methods of managing Achilles tendon contractures in boys with DMD. One group received passive stretching, while the second group received stretching and below-knee splints to wear at night. At the 30-month follow-up, the boys who received the night splinting intervention demonstrated a 23% decrease in the expected Achilles tendon contracture development, while the boys receiving passive stretching alone demonstrated the expected level of contracture development. These researchers also suggest that increased contracture of this tendon is an important factor leading to the loss of ambulation.

Clinicians have been confused about whether they should include strengthening activities in the plan of care for individuals with DMD. There is both concern about whether certain types of strengthening exercises can increase muscle injury, pain, and fatigue as well as recognition that disuse atrophy occurs with increasing sedentary behavior.[36] Currently, there is no evidence indicating that muscle strengthening exercises result in *increased* strength in the DMD population. In 2002, Kilmer[37] identified multiple challenges in interpreting studies using exercise training in individuals with neuromuscular disease. In the three studies reviewed, resistance exercise in individuals with rapidly progressive neuromuscular diseases such as DMD did not result in increased muscle strength. However, it should be considered that no change in strength is a positive result in this population. In 2010, the first prospective randomized controlled trial (RCT) was undertaken to address the efficacy of a strengthening program in 30 boys (7-13 years old) with DMD.[38] The study, titled "No Use is Disuse," examined the effects of two interventions: dynamic leg and arm training for ambulatory boys and those recently wheelchair dependent and functional training with arm support for those who had been confined to a wheelchair for several years. Subjects were randomized into two groups. The intervention group participated in assistive bicycle training of arms and legs for 6 months and the control group participated in the same protocol after a waiting period of 6 months. Although there were no group differences on the assisted 6-minute cycling test (A6MCT), the intervention group *maintained* their total MFM score, while the control group experienced a significant decrease in their MFM score.[39] Results of this RCT support the use of

assistive bicycle exercise of legs and arms to delay the progressive weakness and functional loss characteristic of DMD disease progression.

The importance of prolonging ambulation in the DMD population is well documented. Once ambulation ceases, muscle weakness, additional contractures, scoliosis, and respiratory complications develop with a gradual loss of functional skills. The physical therapist should perform an appropriate baseline assessment and encourage ambulation. Specific notes should be taken regarding ambulation frequency, distance, falls, pain, endurance and energy conservation, and stair and ramp negotiation. Adjustment recommendations to improve task completion safely and effectively should be made accordingly. Teamwork is crucial with this young male, his family, educators, and others to participate in making recommendations for reasonable expectations as well as to prepare him for wheeled mobility, environmental adaptations, and modifications.

Since death usually results from respiratory deficiency, the physical therapist must address the respiratory needs of the individual with DMD. Breathing and coughing exercise training and treatment may be important physical therapy interventions. Glossopharyngeal breathing ("frog breathing") is a type of breathing exercise that requires gulping air repeatedly to increase air volume into the lower airways. This technique often prolongs the use of a ventilator during the day and, once on a ventilator, decreases ventilator-assisted breaths. The physical therapist should be aware of the research regarding respiratory options such as the use of NIPPV and make referrals to experts (*e.g.*, respiratory therapist) when this type of support is required for optimal ventilation.[40]

The key to streamlining the individual's transition to less independent stages of mobility is anticipatory planning. This can be done using assistive technology, adapting and modifying the home, school, and, if possible, the community. The physical therapist should be a critical part of the individual's rehabilitation team in decisions regarding orthoses, daytime and nighttime positioning, and mobility including wheelchair and seating systems. Home and community modifications may include those to doors and rooms, and the addition of ramps. Environmental controls such as remote control devices and lifts should be considered. Access to communication and/or communication technology is crucial. The therapist should develop and utilize an access checklist so that this young individual will be able to participate in his community. Transportation needs should be reviewed *before* they are needed. The therapist should always actively participate in and be prepared to make recommendations during family and team meetings.

Evidence-Based Clinical Recommendations

SORT: Strength of Recommendation Taxonomy

A: Consistent, good-quality patient-oriented evidence
B: Inconsistent or limited-quality patient-oriented evidence
C: Consensus, disease-oriented evidence, usual practice, expert opinion, or case series

1. The use of systemic glucocorticoids prolongs ambulation and quality of life in individuals with Duchenne muscular dystrophy. **Grade B**

2. Scores on the Egen Klassification Scale can predict the need for ventilatory support and ongoing loss of physical function in the DMD population. **Grade B**

3. Assistive bicycle exercise of the legs and arms delays the progressive weakness and functional loss characteristic of DMD disease progression. **Grade B**

COMPREHENSION QUESTIONS

11.1 Which distinctive examination sign may be associated with the diagnosis of DMD?

A. Babinski's

B. Thomas test

C. Gowers'

D. Homan's

11.2 Which of the following is appropriate to assess function and participation in the DMD population?

A. Timed Up and Go

B. Range of motion

C. Functional Reach Test

D. Egen Klassification Scale

11.3 Based on the young male in the case study, which of the following represent the most critical interventions?

A. Preserve functional upper extremity use, monitor for worsening scoliosis and decreased respiratory function

B. Preserve lower extremity use, stretching, accessing the environment

C. Wheelchair mobility, home adaptations

D. Emphasize re-acquiring ambulation within his home

ANSWERS

11.1 **C.** The Gowers' sign is a hallmark of DMD. Babinski's is a sign of neurological damage (option A). The Thomas test is a test of hip flexor tightness (option B). The Homan's sign is a positive result on a test that has historically been used to assess for a deep vein thrombosis (option D).

11.2 **D.** Options A, B, and C are impairment level measures. Option D contains functional measures for this population.

11.3 **A.** Options B and C are important but were already in place for this individual. Option D is not realistic given his medical diagnosis.

REFERENCES

1. Emery AE. Population frequencies of inherited neuromuscular diseases—a world survey. *Neuromuscul Disord.* 1991;1:19-29.

2. Ciafaloni E, Fox DJ, Pandya S, et al. Delayed diagnosis in duchenne muscular dystrophy: data from the Muscular Dystrophy Surveillance, Tracking, and Research Network (MD STARnet). *J Pediatr.* 2009;155:380-385.

3. Dubowitz V. *Muscle Disorders in Childhood.* Philadelphia, PA: W.B. Saunders; 1978.

4. Emery AE. *Duchenne Muscular Dystrophy.* 2nd ed. New York: Oxford University Press; 1993.

5. Anderson JL, Head SI, Rae C, Morley JW. Brain function in Duchenne muscular dystrophy. *Brain.* 2002;125:4-13.

6. Bushby K, Finkel R, Birnkrant DJ, et al. Diagnosis and management of Duchenne muscular dystrophy, part 1: diagnosis, and pharmacological and psychosocial management. *Lancet Neurol.* 2010;9:77-93.

7. Moxley RT 3rd, Pandya S, Ciafaloni E, Fox DJ, Campbell K. Change in natural history of Duchenne muscular dystrophy with long-term corticosteroid treatment: implications for management. *J Child Neurol.* 2010;25:1116-1129.

8. Lebel DE, Corston JA, McAdam LC, Biggar WD, Alman BA. Glucocorticoid treatment for the prevention of scoliosis in children with Duchenne muscular dystrophy: long-term follow-up. *J Bone Joint Surg Am.* 2013;95:1057-1061.

9. Raphael JC, Chevret S, Chastang C, Bouvet F. Randomised trial of preventive nasal ventilation in Duchenne muscular dystrophy. French Multicentre Cooperative Group on Home Mechanical Ventilation Assistance in Duchenne de Boulogne Muscular Dystrophy. *Lancet.* 1994;343:1600-1604.

10. Simonds AK, Muntoni F, Heather S, Fielding S. Impact of nasal ventilation and survival in hypercapnic Duchenne muscular dystrophy. *Thorax.* 1998;53:949-952.

11. Kohler M, Clarenbach CF, Bahler C, Brack T, Russi EW, Bloch KE. Disability and survival in Duchenne muscular dystrophy. *J Neurol Neurosurg Psychiatry.* 2009;80:320-325.

12. Bushby K, Finkel R, Birnkrant DJ, et al. Diagnosis and management of Duchenne muscular dystrophy, part 2: implementation of multidisciplinary care. *Lancet Neurol.* 2010;9:177-189.

13. Bendixen RM, Senesac C, Lott DJ, Vandenborne K. Participation and quality of life in children with Duchenne muscular dystrophy using the International Classification of Functioning, Disability and Health. *Health Qual Life Outcomes.* 2012;22:10-43.

14. Brooke MH, Griggs RC, Mendell JR, Fenichel GM, Shumate JB, Pellegrino RJ. Clinical trial in Duchenne dystrophy. I. The design of the protocol. *Muscle Nerve.* 1981;4:186-197.

15. Florence JM, Pandya S, King WM, et al. Intrarater reliability of manual muscle test (Medical Research Council Scale) grades in Duchenne's muscular dystrophy. *Phys Ther.* 1992;72:115-122.

16. Scott E, Mawson SJ. Measurement in Duchenne muscular dystrophy: considerations in the development of a neuromuscular assessment tool. *Dev Med Child Neurol.* 2006;48:540-544.

17. Pandya S, Florence JM, King WM, Robison JD, Oxman M, Province MA. Reliability of goniometric measurements in patients with Duchenne muscular dystrophy. *Phys Ther.* 1985;65:1339-1342.

18. Aras B, Aras O, Karaduman A. Reliability of balance tests in children with Duchenne muscular dystrophy. *Sci Res Essays.* 2011;6:4428-4431.

19. Blakeney J, Johnston R. Seating. In: Stone K, Tester C, Howarth A, et al., eds. *Occupational Therapy and Duchenne Muscular Dystrophy.* Hoboken, NJ: John Wiley & Sons Inc; 2007.

20. McDonald CM, Henricson EK, Han JJ, et al. The 6-minute walk test as a new outcome measure in Duchenne muscular dystrophy. *Muscle Nerve.* 2010;41:500-510.

21. McDonald CM, Henricson EK, Abresch T, et al. The 6-minute walk test and other clinical endpoints in Duchenne muscular dystrophy: reliability, concurrent validity, and minimal clinically important differences from a multicenter study. *Muscle Nerve.* 2013;48:357-368.

22. Hiller LB, Wade CK. Upper extremity functional assessment scales in children with Duchenne muscular dystrophy: a comparison. *Arch Phys Med Rehabil*. 1992;73:527-534.

23. Vignos PJ Jr, Spencer GE Jr, Archibald KC. Management of progressive muscular dystrophy in childhood. *JAMA*. 1963;184:89-96.

24. Barr AE, Diamond BE, Wade CK, et al. Reliability of testing measures in Duchenne or Becker muscular dystrophy. *Arch Phys Med Rehabil*. 1991;72:315-319.

25. Berard C, Payan C, Hodgkinson I, Fermanian J; MFM Collaboration Study Group. A motor function measure for neuromuscular diseases. Construction and validation study. *Neuromuscul Disord*. 2005;15:463-470.

26. Vuillerot C, Girardot F, Payan C, et al. Monitoring changes and predicting loss of ambulation in Duchenne muscular dystrophy with the Motor Function Measure. *Dev Med Child Neurol*. 2010;52:60-65.

27. Vuillerot C, Payan C, Girardot F, et al. Responsiveness of the motor function measure in neuromuscular diseases. *Arch Phys Med Rehabil*. 2012;93:2251-2256.

28. Steffensen B, Hyde S, Lyager S, Mattsson E. Validity of the EK scale: a functional assessment of non-ambulatory individuals with Duchenne muscular dystrophy or spinal muscle atrophy. *Physiother Res Int*. 2001;6:119-134.

29. Lyager S, Steffensen B, Juhl B. Indicators of need for mechanical ventilation in Duchenne muscular dystrophy and spinal muscular atrophy. *Chest*. 1995;108:779-785.

30. Msall ME, DiGaudio K, Rogers BT, et al. The Functional Independence Measure for Children (WeeFim). Conceptual basis and pilot use in children with developmental disabilities. *Clin Pediatr*. 1994;33:421-430.

31. Haley SM, Coster WJ, Ludlow LH, Haltiwanger JT, Andrellos PJ. *Pediatric Evaluation of Disability Inventory: Development, Standardization and Administration Manual*. Boston, MA: Trustees of Boston University;1992.

32. Enderle J, Severson S. *Enderle-Severson Transition Rating Scales*. 3rd ed. Moorhead, MN: ESTR Publications; 2003.

33. Davis SE, Hynan LS, Limbers CA, et al. The PedsQL in pediatric patients with Duchenne muscular dystrophy: feasibility, reliability and validity of the Pediatric Quality of Life Inventory Neuromuscular Module and Generic Core Scales. *J Clin Neuromuscul Dis*. 2010;11:97-109.

34. Bakker JP, de Groot IJ, Beckerman H, de Jong BA, Lankhorst GJ. The effects of knee-ankle-foot orthoses in the treatment of Duchenne muscular dystrophy: review of the literature. *Clin Rehabil*. 2000;14:343-359.

35. Hyde SA, Fløytrup I, Glent S, et al. A randomized comparative study of two methods for controlling Tendo Achilles contracture in Duchenne muscular dystrophy. *Neuromuscul Disord*. 2000;10:257-263.

36. Angelini C, Tasca E. Fatigue in muscular dystrophies. *Neuromuscul Disord*. 2012;22:S214-S220.

37. Kilmer DD. Response to resistive strengthening exercise training in humans with neuromuscular disease. *Am J Phys Med Rehabil*. 2002;81:S121-S126.

38. Jansen M, de Groot IJ, van Alfen N, Geurts AC. Physical training in boys with Duchenne Muscular Dystrophy: the protocol of the No Use Is Disuse study. *BMC Pediatr*. 2010;10:55.

39. Jansen M, van Alfen N, Geurts AC, de Groot IJ. Assisted bicycle training delays functional deterioration in boys with Duchenne muscular dystrophy: the randomized controlled trial "no use is disuse." *Neurorehabil Neural Repair*. 2013;27:816-827.

40. Bach JR, Bianchi C, Vidigal-Lopes M, Turi S, Felisari G. Lung inflation by glossopharyngeal breathing and "air stacking" in Duchenne muscular dystrophy. *Am J Phys Med Rehabil*. 2007;86:295-300.

Developmental Coordination Disorder

Phyllis Guarrera-Bowlby

A 6-year-old child is referred for a physical therapy evaluation to determine eligibility for school-based services secondary to coordination difficulties and inability to keep up with her peers. She has not had any major illnesses or significant hospitalizations. The parents report that early motor milestones were on time, but their daughter has always been clumsy. The child is currently in a regular education kindergarten classroom with typically developing peers. The physical therapist is to examine, evaluate, and make recommendations for the plan of care under the Individualized Education Program (IEP; see Case 7). The child is in an inclusive classroom in her local school district. Considering her age, she makes good eye contact and interacts appropriately with the therapist. Upon examination, the therapist finds slight hypotonia throughout the trunk and bilateral upper and lower extremities without any signs of hyperactive deep tendon reflexes or clonus. She demonstrates significant associated reactions (especially in the head and face) and has difficulty with tasks such as handwriting. During handwriting, the associated reactions include tongue protrusion and opposite hand fisting and head movements corresponding to the letters being written (*e.g.*, when writing a "z," her head moves in a zig-zag motion). When she is assessed in the quadruped position, she demonstrates an increased influence of the asymmetric tonic neck reflex (ATNR) and the symmetric tonic neck reflex (STNR). She has difficulty with diadokinetic movements in upper and lower extremities. The child has also had challenges with static balance skills such as standing on one foot and dynamic balance skills such as stair negotiation and jumping skills. She ascends and descends stairs using an alternating pattern and a railing. When asked to descend stairs without a railing, she uses a non-alternating pattern. When asked to skip, she utilizes a non-alternating pattern similar to galloping. She has difficulty walking on a straight line especially backwards. She can kick a slowly moving ball with her right foot better than her left. She can throw a ball with good accuracy, but is only able to catch a tennis ball one out of five times. Proximal stability is poor with all gross and fine motor skills. When writing, she has to keep her elbow against her trunk or against the table to steady her lines. She is able to accurately copy and construct structures with blocks with assistance for aligning the blocks. In the quadruped position, she can only lift one extremity at a time and uses significant lumbar lordosis to do so. She is able to assume the half-kneeling position, but falls with external perturbations. She has not had any other formal medical or occupational therapy evaluations at the time of this initial physical therapy examination. There is adaptive physical education available at her school. The child's parents are motivated to learn about her condition and interested in carrying out home program recommendations.

▶ Based on the clinical presentation, what are potential diagnoses to rule out?
▶ How does the school environment modify the therapist's examination priorities?
▶ Are the child's skills delayed enough to qualify for physical therapy services within the school system?
▶ How would the child's contextual factors influence or change your patient/client management?

KEY DEFINITIONS

ASSOCIATED REACTIONS: Involuntary movements that occur when a person is engaged in difficult or resisted movement; observed in typically developing children up to the age of 8 years. After this time, these movements indicate central nervous system (CNS) damage.

COGNITIVE ORIENTATION TO DAILY OCCUPATIONAL PERFORMANCE (CO-OP) PROGRAM: Program designed to remediate motoric skills in children with developmental coordination disorder by incorporation of motor learning concepts and dynamic systems framework[1]

DIADOKINETIC MOVEMENTS: Rapidly alternating movements such as supination-pronation, tapping toes, or verbally repeating "pa-ta-ka"; inability to perform these movements indicates CNS injury.

DYSPRAXIA: Impairment in the ability to perform coordinated movement

Objectives

1. Identify the diagnostic criteria for developmental coordination disorder (DCD).

2. Rule out other conditions that may present similarly to DCD.

3. Choose appropriate examination tools to determine the extent of coordination deficits.

4. Recognize the various subtypes of DCD.

5. Choose effective interventions and a plan of care based on current evidence and client presentation.

Physical Therapy Considerations

PT considerations for management of the young child with DCD in the educational setting:

▶ **General physical therapy plan of care/goals:** Initiation of educationally based services; maximize independent mobility and physical function, activity, and participation; minimize secondary impairments; referral to other specialists, as indicated

▶ **Physical therapy interventions:** Coordination and communication with parent, IEP team, medical team; patient-related instruction (targeted toward parents and other caregivers) regarding gross motor skill acquisition (such as additional practice and breaking tasks into smaller steps) and safety; direct services, as needed

▶ **Precautions during physical therapy:** Close positioning of physical therapist to the child during training of difficult/new gross motor skills; safety monitoring during all movement due to potential impulsivity of the child

► **Complications interfering with physical therapy:** Parents and school staff need to learn about diagnosis and implications and how best to help this child learn, play, and gain age-appropriate gross motor skills

Understanding the Health Condition

Developmental coordination disorder (DCD) is a medical condition that is characterized as difficulty in a multitude of gross and fine motor skills. According to the Diagnostic and Statistical Manual of Mental Disorders, 4th Edition, Text Revision (DSM-IV-TR) diagnostic criteria 315.40,[2] four criteria need to be fulfilled for a formal diagnosis of DCD to be considered. First, performance in daily activities requiring motor coordination must be substantially below average taking into consideration the individual's age and intellectual level. Second, the motoric disturbance must significantly interfere with academic performance and/or activities of daily living (ADLs). Third, all other conditions causing coordination problems must be ruled out, including cerebral palsy (CP) and pervasive developmental disorders. Finally, if the child has cognitive limitations, the child's coordination difficulties must be significantly more immature than the developmental cognitive level of the child. DCD can co-occur with neurobehavioral disorders including attention deficit hyperactivity disorder (ADHD) and attention deficit disorder (ADD). The Diagnostic and Statistical Manual of Mental Disorders, 5th Edition (DSM-V),[3] adds the criterion that the onset is seen in early development, but notes that frequently the diagnosis is not given until after 5 years of age. Previously, autism spectrum disorder was an exclusion criterion, but now the child can present with both conditions provided that the coordination difficulties are not attributable to the autistic behaviors.

Children with DCD are frequently referred to physical therapy when they enter the school system due to their difficulties in academic performance and motoric function when compared to their peers. When the coordination problems are more significant and the child is having difficulty acquiring early motor milestones, the child may enter into the early intervention system. When the child is referred for an evaluation, it is critical that the physical therapist quantify the degree of motor involvement in order for the child to be eligible for school services. It is also important for the physical therapist to gather information during the examination that would contribute to an alternative medical diagnosis such as CP or pervasive developmental disorder.

Over the years, DCD has had multiple names such as clumsy child syndrome or developmental dyspraxia. DCD was a term endorsed at an International Consensus Meeting in London, Ontario, in 1994.[4] The consistent incidence of this disorder is 5% to 6%, but has been reported as high as 19% in Greece.[5] DCD is more common in males with reported ratios ranging from 2:1 to 7:1.[5] Although the etiology of DCD lies within the CNS, the specific pathology is largely unknown. Magnetic resonance imaging (MRI) and other medical testing are primarily used to rule out conditions such as tumors or CP. DCD is suspected to be a perinatal acquired brain dysfunction because a larger percentage of infants born prematurely are diagnosed with this condition. Due to the strong association with perinatal issues, some researchers[6] question whether DCD is on a continuum with CP and suggest that the two conditions may share similar dysfunctional pathways. There is also considerable overlap with children with joint hypermobility condition[7] (see Case 27). Therefore, it is important that this diagnosis be considered when performing the physical therapy assessment.

Because individuals with DCD present with a wide array of impairments, there have been attempts to classify these children into subgroups.[8,9] Sensorimotor dysfunction is the category with the highest incidence of comorbid conditions such as dyslexia, attention deficits, and hyperactivity. When the children were grouped according to neuropsychological testing,[8] researchers found three clusters: (1) ideomotor dyspraxia with movement deficits, problems with imitation, dynamic balance, and handwriting; (2) visual spatial and visual construction dyspraxia and deficits in both visual motor skills and handwriting; and (3) mixed dyspraxia (global deficit categories including the signs observed in the prior two groups and additional significant coordination problems between the limbs). Green et al.[9] attempted to determine if subgrouping the DCD diagnosis affected the outcomes of children with DCD after participation in the CO-OP program. The investigators divided the groups of children into five clusters based on evaluation using several scales including the Movement ABC (M-ABC), Developmental Test of Visual-Motor Integration (VMI), and the Clinical Observations of Motor and Postural Skills (COMPS). The five clusters included: (1) strongest performance in perceptual motor skills, (2) strongest performance in perceptual and fine motor skills, (3) particular deficits in static and dynamic balance, (4) deficits in perceptual and fine motor tasks, and (5) deficits in all areas. Overall, one-third of children demonstrated minimal or no progress after participation in the CO-OP program. Children with visual perceptual problems had the poorest outcomes and those with a comorbid diagnosis such as ADD were less likely to make progress. However, a third of these children with comorbid conditions made progress. A correlational analysis indicated that better verbal ability scores based on intellectual testing were significantly associated with better progress with therapeutic intervention.

The World Health Organization's International Classification of Functioning, Disability and Health (ICF) model[10] allows clinicians to classify deficits based on body structures and functions, activity limitations, and participation in activities at home and in the community. For the child with DCD, the body structures and functions classification includes impairments with visual-spatial motor control and deficits in adaptive postural control. Visual-spatial motor control includes movements directed in and outside of the child's personal space. Adaptive postural control includes poor integration of sensory information in sensory conflict situations and control in static and dynamic balance activities.[11] Children with DCD have difficulty with obstacle crossing and controlling momentum of their center of mass.[12] Laufer et al.[13] discovered that children with DCD had higher postural sway and more center of pressure (COP) amplitude variability than typically developing children. This variability in COP amplitude increased during dual-task conditions such as verbal naming of simple objects (*e.g.*, ball, table) while standing on a firm or compliant surface. Children with DCD tend to prioritize the cognitive task over the postural task in such dual-task paradigms. Fong et al.[11] have found sensory deficits on tests such as the Sensory Organization Test (SOT), especially when sensory inputs were degraded or absent. In addition, children with DCD demonstrate "soft" neurological signs such as mirror movements (associated reactions), slight hypotonia, and persistence of primitive reflexes.

Movement deficits in children with DCD include immature and slow movements, especially distal movements. These slow distal movements often manifest as poor handwriting. Children with DCD have more variability in gait and running skills, suggesting difficulty controlling the lower extremities.[14,15] Diamond et al.[15] found that ankle propulsion was decreased in children with DCD compared to their peers. Children with DCD also have difficulty with intersegmental control as seen with ball-catching activities. Przysucha and Maraj[16] found that children with DCD had the most difficulty coordinating their arms and trunk in order to adjust their bodies to intercept the ball and had poor temporal control of their grasp. Lateral ball catching was the most difficult task for these children because the task requires more coordination of all body segments. To catch the laterally thrown ball, children with DCD either stayed still or over-adjusted in their attempts.

Children with DCD have memory issues including visual-spatial, verbal working memory, and motor imagery. Asonitou et al.[17] found that cognitive deficits in planning, attention, and simultaneous processing were associated with poor performance of gross motor skills assessed via standardized tools. Wilson et al.[18] summarized the research related to performance deficits and concluded that the fundamental problem is a disruption in predictive control of action. Children with DCD demonstrate impaired functional performance across gross motor, fine motor, and self-help skills. In their review, Wilson et al.[18] attribute motoric deficits in DCD to an inability to develop stable coordination patterns.

There is evidence that children with DCD participate less in physical and social activities in the home, school, and community, including organized sports.[19] Evidence suggests that the motoric and coordination deficits remain at least into adolescence in 50% to 70% of these children.[4] In personal factors, deficits include feelings of inadequacy, decreased self-esteem, and limited coping strategies.[19] Children with DCD have difficulties at home and school,[20] causing increased parental concerns about long-term motor and academic difficulties and limited acceptance with their peers.[21] These children are at higher risk of being sedentary with subsequent decreased fitness and cardiovascular health, as well obesity.[5] The effect of successful participation can build confidence in these children and enable them to try new activities.

Adults who were diagnosed with DCD in childhood have cognitive and motoric difficulties that continue to affect their daily lives. They have higher rates of depression and anxiety than their peers and lower rates of employment and life satisfaction.[22] Driving an automobile is a new motoric skill typically acquired during adolescence. Interviews with adolescents and adults with DCD reveal that fewer learn to operate a motor vehicle than their peers. Those who ultimately do learn to drive have more difficulty acquiring the skill due to deficits in visual-motor skills that impair distance estimation and the ability to park.[23]

In children with DCD, there are indications of mild cerebral dysfunction or global dysfunction in the brain regions involved with motoric control.[24] Specific areas that have been implicated include the parietal lobe and cerebellum along with their respective pathways. Impaired imagery and inadequate development and updating of internal representations have also been proposed.[25] The development of these internal representation models is crucial in order to adjust movements while the particular goal-directed activity is occurring. Without accurate internal representation models, the child is limited to motor control feedback, which prevents correction *during* the movement due to delays in neurological processing. Wilson et al.[25] have recommended that children with DCD be trained to use both the internal feedback (kinesthetic or feel of the movement) and external imagery (watching from another person's perspective) in order to develop the formation of these internal representation models. In some children with DCD, cerebellar dysfunction has been implicated due to the noted deficits in automatization of skills[24] and in learning new skills.[26]

Physical Therapy Patient/Client Management

The school system team includes the teacher(s), other professionals such as the occupational therapist and speech-language pathologist, and the family unit. Other medical professionals are critical in making the final diagnosis of DCD and ruling out other conditions. The physical therapist can offer essential information to the team regarding deficits in gross motor skills and identification of neurological signs that can assist in an appropriate diagnosis and treatment plan. Missiuna et al.[27] found that with education from other healthcare professionals about the motoric deficits and diagnostic criteria associated with DCD, physicians were more likely to identify children with significant problems on their caseloads. It is unknown whether this education had a prospective effect on the referral for those children with milder presentations. Children with DCD do not outgrow the condition and will need assistance to identify appropriate fitness plans and strategies to cope with their attempts to participate at levels equivalent with peers.

Examination, Evaluation, and Diagnosis

The physical therapy examination includes assessment of impairments including active and passive range of motion (ROM), muscle strength, muscle tone, primitive reflexes, and overall coordination. The school-based physical therapist must also assess the child's gross motor skills to determine the degree of delay present in order to determine if the child qualifies for school-based services. The physical therapist may be the first healthcare professional to see the child and will need to screen and/or assess fine motor skills to determine if there is a need for referral to other healthcare professionals (*e.g.*, occupational therapist).

During the examination, the physical therapist collects data to assist in ruling out other diagnoses.[28] Children with DCD typically present with soft neurological signs, such as associated reactions and retention of primitive reflexes (*e.g.*, ATNR, STNR). Children who present with more significant neurological findings may have other related diagnoses including CP. Progressively worsening functional findings (decreasing strength, change in muscle tone, and/or loss of gross motor skills) would be more indicative of progressive disorders such as muscular dystrophy or spinal muscular atrophy. Past medical history including brain trauma or concussion would indicate signs of a traumatic brain injury. Abnormal social behaviors including a lack of eye contact, delayed or stereotypic language, and/or repetitive non-purposeful play regimes could indicate an autistic spectrum disorder.

Physical therapists have a choice of standardized motor skills tests to assess gross and fine motor delays in children with DCD. However, local agencies may dictate the use of a specific school district–chosen standardized tool(s) to assess children in either early intervention or school-based settings. A recent review[29] indicates that the most consistently used tools for assessment include the **Movement Assessment Battery for Children, Second Edition (MABC-2)**[30] and the Test of Gross Motor Development, Second Edition (TGMD-2).[31] These tools assess skills that are achievable for 3- to 10-year-old children (TGMD-2) and 4- to 12-year-old children (MABC-2). Both tests have good psychometric properties, including reliability and validity.[29] The MABC-2 has been used more frequently with children with DCD, while the TGMD-2 has primarily been used with typically developing children. In addition, the MABC-2 is the only measure with research showing its responsiveness to change in this population.[29] Some researchers[32] question the use of the MABC-2 as the gold standard for identification of DCD and cautioned using this tool in isolation secondary to limited support for its reliability and validity. Other motor tools available to physical therapists to assess gross and fine motor skills in children with DCD include the Peabody Developmental Motor Scales, 2nd edition (PDMS-2)[33] and the Bruininks-Oseretsky Test of Motor Proficiency (BOT-2).[34] The PDMS-2 is appropriate to use when the child's skills are in the 0- to 6-year-old level. The BOT-2 is the only tool with norms for children older than 12 years. Drawbacks of the BOT-2 tool include set-up time (unless the set-up can be left intact, which is difficult for the traveling school therapist) and high demands for attention since many tasks require multi-step directions often beyond the capabilities of the child with DCD, especially those with the comorbidity of ADD. Each of the tests mentioned includes assessment of gross and fine motor skills, except for the TGMD-2 that primarily assesses gross motor and ball-handling skills. While the total scores on these tests are helpful to determine if the child is eligible for related services, the sub-test profiles are helpful to determine the specific deficits for the child.[35]

Physical therapists may also choose to use specific impairment-based tests that include an assessment of sensory integration (SI) such as the Sensory Integration and Praxis test (SIPT),[4,29] the SOT,[11] or the Clinical Test of Sensory Interaction and Balance (CTSIB or "foam and dome").[4,36]

Screening questionnaires can be used for cost-effectiveness and to assess the impact of the condition on the child, family, and classroom staff. The Developmental Coordination Disorder Questionnaire (DCDQ) and the Developmental Coordination Disorder Questionnaire-Revised (DCDQ-R) are questionnaires specific to DCD. The MABC checklist is a teacher questionnaire which has lower sensitivity than the DCDQ-R[4] and limited correlation with the MABC performance score ($r = 0.51$). In addition, many children with motoric issues were not identified when only the MABC checklist was utilized. One self-efficacy tool that has been used with this population is the Children's Self-Perceptions of Adequacy in and Predilection for Physical Activity (CSAPPA) scale.[37] The CSAPPA tool has good reliability and fair to good validity. For general physical activity and fitness levels, accelerometry can be used reliably with children with DCD with and without ADHD.[38]

Plan of Care and Interventions

The physical therapy plan of care includes consideration of the child's entire therapeutic intervention and prioritization of critical components in order to address the child's significant motoric delays. There may be times when the requisite amount of physical therapy can negatively impact educational issues for the child. At these times, the team may decide to provide certain therapies on a consultation service, while other therapies are prioritized as more germane to the child's current level of functioning. For this 6-year-old child, her handwriting issues may be more critical to address. Therefore, school-based occupational therapy may be prioritized. Alternatively, the gross motor coordination deficits may be prioritized based on difficulties moving in the environment, specifically in physical education class and at recess.

Physical therapy intervention is more beneficial for the motor performance of children with DCD than no physical therapy intervention.[5,39] The diverse interventions available for these children can be divided into two general theoretical-based categories: process or deficit-oriented interventions (*e.g.*, neurodevelopmental treatment [NDT], SI) and task-oriented interventions.[5,39] The evidence for the efficacy of process-oriented interventions is considered weak. While process-oriented interventions provide some benefits, there is limited carryover to functional skills. In contrast, the evidence is stronger for the efficacy of task-oriented interventions, suggesting that functionally based activities should be included in the therapy plan of care.[4]

Process-oriented approaches propose to remediate the underlying cause of the motor problems. NDT is an intervention approach that primarily involves handling skills, but also incorporates motor learning concepts. For example, if a child with DCD is having particular problems with altering her inefficient movement patterns, it may be helpful to physically guide her through alternative patterns to assist in widening her repertoire. Since these children have poor balance, gymnastic ball activities may be helpful to improve balance and core stability. Poor proprioception and kinesthesia and visual-perceptual deficits may be addressed by sensory integration techniques to help the child utilize sensory information to improve gross and fine motor skills. The therapist must keep in mind that these impairment-level interventions need to be paired with functional training since these children often do not generalize these gains and integrate them into other motor skills.[4]

Task-oriented approaches integrate components from motor learning paradigms. Practice of task-specific activities with the provision of appropriately timed feedback is a key component of motor learning.[4] Therapists in pediatric settings frequently use these concepts since children are less willing to perform exercises.

The Cognitive Orientation to Daily Occupational Performance (CO-OP) program[1] is an organized program that has been designed to incorporate motor learning concepts and a dynamic systems framework to remediate motoric skills in children with DCD. The program starts with an assessment of motor skills and the prioritization of a maximum of three key skills in conjunction with the child and parents. The therapist is critical in analyzing the prioritized skills and determining the key roadblocks in attaining the chosen skills. While the CO-OP program was primarily designed with short bursts of intensive intervention (10 sessions) outside of the school setting, the skill prioritization can revolve around a particular setting (e.g., skills necessary to be successful in the school environment). The skills are then practiced over ten sessions with each session focused on one to two of those skills. After teaching the child how to utilize the "plan, goal, do, and check" procedure, the therapist guides the child to develop self-assessment strategies. This process sets up the child to continue this process beyond the direct intervention period when she approaches new tasks she would like to acquire in the future. The therapist may provide the child with additional strategies to expand her repertoire of choices for attempting motor skills. For example, if the child is only using an underhand throw, the therapist may suggest trying an overhand throw and having the child assess her success. For multi-step or sequential skills, the therapist can assist with the development of mnemonics or scripts to help the child remember the sequence of activities. For example, when tying shoes, the child may utilize a rhyme or song to remember the correct sequence of steps. There is a huge emphasis on self-discovery, meaning that the therapist asks questions as opposed to providing answers for the child and then coaches the child rather than guiding her through the skill. There is still a place for therapist demonstration of a skill to enable the child to assess the skill in an external versus internal viewpoint of performance. For example, the therapist may emphasize a component of the skill that is critical to the child's success in order to make it easier for her to see and determine how it impacts the overall skill performance. Other individuals involved with the child must understand the training program in order to provide the child with additional practice outside of the direct therapy sessions. Parents are essential in helping the child with skill practice and teachers can assist the child with transitioning these skills into other settings that incorporate generalization for these children. The CO-OP manual[1] is an excellent resource and additional resources are provided on a DVD for therapeutic use. After intervention with this approach, children continue to self-monitor performance and utilize cognitive strategies. The development of the self-assessment skills can lead to generalization and transfer to other tasks outside of the therapy situation, though this has only been studied over short post-intervention periods (<1 year).[40]

An alternative to direct therapy services is a school health service model developed in Canada called Partnering for Change (P4C) in which the attention is directed to the educators and parents as the collaborators and coaches for children with DCD. In P4C, the school is the client rather than an individual student. The program includes relationship and trust building with the school staff and education to expand the teachers' skills and to enable their effectiveness with coaching to assist in the child's self-discovery processes. While the research has primarily related to feasibility,[41,42] initial reactions of occupational therapists and teachers involved with this program were positive and were effective in increasing teacher knowledge and capacity to work with this population. As a result of participation in this training program, teachers changed their classrooms and instructional strategies.[41] P4C is similar to the intention of the Response to Intervention (RTI)[42] program, which is a multi-tier approach that aids in the early identification of students with behavioral and learning needs. Because of this similarity and the wide use of RTI, there may be earlier identification of these children and decreased need for direct services, and teachers may be better prepared to accommodate the needs of these children. This process also involves the parents since these strategies should be reinforced at home. Toglia et al.[43] provided an overview of cognitive strategies and a clinical reasoning tool that is helpful to determine which cognitive strategies to utilize for a particular child.

Group-based work[44-46] also appears successful with this population. In two studies, Pless and colleagues[44,45] utilized physical education teachers to administer gross motor activity sessions. They found improvements in self-efficacy,[45] but no differences in MABC scores except for children with borderline DCD.[44] Hung et al.[46] found that motor skill training improved MABC scores and there were no differences in individual- versus group-based training, suggesting that group-based training may be preferable due to its cost-effectiveness.

Motor imagery and virtual reality (VR) are methods that can provide additional practice and home programming in children with DCD. Williams et al.[47] looked at the ability of children to perform motor imagery. While children with severe impairments may be unable to use motor imagery, those children who could successfully use motor imagery had the greatest benefit.[48] Two studies have utilized off-the-shelf gaming: PlayStation EyeToy over ten sessions with 4- to 6-year-old children[49] and the Wii Fit over 12 sessions with 7- to 11-year-old children.[50] Both studies revealed improvement on gross motor assessment, especially in balance components with some loss of skills without continued intervention. Although some children (~50%) improved on the BOT-2, the researchers could not determine the characteristics of the children who made improvements due to the small sample size. In a VR system, Snapp-Childs et al.[51] trained manual tracing skills using a haptic (touch technology) VR device that provided either assistance and/or friction to the pathway over one session. Children with DCD benefited more from the VR training than typically developing children and were able to approach the performance of typically developing children.

For parental training, a new tele-intervention[52] has been designed and conducted with a physical therapist that instructed parents how to teach their child shoelace tying and bicycle riding for 11 children. Materials via DVD, computer blogs and emails, and weekly phone calls from the physical therapist assisted the parents with teaching the skills. In this study, there were no changes on the DCD-Q, but three out of seven children improved on the MABC.[52]

Sports-based activities (taekwondo,[53] soccer,[54] table tennis[55]) have also been used to help improve motor skills in children with DCD. Taekwondo provided daily for 3 months improved sensory organization and balance. The soccer and table tennis interventions (10 weeks for both activities; 3 times per week for table tennis and 5 times per week for soccer) both improved attention skill and scores on the MABC for the training group compared to the control group.

In conclusion, task-oriented training is the optimal method of intervention delivered through either individual- or group-based interventions. Throughout the training, the child with DCD should be encouraged to self-assess and develop coping strategies in order to learn new skills after the therapeutic period. Children should be encouraged to become more active via sports-type activities in order to promote life-long fitness. Therapists can assist and guide the child toward sports in which the child may be ultimately successful.

Evidence-Based Clinical Recommendations

SORT: Strength of Recommendation Taxonomy

A: Consistent, good-quality patient-oriented evidence
B: Inconsistent or limited-quality patient-oriented evidence
C: Consensus, disease-oriented evidence, usual practice, expert opinion, or case series

1. The Movement Assessment Battery for Children, Second Edition (MABC-2) is the most appropriate standardized assessment tool to use in evaluating the gross motor skills in children with DCD. **Grade B**

2. Physical therapy interventions improve the motor performance of children with DCD. **Grade B**

3. Motor learning models, such as task-oriented training, demonstrate consistent beneficial effects for children with DCD. **Grade C**

COMPREHENSION QUESTIONS

12.1 Which subtype of DCD explains *most* of motoric difficulties demonstrated by the child in this case?

A. Fine motor deficits

B. Visual perceptual deficits

C. Mixed dyspraxia

D. Constructional dyspraxia

12.2 Which of the following is the *most* appropriate tool for the physical therapist to choose to determine the extent of this child's functional delays?

A. TGMD-2

B. MABC-2

C. PDMS-2

D. BOT-2

12.3 What is the *most* effective intervention strategy given this child's clinical presentation and personal and environmental factors?

A. NDT

B. Sensory integration

C. Core stability training

D. CO-OP

ANSWERS

12.1 **C.** She has gross motor difficulties along with fine motor control deficits, making mixed dyspraxia the best option. She is able to construct structures, ruling out basic visual perceptual and constructional deficits (options B and D). She has difficulty with control of all the extremities, especially with complex motoric activities and not just fine motor deficits (option A).

12.2 **B.** Given her presentation of fine and gross motor deficits, the MABC-2 is the best and most researched tool for this population. The TGMD-2 (option A) only provides information on gross motor and ball skill activities. Since she has not had an occupational therapy evaluation, it would be beneficial to determine the extent of fine motor problems for the school team and appropriate referral. The PDMS-2 and the BOT-2 (options C and D) assess gross and fine motor function, but have not been used as diagnostic tools as much as the MABC-2.

12.3 **D.** While any therapy is more effective than no therapy, systematic reviews of interventions with this population support the use of task-oriented training, which are concepts that are incorporated in the CO-OP program. With the family's motivation to be involved, this program can be incorporated into the home program and is one of the key concepts in this program. NDT, sensory integration, and core stability fall under the category of process-oriented types of interventions.

REFERENCES

1. Polatajko H, Mandich A. *Enabling Occupation in Children: The Cognitive Orientation to Daily Occupational Performance (CO-OP) Approach.* Ottawa: CAOT Publications ACE; 2004.

2. American Psychiatric Association. *Diagnostic and Statistical Manual of Mental Disorders.* 4th ed, Text Revision. Washington, DC: American Psychiatric Association; 2000.

3. American Psychiatric Association. *Diagnostic and Statistical Manual of Mental Disorders.* 5th ed. Washington, DC: American Psychiatric Association; 2013.

4. Blank R, Smits Engelsman B, Polatajko H, Wilson P. European Academy for Childhood Disability (EACD): recommendations on the definition, diagnosis and intervention of developmental coordination disorder (long version). *Dev Med Child Neurol.* 2011;54:54-93.

5. Zwicker JG, Missiuna C, Harris SR, Boyd LA. Developmental coordination disorder: a review and update. *Eur J Paediatr Neurol.* 2012;16:573-581.

6. Pearsall-Jones JG, Piek JP, Levy F. Developmental coordination disorder and cerebral palsy: categories or a continuum? *Hum Mov Sci.* 2010;29:787-798.

7. Kirby A, Sugden D, Purcell C. Diagnosing developmental coordination disorders. *Arch Dis Child.* 2014;99:292-296.

8. Vaivre-Douret L, Lalanne C, Ingster-Moati I, et al. Subtypes of developmental coordination disorder: research on their nature and etiology. *Dev Neuropsychol.* 2011;36:614-643.

9. Green D, Chambers ME, Sugden DA. Does subtype of developmental coordination disorder count: is there a differential effect on outcome following intervention? *Hum Mov Sci.* 2008;27:363-382.

10. World Health Organization (WHO). International Classification of Functioning, Disability and Health (ICF). 2014. www.who.int/classifications/icf/en/. Accessed September 15, 2014.

11. Fong SS, Lee VY, Pang MY. Sensory organization of balance control in children with developmental coordination disorder. *Res Dev Disabil.* 2011;32:2376-2382.

12. Deconinck FJ, Savelsbergh GJ, DeClercq D, Lenoir M. Balance problems during obstacle crossing in children with developmental coordination disorder. *Gait Posture.* 2010;32:327-331.

13. Laufer Y, Ashkenazi T, Josman N. The effects of a concurrent cognitive task on the postural control of young children with and without developmental coordination disorder. *Gait Posture.* 2008;27:347-351.

14. Rosengren KS, Deconinck FJ, Diberardino LA 3rd, et al. Differences in gait complexity and variability between children with and without developmental coordination disorder. *Gait Posture.* 2009;29:225-229.

15. Diamond N, Downs J, Morris S. "The problem with running"—comparing the propulsion strategy of children with developmental coordination disorder and typically developing children. *Gait Posture.* 2014;39:547-552.

16. Przysucha EP, Maraj BK. Movement coordination in ball catching: comparison between boys with and without developmental coordination disorder. *Res Q Exerc Sport.* 2010;81:152-161.

17. Asonitou K, Koutsouki D, Kourtessis T, Charitou S. Motor and cognitive performance differences between children with and without developmental coordination disorder (DCD). *Res Dev Disabil.* 2012;33:996-1005.

18. Wilson PH, Ruddock S, Smits-Engelsman B, Polatajko H, Blank R. Understanding performance deficits in developmental coordination disorder: a meta-analysis of recent research. *Dev Med Child Neurol.* 2013;55:217-228.

19. Batey CA, Missiuna CA, Timmons BW, Hay JA, Faught BE, Cairney J. Self-efficacy toward physical activity and the physical activity behavior of children with and without developmental coordination disorder. *Hum Mov Sci.* 2014;36:258-271.

20. Wang TN, Tseng MH, Wilson BN, Hu FC. Functional performance of children with developmental coordination disorder at home and at school. *Dev Med Child Neurol.* 2009;51:817-825.

21. Stephenson EA, Chesson RA. 'Always the guiding hand': parents' accounts of the long-term implications of developmental co-ordination disorder for their children and families. *Child Care Health Dev.* 2008;34:335-343.

22. Kirby A, Williams N, Thomas M, Hill EL. Self-reported mood, general health, wellbeing and employment status in adults with suspected DCD. *Res Dev Disabil.* 2013;34:1357-1364.

23. Kirby A, Sugden D, Edwards L. Driving behaviour in young adults with developmental coordination disorder. *J Adult Dev.* 2011;18:122-129.

24. Visser J. Developmental coordination disorder: a review of research on subtypes and comorbidities. *Hum Mov Sci.* 2003;22:479-493.

25. Wilson PH, Maruff P, Ives S, Currie J. Abnormalities of motor and praxis imagery in children with DCD. *Hum Mov Sci.* 2001;20:135-159.

26. Cantin N, Polatajko HJ, Thach WT, Jaglal S. Developmental coordination disorder: exploration of a cerebellar hypothesis. *Hum Mov Sci.* 2007;26:491-509.

27. Missiuna C, Gaines R, McLean J, DeLaat D, Egan M, Soucie H. Description of children identified by physicians as having developmental coordination disorder. *Dev Med Child Neurol.* 2008;50:839-844.

28. Missiuna C, Gaines R, Soucie H. Why every office needs a tennis ball: a new approach to assessing the clumsy child. *CMAJ*. 2006;175:471-473.

29. Slater LM, Hillier SL, Civetta LR. The clinimetric properties of performance-based gross motor tests used for children with developmental coordination disorder: a systematic review. *Pediatr Phys Ther*. 2010;22:170-179.

30. Henderson SE, Sugden DA, Barnett A. *Movement Assessment Battery for Children-2 Examiner's Manual*. 2nd ed. Oxford: Pearson; 2007.

31. Ulrich DA. *Test of Gross Motor Development-2*. 2nd ed. Austin, TX: Pro-Ed; 2000.

32. Venetsanou F, Kambas A, Ellinoudis T, Fatouros I, Giannakidou D, Kourtessis T. Can the movement assessment battery for children test be the "gold standard" for the motor assessment of children with developmental coordination disorder? *Res Dev Disabil*. 2011;32:1-10.

33. Folio M, Fewell R. *Peabody Developmental Motor Scales Examiner's Manual*. 2nd ed. Austin, TX: Pro-Ed; 2000.

34. Bruininks R, Bruininks B. *Bruininks-Oseretsky Test of Motor Proficiency-Second Edition Manual*. Circle Pines, MN: AGS Publishing; 2005.

35. Wilson PH. Practitioner review: approaches to assessment and treatment of children with DCD: an evaluative review. *J Child Psychol Psychiatry*. 2005;46:806-823.

36. Cherng RJ, Hsu YW, Chen YJ, Chen JY. Standing balance of children with developmental coordination disorder under altered sensory conditions. *Hum Mov Sci*. 2007;26:913-926.

37. Hay JA, Hawes R, Faught BE. Evaluation of a screening instrument for developmental coordination disorder. *J Adolesc Health*. 2004;34:308-313.

38. Baerg S, Cairney J, Hay J, Rempel L, Mahlberg N, Faught BE. Evaluating physical activity using accelerometry in children at risk of developmental coordination disorder in the presence of attention deficit hyperactivity disorder. *Res Dev Disabil*. 2011;32:1343-1350.

39. Smits-Engelsman BC, Blank R, van der Kaay AC, et al. Efficacy of interventions to improve motor performance in children with developmental coordination disorder: a combined systematic review and meta-analysis. *Dev Med Child Neurol*. 2013;55:229-237.

40. Hyland M, Polatajko HJ. Enabling children with developmental coordination disorder to self-regulate through the use of Dynamic Performance Analysis: evidence from the CO-OP approach. *Hum Mov Sci*. 2012;31:987-998.

41. Missiuna C, Pollock N, Campbell WN, et al. Use of the Medical Research Council Framework to develop a complex intervention in pediatric occupational therapy: assessing feasibility. *Res Dev Disabil*. 2012;33:1443-1452.

42. Missiuna CA, Pollock NA, Levac DE, et al. Partnering for change: an innovative school-based occupational therapy service delivery model for children with developmental coordination disorder. *Can J Occup Ther*. 2012;79:41-50.

43. Toglia JP, Rodger SA, Polatajko HJ. Anatomy of cognitive strategies: a therapist's primer for enabling occupational performance. *Can J Occup Ther*. 2012;79:225-236.

44. Pless M, Carlsson M, Sundelin C, Persson K. Effects of group motor skill intervention on five-to-six-year old children with developmental coordination disorder. *Pediatr Phys Ther*. 2000;12:183-189.

45. Pless M, Carlsson M, Sundelin C, Persson K. Pre-school children with developmental coordination disorder: self-perceived competence and group motor skill intervention. *Acta Paediatr*. 2001;90:532-538.

46. Hung WW, Pang MY. Effects of group-based versus individual-based exercise training on motor performance in children with developmental coordination disorder: a randomized controlled study. *J Rehabil Med*. 2010;42:122-128.

47. Williams J, Thomas PR, Maruff P, Wilson PH. The link between motor impairment level and motor imagery ability in children with developmental coordination disorder. *Hum Mov Sci*. 2008;27:270-285.

48. Wilson PH, Thomas PR, Maruff P. Motor imagery training ameliorates motor clumsiness in children. *J Child Neurol*. 2002;17:491-498.

49. Ashkenazi T, Weiss PL, Orian D, Laufer Y. Low-cost virtual reality intervention program for children with developmental coordination disorder: a pilot feasibility study. *Pediatr Phys Ther*. 2013;25:467-473.

50. Hammond J, Jones V, Hill EL, Green D, Male I. An investigation of the impact of regular use of the Wii Fit to improve motor and psychosocial outcomes in children with movement difficulties: a pilot study. *Child Care Health Dev*. 2014;40:165-175.

51. Snapp-Childs W, Mon-Williams M, Bingham GP. A sensorimotor approach to the training of manual actions in children with developmental coordination disorder. *J Child Neurol*. 2013;28:204-212.

52. Miyahara M, Butson R, Cutfield R, Clarkson JE. A pilot study of family-focused tele-intervention for children with developmental coordination disorder: development and lessons learned. *Telemed J EHealth*. 2009;15:707-712.

53. Fong SS, Tsang WW, Ng GY. Taekwondo training improves sensory organization and balance control in children with developmental coordination disorder: a randomized controlled trial. *Res Dev Disabil*. 2012;33:85-95.

54. Tsai CL, Wang CH, Tseng YT. Effects of exercise intervention on event-related potential and task performance indices of attention networks in children with developmental coordination disorder. *Brain Cogn*. 2012;79:12-22.

55. Tsai CL. The effectiveness of exercise intervention on inhibitory control in children with developmental coordination disorder: using a visuospatial attention paradigm as a model. *Res Dev Disabil*. 2009;30:1268-1280.

Autism Spectrum Disorder: Motor Concerns

Beth Ennis

CASE 13

A 3-year-old male presents with a diagnosis of pervasive developmental disorder, not otherwise specified (PDD-NOS), autism spectrum disorder (ASD) to an outpatient clinic for evaluation. He was born full term, but had difficulty nursing as a child, and was mildly behind in his motor milestone acquisition. While he is able to walk, his mother reports that he has difficulty with balance, does not like to explore much, and is not climbing or jumping. She also states that he has difficulty with eye contact, rarely smiles, and is not making many sounds. She would like to know if her son would benefit from physical therapy services to address his current delays.

▶ What are the most appropriate tests and measures to be used?
▶ What are the most appropriate physical therapy interventions?
▶ What aspects of his diagnosis should be taken into consideration when planning a treatment session that would differ from a child with balance issues alone?
▶ Identify potential referrals to other medical team members.

KEY DEFINITIONS

AUTISM SPECTRUM DISORDER (ASD): Umbrella classification for autism that encompasses all levels of severity, with characteristics defined by the Diagnostic and Statistical Manual of Mental Disorders V (DSM-V)[1]; typically, the most impaired functioning is in social and language skills.

PERVASIVE DEVELOPMENT DISORDER, NOT OTHERWISE SPECIFIED (PDD-NOS): Classification used for children with "atypical autism"; individuals display some of the characteristics of typical autism, but demonstrate different onset, severity, or lack some characteristics of classic autism. This has changed under the implementation of DSM-V and this diagnosis is included under the diagnosis of ASD, with a severity level defined.[2]

STEREOTYPY: Ritualistic movement pattern or behavior; when seen in children with a diagnosis of ASD, these movement patterns are considered secondary to the diagnosis.

Objectives

1. Understand the typical motor issues that often present in a child with ASD.

2. List two reliable and valid tools that can be used to measure successful outcomes for children with ASD.

3. Discuss effective interventions for improving body functions and structure and activity limitations in children diagnosed with ASD.

4. Consider methods of therapy service delivery that may be beneficial for children with ASD.

Physical Therapy Considerations

PT considerations for the young child with ASD:

▶ **General physical therapy plan of care/goals:** Address bilateral coordination, balance, and motor planning of movement to allow for typical development of skills and age-appropriate participation.

▶ **Physical therapy interventions:** Developmental activities addressing balance and coordination; gait training; aquatics for proprioception and strengthening; parent education on incorporating activities throughout daily routine

▶ **Precautions during physical therapy:** Be aware of the child's sensory system and tendencies toward overstimulation; some children have difficulty transitioning between activities, so cues and warnings may be needed.

▶ **Complications interfering with physical therapy:** Some children have difficulty with various sensory stimuli, becoming overwhelmed by sounds, visual input, and/or tactile stimuli, causing them to "shut down" and not be able to participate in therapy.

Understanding the Health Condition

Autism spectrum disorder (ASD) is the most rapidly growing diagnostic category in childhood (approximately 1/88 children in the United States), although it is unclear if this is due to increased identification or a true increase in the prevalence.[2] There is no specific cause for autism, but studies have identified risk factors such as advanced parental age, sex of the child (males have a higher incidence), family history, and other diagnoses. Families with a child with a diagnosis on the autism spectrum are also more likely to have another child diagnosed. Common comorbidities in children with a diagnosis of ASD are fragile X, tuberous sclerosis, Tourette syndrome, epilepsy, and prematurity.[2]

While autism is classically thought of as a diagnosis that impacts children's language skills and social interactions, a growing body of literature is demonstrating its impact on motor skills, often *before* language and social delays are noted. Children with ASD have been noted to have difficulty with symmetrical movements, head lag in infancy, motor coordination deficits, low muscle tone, and apraxia. While most children receive a diagnosis by age 2 or 3 due to difficulties with language or social functioning, recent research has identified motor issues that can be early indicators for risk of diagnosis of a disorder on the spectrum. One prospective study identified head lag in infancy as an indicator of factors like low tone and poor postural control, that later correlated with a diagnosis of ASD.[3] Other studies show links between motor delay in infancy and language skills at 18 months,[4] time spent in functional play in infancy and later diagnosis with ASD,[5] and visual and motor atypicalities in infants who are diagnosed with ASD prior to the age of 2 years.[6] These studies are influencing clinicians to redefine the characteristics of children with ASD to include delays in motor skills and play skills along with the well-recognized delays in cognitive, social, and language skills in the definition of ASD. The child's motor difficulties often add to the isolation imposed by difficulties with language and social skills. Physical therapy interventions can be used to address not only the motor impairments, but also the participation restrictions caused by these impairments.

Children with ASD can be taking medications for behavioral issues, hyperactivity, and/or depression. Physical therapists should be aware of their indicated effects as well as common adverse drug reactions (ADRs). The most common medications taken to mitigate irritability and aggression are risperidone (Risperdal) and aripiprazole (Abilify). The ADRs that can negatively impact participation in therapeutic activities include sleepiness, constipation, and weight gain.[7] Medications for hyperactivity are only indicated with a dual diagnosis of attention-deficit/hyperactivity disorder (ADHD)[7]; if these drugs are used, therapists should closely monitor vital signs and body mass index (BMI) and discuss any out of range findings for age and sex with the primary care physician. Medication to treat depression is generally given as a last resort because there are few studies investigating their use in children with ASD and the ADRs may outweigh the benefits.[7]

Physical Therapy Patient/Client Management

Physical therapy management of the child with ASD depends on the body structures and functions and activities that are affected. Evaluating each child based on expected developmental milestones, along with a complete history from the family, provides the therapist with the information to begin working with the child on his areas of need. Often, speech pathologists, applied behavioral analysis therapists, and occupational therapists are involved in the care of children with ASD for language, behavior, and sensory concerns. It is important for the physical therapist to communicate with other team members regarding strategies that are successful in allowing the child to increase engagement and participation. Working with other team members is critical because consistency makes learning easier for children with ASD. Given the sensory and perceptual issues often present in children with ASD and their preference for consistency and routine, modifications to service delivery may need to be made. Working with the family to decrease the isolation they may be feeling is also important. Activities can be chosen that are not only therapeutically beneficial, but also helpful for re-integrating the child and family back into the community.

Examination, Evaluation, and Diagnosis

The age of the child determines the specific dysfunctions that are present. However, a complete history can provide insight into the currently observed skills and delays. Often, children later diagnosed with ASD had low muscle tone at birth or difficulty nursing, but did well with the bottle. Many show asymmetries in movement and difficulty with visual attention.[8,9] If the child being evaluated already has a diagnosis of ASD, as is the case with this patient, skills related to bilateral coordination, distal strength, and eye-hand coordination that are appropriate for his age should be assessed.

Outcome measures for motor performance are often used with children with ASD. While some tests have norms for these children, others do not. It is suggested that the selection of the motor assessment not be based on the medical diagnosis, but rather on the *reason* for assessment, whether that is classification, identification, or treatment planning.[10] It has been recommended that when a child is out of the age range for a tool, the raw score should be used and not the standard score. This allows the therapist to show progress, but not compare to normative values.[10]

The **Movement Assessment Battery for Children, Second Edition (MABC-2)** assesses gross and fine motor skills in children in three different age bands (3-6 , 7-10, and 11-16 years). There are eight tasks in each age range and major areas assessed include balance (static and dynamic), ball skills, and manual dexterity.[11] In a study with 30 children with ASD (3-16 years old), their performance on the MABC-2 showed that they were delayed in all three major areas of the MABC-2 compared to age-matched typically developing peers.[12] Another study using the MABC-2 in 101 children with ASD (10-14 years old) showed that 79% showed delays in motor skills and the severity was correlated with lower IQ.[13] Studies of the MABC-2 have shown good reliability and validity, especially in the first age band, which is where the child in this case would fit.[14-16]

The **Bruininks-Oseretsky Test of Motor Proficiency, Second Edition (BOT-2)** uses eight subtests to measure gross and fine motor performance, bilateral coordination, balance, running speed, strength, agility, and manual dexterity in children from

4 to 21 years of age.[17] A 2007 review by Deitz et al.[18] reported that while reliability and validity of the BOT-2 are good, the test is long and can be complicated to score. However, studies comparing the performance of typical children to that of age-matched children with delays—including a group with ASD—have identified significant differences in scores, demonstrating that the tool is valid for identifying motor differences in children with diagnoses.[18] Since this child is currently 3 years old, the BOT-2 would not be appropriate to administer at this time.

There are several tools discussed in the literature that can be used for assessment of participation in children with ASD. One tool that has been shown to have good test-retest reliability when used with children with high-functioning autism is the Children's Assessment of Participation and Enjoyment/Preference for Activities of Children.[19] It may also be useful for older children to assess recreational participation.[20] Although the child in this case is not old enough to benefit from the use of this tool (low end of age range is 6 years), the therapist should be aware of this tool as the child ages.

Plan of Care and Interventions

The plan of care and treatment is based on the specific presentation of the child, the child and family's goals and priorities, and the identified barriers to activities and participation. Goals should focus on activities and participation limitations that are isolating the child and not allowing him to fully participate in activities in which his peers are engaging. Treatment should include meaningful and age-appropriate activities. Since multiple forms of simultaneous input may be overwhelming for the child with ASD, the therapist may choose strategies such as modeling, video modeling, or tactile cueing with limited verbal cueing.

Generally, issues related to strengthening, coordination, and functional play are addressed in a variety of ways. Early literature addressing treatment in children with ASD focused on language and social skills, highlighting the role of working with a speech language pathologist (SLP) and an applied behavioral analyst (ABA).[21] Currently, literature is emerging that recommends addressing coordination, perceptual motor concerns, and play, as well as addressing the links between movement and cognition.[5] Using strategies such as rhythm and music to encourage movement could be beneficial for some children with ASD.[22] Studies have shown that using a rhythmic beat, metronome, or music with a steady pulse can help children with ASD to coordinate movement. For example, for the current 3-year-old patient, the therapist could work on jumping or climbing activities using music with a strong 4/4 beat, or cueing using strong rhythmic words like "go, go, go" to help coordinate each arm movement or foot placement. To encourage continuity, the therapist should discuss treatment strategies with the child's SLP or ABA therapist.

Many children with ASD are receiving **complementary and alternative treatments** (CATs) such as vitamins, melatonin, and specialized diets (*e.g.*, gluten and casein-free). They may also be receiving services such as craniosacral therapy, massage therapy, and auditory integration training from other providers. While physical therapists are not experts in every available CAT, they should be aware of literature regarding these interventions because families may ask for opinions on the current research. In a recent review of research on CATs for ASD, the authors offered several clinical recommendations, emphasizing that families often experiment with many alternative interventions because their children have not responded to evidence-based interventions and/or parents are concerned about the adverse effects of medications.[23] Despite the growing body of research on CATs, the authors concluded that studies vary greatly in sample size and outcomes and many of the randomized control trials (RCTs) lack positive effects or do not provide sufficient evidence to make a judgment about the efficacy of the particular treatment.[23] Based on interventions tested in RCTs that have shown positive results, the authors recommended that clinicians could consider melatonin, multivitamins, massage therapy, acupuncture, exercise, music therapy, or animal-assisted therapy for short-term, monitored trials.[23] Diets such as gluten-free (GF), casein-free (CF), or GFCF combined were not supported in clinical trials,[23-25] although some families report some benefit.

Two specific types of intervention that have gained popularity are aquatics and riding programs. Several studies have used **aquatics as a treatment modality** for children with ASD from 12 months through teen years.[26-29] After several weeks of either group or individual sessions, improvements were noted in swimming skills, movement skills, eye contact, and vocalization. Hypotheses behind the efficacy of aquatics revolve around the properties of water that provide a safe and sensory-rich environment for movement and body awareness, resistance for a strengthening component, and water play being fun. Anecdotally, children who were averse to water (*i.e.*, did not like baths or showers) report enjoying time in the pool and swimming under the water and demonstrate improved engagement during the experience.

Therapeutic riding and hippotherapy programs are increasingly popular and their success may be related to the social aspect of having the animal as a part of the experience. One study investigated the effects of therapeutic riding in 24 children with ASD. After 3 and 6 months of riding, participants showed improved scores on the Childhood Autism Rating Scale (CARS), an observational tool used to identify children with autism based on severity of symptoms.[30] Another study that simulated riding with equipment also showed gains over a 20-week period that was sustained for 6 months.[31]

The therapist working with a child with ASD must consider the child's functional level and how he processes information. Children with ASD are often overwhelmed with multisensory information; providing verbal cueing along with demonstration and tactile cueing, followed by consistent verbal feedback, could be overwhelming to the child. Simple commands, modeling, and allowing time for the child to process are examples of strategies that could be used. Some children with ASD like deep pressure, while others are averse to all types of touch. Therefore, the therapist should be aware of the child's specific perceptual processes when developing treatment strategies. Repetitive practice with small changes can help the child to generalize the skill across situations, but large changes in task may make skill acquisition more difficult.

Evidence-Based Clinical Recommendations

SORT: Strength of Recommendation Taxonomy

A: Consistent, good-quality patient-oriented evidence
B: Inconsistent or limited-quality patient-oriented evidence
C: Consensus, disease-oriented evidence, usual practice, expert opinion, or case series

1. The Movement Assessment Battery for Children, Second Edition (MABC-2) and the Bruininks-Oseretsky Test of Motor Proficiency (BOT-2) are reliable tools that are appropriate to assess motor skills in children with autism spectrum disorder. **Grade A**

2. Select complementary and alternative treatments (CATs) such as melatonin, multivitamins, massage therapy, acupuncture, exercise, music therapy, or animal-assisted therapy appear safe and may improve aspects of behavior in children with ASD. **Grade B**

3. Aquatic therapy improves motor skills and social interaction in children with ASD. **Grade B**

COMPREHENSION QUESTIONS

13.1 Motor impairments in children with ASD typically include all of the following, except:

   A. Low muscle tone

   B. Early difficulty with head control

   C. Early asymmetries in use of arms

   D. Spasticity

13.2 A valid and reliable outcome measure for evaluating bilateral coordination in children with ASD is:

   A. Childhood Autism Rating Scale (CARS)

   B. Bruininks-Oseretsky Test of Motor Proficiency (2nd edition; BOT-2)

   C. Movement Assessment Battery for Children, Second Edition (MABC-2)

   D. Children's Assessment of Participation and Enjoyment/Preference for Activities of Children

13.3 Treatments that are proving effective for children with ASD in improving motor functioning include all of the following except:

   A. Hippotherapy

   B. Aquatics

   C. Repetitive play activities

   D. Antidepressants

ANSWERS

13.1 **D.** Spasticity would indicate an upper motor neuron disorder that is typically not present in children with ASD. Any or all of the other three impairments could be present.

13.2 **B.** The Bruininks-Oseretsky Test of Motor Proficiency (2nd edition; BOT-2) measures not only bilateral coordination, but also gross and fine motor performance, balance, running speed, strength, agility, and manual dexterity. The CARS (option A) is an observational rating scale. The MABC-2 (option C) evaluates movement skills, but does not specifically address bilateral coordination. The Children's Assessment of Participation and Enjoyment/Preference for Activities of Children (option D) evaluates the participation level of the International Classification of Functioning, Disability and Health (ICF), whereas bilateral coordination is at the functional limitation level.

13.3 **D.** There are no good studies evaluating the effectiveness of antidepressant use in children with ASD. Current recommendations are that these medications should be a last resort, after other better-supported interventions.

REFERENCES

1. American Psychiatric Association. *Diagnostic and Statistical Manual of Mental Disorders.* 5th ed. Arlington, VA: American Psychiatric Association; 2013.

2. Centers for Disease Control and Prevention. Autism spectrum disorder: data and statistics. http://www.cdc.gov/ncbddd/autism/data.html. Accessed September 17, 2014.

3. Flanagan JE, Landa R, Bhat A, Bauman M. Head lag in infants at risk for autism: a preliminary study. *Am J Occup Ther.* 2012;66:577-585.

4. Bhat AN, Galloway JC, Landa RJ. Relation between early motor delay and later communication delay in infants at risk for autism. *Infant Behav Dev.* 2012;35:838-846.

5. Lobo MA, Harbourne RT, Dusing SC, McCoy SW. Grounding early intervention: physical therapy cannot just be about motor skills anymore. *Phys Ther.* 2013;93:94-103.

6. Zwaigenbaum L, Bryson S, Lord C, et al. Clinical assessment and management of toddlers with suspected autism spectrum disorder: insights from studies of high-risk infants. *Pediatrics.* 2009;123:1383-1391.

7. Baribeau DA, Anagnostou E. An update on medication management of behavioral disorders in autism. *Curr Psychiatry Rep.* 2014;16:1-13.

8. Bhat AN, Landa RJ, Galloway JC. Current perspectives on motor functioning in infants, children, and adults with autism spectrum disorders. *Phys Ther.* 2011;91:1116-1129.

9. Lane A, Harpster K, Heathcock J. Motor characteristics of young children referred for possible autism spectrum disorder. *Pediatr Phys Ther.* 2012;24:21-29.

10. Staples KL, MacDonald M, Zimmer C. Assessment of motor behavior among children and adolescents with autism spectrum disorder. *Int Rev Res Dev Disabil.* 2012;207:179-214.

11. Henderson SE, Sugden DA. *Movement Assessment Battery for Children.* London: Psychological Corporation; 1992.

12. Liu T, Breslin CM. Fine and gross motor performance of the MABC-2 by children with autism spectrum disorder and typically developing children. *Res Autism Spect Disord.* 2013;7:1244-1249.

13. Green D, Charman T, Pickles A, et al. Impairment in movement skills of children with autistic spectrum disorders. *Dev Med Child Neurol.* 2009;51:311-316.

14. Schoemaker MM, Niemeijer AS, Flapper BC, Smits-Engelsman BC. Validity and reliability of the Movement Assessment Battery for Children-2 Checklist for children with and without motor impairments. *Dev Med Child Neurol.* 2012;54:368-375.

15. Valentini NC, Ramalho MH, Oliveira MA. Movement Assessment Battery for Children-2: translation, reliability, and validity for Brazilian children. *Res Dev Disabil.* 2014;35:733-740.

16. Wuang YP, Su JH, Su CY. Reliability and responsiveness of the Movement Assessment Battery for Children-Second Edition Test in children with developmental coordination disorder. *Dev Med Child Neurol.* 2012;54:160-165.

17. Bruininks R, Bruininks B. *Bruininks-Oseretsky Test of Motor Proficiency, Second Edition (BOT2).* Circle Pines, MN: AGS Publishing; 2005.

18. Deitz JC, Kartin D, Kopp K. Review of the Bruininks-Oseretsky test of motor proficiency, (BOT-2). *Phys Occup Ther Pediatr.* 2007;27:87-102.

19. King GA, Law M, King S, et al. Children's Assessment of Participation and Enjoyment (CAPE) and Preferences for Activities of Children (PAC). *Development.* 2004;33:28-39.

20. Potvin MC, Snider L, Prelock P, Kehayia E, Wood-Dauphinee S. Children's assessment of participation and enjoyment/preference for activities of children: psychometric properties in a population with high-functioning autism. *Am J Occup Ther.* 2013;67:209-217.

21. Rogers SJ. Empirically supported comprehensive treatments for young children with autism. *J Clin Child Psychol.* 1998;27:168-179.

22. LaGasse AB, Hardy MW. Rhythm, movement, and autism: using rhythmic rehabilitation research as a model for autism. *Front Integr Neurosci.* 2013;7:19

23. Lofthouse N, Hendren R, Hurt E, Arnold LE, Butter E. A review of complementary and alternative treatments for autism spectrum disorders. *Autism Res Treat.* 2012;2012:870391.

24. Elder JH, Shankar M, Shuster J, Theriaque D, Burns S, Sherrill L. The gluten-free, casein-free diet in autism: results of a preliminary double blind clinical trial. *J Autism Dev Disord.* 2006;36:413-420.

25. Millward C, Ferriter M, Calver S, Connell-Jones G. Gluten- and casein-free diets for autistic spectrum disorder. *Cochrane Database Syst Rev.* 2008;2:CD003498.

26. Fragala-Pinkham MA, Haley SM, O'Neil ME. Group swimming and aquatic exercise programme for children with autism spectrum disorders: a pilot study. *Dev Neurorehabil.* 2011;14:230-241.

27. Ennis E. The effects of a physical therapy-directed aquatic program on children with autism pectrum disorders. *J Aquatic Phys Ther.* 2011;19:4-10.

28. Getz M, Hutzler Y, Vermeer A. Effects of aquatic interventions in children with neuromotor impairments: a systematic review of the literature. *Clin Rehabil.* 2006;20:927-936.

29. Oriel KN, Marchese VG, Shirk A, Wagner L, Young E, Miller L. The psychosocial benefits of an inclusive community-based aquatics program. *Pediatr Phys Ther.* 2012;24:361-367.

30. Kern JK, Fletcher CL, Garver CR, et al. Prospective trial of equine-assisted activities in autism spectrum disorder. *Altern Ther Health Med.* 2011;3:14-20.

31. Wuang YP, Wang CC, Huang MH, Su CY. The effectiveness of simulated developmental horse-riding program in children with autism. *Adapt Phys Activ Q.* 2010;27:113-126.

Anterior Neck Burn

Meri Goehring

A previously healthy 3-year-old boy was taken to the emergency department by ambulance. The child had tipped a pan off the stove and hot grease poured over his chin and anterior neck. He sustained thermal injury due to a scald burn with a mix of superficial, superficial and deep partial thickness, and full thickness burn depth. The parents immediately called 911. While waiting for the ambulance to arrive, the mother attempted to put a towel moistened with ice water over the wound but the child vigorously resisted any attempt to touch the burned area. She then poured honey over the wound. When the ambulance arrived, the mother told the emergency medical technicians that she had heard that honey was good for burns. While en route to the hospital, intravenous fluids were begun and the child received a low dose of morphine for pain control. The emergency department physician consulted the wound care nurse, but this incident occurred early Saturday morning and the wound care nurse would not be available to provide a consultation until Monday. The physician ordered physical therapy for immediate examination of the type and size of burn as well as treatment of the burn with recommendations for dressings. There was also an order for whirlpool treatment to clean the wound. The emergency department physician informed the physical therapist that the child will be airlifted to a verified burn center after initial physical therapy examination and treatment. The parents are distraught because they had been encouraging the child to participate in cooking on other occasions and felt that their neglect of the child caused the burn to occur. They are very concerned about the child's welfare and have many questions regarding the healing process and the treatments involved.

- ▶ What are the examination priorities?
- ▶ Is there any indication of abuse in this case?
- ▶ How can the level of pain and function best be examined with this child?
- ▶ Is whirlpool an appropriate treatment modality at this time?
- ▶ What are appropriate outcome measures, assuming the child may be going to a burn unit?
- ▶ Describe the physical therapy plan of care.

KEY DEFINITIONS

BURN CLASSIFICATION: Burn injuries are classified by etiology, depth, and size of the burn.

DEEP PARTIAL THICKNESS BURN: Epidermis and papillary and reticular layers of dermis involved; wound is typically moist, painful, swollen, and red; if deeper, wound can appear pale or white; commonly heals within 21 to 35 days, though often needs grafting; may cause scarring[1]

DONOR SITE: Area of unburned healthy skin that is harvested and grafted onto burned area; skin is typically harvested using a surgical instrument known as a dermatome, but newer instruments are being investigated that assist with skin harvesting and do not require surgery.[2]

EXCISION OF BURN WOUND: Surgical procedure of removing eschar, which must be done to help prepare wound bed for skin grafting

FULL THICKNESS BURN: Epidermis and all dermal layers involved with potential damage to subcutaneous fat, but not to fascia or muscle; wound is dry, firm, and leathery and can range from white or pale yellow to dark red or black; wound is not painful since nerve endings are destroyed, but surrounding healthy or less burned tissue may be painful; often takes several weeks to heal and usually requires skin grafting; scarring expected

SKIN GRAFT: Section of skin that is surgically removed from a non-burned, healthy area of the body to cover an area of burned skin that has been prepared for the graft; harvested graft usually contains only the epidermis and papillary dermis (*i.e.*, superficial partial thickness graft or split-thickness graft); a full thickness skin graft includes the epidermis and entire dermal layer. Because the harvested area will also need grafting, full thickness grafts are typically limited to small areas. Temporary skin grafts include skin harvested from another species (*i.e.*, pig) or from a human cadaver.

SUBDERMAL BURN: Epidermis, dermis, subcutaneous fat as well as fascia, muscle, and deeper tissue (muscles, nerves, bones) may be involved; appearance is variable depending on cause; damaged tissue is not painful, but surrounding tissues may be painful; takes several weeks or longer and requires surgical intervention and/or skin grafting; scarring expected

SUPERFICIAL BURN: Only epidermal layer of skin involved (*e.g.*, sunburn without blisters); wound is typically dry, red, painful, and presents with minimal edema; commonly heals within 2 to 5 days without scarring

SUPERFICIAL PARTIAL THICKNESS BURN: Epidermis and papillary layer of dermis involved; wound is typically moist, red, blistered, and painful, and presents with some edema; commonly heals within 7 to 14 days without scarring

Objectives

1. Identify the most reliable method of evaluating the size and type of burn in children.
2. Describe the optimal method for cleaning a neck wound in a young child.

3. Identify the most appropriate methods of positioning and handling the awake or sleeping child with a burn.

4. Identify a reliable and valid method of determining a young child's level of pain.

Physical Therapy Considerations

PT considerations during management of the young child with an anterior neck burn:

► **General physical therapy plan of care/goals:** Promote healing; prevent/minimize loss of range of motion (ROM), strength, and aerobic functional capacity; maximize physical function and safety; minimize secondary impairments such as infection and/or excessive scarring; return to daily functional activities including play and a reasonable home exercise program that can be incorporated into daily care of the child; optimize parent and/or caregiver education and health-related quality of life

► **Physical therapy interventions:** Family/caregiver education regarding burn wounds and the healing process, risk of infection and procedure for dressing changes, risk of contracture and scarring, proper hygiene and wound management, proper handling of child including positioning for carrying, sleeping, and meals; multidisciplinary communication, especially hand-off of information to other healthcare professionals

► **Precautions during physical therapy:** Use of proper infection control techniques; monitor skin during wound care; maintain safety of child during positioning and dressing changes to prevent excessive pain and/or additional injury (*e.g.*, falls, bruising)

► **Complications interfering with physical therapy:** Infection; respiratory problems due to location of burn; emotional distress of child and family/caregivers

Understanding the Health Condition

Scald burns result from contact with hot liquids or steam. This type of burn can occur due to immersion of the body in a liquid or from splashing, pouring, or spilling hot liquid on the body. Scald burns are the most common burns in children 5 years of age and younger.[3] The pattern of a scald burn should match the parent or caregiver's description of the scalding incident because a lack of correspondence suggests the possibility of abuse.[3] Abuse by burning may comprise 6% to 20% of all child abuse cases in the United States.[4] Scald burns are often accidental and occur on the head, neck, or trunk when a hot liquid falls from a higher surface and spills over the child. Accidental burns are often patchy with mixed burn depths as the child quickly withdraws from the heat source. Distinguishing between accident and abuse can be difficult as both inflicted and accidental splash and spill burns have irregular margins and variable depths.[3] It is important that every healthcare provider listens carefully to the description of the accident as given by the observer and/or caregiver. The description of the injury should match the injury. Information that is not consistent with the injury may indicate an intentionally inflicted burn.

There are many physiologic changes that occur after a burn. Anticipated changes include cardiovascular effects, increased metabolism, increased risk of infection, and pulmonary complications, as well as pain and associated anxiety. Cardiovascular effects are primarily caused by a fluid shift from the vascular system to the skin and tissues surrounding the burn, resulting in edema. This fluid shift occurs primarily in the first 24 hours after the burn injury. Typically, intravenous fluids are given during this period to reduce the resulting hypovolemia that occurs as body water moves from intravascular to extravascular tissues.[1] Although extra fluid [2-4 mL/kg/percentage of total body surface area (TBSA) burned using the Parkland formula[5]] can be critical to maintain blood pressure in burns, intravenous fluid also contributes to the edema, therefore careful observation of circumferential burns is important to ensure that circulation is not compromised. Metabolic rate increases after a burn because of the body's attempt to initiate healing and reduce bacterial load. Heart rate elevates to adequately manage reduced vascular volume and to meet increased cardiac output demands. As a result, caloric needs are increased. It is common for a dietician to be a part of the team to determine appropriate caloric intake; blood work is often used to ensure adequate levels of protein and/or specific vitamins or minerals (e.g., vitamin E, zinc). With damage or loss of skin, the body's primary external defense to infection is breached. Thus, there is a high risk of infection in individuals with burns. The surface of the burn wound is an avascular, warm, protein-laden environment that is ideal for microbial propagation.[1] Necrotic tissue on the wound surface also impedes oxygen delivery and prolongs healing. If there are comorbid issues such as respiratory complications and/or increased metabolism, there may be a decreased immune response from the burn victim. If there is an infection, healing times are longer and scarring is more likely. Infections at the burn surface can lead to systemic infections requiring pharmacologic interventions that often cause adverse effects. Therefore, prevention of infections is key in burn care; a clean wound provided with the optimal environment to heal as quickly as possible is the best prevention against infection. Environmental control measures include use of standard precautions, appropriate wound care, antimicrobial topical agents (if indicated), sterile debridement tools and dressings, and clean linens. However, infections can also come from microorganisms on the patient (e.g., from normal flora on undamaged skin) and are common even when strict environmental control procedures are consistently followed.

Physical Therapy Patient/Client Management

A multidisciplinary team can best manage a child with a wound or burn. The American Burn Association has specified that children with burns who are initially treated in hospitals without qualified personnel or equipment for the care of children should be transferred to a verified burn center.[6] In this case, the team would include physicians, nurses, physical therapist (and possibly a physical therapist assistant), occupational therapist, dietician, and a social worker. One of the nurses or therapists may have a specialization in wound or burn care, but this is not always the case. Other possible team members include physician assistant, surgeon, and psychologist. A religious or spiritual leader (*e.g.*, rabbi, priest, minister) may also be a member of the team. The therapist should be aware of the specific needs of children and use examination and evaluation tools that are age-appropriate. Even when the child is medically unstable due to pain, the extent and location of the burn, and careful administration of intravenous fluids, it is essential to involve and educate the parents. The therapist works with the family to inform them of the plan of care and potential healing times for the burn. In this case, the foremost goal for the therapist is to examine and treat the burn itself and provide a clean wound bed while keeping the child as medically stable as possible. Proper wound care and medical management takes priority in the initial stages of burn care. Once the child is medically stable, the therapist becomes more involved in observing the child's functional movement and impairments. As the child nears hospital discharge, therapists will be involved in educating parents and/or other providers such as home health physical therapists and/or nurses on: wound management (*e.g.*, dressing changes), ROM activities, the function, fit, and use of pressure garments (if indicated), positioning, transfers, and scar management.

Examination, Evaluation, and Diagnosis

Since this child will be airlifted to a verified burn center later that day, all decisions and treatments need to be made in an organized and efficient manner in order to provide the best care. The immediate need is to **evaluate and treat** to provide optimal pain relief and prevent unnecessary wound exposure that could lead to infection. History taking should focus on determining how the burn injury occurred. The parents in this case expressed a clear and precise description of how the injury occurred that corresponded with the location of the burn, making abuse less likely.[3] Prior to the physical therapy examination, the child would have already been assessed for problems with airway, breathing, or circulation. The medical condition of the child must be monitored at all times. Temperature, heart rate, respiratory rate, blood pressure, and oxygen saturation levels should be monitored and recorded. Any first aid rendered prior to arrival at the emergency department should be documented. In this case, the therapist noted the mother's use of honey over the wound. General observation of the child should include whether he is in generally good condition (*e.g.*, cleanliness of his hair, nails, and clothing). In addition, the physical therapist should ask whether the child has reached the normal developmental milestones for his age. Last, the therapist should note whether the child is crying, withdrawn, whimpering, or calm. Since the emergency department physician specifically asked for whirlpool to clean the burn wound, the therapist needs to evaluate the appropriateness of this intervention at this time and discuss any recommendations with the rest of the team. Timing of burn care, including the physical therapy examination, should be carefully coordinated with the administration of pain medications.

There are two classic ways to measure the extent, or TBSA, of the burn. The first is the Rule of Nines, which is often used for a quick estimate and in triage situations. This method estimates the surface area of the body by dividing the body into 11 different areas, each equal to 9% with the final 1% for the genitalia. The second method to calculate TBSA is by using the Lund-Browder chart. This method is more time-consuming than the Rule of Nines; however, it accounts for the different shape and size of body segments based on age. This method is thought to provide a more accurate estimation of the size of the burn and is recommended for use with children.[1] Newer computer-aided systems are being developed that may result in improved precision and accuracy in determining TBSA.[7] The physical therapist may be the person to estimate the size of the burn when other available health care professionals such as a wound/ostomy nurse or physician who are trained to do so are not available.

The depth of the burn is determined by visual inspection. Different depths of tissue damage must be documented. The tissue depth categorizes the burn wound as superficial, superficial partial thickness, deep partial thickness, full thickness, or subdermal. Photography can be of great assistance to document wound size, color, depth, and extent. It also allows the therapist to carefully inspect the wound, since it can be very difficult to get a small child to remain still for a thorough visual inspection especially when he is in pain. For the physical therapist, it is critical to evaluate the *distribution* of a burn injury across any joints. In this case, the burn covers the anterior surface of the neck, crossing multiple joints of the cervical spine. The physical therapist should help adequately position the child (in neutral or slight cervical extension) to help prevent the development of contractures. Later, the physical therapist provides recommendations for splinting in coordination with other health care professionals (*e.g.*, occupational therapist) and provides adequate ROM across the burned joints.

Evaluation of pain is especially important with burn injuries. Since this child is 3 years old, it is unlikely he will be able to rate his pain on a standard verbal pain scale. Children often lack the verbal and cognitive skills necessary to provide a good description of their pain. Therefore, behavioral and physiologic measures are recommended. The **Face, Legs, Activity, Cry, Consolability (FLACC) scale** is a well-established behavioral pain assessment tool that can be very useful with children between the ages of 2 months and 7 years. This scale consists of the five categories in its name and provides a simple and consistent method of pain assessment. Each category is scored between 0 and 2; the total score is between 0 and 10, with 0 indicating the least pain and 10 the most pain. For example, in the Activity category, a score of 1 indicates the child is lying quietly, normal position, and moves easily, whereas a score of 2 indicates squirming, shifting back and forth, and tense. A score of 1 would be given for a child who is arched, rigid, or jerking. The FLACC scale is reliable and valid in critically ill children unable to self-report pain.[8]

Plan of Care and Interventions

The main goals of treatment are to prevent infection, restore function to the burned area, and promote full physical, psychologic, and emotional recovery from the burn. First, the therapist must decide the appropriateness of the whirlpool intervention ordered by the physician to clean the burn wound that is covered in honey. If it is determined that whirlpool is inappropriate for this patient, the therapist must decide on the best way to clean and debride the wound. Whirlpool is a form of non-selective debridement that can be used to help remove loosely adherent necrotic tissue, surface bacteria, and foreign debris. In order to completely access the burns, this child would need to be immersed into the whirlpool up to neck level. This would make whirlpool treatment less safe as the child is at risk of getting his head underwater and/or swallowing water. Whirlpool is also contraindicated in individuals who are incontinent of bowel and/or bladder.[9] Although a 3-year-old child may be toilet trained, it is doubtful that he has complete bowel and bladder control, especially in the face of such a painful event. Furthermore, there is an increased risk of infection with whirlpool hydrotherapy due to cross-contamination.[10,11] The physical therapist decided that the risks of infection and difficulty with safe positioning outweighed the benefits of using the whirlpool to clean and debride the wound. **Common practice in most burn centers is to shower off the wound using tap water**[9] between 92°F and 98°F. An alternative is pulsed lavage, which involves the regular, automatic interruption of fluid flow with a hand-held device that regulates the irrigation pressure. Negative pressure suction occurs simultaneously to remove the irrigation liquid. Typically, the irrigation is performed with saline. Pulsed lavage is often indicated in wounds that have deep areas or tunneling, or a large amount of necrotic tissue to remove. However, there is no evidence to indicate that this type of wound cleaning and debridement is safe on the more inherently fragile skin of a child. Another option is the use of non-contact, low-frequency ultrasound. This device often uses a low-pressure saline spray. However, there is also no evidence to support use of low-frequency ultrasound in children. Therefore, the therapist chose to clean and mechanically debride the wound with saline-soaked gauze by gently wiping the area to remove the honey and any necrotic tissue. It should be emphasized that this type of manual mechanical debridement must be done gently so no further tissue damage is caused.

After cleaning and debridement, a decision needs to be made regarding the type of topical ointment and dressings used to cover the wound. This should be performed in cooperation with the physician and nursing staff. Dressings must absorb drainage, protect the wound from trauma, allow ROM and function of the entire neck, and control edema. Topical antimicrobial ointments covered with secondary dressings are often the treatment of choice with burn wounds. This is because prevention of infection is important with these open areas. Silver sulfadiazine (Silvadene) cream is the most commonly used topical antibacterial because it is effective against a large number of bacteria.[9] The disadvantage of this cream is that it is somewhat difficult to remove from the wound during dressing changes. However, since this child will be transported to a burn center, the therapist determined that adequate resources would be available to provide further cleaning as needed. Next, the therapist chose a dressing to cover the cream and keep the wound moist. Xeroform, a sterile nonadherent bismuth- and petrolatum-impregnated gauze, is a good choice because it has added bacteriostatic effects. This was placed over the Silvadene cream and the entire area was covered loosely with rolled gauze. Lightly wrapped elastic bandages or surgical netting that goes over the top of the head can be used to keep the dressings in place over the chin, since the chin is difficult to effectively cover with gauze. If surgical netting is used, this should be changed with each dressing change. If elastic bandages are used, these can be hand washed and dried flat and kept away from sunshine. Every effort should be taken to keep the child from removing the dressings, which may entail use of hand mitts at night or when the child is unattended for short periods. Positioning and exercise are also very important to the burn victim. Since the patient is imminently being transferred to a burn center, these are not the foremost goals. Once the child reaches the burn center, therapists in that facility will address contracture prevention by keeping the child's neck positioned in slight cervical extension and emphasizing movement of the affected area once the child is medically stable.

Beginning at this early stage, communication with the parents is important. The parents need to be informed of the pain-reducing efforts undertaken by the healthcare team and how they can be involved as much as possible. Even when the child is medically unstable due to medication-induced sedation and/ or the need for careful intravenous fluid management, involving the parents can enhance recovery and promote empowerment. It is important to provide clear, concise information regarding how the wound needs to be cleaned and dressed because the parents will need to perform cleaning and dressing changes once the child returns home. Information regarding what may happen in the burn center, what to expect in terms of healing times, and the prognosis for recovery can help reduce anxiety.[12]

Evidence-Based Clinical Recommendations

SORT: Strength of Recommendation Taxonomy

A: Consistent, good-quality patient-oriented evidence
B: Inconsistent or limited-quality patient-oriented evidence
C: Consensus, disease-oriented evidence, usual practice, expert opinion or case series

1. Immediate priorities in children with burns include evaluation and treatment to provide optimal pain relief and prevent unnecessary wound exposure that could lead to infection. **Grade C**

2. The Face, Legs, Activity, Cry, Consolability (FLACC) scale is an established behavioral pain assessment tool that is reliable and valid in critically ill children unable to self-report pain. **Grade B**

3. For wound cleaning and debridement of an anterior neck burn in a young child, tap water or saline with gentle mechanical gauze debridement is an optimal choice over submersion in a whirlpool. **Grade C**

COMPREHENSION QUESTIONS

14.1 Which of the following statements regarding burns in children is *most* accurate?

A. Abuse by burning comprises approximately 50% to 70% of all child abuse cases.

B. Scald burns are the most common cause of burns in children age 12 years and younger.

C. Caregiver incident description that does not match the burn pattern may suggest abuse.

D. The Lund-Browder chart estimates burn size by dividing the body into 10 areas, each representing 10% of the body surface area.

14.2 Which statements is *not* accurate regarding infected burns?

A. Healing times will be longer.

B. There is an increased risk of scarring.

C. There is an increased risk of systemic problems.

D. Surgery will be needed to clean the burn.

14.3 What is the best water temperature to clean a burn wound?

A. 98.6°F

B. 94°F

C. 78°F

D. 100°F

ANSWERS

14.1 **C.** Caregiver incident description should match the burn injury or abuse may be involved. Abuse by burning comprises only 6% to 20% of burn injuries in children (option A). Scald burns are most common at age 5 years and younger, not 12 years and younger (option B). The Lund-Browder chart allows the burn to be estimated by percentage of body part based on age (option D).

14.2 **D.** With infected burns, healing time may be longer, the risk of scarring is increased, and the risk for systemic infection increases. Infected burns do not necessarily mean that surgery is needed.

14.3 **B.** The correct water temperature for cleaning the wound should be between 92°F and 98°F.

REFERENCES

1. Sussman C, Bates-Jensen B. *Wound Care*. 4th ed. Philadelphia, PA: Lippincott, Williams and Wilkins; 2012:401-411.

2. Laxmisha C, Thappa DM. Surgical Pearl: gloved finger as a transport platform for epidermal graft of suction blister. *J Am Acad Dermatol*. 2007;57:S118-S119.

3. Ermertcan AT, Ertan P. Skin manifestations of child abuse. *Indian J Dermatol Venereol Leprol.* 2010;76:317-326.

4. Hight DW, Bakalar HR, Lloyd JR. Inflicted burns in children: recognition and treatment. *JAMA.* 1979;242:517-520.

5. Bak Z, Sjoberg F, Eriksson O, Steinvall I, Janerot-Sjoberg B. Hemodynamic changes during resuscitation after burns using the Parkland formula. *J Trauma.* 2009;66:329-336.

6. Burn Center Referral Criteria. http://www.ameriburn.org/BurnCenterReferralCriteria.pdf. Accessed August 27, 2014.

7. Giretlehner M, Dirnberger J, Owen R, Haller HL, Lumenta DB, Kamolz LP. The determination of total burn surface area: how much difference? *Burns.* 2013;29:1101-1113.

8. Voepel-Lewis T, Zanotti J, Dammeyer JA, Merkel S. Reliability and validity of the face, legs, activity, cry, consolability behavioral tool in assessing acute pain in critically ill patients. *Am J Crit Care.* 2010;19:55-61.

9. Myers BA. *Wound Management: Principles and Practice.* 3rd ed. Upper Saddle River, NJ: Pearson; 2012:321-346.

10. Stanwood W, Pinzur MS. Risk of contamination of the wound in a hydrotherapeutic tank. *Foot Ankle Int.* 1998;19:173-176.

11. Hollyoak V, Boyd P, Freeman R. Whirlpool baths in nursing homes: use, maintenance, and contamination with Pseudomonas aeruginosa. *Commun Dis Rep CDR Rev.* 1995;5:R102-R104.

12. Hollywood E, O'Neill T. Assessment and management of scalds and burns in children. *Nurs Child Young People.* 2014;26:28-33.

Palmar Hand Burn

David John Lorello

The patient is a 2-year-old female, who sustained a 1% total body surface area (TBSA) deep partial thickness burn to the left palm, left lateral thumb, and the volar surface of the middle and distal phalanx of digits 2 to 4 (Fig. 15-1). The patient sustained the burns when she placed her hand on the surface of a glass-covered fireplace. Current plans are to treat the injury conservatively with twice daily dressing changes of silver sulfadiazine cream, gauze, and burn netting. The physical therapist is examining the patient in the emergency department prior to the patient's admission to the hospital.

▶ What are the examination priorities?
▶ Based on her health condition, what do you anticipate will be contributors to activity limitations?
▶ What are the most appropriate physical therapy interventions?
▶ Describe a physical therapy plan of care based on each stage of wound healing.

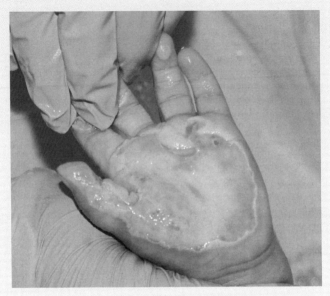

Figure 15-1. 1% total body surface area (TBSA) deep partial thickness burn to the left palm, left lateral thumb, and the volar surface of the middle and distal phalanx of digits 2 to 4. The burn is blistered and peeling, and mottled white in color with some yellow eschar present. The burn appears wet because the photo was taken during a dressing change and had just been cleaned.

KEY DEFINITIONS

AUTOGRAFT: Skin that is taken from an unburned area of the patient and transplanted to cover an injured area of the same patient

CONTRACTURE: Loss of range of motion (ROM) over a joint

SILVER SULFADIAZINE: Also known as Silvadene, or AgSD; broad-spectrum antimicrobial topical cream often used for treating burn wounds; effective against gram-negative and gram-positive bacteria; short-term effectiveness and typically needs to be changed twice per day

Objectives

1. Describe the classification of burn injuries.
2. Understand burn wound physiology, including systems affected and the phases of wound healing.
3. Describe the appropriate plan of care for each phase of wound healing.

Physical Therapy Considerations

PT considerations during management of the toddler with a palmar hand burn:

▶ **General physical therapy plan of care/goals:** Prevent loss of ROM/contracture; achieve pre-injury level of strength and maximize functional independence with activities of daily living (ADLs)

▶ **Physical therapy interventions:** ROM exercises, stretching, splinting and positioning, resistive exercise, training in ADLs, patient and family education regarding exercise and splint-wearing schedule

▶ **Precautions during physical therapy:** Postsurgical limitations, if applicable

▶ **Complications interfering with physical therapy:** Compartment syndrome, hypertrophic scarring

Understanding the Health Condition

Although the hand constitutes a small percentage of the overall total skin surface area (<3%), there is an inherent potential for permanent functional deficits as a result of a hand burn. For this reason, the American Burn Association has designated burns that involve the hands as one of their referral criteria for who should be transferred to a verified burn center.[1] For the therapist treating patients with burn injuries, it is helpful to consider the hand as an "organ" of the body consisting of thin, highly mobile skin on the dorsal surface, thicker, sensory-enriched skin on the palmar surface, and a delicately balanced musculotendinous system.[2] Burn injuries to these areas can have significant damaging effects for the patient. The treating therapist should have a thorough knowledge of the anatomy and physiology of the integumentary system, wound healing, and wound care.

In 2013, the National Burn Repository (NBR) reported that approximately 52,000 children (0-15.9 years old) sustained burn injuries between the years 2003 and 2011 that required inpatient treatment at a specialized burn center.[3] This statistic does not include those individuals that did not require hospital admission and were treated on an outpatient basis. According to the NBR, 75% of the individuals treated by burn centers are treated as outpatients. For children ages 0 to 4.9 years, the majority of these burns were caused by scalding, closely followed by contact with hot objects. It is not until the ages of 5 to 15.9 years when flame burns are the most prevalent. It is not surprising that scald and contact burns are most common for this very young population because this is the time when children are exploring their world and often reach out and grab or touch things they should not.[4] This exploratory behavior in combination with slower reflexes and thinner skin puts young children at risk for more severe burns at lower temperatures.[4-6]

As the largest organ of the body, the skin protects the body from infection and injury, prevents the loss of body fluid, regulates body temperature, receives external stimuli, serves as an indicator of internal events (e.g., erythema seen in the skin as a result of infection), and helps to determine one's identity. Burn injuries can cause a loss to some or all of these functions.

Knowledge of epidermal and dermal skin layers helps determine how to classify the depth of a burn injury. The skin is composed of the epidermis, dermis, and the subcutaneous tissue beneath which are fascia, muscles, tendons, ligaments, nerves, bone, and organs. The most superficial layer, the epidermis, has a thickness that varies from 0.05 mm to 1.5 mm. This avascular structure receives its necessary cellular nutrients from the vascular plexus within the deeper dermis.[7,8] There are five layers within the epidermis: stratum corneum, stratum lucidum (found only in the palms of the hand and soles of the feet), stratum granulosum, stratum spinosum, and stratum basale.[7-9] The deepest layer of the epidermis, the stratum basale, contains the keratinocytes that produce the protective protein keratin. Other important cells within the epidermis are melanocytes, Merkel cells (mechanoreceptors that provide information on light touch), and Langerhans cells (dendritic cells that regulate immune responses in the skin).[7-10]

Important structures within the epidermis include hair follicles (lined with epithelium that are continuous with the epidermis), sebaceous glands (contained within the hair follicle and produce sebum that lubricates the skin and hair), and sudoriferous glands (secrete sweat to assist the body in dissipating heat and cooling the body).[7-9] The basement membrane is an area of connective tissue between the epidermis and dermis that acts as scaffolding where ridges in the epidermis fit within projections in the dermis. This series of ridges and projections are known as rete pegs and dermal papillae, respectively; the rete pegs anchor the dermis to the epidermis to prevent shearing forces.[7-9]

Beneath the epidermis is the thicker dermis. It can range in thickness from 2 mm to 4 mm. It is a highly vascularized layer providing nutrition to both the dermis and epidermis. The dermis consists of two distinct layers. The papillary dermis is the top layer and it conforms to the epidermis. The deeper, thicker layer is the reticular dermis that contains collagen bundles that provide the skin with its extensibility.[7-9] Important structures within the dermis include smooth muscle that causes hair follicles to elevate (*i.e.*, goose bumps), blood vessels that provide nutrition and help in thermoregulation, lymphatic vessels, and afferent nerve fibers that supply sensory information on temperature, pain, touch, itch, and pressure.[7-9] Beneath the dermis is a subcutaneous layer consisting of connective tissue and adipose tissue that provides energy, cushioning, and insulation to deeper structures.[7-9]

Burn injuries are classified based on the mechanism, depth, and size of the injury. The six primary mechanisms of injury are scald, flame, contact, chemical, electrical, and radiation. Knowing the mechanism of injury can help give a physical therapist clues as to how severe an injury may be. Mechanisms that generate higher temperatures will cause greater injury. For example, skin exposed to water at 158°F for 1 second can cause a deep partial thickness burn.[11] Hot grease can typically be greater than 350°F.[8] Oils and melted sugars can remain at higher temperatures for longer periods of time than plain water. Therefore, soups, broths, and coffees may cause deeper burns than hot water.[12,13]

Classification of burn depth is based on how much destruction the burn causes to the epidermis, dermis, and/or underlying structures. These classifications are known as superficial, superficial partial thickness, deep partial thickness, and full thickness.[14] Superficial burns only involve the epidermis. The skin appears red with no blistering. It can take 3 to 7 days to heal as the outer epidermal cells peel away. An example of this type of burn would be a painful sunburn.[14-16] Superficial partial thickness burns involve the entire epidermis as well as the papillary (top) layer of the dermis. The appearance is red, moist, and weepy. Blisters may be present. The wound blanches easily. These are extremely painful burns because nerve endings in the dermis are exposed or damaged. Since the deeper structures of the dermis are intact, the superficial partial thickness wound typically heals within 7 to 21 days with minimal scarring.[14-16] A deep partial thickness burn involves not only the epidermis and papillary layers of the dermis, but also the reticular layer of the dermis. It can appear mottled white, pink, or deep red. Blisters are large, and the burn can still be very painful, since many nociceptors remain intact. Because some hair follicles and sebaceous glands remain undamaged, the wound may be able to re-epithelialize. However, if the burn is large, or is predicted to take longer than 21 days to heal, a physician may consider skin grafting to achieve faster wound closure. Deep partial thickness burns are at risk for hypertrophic scarring and contracture. With poor nutrition or infection, these burns are at risk of converting to full thickness.[14-16] Full thickness burns involve the epidermis, the entire dermis, and the subcutaneous tissue. They appear white, yellow, or brown, charred, and/or leathery. Because all of the blood vessels have thrombosed and the nociceptors and other skin receptors have been destroyed by the burn injury, the wound is dry and there is little to no pain. Since the hair follicles are destroyed, any remaining hairs will pull out easily. If the wound is very small, it may be allowed to heal on its own by epithelial in-growth, but most often these wounds require surgical debridement and skin grafting. Full thickness wounds are also at risk for hypertrophic scarring and contracture.[14-16] Subdermal burns are burns that extend deep past the dermis into the underlying structures such as fat, muscle, and bone.[9] These burns are often difficult to treat and require extensive surgical intervention including debridement, grafting, and sometimes amputation.[9]

In addition to the depth of a burn, the percentage of TBSA of a burn must be calculated. Only areas of partial thickness and full thickness injury are included in the calculation. Methods of calculating TBSA include the Rule of Nines and the Lund-Browder classification.[9] The Rule of Nines is a simple way to calculate TBSA, but this method is not accurate when calculating the TBSA of a burn of a child or infant. The Lund-Browder classification system is a more accurate system of calculating TBSA with infants and children because it accounts for the fact that a child's head represents a larger area and the lower limbs a smaller area than in an adult.[9]

Wound healing can be divided into three phases: inflammatory, proliferative, and remodeling/maturation.[9] The inflammatory phase begins at the time of injury and can last 2 to 5 days. There is an immediate vascular response: vasoconstriction to stop bleeding shortly followed by vasodilation to bring nutrients to the surrounding tissues.[9,17-19] There is also a cellular response in which neutrophils and macrophages begin to rid the wound of bacteria and foreign debris. The wound is characterized by redness, edema, warmth, pain, and decreased ROM.[9,17,18] The proliferative phase begins around the 3rd to 5th day after injury and can last up to 3 weeks. It is characterized by angiogenesis (formation of new blood vessels), granulation tissue formation (fibroblasts enter the wound and produce extracellular matrix of collagen and elastin, appearing as moist, red tissue within the wound bed), wound contraction (myofibroblasts pull wound margins together), and epithelialization (keratinocytes at wound margins and within hair follicles migrate across the wound).[9,17-19] The end of epithelialization marks the beginning of the remodeling/maturation phase. This final phase can last from 6 months to 3 years. During this time, collagen bonds strengthen and fibers align more parallel in formation. New collagen is being created in the wound, while older collagen is being removed (collagen turnover). Collagen synthesis should be equal to collagen degradation during this phase—leaving a flat, pliable scar. If collagen synthesis is greater than collagen degradation, then hypertrophic scarring can occur.[9,18]

All phases of wound healing require oxygen. Burns develop necrotic tissue on the wound surface that impedes oxygen delivery, supports bacteria, encourages infection, and prolongs healing. More superficial burns can be healed using a variety of different wound dressings that simply need to provide a clean and moist healing environment. Full thickness burns typically require surgical removal. When it is determined that a burn wound will take longer than 21 days to heal, surgical intervention is required because these burns are at an increased risk for hypertrophic scarring and contracture.[20] Removal of eschar through tangential excision allows a surgeon to preserve underlying tissue.[15,17,18] In tangential excision, the surgeon debrides thin layers of burned tissue until healthy, viable tissue is reached.[15,18] Once the burned tissue has been removed, the wound needs to be covered by new skin. Sometimes the excised wound bed is not healthy enough to accept the patient's own skin, or with larger TBSA burns, the patient may not have enough unburned skin to cover the large surface area of injury. In these instances, temporary grafts are used. Cadaver skin (known as allograft or homograft) or porcine skin (xenograft) may be used until a donor site (area of unburned skin) is available or when the wound is healthy enough to graft with the patient's own skin (autograft).[9,15,17,18]

In addition to length of time to heal, other factors increase a patient's risk for abnormal scarring. Infection, young age, darker pigmented skin, burn location (sternum, upper back, and shoulder), and areas of tension (shoulder and upper back) are all risk factors for hypertrophic scars.[20] To decrease the likelihood of hypertrophic scarring, the hand is one of the areas that is autografted as soon as possible. For dorsal hand burns, the surgeon typically uses a split-thickness skin graft (contains the epidermis and a small layer of dermis[21]). If enough unburned skin is available (e.g., a small TBSA burn), the surgeon will use a sheet graft.[5] A sheet graft is an autograft that is not altered in any way after it is harvested. If there is not enough skin available, the harvested skin will be meshed with a mechanical meshing instrument. When available, it is always best to use a sheet graft because sheet grafts have a better cosmetic appearance and are less likely to develop contracture.[17,22] For palmar burns or isolated finger burns, the burn surgeon may elect to utilize a full-thickness graft.[4,5,23,24] A full-thickness graft contains the epidermis and entire dermis.[21] The full-thickness portion of skin is taken from an area with excess skin, like the groin, so that the donor area can be primarily closed with the use of sutures.[9,21]

Physical Therapy Patient/Client Management

A successful outcome for the patient depends on a team effort to ensure timely healing. The burn team consists of the patient and her family, general and plastic surgeons, physician extenders such as physician assistants and nurse practitioners, nurses, dieticians, clinical pharmacologists, respiratory therapists, child life specialists, physical and occupational therapists, speech language pathologists, psychologists, case managers, social workers, and researchers. Although the entire burn team may not be involved in individuals with smaller burns, it is important for the physical therapist to communicate with the team if needs arise, so that appropriate timely intervention can be initiated. Physical therapy examination is often initiated within 24 hours of admission to the hospital. Treatments begin immediately thereafter, and a plan of care is formulated for every phase of wound healing. Management includes preventing loss of ROM, strengthening, and maximizing independence with ADLs. Treatments can include therapeutic exercise, splinting, and functional activities. Therapy goals and interventions are influenced and frequently modified by surgical management and the phases of wound healing.

Examination, Evaluation, and Diagnosis

Prior to seeing the patient for the first time, it is important for the physical therapist to do a thorough chart review. It is important to know the mechanism of injury, TBSA, location, and depth of the burns. This helps the physical therapist have an idea of what to expect before entering the patient's room. The physical therapist should learn if there were any surgical procedures performed since admission to the hospital. A recent or impending surgery will give immediate clues that the burn is deep enough that it will not heal on its own. Patients with circumferential burns to an extremity are at risk for compartment syndrome. One of the first systemic responses to burn injury is the development of edema. When edema forms beneath inelastic burn eschar, circulatory compromise may occur. This can lead to damage or death to underlying muscle and nerve. If compartment syndrome is confirmed, the patient may have to undergo an escharotomy or fasciotomy. An escharotomy is a surgical intervention whereby the surgeon makes an incision through the eschar to relieve pressure.[4] A fasciotomy is a surgical intervention in which the incision is made through the fascia to relieve pressure.[4] Whereas the dorsal surface of the hand has thin, flexible skin that allows for expansion from edema, the palmar surface has limited room, which places it at greater risk for compromise.[5] The therapist should also learn whether there is significant past medical history, pre-injury level of mobility, and social history including family dynamics and school environment. It is important to speak with the patient's nurse before entering the room. Nurses are invaluable sources of information. Sometimes not all of the information makes it into the chart and the therapist can learn pertinent things about the patient and her family.

Of utmost importance, the physical therapist must learn the patient's current medication regimen for decreasing pain and how well the patient's pain is being controlled. Typically, the patient will have medications for background pain, breakthrough pain, and procedural pain. Common medications prescribed include: opioid analgesics (morphine, oxycodone, fentanyl, hydromorphone, methadone), benzodiazepines (midazolam, lorazepam), and anesthetic agents (ketamine, propofol) that can be used for procedural sedation.[25,26] Controlling the patient's pain throughout her stay is important not only for the relationship between the therapist and the patient, but also for the nurse-patient, nurse-therapist, family-patient, and family-therapist relationships. Occasionally, it takes time to achieve the correct analgesia. The nurse may indicate that the patient is in too much pain to be evaluated by the therapist. If the patient is in too much pain with only the background pain medications administered, it may be appropriate to hold the initial physical therapy evaluation until procedural medications can be administered. If the physical therapist can learn when the patient is going to have a dressing change later in the day, this is an excellent opportunity to assess ROM while the patient is under maximal analgesia. Ultimately, the burn injury will need to be assessed with the dressings removed. Once all this information has been gathered, the physical therapist can begin the examination.

The first step is to assess whether the patient is alert and able to follow commands. If the patient's dressing change does not correspond with the time of the evaluation, the physical therapist can get a thorough history from the patient's family regarding the mechanism of injury, past medical history, hand dominance, and family and social support network. Examination of active ROM (AROM) for joints *unaffected* by the burn injury can be done at this time, as well as a cursory assessment of the child's gross/fine motor, language, and social development. When dealing with an older child, if the injured hand is completely covered by dressings, the therapist can ask age-appropriate questions regarding intactness of sensation in her burned hand. The therapist should specifically ask if she feels any numbness or tingling because these can be symptoms of compartment syndrome and should be brought to the attention of the medical team immediately. For infants, toddlers, or young children that are too young to provide information, the therapist can palpate pulses distal to the injury and check the digits for capillary refill and temperature for signs of circulatory compromise. The physical therapist will need to return to complete the evaluation when the dressings are removed.

There are three critical reasons why the burned hand must ultimately be evaluated with the dressings removed. First, accurate ROM cannot be measured with the dressings in place. Second, for those patients with burns to the dorsum of the hand, the dorsal skin is very thin and the extensor tendons lay just beneath. Pressure exerted from the dressings and from the edema can cause damage to these delicate structures resulting in permanent injury such as a boutonniere deformity. Last, the therapist can visually identify joints that the burns have crossed, which are potential structures for contracture development during healing. The therapist should assess AROM and passive range of motion (PROM) during the patient's dressing change. On the involved extremity, ROM measurements should be taken for joints affected by the burn and for those unaffected as well. Sensation testing (e.g., light touch/pinprick) of any intact skin of the hand is also assessed. Initial physical therapy goals are based on a number of factors including the phase of wound healing, extent and depth of burn, patient's current health status, age, and physical and mental condition. Goals will change frequently based on surgical procedures because the patient's status and postsurgical movement restrictions change often. The foremost goal will be to prevent loss of ROM. Other goals include maintaining the patient's pre-injury level of strength and ensuring she is meeting all developmental milestones.

Plan of Care and Interventions

In the initial inflammatory phase (2-5 days from time of injury), edema control is one of the primary goals. If the patient has been admitted to the hospital promptly after injury, she is in the inflammatory phase of wound healing and edema will be present. The patient's affected hand should be elevated above the level of the heart and the family should be educated regarding edema prevention and requisite elevated positioning. The affected extremity can be positioned using pillows or foam wedges. Even stuffed animals can be utilized to keep the extremity elevated. Active flexion of the metacarpophalangeal joints (MCPs) and active abduction and adduction of the fingers should be initiated because the muscle pump action provided from these motions helps reduce edema.[2,27,28] Because young children are unable to understand the importance of ROM and perform a regimented exercise program, a variety of play techniques can be used to simulate most, if not all, patterns of motion of the hand. Often in hospitals with a pediatric department, a licensed child life specialist is available and can assist in creating activities that simulate the patterns of motion the therapist wants to achieve. Omar et al.[29] compared the outcomes in children with hand burns who performed rote exercises during treatment sessions with those who performed purposeful activities (i.e., play) that they enjoyed during treatment sessions. They found that children who were allowed to play using their burned hand during treatment sessions had less severe pain after treatment and had significantly larger improvements in total active motion than those that performed rote exercise. Both nursing staff and the majority of parents

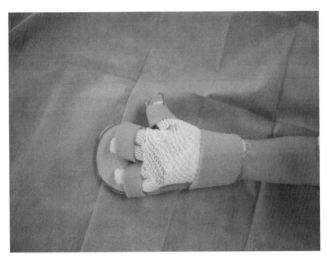

Figure 15-2. Example of a type of dorsal hand extension splint for a palmar burn. Note that the wrist, palm, and fingers are kept in neutral to full extension, with the thumb in radial abduction. The therapist chose to strap fingers 2-3 and 4-5 to prevent flexion of the IP joints.

also felt that having the child perform purposeful activities was more effective in distracting them from the source of pain.

ROM exercises, positioning, and splinting are important modalities to prevent loss of ROM or contractures associated with burn injury. The most important motion that the patient with a palmar burn will need to achieve and maintain is full extension of the palm and the fingers. This may be difficult for a young child to achieve. Splints will need to be utilized to ensure the tissue heals in an elongated position to prevent contracture. There are many different protocols for splinting a palmar burn.[2,24,27,30-32] Our facility aggressively splints palmar burns with the wrist, palm, and fingers kept in neutral to full extension with the thumb in radial abduction using a dorsal extension splint (Fig. 15-2). Some patients are even placed in slight MCP hyperextension. This position flattens the palmar arches and keeps the fingers extended to prevent any deformity as the wound begins to contract.[2] Patients are splinted immediately following the application of dressings in our burn emergency department. The splint is only removed for dressing changes, therapy sessions, and for scheduled play sessions; the patient may spend 23 hours per day splinted. The hand is splinted until well into the maturation phase of healing when it has been determined that contracture is no longer a risk. To prevent any maceration of the wound from a combination of the splint and the dressing, the dorsal aspect of the hand is splinted. Splints can be held in place with foam straps, cohesive bandages such as Coban or Co-Flex, or even elastic bandages. The method of application depends upon the treating therapist, the patient, and her family, who will ultimately be responsible for donning and doffing the splint for a 2-year-old toddler. For infants, toddlers, and young children who are prone to removing splints, the therapist can cover the hand and splint in a hospital sock. Once the hand is covered in the sock, it is out of sight and hopefully out of mind.

From about the third or fifth day post-burn until approximately 3 weeks post-burn, the patient is in the proliferative phase of wound healing. During this time, eschar is being removed from the burn either surgically or during the dressing changes. The physical therapist should continue treating the patient during dressing changes in order to visualize the tissue. Every effort should be made for the patient to perform all ROM actively. If the patient cannot tolerate ROM because the pain is not well controlled, the physical therapist can take advantage of seeing the patient in the operating room to perform PROM when the patient is unconscious or provide therapy interventions during procedural sedation. It is not uncommon in the acute care setting for procedural sedation to be ordered and performed solely for the purpose of ROM exercises. Procedural sedation, sometimes referred to as conscious sedation, is when analgesics and sedatives are administered by the medical team to minimize pain and awareness but preserve spontaneous respiration during a therapeutic intervention.[33] Several studies have looked at the use of **multimodal distraction** during dressing changes and procedures as a form of pain reduction.[34-36] Multimodal distraction utilizes hand-held technology that the patient can engage with during painful procedures.[35] In addition to a reduction in pain and anxiety,[34-36] Brown et al.[36] found that children using multimodal distraction during dressing changes had significantly faster healing times. Regardless of the method used to achieve ROM, aggressive PROM and stretching (*i.e.*, beyond normal range) should be avoided during the proliferative phase because some have theorized that damage to granulation tissue during stretching prolongs inflammation and may lead to hypertrophic scarring.[20,37-39]

In addition to guiding ROM exercises during the dressing changes, the physical therapist should progress exercises and practice functional play activities with the involved hand. During periods of rest, the patient's hand should be placed in the dorsal extension splint. Once it was determined that the patient's wound was uninfected, had an adequate blood supply, and it was predicted that it would not heal independently within 21 days, the surgeon elected to cover the wound with a skin graft. Immediately prior to the surgery, the physical therapist should be present to perform PROM to the hand, as this is the last opportunity for the hand to be mobilized until the graft has adhered. The physical therapist should also be involved with determining the optimal positioning of the wound bed for graft application to allow full functional ROM postoperatively. The graft is often attached with sutures and an occlusive petroleum gauze dressing is placed over the graft to keep it moist. In our burn center, the physical therapist is present in the operating room to wrap the fingers and hand with cohesive bandages immediately after surgery. Cohesive bandages inhibit edema and fluid collection underneath the graft. After application of the cohesive bandages, a new dorsal extension splint must be fabricated to maintain tissue length during graft healing and to accommodate any changes in the size of the hand because of decreases in edema and the amount of dressings. During the 5 days while the patient's hand is immobile in order to allow the sheet graft to adhere, other non-grafted joints should be exercised so the patient maintains strength and endurance. The physical therapist must ensure that the patient and her family keep her grafted hand elevated during all activities.

On postoperative day (POD) 2, the dressings are removed so that the graft can be visually inspected. If a split-thickness skin graft was utilized, any areas of fluid that have collected beneath the graft are evacuated because fluid acts as a barrier that prevents adherence between the graft and the wound bed. New dressings are then applied to the hand and the splint is put back on. If it is determined that the graft is well vascularized and adhered on POD 5, active exercises with the grafted hand can be resumed. ROM should begin with the dressings removed to prevent any shearing caused by the cohesive bandages. The patient is placed in less restrictive dressings to continue to keep the graft moist while allowing greater movement. The splint schedule remains the same (*i.e.*, ~ 23 hours/day). Exercise can be initiated and should include ROM for individual joints as well as composite flexion and extension exercises. The patient and the patient's family should work up to performing exercises 5 times per day. Once the patient's pain is adequately controlled and the family has the ability to perform the dressing changes independently, discharge planning will commence. The patient should have a home exercise program (HEP) in place, as well as a splint-wearing schedule. Prior to discharge, outpatient therapy should be arranged by the case manager or the social worker.

After hospital discharge, the patient's burn is usually in the maturation phase of healing. This phase lasts an average of 1.5 years, but can be as long as 3 years. At this time, the patient is most often seen in the outpatient setting for exercise, ROM, splinting, and scar management. The primary goals in this phase are full AROM and normal strength of the hand, independent performance of ADLs, and the presence of a flat, pliable scar. Common hand deformities after a palmar burn that occur during this phase include the palmar cupping deformity (Fig. 15-3) and flexion contractures of the MCP and IP joints (Fig. 15-4). These deformities often occur when splints are not used at home, therapy is not initiated early enough, therapy is not done frequently enough, or if patients are noncompliant with the physical therapy plan of care.[2,20,27,28,40]

Hypertrophic scarring can limit ROM and cause joint contractures and extreme pain. The prevalence of hypertrophic scarring in burn survivors is between 32% and 72%.[41] Risk factors include young age, longer time to heal (>21 days), darker pigmented skin, burn wound infection, and area of the body burned (neck and upper extremity).[41-44] Various modalities may influence, prevent, or decrease hypertrophic scarring after a burn. These include pressure therapy, scar massage, and silicone gel. **Pressure therapy** (provided by the use of pressure garments and custom inserts) is often used for the prevention and/or control of burn scars. It has been suggested that pressure therapy limits collagen synthesis and promotes realignment of collagen already present in the scar by restricting the supply of blood, oxygen, and nutrients to the scar tissue.[45] Engrav et al.[46] evaluated the effectiveness of pressure garment therapy over a 12-year period and found that scars were significantly softer, thinner, and had improved clinical appearance, but this effect was only observed with scarring that was moderate to severe. The authors recommended custom pressure garments be used for: deep partial thickness burns that have healed spontaneously over weeks, burns in children and young adults, burns in individuals with darker pigmented skin, and in instances where vascular support or protection is needed.[46] Our facility initiates pressure therapy once the

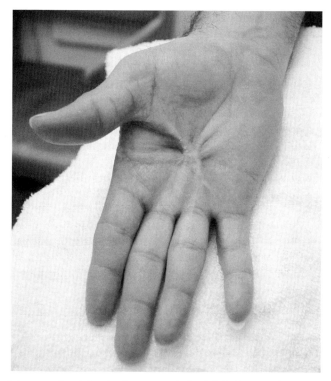

Figure 15-3. Palmar cupping deformity that occurred after full-thickness grafting to the palm when the patient refused to wear the splint prescribed by the physical therapist. Note scar in center of palm that is pulling the tissue toward the center.

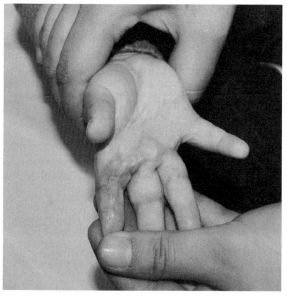

Figure 15-4. Flexion contractures of the MCP and IP joints of digits 2 and 3, and hypertrophic scarring at the MCP joint of the index finger.

graft is fully adhered and no open areas remain. An off-the-shelf interim glove is used. In addition to providing pressure on the graft, the interim glove helps prevent edema in the hand. After 2 weeks, the patient is measured for custom pressure garments. The patient's family is advised to have the patient wear the garment 23 hours per day and should remove it only for bathing and scar massage. It is important that sunscreen is applied to the skin underneath the pressure garments because newly grafted skin can sunburn easily and will be permanently discolored due to sun exposure. Massage has also been advocated in the treatment of hypertrophic scarring. Massage has been thought to encourage collagen remodeling, decrease itching, desensitize the scar, and provide moisture and pliability through the use of moisturizers.[20,37-39] Studies in patients with burn injuries have shown that scar massage decreases itching and pain and improves anxiety and depression.[37-39] **Silicone gel** is another modality frequently used in the treatment of hypertrophic scars. The exact mechanism of action is unknown, although it has been hypothesized that silicone works by increasing scar hydration, increasing pressure on the scar, and increasing the temperature of the scar.[47-49] A 2013 Cochrane review evaluated the evidence regarding the use of silicone gel sheeting for preventing and treating hypertrophic and keloid scars. The authors determined that there is weak evidence to support the use of silicone gel sheeting.[50] While there were studies that demonstrated improvements in scar height and color with the use of silicone, the authors felt that these studies were of poor quality and subject to bias.[50] Our facility recommends use of silicone gel sheeting on hypertrophic scars for 12 hours per day. If the patient has been issued pressure garments, the silicone gel sheeting is worn beneath the garments. If the patient does not have garments, the silicone gel sheeting is held in place using tape or cohesive bandages.

Finally, education is paramount during this phase of healing. The child will need a HEP that builds upon what has been learned during therapy sessions. In addition to exercise, the patient and her family need instruction and education regarding use of splints, pressure garments, and silicone, if those modalities are utilized. It is important for the physical therapist to begin education and instruction early in the rehabilitation and reinforce it throughout the entire plan of care.

Evidence-Based Clinical Recommendations

SORT: Strength of Recommendation Taxonomy

A: Consistent, good-quality patient-oriented evidence
B: Inconsistent or limited-quality patient-oriented evidence
C: Consensus, disease-oriented evidence, usual practice, expert opinion, or case series

1. Range of motion exercises, positioning, and splinting are important modalities to prevent loss of ROM or contractures associated with burn injury. **Grade C**

2. Multimodal distraction can be utilized during dressing changes and procedures to reduce pain and anxiety and improve healing. **Grade B**

3. Pressure garments worn 23 hours per day in the maturation phase of wound healing minimize hypertrophic scarring. **Grade B**

4. Silicone gel sheets worn 24 hours per day decrease thickness, pigmentation, pain, vascularity, and itching and increase the pliability of hypertrophic scars. **Grade B**

COMPREHENSION QUESTIONS

15.1 A patient with a burn wound that appears moist, red, weepy, and extremely painful most likely has a depth of burn that can be classified as:

A. Superficial

B. Superficial partial thickness

C. Deep partial thickness

D. Full thickness

15.2 Tissue tightness from a palmar burn can lead to which of the following deformities?

A. Boutonniere deformity

B. Swan neck deformity

C. Palmar cupping deformity

D. Mallet finger

15.3 Which of the following does *not* increase the risk of developing hypertrophic scarring?

A. Burns of superficial depth

B. Darker pigmented skin

C. Younger age

D. Aggressive stretching

ANSWERS

15.1 **B.** Superficial partial thickness burns involve the entire epidermis as well as the papillary layer of the dermis. The appearance is red, moist, and weepy. Blisters may be present. The wound will blanch easily.

15.2 **C.** A palmar cupping deformity is often seen with burns to the palm, as the scar tissue begins to contract. To counteract the pull of the scar tissue, the hand and fingers must be placed in extension.

15.3 **A.** The following factors contribute to increased risk of hypertrophic scarring: deeper burns, younger age, infection, healing > 21 days, darker pigmented skin, tension on the wound from aggressive stretching, and location of burn.

REFERENCES

1. Guidelines for the Operation of Burn Centers. http://www.ameriburn.org/Chapter14.pdf. Accessed November 20, 2014.

2. Howell JW. Management of the acutely burned hand for the nonspecialized clinician. *Phys Ther.* 1989;69:1077-1090.

3. 2013 National Burn Repository. http://www.ameriburn.org/2013NBRAnnualReport.pdf. Accessed November 20, 2014.

4. Feldmann ME, Evans J, O SJ. Early management of the burned pediatric hand. *J Craniofac Surg.* 2008;19:942-950.

5. Palmieri TL. Initial management of acute pediatric hand burns. *Hand Clin.* 2009;25:461-467.

6. Choi M, Armstrong MB, Panthaki ZJ. Pediatric hand burns: thermal, electrical, chemical. *J Craniofac Surg.* 2009;20:1045-1048.

7. Falkel JE. Anatomy and physiology of the skin. In: Richard RL, Staley MJ, eds. *Burn Care and Rehabilitation Principles and Practice.* Philadelphia, PA: FA Davis; 1994:10-28.

8. Pham TN, Gibran NS, Heimbach DM. Evaluation of the burn wound. In: Herndon DN, ed. *Total Burn Care.* 3rd ed. Philadelphia, PA: Elsevier; 2007:119-126.

9. Myers BA. *Wound Management: Principles and Practice.* Upper Saddle River, NJ: Prentice Hall; 2012.

10. Kaplan DH, Jenison MC, Saeland S, Shlomchik WD, Sclomchik MJ. Epidermal langerhans cell-deficient mice develop enhanced contact hypersensitivity. *Immunity.* 2005;23:611-620.

11. Katcher ML. Scald burns from hot tap water. *JAMA.* 1981;246:1219-1222.

12. Warner RM, Wilson Y, Chester DL. Cooling properties of everyday liquids. *Burns.* 2012;38:1186-1191.

13. Shalom A, Bryant A, Smith-Meek M, Parsons LR, Munster A. Noodles stay hotter longer. *J Burn Care Res.* 2007;28:474-477.

14. Bessey PQ. Wound care. In: Herndon DN, ed. *Total Burn Care.* 3rd ed. Philadelphia, PA: Elsevier; 2007:127-135.

15. Muller M, Gahankari D, Herndon DN. Operative wound management. In: Herndon DN, ed. *Total Burn Care.* 3rd ed. Philadelphia, PA: Elsevier; 2007:177-195.

16. Johnson C. Pathologic manifestations of burn injury. In: Richard RL, Staley MJ, eds. *Burn Care and Rehabilitation Principles and Practice.* Philadelphia, PA: FA Davis; 1994:29-48.

17. Greenhalgh DG, Staley MJ. Burn wound healing. In: Richard RL, Staley MJ, eds. *Burn Care and Rehabilitation Principles and Practice.* Philadelphia, PA: FA Davis; 1994:70-102.

18. Miller SF, Staley MJ, Richard RL. Surgical management of the burn patient. In: Richard RL, Staley MJ, eds. *Burn Care and Rehabilitation Principles and Practice.* Philadelphia, PA: FA Davis; 1994:177-197.

19. Sussman C, Bates-Jensen BM. *Wound Care: A Collaborative Practice Manual for Physical Therapists and Nurses.* Gaithersburg, MD: Aspen Publishers; 2011.

20. Richard RL, Staley MJ. Scar management. In: Richard RL, Staley MJ, eds. *Burn Care and Rehabilitation Principles and Practice.* Philadelphia, PA: FA Davis; 1994:380-418.

21. Andreassi A, Bilenchi R, Biagioli M, D'Aniello C. Classification and pathophysiology of skin grafts. *Clin Dermatol.* 2005;23:332-337.

22. Greenhalgh DG. Wound healing. In: Herndon DN, ed. *Total Burn Care.* 3rd ed. Philadelphia, PA: Elsevier; 2007:578-595.

23. Scott JR, Costa BA, Gibran NS, Engrav LH, Heimbach DH, Klein MB. Pediatric palm contact burns: a ten-year review. *J Burn Care Res.* 2008;29:614-618.

24. Sheridan RL, Baryza MJ, Pessina MA, et al. Acute hand burns in children: management and long-term outcome based on a 10-year experience with 698 injured hands. *Ann Surg.* 1999;229:558-564.

25. Meyer WJ, Patterson DR, Jaco M, Woodson L, Thomas C. Management of pain and other discomforts of burn patients. In: Herndon DN, ed. *Total Burn Care.* 3rd ed. Philadelphia, PA: Elsevier; 2007:797-818.

26. Richardson P, Mustard L. The management of pain in the burns unit. *Burns.* 2009;35:921-936.

27. Moore ML, Dewey WS, Richard RL. Rehabilitation of the burned hand. *Hand Clin.* 2009;25:529-541.

28. Grigsby deLinde L, Knothe B. Therapist's management of the burned hand. In: Hunter JM, Macklin EJ, Callahan AD, eds. *Rehabilitation of the Hand and Upper Extremity.* St. Louis, MO: Mosby; 2002:1492-1526.

29. Omar MT, Hegazy FA, Mokashi SP. Influences of purposeful activity versus rote exercise on improving pain and hand function in pediatric burn. *Burns.* 2012;38:261-268.

30. Schwanholt C, Daugherty MB, Gaboury T, Warden GD. Splinting the pediatric palmar burn. *J Burn Care Rehabil.* 1992;13:460-464.

31. Barret JP, Desai MH, Herndon DN. The isolated burned palm in children: epidemiology and long-term sequelae. *Plast Reconstr Surg.* 2000;105:949-952.

32. Duncan RM. Basic principles of splinting the hand. *Phys Ther.* 1989;69:1104-1116.

33. Brown TB, Lovato LM, Parker D. Procedural sedation in the acute care setting. *Am Fam Physician.* 2005;71:85-90.

34. Miller K, Rodger S, Bucolo S, Greer R, Kimble RM. Multi-modal distraction. Using technology to combat pain in young children with burn injuries. *Burns.* 2010;36:647-658.

35. Miller K, Rodger S, Kipping B, Kimble RM. A novel technology approach to pain management in children with burns: a prospective randomized controlled trial. *Burns.* 2011;37:395-405.

36. Brown NJ, Kimble RM, Rodger S, Ware RS, Cuttle L. Play and heal: randomized controlled trial of Ditto™ intervention efficacy on improving re-epithelialization in pediatric burns. *Burns.* 2014;40:204-213.

37. Field T, Peck M, Krugman S, et al. Burn injuries benefit from massage therapy. *J Burn Care Rehabil.* 1998;19:241-244.

38. Field T, Peck M, Hernandez-Reif M, Krugman S, Burman I, Ozment-Schenck L. Postburn itching, pain, and psychological symptoms are reduced with massage therapy. *J Burn Care Rehabil.* 2000;21:189-193.

39. Patino O, Novick C, Merlo A, Benaim F. Massage in hypertrophic scars. *J Burn Care Rehabil.* 1999;20:268-271.

40. Schneider JC, Holavanahalli R, Helm P, O'Neil C, Goldstein R, Kowalske K. Contractures in burn injury part II: investigating joints of the hand. *J Burn Care Res.* 2008;29:606-613.

41. Lawrence JW, Mason ST, Schomer K, Klein MB. Epidemiology and impact of scarring after burn injury: a systematic review of the literature. *J Burn Care Res.* 2012;33:136-146.

42. Gangemi EN, Gregori D, Berchialla P, et al. Epidemiology and risk factors for pathologic scarring after burn wounds. *Arch Facial Plast Surg.* 2008;10:93-102.

43. Deitch EA, Wheelahan TM, Rose MP, Clothier J, Cotter J. Hypertrophic burn scars: analysis of variables. *J Trauma.* 1983;23:895-898.

44. Baker RH, Townley WA, McKeon S, Linge C, Vijh V. Retrospective study of the association between hypertrophic burn scarring and bacterial colonization. *J Burn Care Res.* 2007;28:152-156.

45. Macintyre L, Baird M. Pressure garments for use in the treatment of hypertrophic scars: a review of the problems associated with their use. *Burns.* 2006;32:10-15.

46. Engrav LH, Heimbach DM, Rivara FP, et al. 12-year within-wound study of the effectiveness of custom pressure garment therapy. *Burns.* 2010;36:975-983.

47. Slemp AE, Kirschner RE. Keloids and scars: a review of keloids and scars, their pathogenesis, risk factors, and management. *Curr Opin Pediatr.* 2006;18:396-402.

48. Wolfram D, Tzankov A, Pülzl P, Piza-Katzer H. Hypertrophic scars and keloids: a review of their pathophysiology, risk factors, and therapeutic management. *Dermatol Surg.* 2009;35:171-181.

49. Bloemen MC, van der Veer WM, Ulrich MM, van Zuijlen PP, Niessen FB, Middelkoop E. Prevention and curative management of hypertrophic scar formation. *Burns.* 2009;35:463-475.

50. O'Brien L, Jones DJ. Silicone gel sheeting for preventing and treating hypertrophic and keloid scars. *Cochrane Database Syst Rev.* 2013 Sep 12;9:CD003826.

Portions of this case have been modified from Jobst EE. *Physical Therapy Case Files: Acute Care.* 2013. Cases 26 and 27.

Chronic Wound

Meri Goehring

A 13-year-old female has been admitted to the intensive care unit (ICU) of the hospital with acute systemic illness including acute hemolytic anemia, hypotension, and a poorly healing and painful wound on the posterior right thigh just inferior to the gluteal fold. The wound is bluish-black in color and appears to be covered with hard, black eschar. She reports it is very painful when she touches the area, sits, or moves her right leg, rating it as 8 on a 0 to 10 numeric pain rating scale. At rest, she rates her pain as 3. Her previous medical conditions include tonsillitis and recurrent otitis media (at the age of 4) with tonsillectomy and Eustachian tube surgery at age 6 with full recovery. In the last year, she was given the diagnosis of obesity. She is 5 feet, 2 inches tall and weighs 178 lbs (body mass index 32.6). The subjective history from the physician's note on admission indicates that the patient was camping at Hot Springs National Park in Arkansas and noticed spiders in her sleeping bag in the early morning after waking up in pain from a suspected bug bite. The patient's mother confirms that she saw spiders in the sleeping bag and thinks they may have been brown in color. The mother reports there was a red ring around the wound the day after the bite occurred. However, the mother has not looked at it since that day because her daughter is very shy and does not want her parents looking at the wound. The mother reports she feels terrible about this because now her daughter is very sick and she thought the wound would heal on its own. The physician's impression is that the wound is most likely the result of a brown recluse spider (BRS) bite since other diagnoses have been ruled out. Physical therapy has been ordered for examination and treatment of the patient's wound as well as her function.

- ▶ What examination techniques should be used with this diagnosis?
- ▶ Describe the physical therapy plan of care regarding wound management.
- ▶ How will continuing wound care needs be communicated to other healthcare staff?
- ▶ Identify appropriate referrals to other healthcare professionals.

KEY DEFINITIONS

ACUTE WOUND: A wound caused by surgery or trauma in an otherwise healthy individual

CHRONIC WOUND: Any acute wound whose progression through the phases of wound healing is prolonged or arrested due to underlying conditions, resulting in a failure to heal in the expected timeframe for that particular type of wound

DEBRIDEMENT: Removal of necrotic tissue, foreign material, and/or debris from the wound bed. Categories of debridement are further defined:

Enzymatic: Use of exogenous enzymes to remove devitalized tissue from a wound

Mechanical: Use of force to remove devitalized tissue, foreign material, and/or debris from a wound

Nonselective: Removal of nonspecific areas of devitalized tissue; may include surgical and mechanical debridement

Selective: Removal of specific areas of devitalized tissue using sharp, enzymatic, or autolytic debridement

Sharp: Use of forceps, scissors, or scalpel in a *clean* environment to selectively remove tissue, foreign material, and/or debris from a wound

Surgical: Use of scalpel, scissors, or laser in a *sterile* environment by a physician or podiatrist to remove necrotic tissue, foreign material, and/or debris from a wound

ESCHAR: Black necrotic tissue (may be soft or hard)

INFECTION: Invasion and multiplication of microorganisms within body tissues; wound culture reveals greater than 10^5 microbes per gram of tissue.[1]

NECROTIC: Dead, devitalized tissue adhered to the wound bed

TUNNELLING: Narrow passageway within a wound bed

UNDERMINING: Area of tissue under the wound edges that becomes eroded, resulting in a large wound with a small opening

Objectives

1. Identify a reliable method of evaluating the size of a wound.
2. Identify an optimal method of cleaning and debriding a chronic wound with eschar.
3. Identify appropriate wound dressings to provide a clean and moist healing environment.
4. Understand the medical treatments and how they might affect physical therapy interventions.
5. Identify a valid method of determining the level of pain in a teenager.
6. Describe how to educate the patient and her parents about wound care at home.

Physical Therapy Considerations

PT considerations during management of a teenager with a chronic wound:

▶ **General physical therapy plan of care/goals:** Promote healing; prevent/minimize loss of range of motion (ROM), strength, and aerobic functional capacity; maximize physical function and safety; minimize secondary impairments such as infection and/or excessive scarring; optimize parent and/or caregiver education and health-related quality of life

▶ **Physical therapy interventions:** Wound cleaning, debridement, and dressing; patient/family education regarding wound management, including the wound healing process, risk of infection, procedure for dressing changes, risk of contracture and scarring, and proper hygiene; reasonable home exercise program that can be incorporated into the daily life of a teenager; communication and hand-off of information to other healthcare professionals

▶ **Precautions during physical therapy:** Use of proper infection control techniques; specific precautions with use of indicated modalities; monitor wound for signs of infection and/or maceration of wound bed or surrounding skin; if performing sharp debridement, use of sterile instrument and clean techniques; maintain modesty of teenager during functional activities; monitor for hypotensive episodes due to systemic response/current condition

▶ **Complications during physical therapy:** Local and/or systemic infection, hypotension, emotional distress of teenager or family/caregivers

Understanding the Health Condition

The most common and dangerous spider in the United States is *Loxosceles reclusa*, commonly known as the brown recluse spider (BRS).[2] BRSs live in a circumscribed area of the United States, specifically the south central Midwest (Fig. 16-1). In these areas, where spider populations may be dense, BRSs may be a cause of significant morbidity. The BRS is often misidentified.[3] While variable in size, the body length of a BRS is not greater than half an inch. The abdomen of the BRS is uniformly colored, but varies from cream to dark brown in color. The most distinguishing features are its fiddle or violin shape and the presence of six eyes, instead of eight, like most spiders. The BRS is not an aggressive spider and bites only when threatened or pressed up against an object. It lives in dark, warm, dry places such as under woodpiles, in barns, under boards, or in small corners or crevices. They have also been found in shoes, clothing, bedding, and on furniture.[4]

Bites from several species of spiders can result in localized as well as systemic problems. Some researchers indicate that the only way to truly identify a BRS bite is to correctly identify the spider itself in the act of biting, which is rarely possible.[2] Thus, conclusive evidence that a spider bite is what caused the initial wound and necrosis may be quite difficult to make.[2,5] A partial list of differential diagnoses for BRS bites includes bacterial skin infections such as community-acquired

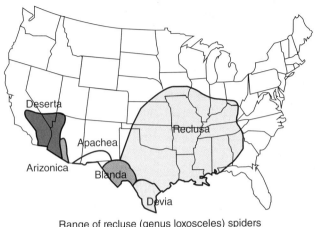

Range of recluse (genus loxosceles) spiders
in the United States

Figure 16-1. Distribution of the Brown recluse spider and other recluse spiders within the United States. (Reproduced with permission from http://spiders.ucr.edu/brs.html.)

methicillin-resistant *Staphylococcus aureus* (MRSA), fungal and viral infections, pyoderma gangrenosum, poison ivy, poison oak, squamous cell carcinoma, localized vasculitis, other types of bites, Lyme disease, chemical burns, and necrotizing fasciitis.[5]

Typically, a bite from a BRS results in pruritus, pain, and erythema within 6 hours. Within 24 hours, an irregular, erythematous ring demarcates the bite. Early signs of necrosis may be seen within 48 to 72 hours. These include a reddish-blue wound that is very painful and covered with hard black or brown eschar.[2] While most BRS bites heal within 3 weeks, rare systemic complications include hemolytic anemia and severe hypotension.[4,5] Medical treatment may include blood transfusions (to treat anemia) and appropriate wound care. Depending on the particular hospital or practice setting, a nurse or physical therapist may be the healthcare professional providing the bedside wound care. Regardless of the level of direct wound care management, the physical therapist is involved in promoting safe and effective wound healing and maximizing functional outcomes.

Physical Therapy Patient/Client Management

A multidisciplinary team can best manage the teenager with a BRS bite that is acutely ill. In this case, the team would include physicians (possibly a plastic surgeon), nurses, physical therapist, occupational therapist, dietician, and a social worker. One of the nurses or therapists could have a specialization in wound care, but this is not always the case. The physical therapist must be aware of the state licensure regulations regarding sharp debridement as well as the specific institution's regulations regarding who is allowed to perform direct wound care. For example, some healthcare facilities stipulate that only registered nurses are to perform wound care, whereas other facilities allow nurses or physical therapists to carry out wound assessment and management. Since the mother reports that this young woman may be extremely modest, extra care should be taken to respect her modesty. The therapist needs to inform the teenager and family regarding the plan of care and potential healing times for the wound. Although this young woman's health is fragile while she is in the ICU, parent involvement and education is still essential at this time. Examination and treatment of the wound and provision of a clean wound bed while keeping the teenager as medically stable as possible is the foremost goal. Once the teenager is considered hemodynamically stable, the therapist will be more involved in assessing her functional movement and impairments. As she nears hospital discharge, the therapist will be involved in educating the parents and home health providers (physical therapy and/or nursing) on dressing changes, ROM activities, positioning, transfers, and scar management.

Examination, Evaluation, and Diagnosis

In this case, the physical therapist needs to examine, evaluate, diagnose, and treat both the teenager's function and the wound itself. If the teenager is not hemodynamically stable, examination and treatment should occur only when the physician has cleared the patient for activity. Certainly, the medical condition of the teenager must be monitored at all times. Temperature, heart rate, respiratory rate, blood pressure, and oxygen saturation levels should be recorded and monitored. During observation, the therapist should note whether the teenager is generally in good physical condition as well as the cleanliness of her hair, nails, and any clothing. The physical therapist will also want to know if the teenager was previously independent in her activities of daily living and her level of activity at home and at school. The therapist should note the teenager's reactions during the subjective assessment. For example, is she crying, withdrawn, or calm? History taking should include questions regarding how the BRS bite occurred and whether the spider was seen. Because the wound is located on a private body part, the therapist must thoughtfully consider the emotions of this young person during examination of the wound. If the patient and/or parents request a female therapist, it will be necessary to accommodate their wishes. However, if the teenager and/or her parents express no discomfort with a male therapist providing the treatment, the male therapist may wish to ask a female healthcare provider and/or family member to be present during examination and treatment of the wound.

Examination of the wound starts with visual inspection and documentation of the dimensions, including differing depths within the wound bed. The therapist must decide how best to measure the surface area of the wound. If the wound has no discernable depth, documentation of width and length may suffice. Two commonly used methods are disposable paper measuring ruler and wound tracing (*i.e.*, tracing the perimeter of the wound margin with a marker onto clear acetate or other film). To measure depth and any undermining of the wound, the therapist places a disposable cotton-tipped applicator into the deepest part of the wound bed. Next, the therapist holds the applicator at the wound margin and places it against a ruler to measure the distance from the base of the wound bed to the wound margin.

For a wound with varying depths, this procedure can be repeated and wound depth ranges documented. Digital photography is an excellent and reproducible method that is often used in combination with wound rulers or tracings. The therapist must determine what type of permission is required *prior* to taking a photograph that will be submitted as part of the electronic medical record. Because the surface of this patient's wound appeared necrotic, debridement must be performed to determine the extent of the necrotic tissue and the true wound dimensions. Since the physician has specifically consulted the therapist for wound management, decisions must be made regarding how to properly clean the wound and debride the hard eschar. Debridement could be done surgically or at the bedside using clean technique with sterile instruments. If the therapist decides that the latter option is feasible, safe, and practical, discussion with the appropriate healthcare professionals must occur prior to implementation of any debridement.

Timing of wound care should always be carefully coordinated with pain medications and evaluation of pain is critical. As the teenager is verbal, she should be able to rate her pain on a standard visual analog scale or numeric pain rating scale. While there is not enough evidence to determine adolescents' preference for either of these types of scales, visual analog scales may be superior for measuring pain intensity for acute procedure-related pain, post-operative, and disease-related pain in children older than 8 years and adolescents.[6] However, her pain may be more thoroughly examined using the **Adolescent Pediatric Pain Tool (APPT)**.[7] The APPT is a multidimensional self-report tool that evaluates not only the intensity of the pain, but also its location (with a body outline diagram) and quality (using 67 pain descriptors). In assessing the quality of the pain, affective, evaluative, sensory, and temporal dimensions are assessed. By assessing other dimensions of pain besides intensity, the therapist may be able to customize multimodal pain management strategies for more effective pain control. The APPT is available in English and Spanish for children and adolescents (8-17 years old) and was modeled after the McGill Pain Questionnaire for adults. It has been found to be valid, reliable, and sensitive for measuring pain in children with a variety of conditions.[7] Although the APPT has not been specifically validated in individuals with pain related to wounds resulting from spider bites, this tool appears to have face validity and may be an ideal choice.

Plan of Care and Interventions

After the examination and evaluation, the physical therapist needs to determine the most appropriate method of wound care. The main goals for treatment are to prevent infection, restore function to the wound area, minimize scarring, and promote full physical and emotional recovery. First, the therapist must decide how best to clean and debride the wound. As with any intervention, choices are based on the benefits, disadvantages, precautions, and contraindications. If the wound requires an excessive amount of debridement, surgical debridement is likely the best option. However, an initial thorough cleaning of the wound is needed to enable the physical therapist to determine whether any further removal of necrotic tissue will be required. To clean the wound, rinsing with water is one option. This will not be effective in this case because rinsing with water will not remove the hard black eschar. An alternative is pulsed lavage. This treatment modality involves the use of a hand-held device to irrigate the wound (with water or saline) using regulated pressure that provides an automatic interruption of fluid flow. Negative pressure suction occurs at the same time to remove the irrigation liquid. Pulsed lavage is often indicated in wounds that have deep portions or tunneling, or a large amount of necrotic skin to remove—common characteristics of wounds caused by BRS bites. Another option for cleaning and debridement is the use of a non-contact, low-frequency ultrasound device with a low-pressure saline spray. Although there is some evidence that non-contact, low-frequency ultrasound enhances healing of a chronic wound, a significant amount of necrotic tissue would not be removed with this modality.[8] For this wound, the therapist decided that the most time-efficient choice to clean and debride would be **initial surgical debridement followed by pulsed lavage and/or sharp debridement** using clean technique and sterile instruments, as needed. Subsequent nonsurgical debridement techniques would be carried out over several treatment sessions at the patient's bedside. It should be emphasized that bedside nonsurgical debridement must be done gently so that damage to healthy tissue is minimized.[9] The goal would be for the patient to have a clean wound bed before leaving the hospital so that further debridement would not need to be performed at home or on an outpatient basis.

After cleaning and debridement, the type of dressings to cover the wound must be chosen. This is performed in cooperation with the physician and nursing staff. Chronic wounds usually require more than one dressing type. Dressings need to absorb drainage, protect the wound from trauma, allow ROM and function of the entire hip and leg area, and control edema. Ideal dressings cover the wound and provide a warm, moist environment to promote healing. Any tunneling or undermining must be filled with gauze. Gauze is available in long, thin, sterile strips that allow the therapist to specifically measure how much gauze is gently packed into the wound. Over the top of the wound, a nonadherent dressing is needed. The most common choice is an impregnated gauze such as a petrolatum-coated gauze or gauze impregnated with a hydrogel.[1,2] A secondary dressing such as a stockinet, elastic bandage (*e.g.*, Ace wrap), or surgical netting is applied over the primary dressings to secure them in place and provide extra protection from trauma. If surgical netting is used, this should be changed with each dressing change. If elastic bandages are used, these can be hand washed and dried flat and away from sunshine. The patient should be given a second set of elastic bandages to wear while the other set is washed and dried. Given the location of the wound, it is critical that the dressings are kept clean during toileting. Every effort should be taken to keep the patient from removing the dressings and every opportunity should be taken to reinforce the necessity of keeping the area clean. Once the wound bed is clean, an option to promote healing is the use of negative pressure wound therapy (NPWT) commonly known as a "wound vac." **Wound vacs** provide a warm, moist environment that encourages increased circulation to the wound, decreases the accumulation of excessive exudate that can inhibit healing, and promotes the formation of granulation tissue.[1] Dressings are changed every 6 to 10 days or more often if there is excess exudate or dressings become soiled. A wound vac is typically the size of a small backpack and has tubing that attaches to the wound itself. This device is portable and would be a good choice for an active teenage girl. An occupational therapist may be helpful in providing suggestions for appropriate clothing and/or any necessary clothing modifications for the wound vac tubing. The occupational therapist can also assist with recommendations related to positioning of the right lower extremity during dressing and bathing.

Exercise and positioning are also very important. At this early stage, mobility is not the foremost goal, but once the teenager becomes medically stable, mobility should be emphasized. The therapist works with the patient to ensure that she is able to independently position herself off of the wound (e.g., left sidelying, use of cut-out wedge to relieve pressure on right posterior thigh for sitting) and transfer without causing shearing forces on the wound. Although the physician's activity orders have stipulated "weightbearing as tolerated" on the right lower extremity, it is likely that the patient will have an antalgic gait due to pain, bulky dressings, and the presence of a wound vac. Therefore, efforts should be made to keep her posturing symmetrical during gait, which may require use of crutches during the painful period. A modified 3-point gait pattern could be used. Prior to hospital discharge, the therapist must ensure that the patient can safely ambulate with crutches on unlevel surfaces and stairs. Last, it is prudent that the patient is evaluated by a dietician during the hospital stay. Wound healing requires adequate protein and minerals. This teenager also has a high BMI for her age, and although weight loss is not the focus of the current hospital admission, the dietician may provide important information to the child and family about the long-term importance of weight control.

Communication with the parents is vital, and it is important that they become involved in her care as much as possible. Information regarding what may happen during surgical debridement, what to expect in terms of healing times, and the prognosis for recovery can also help reduce anxiety. The parents need to be informed of pain-reducing efforts undertaken during their daughter's hospital stay, the need for careful dressing changes that will continue after hospital discharge, positioning to decrease pressure and shear on the wound, and how they can be involved. The therapist should provide clear, concise information regarding how the wound must be cleaned and dressed since the parents will need to be involved in their daughter's care once she returns home.

Evidence-Based Clinical Recommendations

SORT: Strength of Recommendation Taxonomy

A: Consistent, good-quality patient-oriented evidence
B: Inconsistent or limited-quality patient-oriented evidence
C: Consensus, disease-oriented evidence, usual practice, expert opinion or case series

1. The Adolescent Pediatric Pain Tool (APPT) is a valid, reliable, and sensitive tool for measuring pain intensity, location, and quality in children ages 8 to 17 years old. **Grade B**

2. Choices for cleaning and debriding a chronic wound include surgical debridement followed by pulsed lavage and/or sharp debridement using clean technique and sterile instruments. **Grade C**

3. Negative pressure wound therapy promotes healing of chronic wounds by providing a warm, moist environment that encourages increased circulation to the wound, decreases accumulation of excessive exudate, and promotes formation of granulation tissue. **Grade A**

COMPREHENSION QUESTIONS

16.1 Which of the statements below *best* describes the typical characteristics of a brown recluse spider bite?

A. Pruritus, pain, and erythema within 48 hours that worsens over 72 hours

B. An irregular, erythematous ring that demarcates the bite by 24 hours

C. A wound that shows early signs of deep necrosis after 10 to 12 days

D. A white, waxy wound that is not painful to touch or with movement

16.2 What medical complications might arise after a BRS bite?

A. Hypertension, anxiety, heart palpitations

B. Hypovolemia, nausea, vomiting

C. Hemolytic anemia and hypotension

D. Dehydration, diarrhea, and bradycardia

16.3 Once a clean wound bed is established, what would be the *best* choice for continued wound care after a BRS bite?

A. Negative pressure wound therapy

B. Enzymatic debridement

C. Autolytic debridement

D. Surgical debridement

ANSWERS

16.1 **B.** A BRS bite exhibits a characteristic pattern that includes pruritus, pain, and erythema within 6 hours, and an irregular, erythematous ring that demarcates the bite by 24 hours. Early signs of necrosis are seen within 48 to 72 hours. These include a reddish-blue wound that is very painful and covered with hard, black or brown eschar.

16.2 **C.** Hemolytic anemia and severe hypotension are rare medical complications of a BRS bite.

16.3 **A.** Negative pressure wound therapy, or "wound vac," is often applied to chronic wounds after debridement to promote healing by decreasing accumulation of excessive exudate and promoting the formation of granulation tissue. Once the wound bed is clean, no further debridement should occur (options B, C, and D).

REFERENCES

1. Sussman C, Bates-Jensen B. *Wound Care*. 4th ed. Philadelphia, PA: Lippincott, Williams and Wilkins; 2012:401-411.

2. Andersen RJ, Campoli J, Johar SK, Schumacher KA, Allison EJ. Suspected brown recluse envenomation: a case report and review of different treatment modalities. *J Emerg Med*. 2011;41:e31-e37.

3. University of California, Riverside. Spider Research. Brown Recluse ID. http://spiders.ucr.edu/recluseid.html. Accessed November 13, 2014.

4. Rhoads J. Epidemiology of the brown recluse spider bite. *J Am Acad Nurse Pract*. 2007;19:79-85.

5. McDade J, Aygun B, Ware RE. Brown recluse spider (Loxosceles reclusa) envenomation leading to acute hemolytic anemia in six adolescents. *J Pediatr*. 2010;156:155-157.

6. Stinson JN, Kavanaugh T, Yamada J, Gill N, Stevens B. Systematic review of the psychometric properties, interpretability and feasibility of self-report pain intensity measures for use in clinical trials in children and adolescents. *Pain*. 2006;125:143-157.

7. Jacob E, Mack AK, Savedra M, Van Cleve L, Wilkie DJ. Adolescent pediatric pain tool for multidimensional measurement of pain in children and adolescents. *Pain Manag Nurs*. 2014;15:694-706.

8. Driver VR, Yao M, Miller CJ. Noncontact low-frequency ultrasound therapy in the treatment of chronic wounds: a meta-analysis. *Wound Repair Regen*. 2011;19:475-480.

9. Myers BA. *Wound Management: Principles and Practice*. 3rd ed. Upper Saddle River, NJ: Pearson; 2012:321-346.

Congenital Muscular Torticollis

Sarah Stewart
Colleen P. Coulter

CASE 17

A 14-month-old male toddler has arrived for a follow-up visit with a physical thera-pist in a hospital-based outpatient rehabilitation department. The toddler was originally referred to physical therapy at 2 months of age diagnosed by his pediatri-cian with left congenital muscular torticollis (CMT) and right plagiocephaly. At the 1-month well-baby check, the child's mother reported the baby's left head tilt and preference to turn his head to the right. The pediatrician recommended increas-ing prone activity, "tummy time," and a reassessment at the 2-month well-baby check. Because his left head tilt and positional preference persisted, the patient was referred to physical therapy. He was also referred to a cranial remolding pro-gram for evaluation and monitoring of his head shape by a certified orthotist with rec-ommendations for cranial remolding therapy, if and when appropriate. The patient has been treated in physical therapy for a total of 20 sessions over the past 12 months. The duration of treatment was prolonged due to delayed acquisition of rolling and sitting unsupported and due to his decreased tolerance of prone positions and play. Initial weekly sessions tapered to every other week at 4 months of age, and then monthly at 6 months until he started walking. The mother is a stay-at-home caregiver and has been able to perform the recommended interven-tions. At the current visit, the patient presents with his head positioned in midline. He has equal and active cervical motion for lateral flexion and rotation. His passive range of motion (ROM) is equal for lateral flexion and within 5° for cervical rota-tion. His head shape is grossly symmetrical with residual mild facial asymmetries. The therapist observes that the toddler independently ambulates with his upper extremities held in high guard. The mother reports that her son has been walking independently for three weeks. The reason for this visit is that current evidence supports physical therapy follow-up at 12 months of age or after the acquisition of walking in infants diagnosed and treated for CMT.

- ▶ What other health conditions may present with the same physical findings as CMT?
- ▶ What are the red flags that warrant referral to a pediatrician for further diagnostic testing?
- ▶ What are the most appropriate examination tests?
- ▶ Describe the physical therapy plan of care based on the child's age, severity of torticollis, presence of plagiocephaly, and compliance with the home program.

KEY DEFINITIONS

ALBERTA INFANT MOTOR SCALES (AIMS): Developmental tool appropriate for infants from birth through independent walking (0-18 months of age) used to identify gross motor performance of infants compared to norm-referenced peers

BREECH BIRTH: Presentation of the fetus with buttocks or feet first prior to delivery

CRANIAL VAULT ASYMMETRY (CVA): Measurement of cranial asymmetry obtained by comparing the longest and shortest diagonals from the forehead to the posterior skull using the formula $(A - B)/A$, where A is the longest diagonal and B is the shortest diagonal

CRANIOSYNOSTOSIS: Premature closure of cranial sutures; requires immediate referral to a pediatric neurosurgeon

DEVELOPMENTAL DELAY: Delay in the developmental milestones of fine and gross motor, language, cognition, and/or social interaction

DEVELOPMENTAL DYSPLASIA OF THE HIP: Abnormal development or growth of the hip joint that results in subluxation or dislocation of the femoral head in the acetabulum of the pelvis

MUSCLE FUNCTION SCALE: 6-point scale used to measure lateral cervical flexion strength in infants aged 2 months or older

PLAGIOCEPHALY: Deformity of the skull resulting from positioning that is present at birth or develops during the first few months of life

TUBULAR ORTHOSIS FOR TORTICOLLIS (TOT COLLAR): Prefabricated neck orthosis that is custom fit to each child; it is designed to provide a noxious stimulus to the lateral aspect of the skull to promote midline head position.

Objectives

1. Identify signs and symptoms of congenital muscular torticollis (CMT).
2. Identify valid and reliable outcome tools to measure cervical passive ROM and screen gross motor development.
3. Describe when referral to other healthcare professionals is warranted.
4. Describe a physical therapy treatment plan for an individual with CMT.
5. Establish a home program to be completed by a caregiver with specific parameters for dosing (frequency, duration, number of repetitions).
6. Identify discharge criteria for the toddler with CMT.

Physical Therapy Considerations

PT considerations during management of the toddler with CMT:

▶ **General physical therapy plan of care/goals:** Resolution of CMT: no visible head tilt; symmetry of movements in all positions and during transitions; age-appropriate gross motor development; equal active and passive cervical ROM within 5°; duration and frequency of care depends upon severity of the CMT, associated medical and orthopaedic conditions, and parents' ability to perform the exercises

▶ **Physical therapy interventions:** Parent/caregiver education; passive neck ROM with manual stretching, stretching through carrying, holding, and positioning; neck and trunk active range of motion (AROM); trunk and cervical strengthening to promote symmetrical motor development; repositioning and environmental adaptations

▶ **Precautions during physical therapy:** Passive stretching of cervical structures may be contraindicated in certain orthopaedic and neurologic conditions; passive stretching can cause snapping of the sternocleidomastoid muscle (SCM) in 8% of infants[1]

▶ **Complications interfering with physical therapy:** Comorbidities such as plagiocephaly, gastroesophageal reflux, developmental delay, cardiac, and neurologic conditions may affect outcomes; parental noncompliance with therapy and home exercise program; lack of infant cooperation and stranger/separation anxiety can affect infant's tolerance to interventions

Understanding the Health Condition

CMT is a common postural deformity in infants characterized by a unilateral shortening or fibrosis of the SCM resulting in a head tilt toward and rotational deformity away from the involved side. The reported incidence of CMT ranges from 0.3%[2] to 16%[3] of newborns. The development of CMT is positively correlated with larger babies, breech position, decreased intrauterine space, primiparity, male sex,[4] and use of forceps or vacuum extraction during delivery.[5] Milder forms of CMT appear shortly after birth and are associated with positional preference of the head; if left untreated, this condition may result in asymmetrical shortening of the SCM.[1,6] The "Back to Sleep" campaign aimed at decreasing the incidence of sudden infant death syndrome and the resulting decreased time spent in prone have been associated with an increased incidence of CMT and plagiocephaly.[7-9] CMT occasionally presents with side bending and turning to the same side.[10,11] CMT may also be associated with plagiocephaly,[3] hip dysplasia,[12] brachial plexus injuries,[13-15] developmental delay,[13,16] distal extremity deformities, facial asymmetry, and temporomandibular joint dysfunction.[17] Infants with CMT are also at risk for developmental delay.[7,16] Differential diagnoses that may initially present as CMT include musculoskeletal, neurologic, or ocular impairments.[13] Red flags warranting immediate referral to the primary pediatrician include poor visual tracking, abnormal muscle tone, extramuscular masses, or other asymmetries atypical for a diagnosis of CMT; these may be indicative of a congenital, genetic, or neurologic condition.[13]

CMT has been divided into three types based on the severity of the involved SCM: postural, muscular, and SCM nodule (mass). Postural CMT is the mildest form. Individuals with postural CMT have a postural preference with no limitations

Table 17-1	CMT CLASSIFICATION OF SEVERITY	
Grade	**Severity**	**Age of Infant and Cervical Passive Rotation Impairment**
Grade 1	Early mild	Infants in first 3 months of life with only postural or muscle tightness; <15°
Grade 2	Early moderate	Infants between 4 and 6 months of age with muscle tightness; 15°-30°
Grade 3	Early severe	Infants between 4 and 6 months of age with muscle tightness of >30° or SCM mass
Grade 4	Late mild	Infants between 7 and 9 months of age with only postural or muscle tightness of <15°
Grade 5	Late moderate	Infants between 10 and 12 months of age with only postural or muscle tightness of <15°
Grade 6	Late severe	Infants between 7 and 12 months of age with muscle tightness of >15°
Grade 7	Late extreme	Infants after 7 months of age with SCM mass or after 12 months of age with muscle tightness of >30°, presence of SCM mass, or referred after 12 months of age

in active or passive neck ROM.[8] Individuals with muscular CMT have soft tissue restrictions in the SCM and accessory muscles and decreased passive ROM. The last form of CMT is the most severe. With SCM nodule CMT, individuals present with fibrotic thickening of the SCM and passive ROM restrictions.[1] Overall, individuals diagnosed early with postural deformities require less treatment time, while individuals diagnosed later and those with fibrosis in the SCM require a longer duration of treatment and possibly more invasive interventions.[18,19] In 2013, Kaplan et al.[11] developed a CMT classification of severity derived from four key variables: age of diagnosis, date of referral for treatment, type of CMT (postural, muscular, or SCM nodule), and difference in passive cervical rotation. The purpose of this classification was to establish an episode of care and provide treatment recommendations for each severity level. Table 17-1 shows the seven grades of CMT that categorize the severity by age of onset and condition of the affected SCM.[11]

Physical Therapy Patient/Client Management

Management of the infant or toddler with CMT requires collaboration among physical therapist, primary pediatrician, pediatric nurse practitioner, family/caregiver, orthotist, and other specialists involved in the child's care. During the newborn period, infants are referred to the primary pediatrician and/or physical therapist (in states with direct access) by healthcare providers who have observed a positional preference, decreased cervical ROM, movement asymmetries, cranial or facial asymmetry, or SCM mass.[3,20,21] If not diagnosed during the newborn period, pediatricians should refer to physical therapy as soon as signs of movement preferences are detected.[3,20,21] The diagnosis of CMT typically coincides with well-baby checkups at the ages recommended by the American Academy of Pediatrics.[3,22] Physical therapists should refer infants to their primary pediatrician for further testing when evaluation reveals signs inconsistent with CMT (*e.g.*, poor visual tracking, abnormal muscle tone, extramuscular masses) that may be red flags for more serious conditions.[13] Signs and symptoms of developmental dysplasia of the hip (DDH) warrant a referral to an orthopaedist.[12,23,24] The 2013 CMT clinical practice guideline (CPG) from the Section on Pediatrics of the American Physical Therapy Association (APTA) recommends referral back to the physician with **recommendations for consultation with a specialist when:** intensive physical therapy for 4 to 6 weeks does not improve the condition, the patient reaches a plateau within 6 months of treatment with moderate improvement, the infant is older than 12 months on initial examination and presents with facial asymmetry, and/or a 10° to 15° difference persists between right and left sides, or the infant is 7 months or older and presents with an SCM mass.[11] When conservative treatment is not effective, a patient should be referred to a pediatric ophthalmologist (to rule out visual impairments) and an orthopaedic surgeon (for radiographs of the cervical spine to rule out bony anomalies). Thereafter, a patient will be referred to a plastic surgeon or neurosurgeon for more assessment and invasive treatment. Plagiocephaly is often associated with CMT. If plagiocephaly is suspected or if repositioning has not been effective at improving head shape symmetry after 4 to 6 weeks of treatment, or if the infant is 7 months or older at initiation of treatment for CMT, the physical therapist should refer the child to a center specializing in treatment of infants with deformational plagiocephaly.[1,6,11] The patient presented in this case has been monitored by an orthotist for the potential need for cranial remodeling therapy. After observing an abnormal curvature of the spine, the primary pediatrician also referred the patient to a pediatric orthopaedist; however, radiographs revealed normal spinal alignment and the orthopaedist recommended continuing with physical therapy. Table 17-2 outlines the episode of care for the current patient from initiation of physical therapy treatment to discharge.

Table 17-2 EPISODE OF CARE FOR CASE PATIENT FROM INITIATION OF TREATMENT TO DISCHARGE			
Age	Referrals	Results	Interventions
2 months	Pediatrician referred patient to physical therapy for CMT	Grade 3 (early severe CMT)	Weekly therapy with intensive home program
4 months	Referred to orthotist for cranial scan	Cranial vault asymmetry = 8.9 mm, Level 3 (moderate) on Children's Healthcare of Atlanta Plagiocephaly Severity Scale	Repositioning for cranial remolding and follow-up scan
6 months	None		
9 months	Referred to orthopaedist for assessment of thoracic spine alignment Follow-up cranial scan	Radiographs revealed neutral thoracic spine Cranial vault asymmetry = 6.0 mm, Level 2 (mild) on Children's Healthcare of Atlanta Plagiocephaly Severity Scale	Continue with therapy for passive ROM and postural strengthening exercises
14 months	None	Discharge from therapy	Continue with home stretching program 1 to 3 times per day

Examination, Evaluation, and Diagnosis

The physical therapist should obtain medical and developmental history through parent interview before completing an initial screen on the infant with CMT. Case history includes date of birth, sex, birth rank, reason for referral or parental concerns, overall health of the infant, and any other healthcare providers involved in the infant's care.[11] Additional factors that may affect diagnosis and prognosis of CMT are onset of symptoms,[6,25] intrauterine positioning,[21] birth presentation,[6] use of forceps or vacuum suction during delivery,[3,4,14,19] head posture/preference,[3,8,20,24] family history of torticollis,[26] congenital or developmental conditions,[26,27] other known medical conditions,[13,24] achievement of developmental milestones,[16,28] and daily management of the infant. When the physical therapist had initially evaluated the child at 2 months of age, the mother reported that this was her first child and that he was born at 40 weeks of gestation and weighed 8 pounds, 10 ounces. She reported that her baby was "stuck" in one position during the last trimester. Labor was induced and the baby was born vaginally after seven hours of labor. She reported that her child initially slept on his back with his head turned to the right, but cervical rotation improved with treatment. Although rolling was delayed, he was rotating his head in bilateral directions and was able to roll independently onto his belly at 8 months. He also liked to sleep in an infant swing for naps, though she placed him in an upright positioning device at night. The mother stated she positioned the baby in prone several times per day; he tolerated prone for three minutes prior to fussing and crying or falling asleep. Under close supervision, the baby's parents allowed him to sleep in prone for naps. When asked about feeding, the mother reported that she initially attempted breastfeeding and that the baby preferred to nurse on her left breast keeping his head turned to the right. However, feedings were stressful for both mother and child and she began bottle-feeding. She also reported a history of constipation correlated with episodes of increased fussiness. Because of increased vomiting and inconsolable crying after feeding, the infant was diagnosed with gastroesophageal reflux at the 1-month well-baby visit. He was treated with medication and instruction to position upright for 30 minutes after feeding.

Throughout the examination, the physical therapist should be cognizant of any pain or discomfort in the infant.[10,29] Passive stretching may trigger pain; decreasing the intensity of the stretch may decrease pain and muscle guarding.[30] Crying may also be associated with anxiety due to handling, stress, or an unfamiliar environment. To provide reassurance to the parent, the physical therapist should differentiate pain from discomfort or anxiety. The Face, Legs, Activity, Cry, Consolability (FLACC) scale assesses pain and discomfort in infants with CMT and has been validated for children 2 months to 7 years of age.[11,31,32] The FLACC is a nonverbal tool that assesses pain based on behavioral response in five areas on 3-point scale; total score ranges from 0 to 10, with 0 representing no pain. At the beginning and end of the session, the therapist recorded a score of 0/10. During passive cervical rotation and lateral flexion ROM measurements and instruction of the home program to the mother, the therapist noted a FLACC score of 6/10.

The physical therapist should complete a symptoms screen according to APTA guidelines.[33] Results not typical for a diagnosis of CMT may be red flags that require further diagnostic testing. The musculoskeletal screen includes examination of hip joint integrity.[34] The incidence of DDH with CMT ranges from 2.5% to 17%.[4,16] Infants younger than 3 months are screened using the Ortolani and Barlow maneuvers in which the affected hip is either dislocated (Ortolani maneuver) or reduced (Barlow maneuver).[35] Symptoms of DDH in infants older than 3 months include decreased hip abduction of 5° to 10°, asymmetrical gluteal and thigh folds, and a positive Galeazzi sign in which the affected hip presents with a shorter femur.[35]

At 2 months of age, the baby in this case presented with a left head tilt posture with rotation of the chin to the right and prominent and palpable left SCM. Compensatory posturing included left shoulder elevation and shortening of the trunk on the left. Cranial asymmetry was noted with right posterior flattening, left forehead bossing, and right anterior shift of the ear. An anterior view of the infant's face revealed mild facial asymmetry with recession of the left orbit and zygoma and decreased size and height of the left cheek. The therapist screened the infant for DDH using the Ortolani maneuver, which was negative since a click or pop was not detected. Active and passive hip ROM were equal and within functional range. During the neurologic examination, the therapist screens for abnormal tone, atypical reflexes, cranial nerve integrity, brachial plexus injury,[13-15] temperament, motor development,[13,16] cognitive and social development,[36] and vision.[2,37] The infant had normal muscle tone. He demonstrated reflexive standing and stepping and presence of the asymmetric tonic neck reflex (ATNR), which was normal for a 2-month-old. In supine, the baby could focus with his head in midline and he tracked a toy more to the right than to the left. For the integumentary screen, the therapist should specifically examine for symmetry of cervical[10,38] and gluteal skin folds[21,24] as well as skin color and condition. The infant had an increased number of cervical skin folds, which were deeper on the left. The skin within the cervical folds was red with signs of irritation. Gluteal skin folds of the hip were symmetrical. In the cardiorespiratory screen, the therapist assesses coloration, rib cage expansion and clavicle movement,[24,27] respiratory distress,[15,39] and vocalization. The physical therapist noted that the baby was breathing easily with no signs of distress. The mother also reported that her son was healthy, had no history of respiratory infections, and his heart was reported to be normal. Last, the CMT-CPG recommends a gastrointestinal screen that includes assessing for history of gastroesophageal reflux, constipation,[11,15] or a preference to feed to one side.[8] Parental interview revealed a history of gastroesophageal reflux and constipation. The infant was on medication for the reflux and was positioned upright in a swing after feeding where he frequently napped during the day.

The assessment of an infant with CMT includes a comprehensive evaluation of body function and structure.[33] The therapist observes postural alignment of the head, neck, and trunk in all developmentally age-appropriate positions.[3,8,16,25,29] AROM limitations for the extremities and trunk should be documented. In supine, the therapist should note head position relative to midline alignment[3,8,16,21] and rotational preference, hip girdle alignment,[8,21] and facial symmetry. In prone, the therapist can observe alignment of the head and spine, symmetry of the skull, use of extremities, and tolerance to positions. The patient presented with asymmetrical posture in supine, prone, and supported sitting. He demonstrated fair tolerance to prone activity, though he lacked cervical extensor strength. In sitting and standing (as appropriate for age), the physical therapist should assess postural preferences and compensations in the shoulder, trunk, and hip. When available, the use of digital photography is beneficial to establish a baseline image of the infant's posture in supine and for parent education. To document an objective measure of lateral tilt, the therapist can draw a line on the photograph bisecting the acromion processes and draw another line through the midpoint of the eyes.[39] Visual inspection of the patient revealed lateral flexion of the head and rotation of the chin to the right with compensatory left shoulder elevation and side bending of the trunk. Cranial and facial asymmetry was also present.

Active cervical ROM provides a measurement of cervical strength and symmetrical development.[7,40] For infants younger than 3 months, cervical rotation is assessed in supine; for older infants, meaurements are performed with the infant sitting in the therapist's lap.[41] Lateral flexion is assessed for infants older than 2 months using the Muscle Function Scale.[40,42] To perform this, the therapist holds the infant vertically in front of a mirror and tilts him horizontally; head righting is measured according to a 6-point scale.[42] Infants with CMT may present with a difference of 2 to 3 points compared to typically developing infants who have symmetrical strength.[42] The patient in this case was able to visually track a toy in both directions, but active left cervical rotation was limited. In supine, the therapist recorded 90° cervical rotation to the right and only 60° to the left. Active lateral flexion of the head was tested during facilitated rolling to both sides. The baby was able to lift and turn his head to the right when rolling over the right side. However, when rolling over the left side, he was unable to lift his head off the surface or freely turn to the left. The therapist also noted compensatory movements of hiking the left shoulder and left lateral trunk flexion.

In infants, measuring passive cervical ROM with an **arthrodial protractor** is valid and reliable.[40,43] In infants with CMT, measurements made with an arthrodial protractor are more reliable for passive cervical rotation than passive side bending.[43] Passive cervical rotation is measured with the infant in supine with the head in neutral and the nose vertically aligned. With the shoulder stabilized, the therapist rotates the head in the opposite direction. To measure side bending, the therapist stabilizes the shoulders and laterally flexes the head until the ear contacts the shoulder. For this infant, there was a 50° difference in passive cervical rotation (110° to the right; 60° to the left) and a 20° difference in side bending (65°-70° to the left; 45° to the right), indicating a Grade 3 CMT severity classification.[11]

The therapist visually inspects and palpates affected musculature to identify the presence and location of a palpable mass and tight bands, extent of fibrosis, and condition of accessory cervical muscles such as the upper trapezius, levator scapulae, and scalenes that can contribute to the torticollis.[1,44] The condition of the patient's left SCM was tested with the baby supported in supine on his mother's lap with his head turned to the left and laterally flexed to the right in order to place the left SCM on stretch. The right SCM was tested in the opposite fashion. The therapist noted that the patient's left SCM was thicker, deeper, and wider, and presented with increased tightness that felt like a hard fibrous band; the left upper trapezius also felt harder and thicker and the left shoulder was hiked and protracted. The absence of a palpable mass and early intervention of services improves the patient's prognosis for complete resolution of CMT.[1,44] The **prognosis for complete resolution of CMT** is excellent for infants who receive intervention prior to 3 months of age.[4,18,19,30,45]

The therapist performs the craniofacial assessment by observing for symmetry of the skull and facial structures from multiple views.[3,5,17,18,21,46] A vertex view (*i.e.*, from the top) of the cranium should reveal symmetry of the occiput, parietal, and frontal regions as well as ear position. From the frontal view, orbital alignment, cheek size and shape, and jaw structure can be examined. A posterior view confirms ear alignment and allows observation for any widening of the posterior skull. A lateral view allows examination of any abnormal vertical growth in cases of severe plagiocephaly. The clinical classification of plagiocephaly according to Argenta[47] distinguishes five types of plagiocephaly based on severity of asymmetry. Type I only involves occiput flattening. Type II includes an ipsilateral ear shift. Type III progresses to include ipsilateral frontal bossing. Type IV advances to facial asymmetry and type V involves temporal bossing.[47] Quantifying the level of deformity allows the physical therapist to monitor change over time and determine the effectiveness of treatment interventions.[20] This is often accomplished with a 3-dimensional (3D) computerized cranial scanning system that uses a non-invasive laser to scan an infant's head in 1.5 seconds,[48] allowing an orthotist to accurately measure head shape. Cranial scans can be performed with a hand-held scanning device or by placing the infant in a scanner. For this patient, an initial 3D scan at age 5.5 months revealed a cranial vault asymmetry of 8.9 mm. Utilizing Argenta's classification, the patient presented as a type IV. Based on the Children's Healthcare of Atlanta Plagiocephaly Severity Scale,[48] the patient was categorized as a Level 3. Due to the patient's young age, repositioning to prevent pressure on the back of the head was recommended as the first intervention to halt the progression of cranial asymmetry. A follow-up scan completed at 9 months of age revealed a cranial vault asymmetry of 6.0 mm. The patient was then categorized as Level 2 severity.[48] Recommendations were to continue with repositioning and treatment of the CMT. Therefore, cranial remolding therapy was not indicated for treatment in this case.

Activity limitations are assessed by observing the infant in age-appropriate positions for tolerance, symmetry of movement, and age-appropriate motor development. Reliable and standardized tools for assessing motor development in infants include the Test of Infant Motor Performance (TIMP) for infants younger than 4 months and the Alberta Infant Motor Scale[49] (AIMS) for infants 4 to 18 months of corrected age (*i.e.*, age corrected for premature birth). The TIMP has been validated for infants younger than 4 months and the AIMS for infants older than 4 months. The patient demonstrated good tolerance to prone for three minutes during the evaluation before becoming fussy and crying. Because infants with torticollis are typically monitored until the onset of walking, the evaluating physical therapist performed the AIMS on the patient to enable consistent assessment of gross motor development over time. At the initial evaluation at 2 months of age, the patient scored in the 25th percentile. When the patient was discharged at 14 months of age, he scored in the 75th percentile.

Participation can be assessed by observing the parent handling the infant and by the parent's report (*e.g.*, tolerance to position changes, preferential feeding positions, time spent in equipment or positioning devices). While being held, the infant in this case preferred to turn his head to the right with the head tilted to the left. The mother reported that he preferred feeding to the right as well and that he typically fell asleep when placed in prone. For night sleeps, the patient was positioned upright in an infant positioner (*e.g.*, Nap Nanny); for naps, he was placed in an infant swing. The therapist took this opportunity to educate the mother about the American Academy of Pediatrics 2011 recommendations for safe sleep, which state that infants are to sleep on their backs on a firm surface. Car seats and other sitting devices are not recommended for routine sleep and wedges and positioners should not be used.[50]

At 2 months of age, the severity of this patient's CMT would have been classified as Grade 3 (early severe) based on the following presenting characteristics: age at onset of symptoms or diagnosis, age at referral, type of CMT (presence of fibrous bands in SCM without mass/nodule), and 50° of restriction of passive cervical rotation.[11]

Plan of Care and Interventions

The prognosis for an infant with CMT is highly correlated to compliance with the home physical therapy program. Parents are educated on environmental modifications to promote symmetrical cervical ROM and posturing such as alternating the infant's position on the changing table and in the crib to promote active rotation in both directions. Parents are also encouraged to feed infants in both directions. For cranial remolding, recommendations include decreasing the time spent in positioning equipment such as car seats and increasing floor time. Infants who play in the prone position for a total of 60 minutes per day decrease the negative effects of compliance with the Back to Sleep campaign.[51-52]

At the initial evaluation, the therapist set goals for this patient based on the International Classification of Functioning, Disability and Health (ICF) model. For symmetrical body structure and function, goals included: symmetrical passive ROM for cervical rotation and lateral flexion within 5°; symmetrical active rotation to track a toy in supine or supported sitting position to increase visual awareness to affected side; symmetrical righting reaction during rolling; symmetrical cervical skin folds with no evidence of skin breakdown; and patient to tolerate passive stretching activities without increased pain (measured by FLACC scale). Goals aligned with activity included: participation in active prone position with symmetrical use of upper extremities for weightbearing and reaching; demonstration of symmetrical rolling patterns to increase floor mobility; and symmetrical gross motor development with creeping and pulling to stand. For participation goals, the therapist stated that the patient would participate in at least 5 to 10 minutes of prone activity without episodes of fussing 5 times per day and that the mother would complete the home stretching program 5 times per day coinciding with diaper changing.

The duration and frequency for physical therapy is based on the patient's age at referral, severity of CMT, and parental compliance to the recommended treatments. If therapy is initiated within the first 3 months of age, estimated duration for physical therapy treatment is less than 3 months. Infants referred between 3 and 6 months of age are typically treated for 3 to 6 months. Patients with greater fibrotic tissue at the onset of treatment also require a longer treatment duration.[53] Table 17-3 provides the details of the episode of care for this patient. Sessions progressed from weekly, to twice monthly, to monthly, and then consultative until the child was able to independently walk. Progression was based on the patient's achievement of goals that were set at the initial evaluation and during the episode of care as well as the mother's understanding of CMT and compliance with recommended interventions.

Physical therapy interventions address the impairments and limitations documented during the evaluation. The combination of physical therapy and a home program performed by the parent is the most recommended intervention plan for infants diagnosed with CMT.[18,19,29] Initially, physical therapy is recommended weekly; as the CMT resolves, frequency may be decreased to every other week. Following resolution of CMT, infants are monitored every 4 to 6 weeks. An infant may demonstrate increased symptoms during illness or episodes of teething because the asymmetrical posture may be a position of comfort. Secondary to these vulnerable periods and critical periods of growth and motor maturation, the CMT-CPG[11] recommends following an infant with CMT until the initiation of walking or first birthday.

Passive manual stretching is the most common and effective intervention for CMT.[18,19,29] The physical therapist performs manual stretches by passively moving the head in the direction opposite of the preferred posture. Typically, the therapist rotates the SCM toward the affected side and side bends the head away from the affected side. Stretches can be performed in supine and supported sitting in the therapist's lap or through positioning and holding. Carrying the infant in the position opposite of the infant's posture will elongate the affected muscles and promote symmetrical alignment. Carrying stretches are especially beneficial as the infant gets older and less cooperative with passive ROM exercises performed in supine. For this patient, treatment was initiated at the evaluation and included stretching through carrying, positioning, and manual stretching. The therapist instructed the mother to hold the baby in her arms with the infant's left side toward the ground while separating his left ear from his shoulder to stretch out the tighter left side of the neck and trunk. In this position, she can carry her baby and hold him on her lap. The mother was instructed to provide "tummy time" and positioning throughout the day and to limit time spent in the swing and infant seat to 20 to 30 minutes, 1 to 2 times per day. The therapist also instructed the mother in passive stretches to be performed 4 to 5 times per day, with each stretch to be held for a minimum of 30 seconds.

To elongate shortened muscles, the physical therapist facilitates active movement of the neck and trunk during floor time activity and transitional movements such as rolling and righting reactions. During prone activity, the infant works to strengthen extensors of the neck and spine. Active cervical rotation is encouraged

Table 17-3 EPISODE OF CARE FOR CURRENT PATIENT FROM PHYSICAL THERAPY EVALUATION TO DISCHARGE

Age (months)	Frequency of Physical Therapy Sessions	Frequency of Home Program	PROM	AROM Postural Alignment	Condition of Skin Folds	Muscle Function Scale (Strength of Lateral Cervical Flexion)	Pain (FLACC scale)	Activity Development
2	Weekly	5 times per day	*Rotation* R: 110° L: 60° *Lateral flexion* R: 45° L: 65°-70°	*Rotation* R: 90° L: 60° Left lateral tilt and lateral trunk flexion > 75%	Increased redness and depth on left	Facilitated righting reactions sidelying; stronger on left	6/10	25% decreased tolerance to prone (AIMS)
4	Weekly	5 times per day	*Rotation* R: 110° L: 90° *Lateral flexion* R: 60° L: 65°-70°	*Rotation* R: 90° L: 75°	Decreased redness	R: 0/5 L: 4/5	6/10	Prone on forearms Rolling supine to sidelying
6	Every other week	5 times per day	*Rotation* R: 110° L: 95° *Lateral flexion* R: 60° L: 65°-70°	*Rotation* B: 90° Mild L Lateral tilt and lateral trunk flexion	Mild redness in cervical folds	R: 1/5 L: 5/5	4/10	Independent sitting Prone on hands Rolling supine to prone

(Continued)

Table 17-3 EPISODE OF CARE FOR CURRENT PATIENT FROM PHYSICAL THERAPY EVALUATION TO DISCHARGE (CONTINUED)

Age (months)	Frequency of Physical Therapy Sessions	Frequency of Home Program	PROM	AROM Postural Alignment	Condition of Skin Folds	Muscle Function Scale (Strength of Lateral Cervical Flexion)	Pain (FLACC scale)	Activity Development
9	Every other week	3 times per day	*Rotation* R: 110° L: 100° *Lateral flexion* B: 65°	L tilt 50% of time; improved alignment of trunk, increased weightbearing on L pelvis in sitting	Intact	R: 2/5 L: 5/5	0/10	Independent sitting with protective reactions in forward/lateral directions Combat crawling with reciprocal movements
12	Once a month	2-3 times per day	*Rotation* R: 110° L: 105° *Lateral flexion* B: 65°	Neutral alignment of head, trunk, and pelvic girdle	Intact	B: 5/5	4/10[a]	Creeping Pulling to stand Cruising
14	Discharge	2 times per day	Same as 12 months	Same as 12 months	Same as 12 months	Same as 12 months	4/10[a]	Independent walking

Abbreviations: B, bilateral; L, left; R, right.
[a]FLACC score attributed to separation anxiety from mother. Patient immediately calmed when returned to mother.

to the side of limitation; this was achieved by placing toys on the left side to have the infant turn his head to the left.

The physical therapist must also facilitate symmetry with motor development. Infants who demonstrate asymmetrical exploration are at risk for developing delays in early perceptual motor skills, which later correlates to cognition.[36] Therefore, the physical therapist works with the infant to facilitate symmetry with movement patterns during treatment sessions and educates the parents on the infant's limitations in mobility to address in the home. When the patient began rolling at 4 months of age, he demonstrated a preference to roll toward the direction of the affected SCM secondary to decreased cervical rotation. The parents demonstrated excellent compliance with interventions aimed at increasing the infant's body and environmental awareness to his affected side and they worked to facilitate rolling in the opposite direction for symmetrical motor development. When the patient learned to pull to stand at 11 months, he demonstrated increased weightbearing on the left lower extremity due to shortened trunk muscles on the affected side. The mother continued with a carrying stretch to side bend the trunk in the opposite direction and shifted weight to the right lower extremity during supported standing to facilitate symmetrical weightbearing.

Recommendations for frequency of a home exercise program range from 2 to 8 times per day.[18,54] The mother of the current patient was a stay-at-home caregiver and was able to perform exercises 5 times per day, thus increasing the effectiveness of treatment. The patient also participated in active "tummy time" during each wakeful period for an average of 5 times per day and the mother transitioned the infant to sleep in his crib without any positioning device for naps and nighttime sleeps.

Alternative treatment approaches for CMT may be recommended when conservative treatment is not effective, physical therapy services are limited, the infant is unable to tolerate the first intervention,[3] or the infant is older at the time of referral. The most common supplemental interventions are the use of **kinesiological taping**[29,38] **(KT) and the tubular orthosis for torticollis (TOT) collar.**[38,55] KT is a stretchable tape used to inhibit the affected muscle and/or facilitate weakened muscles to promote improved alignment of the neck and spine.[8,29] Infants with skin sensitivities may not tolerate the application of KT. For the current patient, the physical therapist applied a test strip of KT; however, redness appeared after 24 hours of wear. Therefore, KT was not an appropriate intervention for the patient presented. For the infant with a consistent head tilt greater than 5° to 6° and good head control in supported sitting, a TOT collar (Fig. 17-1) may be applied to inhibit movement toward the affected side and facilitate active movement away from the tilted side. It is recommended that the TOT collar be worn during active playtime and when in a highchair, but not when the infant is sleeping or in a car seat.[38]

If conservative treatment is not effective, a patient should be referred to a specialist for more invasive treatment. The most common interventions are botulinum toxin injections or surgical lengthening of the SCM muscle. Surgical recommendations are made following at least 3 months, but more typically, after 6 to 12 months of conservative treatment.[19,20,34,45,54,56] When treatment is initiated in the first few months of age, the incidence of surgery is as low as 5%.[57]

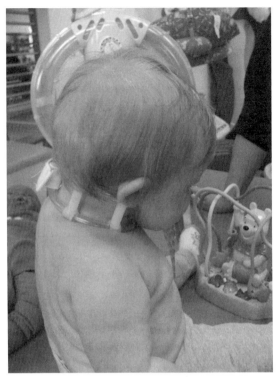

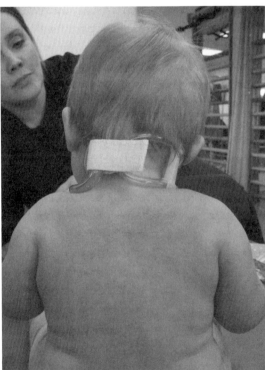

Figure 17-1. Prefabricated tubular orthosis for torticollis (TOT) collar designed to provide a noxious stimulus to the lateral aspect of the skull to promote midline head position.

Resolution of CMT is achieved when the infant: has full passive cervical ROM within 5° of the uninvolved side; presents with midline alignment of head and trunk, symmetrical active movement of the head, neck, trunk, hips, and upper and lower extremities; has achieved age-appropriate motor skills, and the parents have a good understanding of what to monitor as the infant grows to prevent recurrence of CMT. In addition, the physical therapist should monitor the infant diagnosed with CMT for positional preference, symmetry with alignment and movement of head, trunk, hips, and extremities and achievement of gross motor skills for 3 to 12 months or until the initiation of walking. For this patient, the torticollis resolved at 12 months of age, but the patient was monitored until independent walking.

Evidence-Based Clinical Recommendations

SORT: Strength of Recommendation Taxonomy

A: Consistent, good-quality patient-oriented evidence
B: Inconsistent or limited-quality patient-oriented evidence
C: Consensus, disease-oriented evidence, usual practice, expert opinion, or case series

1. An infant with congenital muscular torticollis should be referred to a specialist when: the condition remains the same after 4 to 6 weeks of initial intensive treatment, 6 months of treatment with moderate resolution, the infant is older than 12 months or has a 10° to 15° of restriction in ROM, or the infant is 7 months or older at evaluation and presents with an SCM mass. **Grade B**

2. Measurements of passive cervical ROM made with an arthrodial protractor are reliable and valid in infants; in those with CMT, arthrodial protractor measurements are more reliable for cervical rotation than side bending. **Grade B**

3. The prognosis for complete resolution of CMT is excellent for infants who receive intervention prior to 3 months of age. **Grade A**

4. Passive manual stretching is the most common and effective intervention for CMT. **Grade B**

5. The use of kinesiological taping and the application of the tubular orthosis for torticollis (TOT) collar are effective supplemental treatment approaches when conservative treatment is not effective. **Grade C**

COMPREHENSION QUESTIONS

17.1 Which of the following is *not* typically associated with CMT?

A. Developmental dysplasia of hip (DDH)

B. Fibrosis of the affected sternocleidomastoid muscle

C. Abnormal muscle tone

D. Plagiocephaly

17.2   A 5-month-old infant with a 25° restriction of passive cervical rotation to the left and an SCM mass is referred to physical therapy for treatment of CMT. This patient's CMT would be categorized as:

A. Grade 1—early mild

B. Grade 2—early moderate

C. Grade 3—early severe

D. Grade 4—late mild

17.3   Based on the infant's CMT severity grade and best evidence, which intervention should be included in the initial treatment session?

A. Passive cervical range of motion

B. Facilitation of rolling away from the affected side

C. Active strengthening of the weaker cervical muscles

D. Prone positioning during play

ANSWERS

17.1   **C.** The presence of abnormal muscle tone may be a red flag for a neurologic impairment. It is not consistent with CMT. The treating therapist should refer the patient to a pediatrician or a specialist. DDH is associated with CMT; individuals with hip dysplasia also warrant referral for further diagnostic testing.

17.2   **C.** Based on age of less than 6 months and the presence of SCM mass, the patient would be classified as having Grade 3 (early severe) CMT.

17.3   **A.** The literature supports passive ROM as the first intervention for infants diagnosed with CMT. Passive cervical ROM has been defined in two ways: manual stretching with precise positions for the infant and caregiver and handling and carrying the infant in a manner that incorporates the stretch positions. Active playtime in prone and repositioning is also recommended. Facilitation of gross motor skills should promote symmetrical movement patterns (*i.e.*, movement should be encouraged in both directions, not only to the affected side).

REFERENCES

1. Cheng JC, Wong MW, Tang SP, Chen TM, Shum SL, Wong EM. Clinical determinants of the outcome of manual stretching in the treatment of congenital muscular torticollis in infants. A prospective study of eight hundred and twenty-one cases. *J Bone Joint Surg Am*. 2001;83:679-687.

2. Do TT. Congenital muscular torticollis: current concents and review of treatment. *Curr Opin Pediatr*. 2006;18:26-29.

3. Stellwagen LM, Hubbard E, Chambers C, Jones KL. Torticollis facial asymmetry and plagiocephaly in normal newborns. *Arch Dis Child*. 2008;93:827-831.

4. Cheng JC, Tang SP, Chen TM. Sternocleidomastoid pseudotumor and congenital muscular torticollis in infants: a prospective study of 510 cases. *J Pediatr*. 1999;134:712-716.

5. Chen MM, Chang HC, Hsieh CF, Yen MF, Chen TH. Predictive model for congenital muscular torticollis: analysis of 1021 infants with sonography. *Arch Phys Med Rehabil.* 2005;86:2199-2203.

6. Cheng JC, Tang SP, Chen TM, Wong MW, Wong EM. The clinical presentation and outcome of treatment of congenital muscular torticollis in infants—a study of 1086 cases. *J Pediatr Surg.* 2000;35:1091-1096.

7. Öhman A, Nilsson S, Lagerkvist AL, Beckung E. Are infants with torticollis at risk of a delay in early motor milestones compared with a control group of healthy infants? *Dev Med Child Neurol.* 2009;51:545-550.

8. Boere-Boonekamp MM, van der Linden-Kuiper LT. Positional preference: prevalence in infants and follow-up after two years. *Pediatrics.* 2001;107:339-343.

9. Persing J, James H, Swanson J, Kattwinkel J. Prevention and management of positional skull deformities in infants. American Academy of Pediatrics Committee on Practice and Ambulatory Medicine, Section on Plastic Surgery and Section on Neurological Surgery. *Pediatrics.* 2003;112:199-202.

10. Freed SS, Coulter-O'Berry C. Identification and treatment of congenital muscular torticollis in infants. *J Prosthet Orthot.* 2004;16:S18-S23.

11. Kaplan SL, Coulter C, Fetters L. Physical therapy management of congenital muscular torticollis: an evidence-based clinical practice guideline from the Section on Pediatrics of the American Physical Therapy Association. *Pediatr Phys Ther.* 2013;25:348-394.

12. Tien YC, Su JY, Lin GT, Lin SY. Ultrasonographic study of the coexistence of muscular torticollis and dysplasia of the hip. *J Pediatr Orthop.* 2001;21:343-347.

13. Ballock RT, Song KM. The prevalence of nonmuscular causes of torticollis in children. *J Pediatr Orthop.* 1996;16:500-504.

14. Tatli B, Aydinli N, Caliskan M, Ozmen M, Bilir F, Acar G. Congenital muscular torticollis: evaluation and classification. *Pediatr Neurol.* 2006;34:41-44.

15. Tomczak KK, Rosman NP. Torticollis. *J Child Neurol.* 2013;28:365-378.

16. Schertz M, Zuk L, Zin S, Nadam L, Schwartz D, Bienkowski RS. Motor and cognitive development at one-year follow-up in infants with torticollis. *Early Hum Dev.* 2008;84:9-14.

17. Yu CC, Wong FH, Lo LJ, Chen YR. Craniofacial deformity in patients with uncorrected congenital muscular torticollis: an assessment from three-dimensional computed tomography imaging. *Plast Reconstr Surg.* 2004;113:24-33.

18. Celayir AC. Congenital muscular torticollis: early and intensive treatment is critical. A prospective study. *Pediatr Int.* 2000;42:504-507.

19. Demirbilek S, Atayurt HF. Congenital muscular torticollis and sternomastoid tumor: results of nonoperative treatment. *J Pediatr Surg.* 1999;34:549-551.

20. van Vlimmeren LA, van der Graaf Y, Boere-Boonekamp MM, L'Hoir MP, Helders PJ, Engelbert RH. Risk factors for deformational plagiocephaly at birth and at 7 weeks of age: a prospective cohort study. *Pediatrics.* 2007;119:e408-e418.

21. Stellwagon LM, Hubbard E, Vaux K. Look for the "stuck baby" to identify congenital torticollis. *Contemp Pediatr.* 2004;21:55-65.

22. Hagan JF, Shaw JS, Duncan PM. *Bright Futures: Guidelines for Health Supervision of Infants, Children, and Adolescents.* 3rd ed. Elk Grove Village, IL: The American Academy of Pediatrics; 2008.

23. Hummer CD, MacEwen GD. The coexistence of torticollis and congenital dysplasia of the hip. *J Bone Joint Surg.* 1972;54:1255-1256.

24. Nuysink J, van Haastert IC, Takken T, Helders PJ. Symptomatic asymmetry in the first six months of life: differential diagnosis. *Eur J Pediatr.* 2008;167:613-619.

25. Luxford BK. The physiotherapy management of infants with congenital muscular torticollis: a survey of current practice in New Zealand. *NZ J Physiother.* 2009;37:127-135.

26. Thompson F, McManus S, Colville J. Familial congenital muscular torticollis: case report and review of the literature. *Clin Orthop Relat Res.* 1986;202:193-196.

27. Sönmex K, Turkyilmaz Z, Demirogullari B, et al. Congenital muscular torticollis in children. *J Oto-rhinolaryngol Relat Spec.* 2005;67:344-347.

28. Tessmer A, Mooney P, Pelland L. A developmental perspective on congenital muscular torticollis: a critical appraisal of the evidence. *Pediatr Phys Ther.* 2010;22:378-383.

29. Burch C, Dreyer K, Hudson P, et al. Evidence-based care guideline: therapy management of congenital muscular torticollis. 2009;1-13. http://www.cincinnatichildrens.org/service/j/anderson-center/evidence-based-care/recommendations/topic/.

30. Canale ST, Griffin DW, Hubbard CN. Congenital muscular torticollis. A long-term follow up. *J Bone Joint Surg Am.* 1982;64:810-816.

31. Merkel S, Voepel-Lewis T, Malviya S. Pain assessment in infants and young children: the FLACC scale. *Am J Nurs.* 2002;102:55-58.

32. Merkel SI, Voepel-Lewis T, Shayevitz JR, Malviya S. The FLACC: a behavioral scale for scoring postoperative pain in young children. *Pediatr Nurs.* 1997;23:293-297.

33. American Physical Therapy Association. Guide to Physical Therapist Practice, 2nd ed. *Phys Ther.* 2001;81:1-768.

34. Wei JL, Schwartz KM, Weaver AL, Orvidas LJ. Pseudotumor of infants and congenital muscular torticollis: 170 cases. *Laryngoscope.* 2001;111:688-695.

35. Jesse MW, Leach J. Orthopedic conditions. In: Campell SK, Vander Linden DW, Palisano RJ, eds. *Physical Therapy for Children.* 4th ed. St. Louis, MO: Saunders; 2012:414-445.

36. Lobo MA, Harbourne RT, Dusing SC, McCoy SW. Grounding early interventions: physical therapy cannot just be about motor skills anymore. *Phys Ther.* 2013;93:94-103.

37. Gray GM, Tasso KH. Differential diagnosis of torticollis: a case report. *Pediatr Phys Ther.* 2009;21:369-374.

38. Karmel-Ross K. *Torticollis: Differential Diagnosis, Assessment and Treatment, Surgical Management and Bracing.* Binghamton, NY: Haworth Press, Inc.; 1997.

39. Rahlin M, Sarmiento B. Reliability of still photography measuring habitual head deviation from midline in infants with congenital muscular torticollis. *Pediatr Phys Ther.* 2010;22:399-406.

40. Öhman AM, Beckung ER. Reference values for range of motion and muscle function of the neck in infants. *Pediatr Phys Ther.* 2008;20:53-58.

41. Laughlin J, Luerssen TG, Dian MS. Prevention and management of positional skull deformities in infants. *Pediatrics.* 2011;128:1236-1241.

42. Öhman AM, Nilsson S, Beckung ER. Validity and reliability of the muscle function scale, aimed to assess the lateral flexors of the neck in infants. *Physioth Theory Pract.* 2009;25:129-137.

43. Klackenberg EP, Elfving B, Haglund-Åkerlind Y, Carlberg EB. Intra-rater reliability in measuring range of motion in infants with congenital muscular torticollis. *Adv Physiother.* 2005;7:84-91.

44. Cheng JC, Metreweli C, Chen TM, Tang SP. Correlation of ultrasonographic imaging of congenital muscular torticollis with clinical assessment in infants. *Ultrasound Med Biol.* 2000;26:1237-1241.

45. Burstein FD. Long-term experience with endoscopic surgical treatment for congenital muscular torticollis in infants and children: a review of 85 cases. *Plast Reconstr Surg.* 2004;114:491-493.

46. Hollier L, Kim J, Grayson BH, McCarthy JG. Congenital muscular torticollis and the associated craniofacial changes. *Plast Reconstr Surg.* 2000;105:827-835.

47. Argenta L. Clinical classification of positional plagiocephaly. *J Craniofac Surg.* 2004;15:368-372.

48. Plank LH, Giavedoni B, Lombardo JR, Geil MD, Reisner A. Comparison of infant head shape changes in deformational plagiocephaly following treatment with a cranial remolding orthosis using a noninvasive laser shape digitizer. *J Craniofac Surg.* 2006;17:1084-1091.

49. Darrah J, Piper M, Watt MJ. Assessment of gross motor skills of at-risk infants: predictive validity of the Alberta Infant Motor Scale. *Dev Med Child Neurol.* 1998;40:485-491.

50. Task Force on Sudden Infant Death Syndrome, Moon RY. SIDS and other sleep-related infant deaths: expansion of recommendations for a safe infant sleeping enviroment. *Pediatrics.* 2011;128:1030-1039.

51. Dudek-Shriber L, Zelazny S. The effects of prone positioning on the quality and acquisition of developmental milestones in four-month-old infants. *Pediatr Phys Ther.* 2007;19:48-55.

52. Monson RM, Deitz J, Kartin D. The relationship between awake positioning and motor performance among infants who slept supine. *Pediatr Phys Ther.* 2003;15:196-203.

53. Lee IJ, Lim SY, Song HS, Park MC. Complete tight fibrous band release and resection in congenital muscular torticollis. *J Plast Reconstr Aesthet Surg.* 2010;63:947-953.

54. Cameron BH, Langer JC, Cameron GS. Success of nonoperative treatment for congenital muscular torticollis is dependent on early therapy. *Pediatr Surg Intl.* 1994;9:391-393.

55. Emery C. The determinants of treatment duration for congenital muscular torticollis. *Phys Ther.* 1994;74:921-929.

56. Kozlov Y, Yakovlev A, Novogilov V, et al. SEET—subcutaneous endoscopic transaxillary tenotomy for congenital muscular torticollis. *J Laparoendosc Adv Surg Tech.* 2009;19:S179-S181.

57. Cheng JC, Chen TM, Tang SP, Shum SL, Wong MW, Metreweli C. Snapping during manual stretching in congenital muscular torticollis. *Clin Orthop Relat Res.* 2001;384:237-244.

Osteogenesis Imperfecta

Amanda Stoltz

CASE 18

A 10-year-old boy diagnosed with osteogenesis imperfecta (OI) type IV presents to an outpatient physical therapy clinic with his mother. The child had an unscheduled surgery eight weeks ago to replace the intramedullary rods of bilateral tibias after he stepped down off a step and sustained a left tibial fracture in which the rod bent. Orthopaedic surgeons decided to replace the right tibial rod at the same time to accommodate further growth of the tibia beyond what the rod was adequately supporting. The child initially had bilateral femoral rods inserted when he was 4 years old and tibial rods when he was 6 years old (Fig. 18-1). He has typical features of OI including deformities of the long bones, joint laxity, and short stature. He also has scoliosis and mild bowing of his femurs. He has a leg length discrepancy of three centimeters for which he wears a shoe lift. Bilaterally, he also has moderate radial bowing and lacks 20° of elbow extension. Over his lifetime, the child has had more than ten fractures including vertebral compression fractures and fractures of the right femur, right tibia, left humerus, left radius, and left patella. Prior to the most recent surgery, he complained of bilateral ankle pain when ambulating more than a city block. The boy has been taking bisphosphonates since he was 3 years old, but discontinued the drugs since his surgery. Although it is typically recommended to discontinue bisphosphonate treatment several months *prior* to any surgery that entails osteotomies, this was not possible due to the nature of this unscheduled surgery. The child's family understands that bone healing may be prolonged due to this issue. The patient has a rear-wheeled walker and a lightweight manual wheelchair with elevating leg rests. Over the past year, he has relied more on his walker at home and school due to increased lower leg pain when weightbearing. Previously, he only used the walker when walking outdoors or for community distances. He uses his wheelchair only as needed after a fracture or surgery. The child resides in a single-level home with two steps to enter. Before surgery, he was able to negotiate the two steps in a sideways manner using both hands on the railing. He was independent with all transfers, toileting, and bathing using adaptive equipment. The child was discharged from the

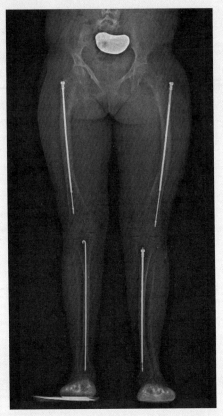

Figure 18-1. Radiograph (standing anteroposterior view) of child with four intramedullary rods in bilateral femurs and tibias.

hospital in bilateral above-knee fiberglass casts with bilateral lower extremity (LE) nonweightbearing precautions. Although he was able to perform sliding board transfers with assistance prior to hospital discharge, his parents have been lifting him for transfers due to upper extremity pain during the transfer. The child was transitioned to below-knee casts six weeks after surgery, though he still had nonweightbearing precautions. The casts were removed two weeks later and his orthopaedic surgeon cleared him to begin mobilizing with physical therapy, weightbearing as tolerated wearing clamshell ankle-foot orthoses (AFOs). In the pool, he is allowed to bear weight without AFOs. The child arrives to the physical therapy clinic two days after cast removal; he has not initiated any weightbearing on his own. Due to marginal bone healing, he must use his walker for at least six weeks. At that time, the surgeon will evaluate a repeat x-ray and reassess weightbearing precautions based on bone healing. The physical therapist has been asked to evaluate the child's strength and readiness for weightbearing and to progress pain-free LE weightbearing for transfers and ambulation. The mother gave the child an over-the-counter analgesic 30 minutes prior to the appointment in anticipation of discomfort with an increase in activity level. The therapist is familiar with this child from previous physical therapy episodes of care for fractures and rodding placement surgery. While the patient admits he is nervous to initiate weightbearing activity, he appears calm. The patient's and mother's long-term goal (6 months) is to walk without an assistive device in the home and at school. Their short-term goals (4 weeks) are to complete independent standing transfers and to tolerate walking household distances using the walker.

- ▶ Based on the patient's diagnosis and prior health condition, what do you anticipate will be contributing factors to activity limitations?
- ▶ What are the examination priorities?
- ▶ What precautions should be taken during the physical therapy examination and interventions?
- ▶ What are the most appropriate physical therapy interventions?
- ▶ Identify psychological factors apparent in this case.

KEY DEFINITIONS

BISPHOSPHONATES: Drug class that helps prevent loss of bone mass by inhibiting osteoclast activity, which in turn decreases bone resorption; used off-label in individuals with OI

BONE MINERAL DENSITY (BMD): Amount of calcium and other mineral matter per unit of skeletal area; measurement is typically used to assess fracture risk and bone health

CLAMSHELL ANKLE-FOOT ORTHOSIS: Brace worn on the lower leg and foot that provides circumferential support with anterior and posterior shell components

DUAL X-RAY ABSORPTIOMETRY (DEXA OR DXA) SCAN: Specialized radiologic technique for measuring BMD using x-rays; radiation exposure during a DXA: Approximately one-tenth of that from a chest x-ray[1]

INTRAMEDULLARY ROD: Long steel or titanium rod surgically inserted into the medullary canal of a long bone in order to add stability to the bone. A rod can be a single solid piece (also called an intramedullary nail) or it can be telescoping. A telescoping rod has a smaller rod inside of a larger hollow rod; the rod is anchored in both ends of the long bone and elongates or "telescopes" as the bone grows.

OSTEOTOMY: Surgical fracture of a bone, typically done to realign a deformed or rotated bone

Objectives

1. Describe typical characteristics of individuals with OI and potential complications associated with OI.

2. Describe the goals and limitations of intramedullary rodding surgery for a child with OI.

3. Understand the potential benefits and limitations of bisphosphonates in the medical treatment of children with OI.

4. Design appropriate short-term and long-term outpatient physical therapy goals for a child with OI who has undergone intramedullary rod revision surgery.

5. Describe the benefits of aquatic therapy as an intervention for post-rodding revision surgery.

6. Design an appropriate home exercise program for a child with OI following rodding revision surgery.

Physical Therapy Considerations

PT considerations during management of the child diagnosed with OI, status/post revision of intramedullary rodding surgery:

▶ **General physical therapy plan of care/goals:** Improve LE strength and endurance; progress standing tolerance and ambulation with and without an assistive device; maximize safe and functional independence; assist with return to prior level of function while minimizing the risk of fractures

▶ **Physical therapy interventions:** Gentle strengthening of the LEs; activities to progress standing tolerance with initiation in pool and progressive weightbearing on land; gait training; stair climbing; home exercise program; patient and family education on the importance of strengthening and how to safely progress weightbearing in order to minimize fracture risk

▶ **Precautions during physical therapy:** No passive twisting, rotating, or forceful range of motion (ROM) in the extremities or trunk due to high fracture risk; pain, weakness, fatigue; close guarding during weightbearing activities to decrease risk of fall or injury; close monitoring of skin when wearing AFOs

▶ **Complications interfering with physical therapy:** Patient discomfort with AFO due to postsurgical LE swelling; pain may limit activity tolerance; patient and parent anxiety regarding potential fractures; upper extremity deformities may increase difficulty in using a walker

Understanding the Health Condition

OI is an inherited disorder that in most cases is caused by an autosomal dominant gene mutation that affects type I collagen production. Type I collagen is the most prevalent collagen type in the body. It makes up the major connective tissue in bones, ligaments, tendons, skin, dentin, corneas, and lungs. In the United States, the prevalence of OI is estimated to be 1 in 20,000 to 50,000 infants, although the prevalence may actually be higher due to frequent underdiagnosis or misdiagnosis.[2] OI was originally classified into four types based on the Sillence criteria[3] of clinical and radiographic presentation and inheritance pattern.[4] Individuals with Type I OI produce normal collagen but have a deficiency in the amount that is produced, whereas individuals with Types II, III, and IV have altered collagen formation that creates a deficient bone matrix. There are now at least eight or more types of OI delineated.[2,4-6] However, OI Types I through IV make up more than 95% of all OI cases.[6] OI is caused by mutations in at least 12 different genes.[6] Because Types V, VI, VII, and VIII do not exhibit Type I collagen mutations, it is not clear if these types will be classified as OI in the future.[7] An initial diagnosis of OI can be made clinically, but a definitive diagnosis is confirmed with genetic testing. The use of DEXA scans has also been useful in the detection of OI.[8] Diagnosing the type of OI in a child is important in order for families to understand prognosis, treatment options, goals, and long-term expectations for their child.[5]

Characteristics of OI include low BMD that results in fragile bones that fracture easily with little or no trauma. Most individuals with OI have resulting bone deformities. While OI does not affect the *rate* of bone healing after fractures (incidental or surgical), healing may be affected by the amount of pre-existing bowing in long bones.[9] Individuals with OI also exhibit joint laxity, weak muscles, blue sclera, poor dentition, hearing loss, easy bruising, excessive sweating, short stature, scoliosis, and fatigue. Cognition is not typically affected as a result of OI. Life expectancy is normal for those with mild to moderate forms of OI; individuals with more severe types have a higher mortality rate related to respiratory compromise, cardiovascular failure (due to severe kyphoscoliosis), neurologic causes (such as brainstem compression), and cranial trauma.[5] Type II OI is typically fatal in the neonatal period. Because children with OI have diverse and complex needs, many different providers are often necessary for comprehensive care. Providers typically include a primary care physician, orthopaedic surgeon, endocrinologist, metabolic geneticist, physical therapist, occupational therapist, and a case manager. A social worker or child life specialist can also be integral to the child's health care. Due to the complex nature of impairments and interventions, children with OI experience many barriers to fully integrating in school and with peers.[10] In addition, families often require emotional support to help meet the needs of their child with OI.[1]

The standard treatment of long bone deformity is surgical placement of a rod through the intramedullary cavity of the bone (often referred to as "rodding").[2,11] Acting as an internal splint, **the rod helps to stabilize and align the bone**, allowing for weightbearing and reducing fracture recurrence at the site.[2,9,10,11] The bone must be large enough in diameter to accommodate placement of the steel or titanium rod into the intramedullary cortex. There are different styles of rods used depending on the child's age, specific needs, and purpose of the surgery. Rodding is typically performed in those with more severe forms of OI and is indicated for a child with significant bowing and recurrent fractures who is initiating standing. The goal of rodding is to decrease pain and reduce the frequency of fractures, which facilitates improvement in gross motor development, function, comfort, and mobility.[2] It is recommended that bilateral limb segments be corrected at the same time.[12] A child may be immobilized in a cast or splint for 6 to 8 weeks after the surgery to allow for sufficient healing. It is not unusual that rods need to be replaced or revised, especially in children who are not near skeletal maturity and still have a significant amount of growth to be gained in the long bones. One retrospective study found that reoperation was performed in 50% of the telescoping rods initially inserted in individuals with OI, with 15% of those reoperations requiring exchange of the rod due to growth of the patient (with rods nearing disengagement).[13]

Bisphosphonates (*e.g.*, pamidronate, alendronate, zoledronate) are a class of drugs that inactivate osteoclasts, thereby decreasing bone resorption. Used to treat children with OI since the early 1990s, the goal of bisphosphonate treatment is to increase BMD, decrease pain and fracture incidence, reduce bone deformity, and improve growth and mobility.[7] While bisphosphonates are intended to increase BMD, the bone matrix of individuals with OI remains composed of defective collagen. BMD is commonly measured by DEXA, which is the gold standard for measuring BMD in adults.[14] In children with OI, bisphosphonates have been shown to increase BMD (as measured by DEXA) of the spine, femoral neck, hip, and tibia.[15,16] Castillo et al.[16] performed a systematic review of eight studies evaluating the effectiveness of bisphosphonates in children with OI. Castillo et al.[16] found that **bisphosphonates increased BMD**; many (but not all) studies demonstrated a reduction in fracture rate. Another systematic review of eight studies (five were the same studies reviewed in Castillo et al.[16]) found that oral and intravenous bisphosphonates increased BMD.[7] However, because their use did not improve function regarding decreased fractures, the authors concluded that more studies investigating bone pain, growth, and quality of life are needed.[7] One study has found that intravenous bisphosphonate significantly improved mobility and grip strength in individuals with severe OI, but did not improve areas of self-care.[17] Seikaly et al.[18] found that oral bisphosphonate treatment did not improve mobility, but improved other quality-of-life measures including self-care and overall well-being (as measured by pain-free days and decreased need for analgesic medications). These authors proposed that such improvements could potentially allow for more effective physical therapy and weightbearing. Despite the documented beneficial effects of bisphosphonates, these drugs do not eliminate fracture risk or the need for rodding surgery in the OI population.[2,19-21] While bisphosphonates have been approved by the Food and Drug Administration for use in other types of bone loss disorders (e.g., Paget's disease), they are currently used "off-label" in children with OI. There are many unanswered questions surrounding the use of bisphosphonates in the OI population including the efficacy of oral versus intravenous administration, which specific medication is optimal, dosing, critical age/s that should be treated, duration of treatment, level of effectiveness for specific types of OI, and long-term effects.[5,7,16,21] There are no established guidelines that answer these questions.[20] Recent recommendations suggest that the use of bisphosphonates should be driven by clinical severity, not solely on bone density measurements.[5,21] Clinical factors considered in the decision making include the extent of long bone deformities, vertebral compression fractures, frequency of fractures, and severity of OI.[12,20] It has also been recommended that bisphosphonates be used as an adjunct to orthopaedic surgery and physical therapy, not as a replacement for these interventions.[20] Bisphosphonates may delay surgical osteotomy healing (but not fracture healing).[2] Therefore, children taking bisphosphonates may be instructed to discontinue use 3 to 4 months prior to a scheduled orthopaedic surgery. They can typically resume the drug 3 to 6 months after surgery. There are no specific recommendations for altering a child's activity level during this drug-free phase because the changes that may occur in bone density during this time have not been thoroughly studied.

The child in this case has Type IV OI. Individuals with OI Type IV are moderately affected (with severity between Type I and Type III) and life expectancy is typically unchanged. Short stature and bowing of the long bones is common and few to multiple fractures are experienced over the lifespan. Most fractures occur before puberty. The prognosis for Type IV OI is good for some form of upright ambulation.[4] Issues that need to be considered in this population are: (1) attenuating the cycle of fracture and immobility; (2) timing of rodding surgery and monitoring deformities, including scoliosis; (3) developing compensations for short stature and fatigue (e.g., lowering work surfaces, keeping frequently used items at a lower level, and using assistive devices/wheeled mobility for community ambulation in order to keep up with peers); (4) choosing appropriate and meaningful age-appropriate exercises; and (5) making decisions about the use of bisphosphonates.

Safe and functional mobility (ambulation or wheeled) for the child with OI is a priority, using adaptive equipment and bracing as necessary. A child with OI and his family members may have increased anxiety and guarding due to potential fractures, which limits the child from integrating fully with his peers.[19] As the child ages, socialization with peers can become increasingly more challenging, especially as the child is unable to participate in higher level and greater impact activities. However, there is a great degree of variability in skills and abilities among individuals with each type of OI. Treatments and goals are guided by patient presentation, focusing on the specific needs of the child, and not based on clinical diagnosis.

Physical Therapy Patient/Client Management

Management of a child with OI who has undergone a rodding revision focuses on progressive weightbearing and functional independent mobility. Gentle, progressive strengthening through isometric and open chain exercises is included. Whenever possible, weightbearing should be initiated in the pool to decrease fracture risk and to allow the child to experience success with low-impact activities. The physical therapist closely monitors pain complaints since this can be an indicator that the bones are being overly stressed; however, pain may also be related to muscle weakness or generalized discomfort with weightbearing. It is important to actively listen to pain complaints, since the child is often familiar with the pain that may indicate a fracture or impending fracture. A pre-verbal child (e.g., younger than 4 years) may not be able to accurately verbalize or localize pain, though his behaviors can be indicators of pain. For example, the child may appear overly irritable or avoid weightbearing or uncomfortable positions. In a verbal child, the therapist should discuss what level of pain is acceptable versus what amount of pain indicates that the activity should be revised or discontinued. Since there are no specific established criteria to assist in determining the level of acceptable pain or discomfort during an activity, the therapist's judgment of when to continue, revise, or stop an activity should be based on a combination of the child's verbal and non-verbal communication.

The child with OI is often guarded with movement due to fear and anxiety of fracture and pain. Maintaining the same treating therapist(s) helps foster rapport, trust, and confidence. Including the child, even at a younger age, in goal setting and treatment planning helps to promote self-advocacy, which is important as the child grows into adulthood. It also allows the child a sense of shared control during therapy sessions. He will likely be more motivated to participate and work toward the end goal when he is included in the process. To increase child participation in this scenario, the therapist can offer choices of activities, challenge the child to "beat" the distance or time that he stood or walked in the pool from the last session, or create other games that promote therapeutic activities, strengthening, and endurance aimed at achieving mutually agreed upon session goals. The therapist may create a tracking grid for exercises and activities to provide a visual aid for the child to highlight his accomplishments, which may provide additional motivation to work on therapy goals in the clinic and home environment.

Examination, Evaluation, and Diagnosis

Prior to seeing the child, the physical therapist should obtain information regarding surgical and fracture history. The therapist should be aware of the postsurgical weightbearing restrictions and any other mobility precautions. Prior to mobilizing the child in any way, the therapist needs to discuss the child's and parent's preferred method of postoperative transfers. It is important to know what current equipment and orthoses the child has, what his level of function and mobility was prior to this most recent surgery, current level of pain and how it is being managed, and what the child's and parent's short-term and long-term goals are. The therapist must also inquire about the design and set-up of the child's home and school environments (*e.g.*, stairs, ramps) as well as any previous participation in physical exercise. If possible, it is helpful for the therapist to investigate previous physical therapy activity likes/dislikes, motivators, fears, degree of compliance with home programs, amount of previous physical therapy-related education provided, and level of needed emotional support. This information can be gathered via chart review, discussion with the child and family, and follow-up with current and previous therapists.

The child may need to take pain medication prior to initiating weightbearing and mobility. It is important to assess pain complaints throughout the examination. When determining if an activity should be revised or discontinued, it is important to listen to and value the child's pain complaint because pain may be an indicator that the child is being challenged beyond what his musculoskeletal system can tolerate. Judicious judgment is necessary in determining when to continue through the pain. A visual analog scale or the Wong-Baker Faces Pain Rating scale[22] can be used to rate the child's pain. The **Wong-Baker Faces Pain Rating scale** has been found to be reliable and valid in children from 3 to 18 years old.[23,24] It uses a picture of six faces ranging in a series from a very happy face ("no hurt" or "0") to a very sad and tearful face ("hurts worst" or "10"). The child is shown the face scale and asked to choose the face that best describes how much he hurts. It has been proposed that the minimal clinically important difference (MCID) on a faces scale is a change of two points, which represents a change of one face.[24] The therapist should also take other factors into consideration, such as: where the pain is located, if pain is diffuse or localized, how stable or unstable the child appears in the activity being performed, if the activity appears challenging or if it is a mastered skill, the child's nonverbal communication (*e.g.*, facial expressions, body language), how tense the child's muscles appear, and the child's respiration rate. The combination of these factors helps determine how the session should progress. In the current case, the child being examined rated his bilateral ankle pain as a 4 on the Wong-Baker Faces Pain Rating scale. He complained of this pain after standing for 10 seconds in waist-deep water with a front-wheeled walker. He also had a grimace on his face, was holding his breath, and held a tense upper body posture with raised shoulders. After assisting him to the chest-deep water, his pain subsided to a 1 on the same scale and he appeared to have a more relaxed posture. The therapist then continued the remainder of the examination in chest-deep water.

The examination priorities are assessment of LE active ROM and strength. This child has been nonweightbearing for 8 weeks and out of below-knee casts for only 2 days. The therapist initiates the evaluation on a mat in a clinic room before transitioning to the pool to complete the examination. To decrease guarding and anxiety around fractures, the therapist should allow the child and parent to demonstrate how they are currently performing transfers by asking them to transfer from the wheelchair to the mat. During therapy sessions, the child and parent should complete all the transfers until the child is comfortable with the therapist. This helps promote trust and avoids injury. Prior to the therapist mobilizing the child, the plan for how the child will be transferred or assisted by the therapist should be mutually agreed upon.

Once on the mat with AFOs removed, the therapist assesses the child's ankle and knee active ROM and LE strength. In general, applying resistance with manual muscle testing to individuals with OI should be avoided to decrease the risk of fracture. The therapist gently supports the leg, following the child's lead through the available knee ROM. The therapist can then examine the child's knee extension strength and hip abduction strength. Knee extension strength can be measured by asking the child to complete a straight leg raise while the therapist lightly supports the limb, observing how well the child can maintain knee extension while lifting the leg. Active knee extension from a sitting position can also be assessed through a supported long-arc quad exercise. Depending on the child's level of comfort, hip abduction strength can be examined in supine or in sidelying with his back supported against the wall. Again, the therapist lightly supports the limb during testing. Unsupported positions on the mat should be avoided. When long sitting, the therapist must ensure that the child's entire leg is resting on the mat; in short sitting, the entire upper leg should be supported on the mat.

Next, the therapist evaluates how much weightbearing the child can tolerate on his LEs. Ideally, tolerance to weightbearing should initially be assessed in the pool. An alternative is to have the child stand with AFOs in the parallel bars for short durations (e.g., 5- to 10-second intervals), while providing careful guarding. The child should be transferred into the pool using a chair lift (AFOs are not used in the pool). Once in the pool, the therapist can assist the child to chest-deep water. The therapist assesses the child's tolerance to standing (with or without a walker at this water level) and gradually moves the child to more shallow water as he tolerates. A standard front-wheeled walker designated for the pool can be used for supported standing in the pool. The child can begin taking steps in the water with a walker. Because this child has been nonweightbearing for the past two months, he is at an increased risk for fractures related to immobilization, weakness, and muscle wasting, in addition to his already fragile bones. The added support of the walker allows more controlled ambulation and balance. In addition to standing and walking, the child's tolerance to general activity and level of fatigue can be assessed. Based on initial evaluation of this patient, the therapist identified two main problems: (1) he cannot tolerate standing in waist-deep water for greater than 10 seconds, and (2) he does not demonstrate the strength or balance to take consecutive steps without the support of a walker in chest-deep water.

Plan of Care and Interventions

Physical therapy interventions should focus on returning the child to his prior level of mobility through gentle strengthening, progressive weightbearing, and endurance training. **Initiating weightbearing in the pool** is optimal for children with OI because the buoyancy of the water lessens the impact on joints and decreases stresses on long bones, allowing a higher degree of activity in a safe environment.[1,10]

In addition, the resistance of the water against the long bones allows a safe and effective means to strengthen muscles while decreasing the risk for fracture.[10]

The first problem the therapist identified was that the child was unable to bear weight in waist-deep water for greater than 10 seconds. Interventions could include progressively increasing standing time in the chest-deep water, initially with a walker and progressing to a flotation device, then without any device. The therapist can instruct the child to perform quadriceps and gluteal isometric muscle contractions during progressions in standing tolerance. Double leg squats and open chain exercises such as supine hip abduction and prone kicking can also be performed in the water to promote strength and endurance for standing. As the child's standing time improves, he can be transitioned to shallower water, again starting with a walker and progressing to no device.

The second identified problem was that the child was unable to ambulate in chest-deep water without a walker. The therapist can guide the child toward increasing ambulation distance with the walker in chest-deep water, progressing to walking with a floatation device and/or no device. The therapist transitions the child to shallower water as he gains strength, endurance, and stability in his gait. Step-ups, side-stepping holding the wall, and backwards walking are other treatment interventions that can be done in varying levels of water to progress the child's ambulation.

When the child demonstrates increased tolerance to standing and walking in waist-deep water, therapy should be transitioned to land-based activities. Weightbearing on land (with AFOs) can be initiated in the parallel bars or with the walker. The therapist must provide close contact support. The child may be more comfortable using a rear-entry walker on land because it is more stable than a front-wheeled walker and does not have to be lifted to turn. However, rear-entry walkers are also heavier to maneuver and require more coordinated steps to transfer in and out. Once transitioned to land-based therapy, the child can continue working on standing tolerance and ambulating with the walker. The orthopaedic surgeon stated that he must use the walker for at least six weeks (when he returns for follow-up). Sit-to-stand activities in the walker and open chain strengthening exercises can be added. It is important to provide rest breaks as needed in order to avoid overly stressing the musculoskeletal system. The child should also be provided with a straightforward home exercise program that he could consistently complete. It may be important for the therapist to be in regular contact with the child's school to ensure good communication with how the child is progressing and to help define the expectations and limitations he may encounter at school. Outpatient physical therapy should continue until the child has met or surpassed his preoperative status.

Evidence-Based Clinical Recommendations

SORT: Strength of Recommendation Taxonomy

A: Consistent, good-quality patient-oriented evidence
B: Inconsistent or limited-quality patient-oriented evidence
C: Consensus, disease-oriented evidence, usual practice, expert opinion, or case series

1. Intramedullary rodding surgery decreases fracture recurrence in long bones and minimizes progression of bowing deformity in children with osteogenesis imperfecta. **Grade A**

2. Bisphosphonates decrease fracture rate in children with OI. **Grade B**
3. The Wong-Baker Faces Pain Rating scale is a reliable and valid tool to assess pain in children between the ages of 3 and 18 years old with a variety of health conditions. **Grade A**
4. Aquatic therapy is an optimal modality for strengthening weak muscles, while protecting fragile bones in children with OI. **Grade C**

COMPREHENSION QUESTIONS

18.1 The *most* appropriate progression from ambulating with a walker to ambulating without an assistive device for the child with OI would be:

   A. Transitioning the child to axillary crutches

   B. Having the child practice taking a few steps at a time with light hand-held assist in a controlled environment

   C. Ensuring that the child can first walk community distances with the walker

   D. Check that the child has at least a 4/5 quadriceps strength as tested with manual muscle test

18.2 A physical therapist is creating a home exercise program for a child with OI who has just begun weightbearing on land following a rodding revision surgery. Which of the following is *not* an appropriate exercise to strengthen the quadriceps for this child?

   A. Sit-to-stand transfers from an elevated surface, using a walker for support

   B. Standing quad sets using a walker for support

   C. Short arc quads

   D. Single leg squats holding a walker for support

18.3 When would it be appropriate to utilize a partial-weightbearing gait therapy device (*e.g.*, LiteGait) as a therapy intervention for a child with OI who has recently begun weightbearing after a rodding surgery?

   A. As an alternative to weightbearing in the pool since a partial-weightbearing gait therapy device can also provide unweighting of the LEs

   B. While ambulating on land instead of using a walker

   C. A child with OI should never be placed in a partial-weightbearing gait therapy device.

   D. To increase standing tolerance prior to ambulating on land

ANSWERS

18.1 **B.** It is generally safer to transition a child with OI from a walker straight to ambulating without an assistive device once he/she is steady and efficient with the walker. Axillary crutches should generally be avoided in children with OI because they place too much strain on the ribcage, axilla, and wrists (option A). Walking short distances without an assistive device does not require the endurance needed for community ambulation (option C). Manual muscle testing with strong resistance should be avoided because it puts the child with OI at risk for fracture (option D).

18.2 **D.** Individuals with OI should not be in positions that may compromise balance or cause rotation of the limb because these cause undue stress on the bone and place the child at risk for falling and fracturing.[1]

18.3 **C.** Individuals with OI should *not* be placed in a partial-weightbearing gait therapy device. Because the harness used must be pulled snug to the torso in order for it to effectively unweight the LEs, it could cause a fracture to the child's ribs or pelvis. In addition, unweighting the child with OI in a harness puts undue stress on the pelvis, which poses a fracture risk at this site.

REFERENCES

1. Osteogenesis Imperfecta Foundation. www.OIF.org. Accessed October 24, 2014.

2. Esposito P, Plotkin H. Surgical treatment of osteogenesis imperfecta: current concepts. *Curr Opin Pediatr.* 2008;20:52-57.

3. Sillence DO, Senn A, Danks DM. Genetic heterogeneity in osteogenesis imperfecta. *J Med Genet.* 1979;16:101-116.

4. Forlino A, Cabral WA, Barnes AM, Marini JC. New perspectives on osteogenesis imperfecta. *Nat Rev Endocrinol.* 2011;7:540-557.

5. Starr SR, Roberts TT, Fischer PR. Osteogenesis imperfecta: primary care. *Pediatr Rev.* 2010;31:54-64.

6. Fitzgerald J, Holden P, Wright H, et al. Phenotypic variability in individuals with type V osteogenesis imperfecta with identical IFITM5 mutations. *J Rare Disorders.* 2013;1:37-42.

7. Philippi CA, Remmington T, Steiner RD. Bisphosphonate therapy for osteogenesis imperfecta. *Cochrane Database Syst Rev.* 2008; Oct 8:CD005088.DOI: 10.1002/14651858.CD005088. pub2.

8. Moore MS, Minch CM, Kruse RW, Harke HT, Jacobson L, Taylor A. The role of dual energy x-ray absorptiometry in aiding the diagnosis of pediatric osteogenesis imperfecta. *Am J Orthop.* 1998;27:797-801.

9. Staheli L, ed. *Pediatric Orthopaedic Secrets.* Philadelphia, PA: Hanley and Belfus, Inc.; 1998.

10. Campbell SK, Palisano RJ, Orlin MN. *Physical Therapy for Children.* 4th ed. Philadelphia, PA: W.B. Saunders Company; 2012.

11. Luhmann SJ, Sheridan JJ, Capelli AM, Schoenecker PL. Management of lower-extremity deformities in osteogenesis imperfecta with extensible intramedullary rod technique: a 20-year experience. *J Pediatr Orthop.* 1998;18:88-94.

12. Shapiro JR, Sponsellor PD. Osteogenesis imperfecta: questions and answers. *Curr Opin Pediatr.* 2009;21:709-716.

13. Nicolaou N, Bowe JD, Wilkinson JM, Fernandes JA, Bell MJ. Use of the Sheffield telescopic intramedullary rod system for the management of osteogenesis imperfecta: clinical outcomes at an average follow-up of nineteen years. *J Bone Joint Surg Am.* 2011;93:1994-2000.

14. Finley L. Evaluating bone mineral density measurement. *Physician Assistant.* 2003;27:17-25.

15. Bishop N, Harrison R, Ahmed F, et al. A randomized, controlled dose-ranging study of risedronate in children with moderate and severe osteogenesis imperfecta. *J Bone Miner Res.* 2010;25:32-40.

16. Castillo H, Samson-Fang L; American Academy for Cerebral Palsy and Developmental Medicine Treatment Outcomes Committee Review Panel. Effects of bisphosphonates in children with osteogenesis imperfecta: an AACPDM systematic review. *Dev Med Child Neurol.* 2009;51:17-29.

17. Land C, Rauch F, Montpetit K, Ruck-Gibis J, Glorieux FH. Effect of intravenous pamidronate therapy on functional abilities and level of ambulation in children with osteogenesis imperfecta. *J Pediatr.* 2006;148:456-460.

18. Seikaly MG, Kopanati S, Salhab N, et al. Impact of alendronate on quality of life in children with osteogenesis imperfecta. *J Pediatr Orthop.* 2005;25:786-791.

19. Astrom E, Jorulf H, Soderhall S. Intravenous pamidronate treatment of infants with severe osteogenesis imperfecta. *Arch Dis Child.* 2007;92:332-338.

20. Rauch F, Glorieux FH. Treatment of children with osteogenesis imperfecta. *Curr Osteoporos Rep.* 2006;4:159-164.

21. Falk MJ, Heeger S, Lynch KA, et al. Intravenous bisphosphonate therapy in children with osteogenesis imperfecta. *Pediatrics.* 2003;111:573-578.

22. Wong DL, Baker CM. Pain in children: comparison of assessment scales. *Pediatr Nurs.* 1988;14:9-17.

23. Keck JF, Gerkensmeyer JE, Joyce BA, Schade JG. Reliability and validity of the Faces and Word Descriptor Scales to measure procedural pain. *J Pediatr Nurs.* 1996;11:368-374.

24. Tomlinson D, von Baeyer CL, Stinson JN, Sung L. A systematic review of faces scales for the self-report of pain intensity in children. *Pediatrics.* 2010;126:168-198.

Spina Bifida

Britta Schasberger

A 10-year-old girl with spina bifida cystica with myelomeningocele has been working with her school-based physical therapist on functional mobility in the school environment. The child presents with a ventriculoperitoneal (VP) shunt and uses bilateral ankle-foot orthoses and forearm crutches to ambulate. She uses a manual wheelchair for longer community distances. She also has a dynamic wheeled prone stander for use at school. Her motor level has been classified as L4 and she is a community ambulator. The child has recently experienced difficulties with ambulation such as decreased speed, decreased foot clearance, and limited endurance. Other impairments include decreased strength and endurance and incontinence. She has recently experienced a growth spurt. She has also demonstrated behavioral challenges during her physical therapy sessions. Specifically, she has a decreased attention span, verbally refuses to participate in sessions, and throws equipment. The physical therapist contacted her parents and pediatrician to discuss the new findings and concerns. Her pediatrician performed an examination and ordered a computed tomography (CT) scan to determine if recent changes in her function and behavior are a result of a VP shunt failure. The CT scan results revealed a functional VP shunt and no changes in the child's ventricles. Each year, the same physical therapist assesses the child's lower extremity strength via a manual muscle test (MMT). On the current MMT, the physical therapist noted a marked decrease in bilateral lower extremity strength. As a result of the therapist's finding, the pediatrician referred her for a magnetic resonance imaging (MRI) scan of the spine, which revealed tethering of her spinal cord. The child underwent surgery to untether the spinal cord and spent three days in the hospital. Three weeks after surgery, she has returned for her first physical therapy session at school.

► What are the most appropriate tests and measures to be used?
► What are the most important priorities of the evaluation?
► What are appropriate physical therapy outcome measures for functional abilities, gait, and muscle strength?
► Identify the most appropriate physical therapy plan of care for this child.
► Identify appropriate referrals to other medical or educational team members.

KEY DEFINITIONS

HYDROCEPHALUS: Abnormal build-up of cerebrospinal fluid (CSF) in and around the brain

HYDROMYELIA: Abnormal amount of CSF in the spinal cord that increases pressure on the nerves and causes weakness

LATEX ALLERGY: Allergic reactions of varying severity to proteins present in natural rubber latex

MENINGES: Membranes covering the brain and spinal cord

MENINGOCELE: CSF and meninges, but no neural elements, protruded through abnormal vertebral opening. Presentation ranges from normal to partial paralysis (or motor impairment) and/or bowel and bladder dysfunction.

MYELOMENINGOCELE: Protrusion of spinal cord and surrounding meninges through abnormal opening in the vertebra; most serious type of spina bifida with most significant health implications

SCOLIOSIS: Lateral curvature of the spine to the left or right. In children with myelomeningocele, scoliosis often results from lack of neuromuscular control.

VENTRICULOPERITONEAL (VP) SHUNT: Tube with valves that is inserted in the brain to permit drainage of CSF to the abdominal cavity

VESICOURETERAL REFLUX: Urine traveling from the bladder back into the kidneys

Objectives

1. Identify the signs and symptoms of spina bifida.

2. Explain the common complications of spina bifida.

3. Identify appropriate, valid, and reliable outcome measures for school function, strength, and mobility.

4. Understand the quality of life and long-term implications of spina bifida and the relevance to physical therapy management.

5. Design an appropriate physical therapy plan of care for a child with spina bifida within a school-based setting.

Physical Therapy Considerations

PT considerations for the school-age child with a diagnosis of spina bifida and post-tethered cord surgery:

▶ **General physical therapy plan of care/goals:** Prevent loss of range of motion (ROM) in upper and lower extremities as well as upper extremity overuse injuries; maximize independent functional mobility; optimize health-related quality of life; maximize health and fitness including strength and aerobic capacity

▶ **Physical therapy interventions:** Patient and family education regarding long-term implications of spina bifida and the risks for obesity, osteoporosis, and urinary tract infections; exercises to maintain ROM and improve strength; functional mobility training (transfers, wheeled mobility, ambulation)

▶ **Precautions during physical therapy:** Decreased cardiorespiratory endurance (higher resting heart rate and increased heart rate during activities); increased risk for fracture secondary to osteoporosis; increased risk for hip dislocation and skin breakdown secondary to decreased sensation; latex allergy; incontinence during exercise; difficulties with thermoregulation; increased risk of falls; increased spasticity with exercise

▶ **Complications interfering with physical therapy:** Illness (*e.g.*, cold, flu, bladder infection); pronounced spasticity, Arnold-Chiari malformation, fracture, pressure sore, tethered cord syndrome, symptomatic hydromyelia, symptomatic hydrocephalus, VP shunt failure

Understanding the Health Condition

Spina bifida is the most common disabling birth defect. It has a worldwide annual incidence of about 1 in 1000.[1] The incidence rate is slightly higher in females than males.[2] The highest incidence rate is in the Hispanic population (4.17 per 10,000) compared to non-Hispanic blacks (2.64 per 10,000) and non-Hispanic whites (3.22 per 10,000).[1]

Spina bifida is a group of congenital disorders characterized by varying degrees of incomplete closure of the embryonic neural tube. The neural tube is formed very early in embryonic development from a small group of cells that create a narrow tube that eventually forms the brain and spinal cord.[3,4] When neural tube formation is disrupted, defects such as spina bifida result. Related neural tube defects include anencephaly (absence of a brain) and encephalocele (malformation of the brain and skull).[5]

The precise etiology of spina bifida has not been identified. Researchers have not been able to pinpoint what causes a failure of the neural tube to close, though a lack of folic acid early in pregnancy is a significant risk factor.[6] Genetic and environmental risk factors have also been identified.[7] Due to folic acid supplementation during pregnancy, the incidence of spina bifida has significantly declined over the past 30 years.[6]

There are three classifications of spina bifida based on presentation of the neural tube defect: spina bifida occulta, spina bifida cystica with meningocele, and spina bifida cystica with myelomeningocele. The latter two classifications are usually diagnosed during pregnancy through prenatal screening tests. If not identified during pregnancy, the defect is visually apparent and diagnosed immediately after the baby is born. Screening tests during pregnancy include maternal blood tests or amniocentesis (extraction of amniotic fluid) that measures the amount of alpha-fetoprotein (AFP) present. High levels of AFP have been correlated with spina bifida.[8] Routine ultrasounds performed during pregnancy may also detect a spinal cord lesion.

Spina bifida occulta is a mild, often asymptomatic, form of spina bifida that is the most challenging to diagnose. "Occulta" is the Latin word for hidden. Although the outer parts of the spinal vertebrae are not completely closed, the openings are so small that there is no herniation of the meninges or nerves of the spinal cord. The skin over the site of the lesion may have a dimple, birthmark, hair, or may even be unremarkable. Children with this form of spina bifida are typically asymptomatic and many are unaware of the disorder.[7] Incidence of spina bifida occulta is estimated to be between 5% and 20% of the general population.[9,10] Although typically considered asymptomatic, there are reports of a potential correlation between nonspecific low back pain and the presence of spina bifida occulta in both children and adults.[11-13]

Spina bifida cystica with meningocele is the least common type of spina bifida.[14] In this form, the meninges protrude through the opening in the vertebra, but there is no spinal cord involvement. Impairments are uncommon, but can include hydrocephalus, lower extremity weakness, and bladder or bowel dysfunction.[7,15,16] There is also an increased incidence of tethered cord syndrome.[15]

Individuals with spina bifida cystica with myelomeningocele (also called meningomyelocele) have the most significant health implications. The spinal cord protrudes through the vertebrae and the skin and presents as a mass of nervous tissue with no overlying covering. The protruding part of the spinal cord is usually damaged or developed incorrectly. Typically, impairments are at and below the level where the spinal cord protrudes through the vertebrae. The extent of the impairments corresponds to the vertebral level of the protrusion. The more cephalad (toward the head) the lesion is, the greater impact on function for the individual. Deficits can range from paralysis (partial or complete) to impairments in gait and mobility. There can be decreased or complete loss of sensation, loss of muscle tone, and impairments in bowel and/or bladder function.[16] In addition, there is a risk of orthopaedic impairments including scoliosis, kyphosis, lordosis, and/or deformities of the hips, knees, or feet. Common complications that occur in conjunction with spina bifida include hydrocephalus and Arnold-Chiari Type II malformations.

There is no cure for the nerve damage caused by spina bifida. To prevent further damage to the nervous tissue and to prevent infection, surgical interventions to close the opening on the back are performed. These are typically performed either on the fetus during the pregnancy or immediately after birth.[17] During the surgical procedure, the spinal cord and its nerve roots are inserted back within the bony spine and covered with meninges.

Hydrocephalus (particularly progressive or symptomatic hydrocephalus) is treated with the placement of a VP shunt to decrease the pressure of increased CSF on the brain. The signs of hydrocephalus are similar to the signs of shunt malfunction, but can vary markedly from individual to individual. The most common sign of shunt failure is headache. Other signs include unusual irritability, excessive and unexplained crying, repeated vomiting, crossed eyes, apnea, swallowing difficulties, seizures, lethargy, or worsening brain function as well as rapid increase in head circumference (growth by more than one standard deviation from the prior measure).[18]

Arnold-Chiari Type II malformation occurs when the cerebellar vermis and a portion of the brainstem descend into the spinal canal. This malformation is present in the majority of individuals with spina bifida cystica with myelomeningocele, but is symptomatic in only about one in three individuals.[19] Symptoms progress over time (*i.e.*, in late childhood or adulthood). Thus, the number of individuals with symptoms is increasing as individuals with spina bifida are living longer. The development of symptoms is correlated with the extent of the Arnold-Chiari malformation. When brain tissue descends into the spinal cord below the level of the fourth cervical vertebrae, serious signs and symptoms are quite likely. These include difficulties with feeding, a weak cry or voice, stiffness or spasticity in the upper extremities, balance impairments, and respiratory difficulties (from inspiratory stridor to insufficient breathing).

Complications due to Arnold-Chiari malformation are the leading cause of mortality in individuals with spina bifida.[18] An MRI scan is used to assess for the presence of an Arnold-Chiari malformation. Medical intervention includes proper shunting of excessive CSF to ensure appropriate intracranial pressure is maintained. In the case of progressive symptomatic Arnold-Chiari malformation, additional surgical interventions are considered such as posterior fossa decompression (to create more space for the cerebellum), spinal laminectomy (to increase the size of the spinal canal), or incision into the dura mater (to examine the brain and spinal cord and create more space for CSF flow).[20]

The second most common cause of a decline in function in children with spina bifida is tethered cord syndrome.[21] Tethered cord syndrome occurs when the spinal cord becomes attached to the spinal column which stretches the spinal cord as the child grows. Symptoms of spinal cord tethering include progressive decline in lower extremity strength, gait and balance impairments, changes in bladder function, and progressive scoliosis.[22] Progressive or worsening symptoms due to tethered cord syndrome are treated surgically.[21,22] The surgical procedure involves gently detaching the spinal cord and/or myelomeningocele from the vertebrae. Once the structures are detached, the wound is closed. After surgery, gait, strength, and spasticity typically improve.[21]

Advances in urologic care in children with spina bifida have decreased mortality and morbidity due to renal failure.[23] Shortly after birth, a complete medical assessment of kidney and bladder function is completed. Children with identified bladder impairments begin early catheterization and medication to ensure emptying of the bladder, in efforts to prevent urinary tract infections and treat kidney reflux.[23,24] Children with spina bifida who are catheterized or have had several bladder or shunt revision surgeries are at high risk for latex allergies because of a cumulative effect of exposure over time.[25]

The most common orthopaedic abnormalities associated with spina bifida are foot deformities.[26] Progressive scoliosis is also common. Improvements in the stabilization of scoliosis through orthopaedic surgery have had a positive impact on morbidity and mortality.[27]

Last, clinicians must be aware of important nonmedical concerns associated with the diagnosis of spina bifida including educational, social, and psychological development. The presence of hydrocephalus and complications related to shunt management has a strong correlation with cognitive dysfunction. Mean IQ scores of children with hydrocephalus and shunt concerns cluster in the 70 to 90 range. In contrast, children with spina bifida with stable or no hydrocephalus have more typical cognitive function with IQ scores in the 100 range.[28] If present, hydrocephalus has a deleterious impact on short-term memory, attention, and organizational skills.[29] Children with spina bifida have impairments in social skill development particularly in the areas of social language and peer interactions.[30]

Prenatal interventions, advances in medical treatment, and earlier access to interventions have all helped decrease morbidity and mortality associated with spina bifida. Children with spina bifida cystica with myelomeningocele who have good muscle strength, average cognitive ability, and are independent in mobility are more likely to be high functioning and possess a better quality of life.[31] The child's functional skills primarily correspond to the anatomical level of the spinal defects. However, research has indicated that functional level was worse than anatomic defect level in almost 50% of individuals with spina bifida, and better than anatomic defect level in almost 15% of individuals.[4] As there is no cure for hydrocephalus or the nerve damage caused by spina bifida, there remain significant needs for long-term follow-up and care for the child with spina bifida.

Physical Therapy Patient/Client Management

Physical therapy management of the child with spina bifida following surgical correction of tethered cord syndrome requires a focus on function within a multidisciplinary approach. The healthcare and school-based team for this child includes her family and primary care pediatrician, and may include any or all of the following: neurosurgeon, orthopaedic surgeon, urologist, outpatient and school-based physical and occupational therapists, and regular and special education teachers. The school-based physical therapist works with the school team in conjunction with the outpatient therapy providers, child, and family to determine the interventions needed to permit the child to participate fully in her educational program. After surgery, school-based physical therapy provision must remain educationally relevant and not focused on traditional postsurgical physical therapy goals. The school-based physical therapist re-evaluates the student to determine whether the tethered cord and subsequent surgery has negatively impacted her abilities to maneuver in the school environment including classrooms, hallways, and stairs, as well as community-based field trips and the outdoor school environment. The physical therapist also ensures that seating and positioning are optimized throughout the day to promote learning and decrease risk of secondary complications (*e.g.*, pressure sores). Physical therapy interventions will likely include a reassessment of the student's equipment needs, muscle strengthening and stretching, transitions and transfer training, gait and wheeled mobility training, and activities for coordination and balance.

Examination, Evaluation, and Diagnosis

The physical therapist conducts a chart review and patient history as the first step in the assessment process. Because this case includes a postsurgical re-evaluation in the school setting, both medical and educational chart reviews are imperative.

Communication with the medical team and family to obtain updates, precautions, or contraindications is also necessary. Typically, the child will remain in the hospital for two to five days after surgery for tethered cord syndrome. Postsurgical pain is usually not a significant factor due to decreased sensation in the incision area. Some surgeons require bed rest for several days postsurgery to minimize the risk of CSF leaking from the incision site.

The physical therapy assessment includes determination of the child's current functional motor level, functional strength, transfers, ambulation, and new equipment needs. The therapist reviews goals related to school mobility and physical therapy from the prior Individualized Education Program (IEP) and, if appropriate, writes new goals. Initially, the physical therapist performs a general screen for muscle strength and the child's ability to perform anti-gravity movements. This will inform the physical therapist whether the noted presurgical weakness was transient or remains after the surgery. There are several functional level classification systems used with children with spina bifida.[32] These include the Spina Bifida Neurological Scale (SBNS),[33,34] and classification systems described by Broughton and colleagues[34] and McDonald and colleagues.[35] If possible, the therapist should use the same system that was used presurgery. To determine the motor level, the physical therapist tests the strength of key muscle groups.[32,35,36] Table 19-1 is an example of key muscle groups to be tested to help determine functional motor level.

Strength testing of the key muscles groups in Table 19-1 should be performed in a cephalocaudal (head-toe) direction. The MMT 6-point scale is commonly used to determine strength and motor level for children with spina bifida.[35,37] In most classification systems, the child receives the grade of the level at which the muscle can be graded a 3 on the 0 to 5 scale. For example, to receive a motor level of L3, a child must have sufficient strength to extend the knee against gravity (i.e., MMT grade of 3 for the quadriceps), but would have a grade of 2 or less for the ankle dorsiflexors. In the interest of efficiency and time, a convention to begin testing three levels above the presurgical motor level is often used. Hand-held dynamometry

Table 19-1 FUNCTIONAL MOTOR LEVEL KEY MUSCLE GROUPS		
Spinal Level	Movement	Muscle Group(s)
C5	Elbow flexors	Biceps, brachialis
C6	Wrist extensors	Extensor carpi radialis longus, extensor carpi radialis brevis
C7	Elbow extensors	Triceps
T1	Small finger abductors	Abductor digiti minimi
L2	Hip flexors	Iliopsoas
L3	Knee extensors	Quadriceps
L4	Ankle dorsiflexors	Tibialis anterior
L5	Long toe extensors	Extensor hallucis longus
S1	Ankle plantar flexors	Gastrocnemius, soleus

is often unavailable in the school setting, but has been shown to have good reliability in the evaluation of muscle function and strength for children with spina bifida.[37]

Light touch and pinprick sensation should be reassessed through the use of cotton balls and a sterilized safety pin, respectively, in each dermatomal level.[38] The identified sensory level will be the most caudal (lowest) intact dermatome for both pin prick and light touch.[32]

Evaluation of ROM should also be completed. Preserving ROM and preventing contractures is critical for health-related quality of life for children with spina bifida.[31] ROM for both upper extremity and lower extremity should be performed in the supine position using a standard goniometer. Particular focus should be placed on shoulder ROM because decreased shoulder ROM has been shown to have a negative impact on effective wheelchair propulsion.[39]

Several standard assessments can be used to evaluate the child with spina bifida. These include the Battelle Developmental Inventory, the Pediatric Evaluation of Disability Inventory (PEDI), and the WeeFIM. The **WeeFIM** is a useful tool to track the impact of functional impairments for children of preschool and young elementary school age.[40] It has been adapted for young children from the Functional Independence Measure (FIM). The WeeFIM is an 18-item, 7-level scale that assesses a child's consistent performance in three primary domains (self-care, mobility, and cognition). It has been specifically validated for use with children with spina bifida[41] and used as an outcome measure of functional ability for children with spina bifida.[41-43]

The PEDI is an outcome measure that has been used to assist with goal setting and to demonstrate improvements in function over time for children with spina bifida. In a study of 63 children with spina bifida, scores on the PEDI provided useful information and a high correlation with function.[44] The PEDI quantifies functional status and change along three dimensions: functional skill level, caregiver assistance, and modifications or adaptations used. It has been shown to have excellent concurrent and construct validity.[45]

The Spina Bifida Health-Related Quality of Life instrument was developed using a relatively large sample population of 329 children and adolescents with spina bifida attending two treatment centers. This instrument has good measurement properties[46,47] and can be used to help define outcomes and the impact of impairment on function.

The child's functional abilities within the school environment must be evaluated. Ambulation with an appropriate assistive device both in empty hallways and during the confusion of classroom transitions should be examined. The ability to navigate the school environment may include stepping over dropped school bags, opening classroom doors, and sidestepping around classmates, desks, and other obstacles. Observational gait analysis should include the time the child takes to cover a set distance in a clear school hallway, within the classroom, and during a class-to-class transition. Finally, gait in the extended school environment (outside recess and transitioning to/from school transportation) should also be assessed. The child in this case was ambulating with forearm crutches prior to surgery. However, a careful reassessment of her current abilities is needed. Consideration must be given to the impact of her decreased strength and endurance on her ability to navigate the school environment as the school day progresses. The therapist will most likely need several sessions to fully determine the child's current abilities since fatigue and limited endurance will impact her ability to complete all of the assessment tasks. Determining if she needs to temporarily use an alternative assistive device or increase wheelchair use while she regains strength and function will be a crucial component to the therapist's assessment and plan.

Classroom seating and the potential need for adaptive seating or standing devices should be evaluated. This requires observation of the student at both the start and the end of the school day when fatigue is present and muscle endurance is compromised. Functional transfers including sit-to-stand and floor-to-stand transfers should be assessed. For this child, that will require assessment of transfers in several classrooms as well as at various times to determine any changes in her functional abilities and as a baseline for ongoing interventions.

The School Function Assessment (SFA; see Case 7) is an additional assessment tool available to objectively describe the impact of the impairments of a child with spina bifida on her independent functioning in the school environment.[48] The SFA includes a detailed assessment of the extent to which the child's impairments impact school-related tasks such as moving around the classroom and school, interacting with peers and teachers, and using classroom materials.

Plan of Care and Interventions

Physical therapy interventions in the school setting primarily address maximizing function within the school environment. The goals must be educationally relevant, objective, and measurable. Interventions include general strengthening as well as ROM and stretching to preserve posture, independent sitting, and limit future contractures. The physical therapist determined that three weeks after surgery to address her tethered cord syndrome, the child in the current case continued to be at her presurgical functional level of L4. However, she demonstrates decreased endurance and strength. She continues to demonstrate decreased foot clearance and gait speed. The therapist's primary focus will be on improving gait to allow her to return to independent school ambulation. To achieve this goal, interventions will focus on strengthening dorsiflexors, knee extensors, and hip flexors. Since surgery, the child needs more assistance going up and down curbs and has decreased endurance in self-propulsion for community distances. **Strengthening activities for the upper extremities** (especially for shoulder flexion/extension and elbow flexion/extension) improve wheelchair mobility, ambulation, and functional activities.[49,50]

Physical therapy services are provided within the classroom to enhance participation in classroom activities. The therapist works on classroom mobility including safe movement around classroom obstacles (backpacks, chairs, and desks). Balance activities within the classroom should focus on unexpected situations (*e.g.*, when a classmate accidentally bumps into the child). To promote independent mobility, therapeutic transfer training must also be included. For this current child, the therapist noted difficulties with sit-to-stand transfers at the end of the school day. Focused practice will emphasize sit-to-stand transfers from classroom chairs and then from the floor. Sample therapeutic activities directly related to practicing the transition from sit to stand that involve peer interaction include Simon Says or Duck

Duck Goose. Initially, the therapist can modify the game by having the child sit on a block or a chair instead of on the floor. Within the classroom environment, therapeutic activities are directed toward sitting balance and pressure relief (seated wheel chair push-ups and weight shifts). Prone stander activities can also improve access to the classroom, balance, and provide weightbearing in standing for osteoporosis prevention and strengthening.

A significant component of the therapy time must be directed toward mobility in the school environment. Safe and effective navigation through school hallways, up ramps, and through doors is critical for educational access. School mobility includes going up and down stairs, over single steps, and up and down curbs. One potential activity for the child in this case might be to have scavenger hunts throughout the school buildings, progressively increasing the distance of the areas that are included, thereby requiring ongoing improvements in school navigation while keeping the activity fun and engaging. These scavenger hunts can involve either wheeled mobility or ambulation with crutches. These variations emphasize practice in transfers, gait, and wheelchair mobility within one fun and functional activity.

The ability to access all areas of the school including the school cafeteria (perhaps with a tray), library, and assembly area should be integrated into physical therapy sessions. The current child had difficulty with walking through the aisles to get to her class during assembly. The therapist initially had her leave early for assembly to avoid navigating around other children. As the child's function improves, the lead-time can be decreased until she is able to walk with her class into the assembly. Last, outdoor school mobility including playground and community mobility for school field trips is a part of the physical therapy intervention plan. It might be necessary for the physical therapist to directly work with the child during a field trip to problem-solve unanticipated concerns and identify appropriate future modifications.

During the physical therapy gait assessment, the therapist noted that the child had decreased gait endurance. In addition to gait training in and throughout the school environment, treadmill training can be used to focus on specific components of gait (e.g., foot clearance) and walking endurance in a controlled environment. In a randomized clinical trial of 34 ambulatory children with spina bifida, a twice per week home-based **treadmill training** program improved gait speed and aerobic fitness.[51] For the current child, the therapist was able to make treadmill training motivational and fun by playing the child's preferred music and referring to the activity as their "walking dance party."

In addition to the direct therapeutic activities and interventions, it is equally important to include education and coordination of the school program with her classroom teacher, any classroom aides, and her family. For this child, the classroom staff needs to be aware of her decreased endurance and resulting need for sitting adaptations (including pressure-relief techniques) and more time for classroom transitions in the later portion of the day. Teaching and supervising the school mobility and positioning programs to ensure safety and independence are critically important. If alternative assistive devices or postural supports during sitting and standing activities are needed, the therapist might need to identify new community mobility needs to her family.

Throughout the plan of care, the physical therapist promotes self-determination and self-awareness to decrease the future risks from secondary complications such as obesity and skin breakdown. It will be important to provide education to the school staff so they are able to identify and eliminate or minimize physical barriers. It is also necessary to help teach her classmates when help is useful and appropriate. It is common for children to want to help their classmates. In this case, classmates offered to push the child in her wheelchair when she returned to class after surgery. The therapist explained that it was important for the child to keep improving her strength to return to full independent mobility and instead encouraged the classmates to be careful with their own bags so as not to create obstacles in the classroom.

Evidence-Based Clinical Recommendations

SORT: Strength of Recommendation Taxonomy

A: Consistent, good-quality patient-oriented evidence
B: Inconsistent or limited-quality patient-oriented evidence
C: Consensus, disease-oriented evidence, usual practice, expert opinion or case series

1. The WeeFIM is a reliable and valid assessment tool that can measure change in function over time in the functional ability of children with spina bifida. **Grade A**

2. Upper extremity strength training programs increase strength and independent wheelchair mobility in children with spina bifida. **Grade B**

3. Treadmill training improves gait speed and aerobic fitness in ambulatory children with spina bifida. **Grade B**

COMPREHENSION QUESTIONS

19.1 Children with spina bifida are at increased risk for all of the following, except

A. Hydrocephalus

B. Urinary tract infections

C. Latex allergy

D. Tuberculosis

19.2 Which of the following is true about ambulation in children with spina bifida?

A. They are never able to ambulate and rely on wheeled mobility to access the community.

B. They can ambulate independently with an assistive device.

C. Their ability to ambulate is dependent on the level of the spinal cord lesion.

D. Their ability to ambulate is related to the presence of hydrocephalus.

ANSWERS

19.1 **D.** Children with spina bifida are not at increased risk from tuberculosis compared to the general population. Hydrocephalus is a known common complication for children with spina bifida, although the exact pathogenesis is unclear. Children with spina bifida have decreased innervation and control of the bladder. Incomplete emptying of the bladder leads to an increased risk for urinary tract infections because residual urine in the bladder can become infected. Latex allergies frequently develop in children with spina bifida due to prolonged exposure to latex products in medical supplies.

19.2 **C.** The ability of children with spina bifida to ambulate is dependent on the level of the lesion in the spinal cord. Children with spina bifida typically have motor impairments below the level of the lesion. These impairments to muscle function may impact the child's ability to move the lower extremities, thereby impacting gait. Some children with spina bifida only use wheeled mobility and do not ambulate (option A). However, this is not true for all children with spina bifida. Similarly, some children with spina bifida use an assistive device. However, many children with spina bifida ambulate without an assistive device (option B). Although hydrocephalus is a significant complication of spina bifida, it does not have a direct impact on a child's ability to ambulate (option D).

REFERENCES

1. Centers for Disease Control and Prevention. Spina bifida homepage. http://www.cdc.gov/ncbddd/spinabifida/data.html. Accessed March 3, 2015.

2. Lary JM, Edmonds LD. Prevalence of spina bifida at birth—United States, 1983-1990: a comparison of two surveillance systems. *MMWR CDC Surveill Summ.* 1996;45:15-26.

3. Lambert HW, Wineski LE, eds. *Lippincott's Illustrated Q&A Review of Anatomy and Embryology.* Philadelphia, PA: Lippincott Williams & Wilkins; 2011.

4. Mitchell LE, Adzick NS, Melchionne J, Pasquariello PS, Sutton LN, Whitehead AS. Spina bifida. *Lancet.* 2004;364:1885-1895.

5. Botto LD, Moore CA, Khoury MJ, Erickson JD. Neural-tube defects. *N Engl J Med.* 1999;341:1509-1519.

6. Williams LJ, Rasmussen SA, Flores A, Kirby RS, Edmonds LD. Decline in the prevalence of spina bifida and anencephaly by race/ethnicity: 1995-2002. *Pediatrics.* 2005;116:580-586.

7. National Institute of Neurological Disorders and Stroke. Spina bifida fact sheet. http://www.ninds.nih.gov/disorders/spina_bifida/detail_spina_bifida.htm. Accessed March 3, 2015.

8. Wald NJ, Cuckle H, Brock JH, Peto R, Polani PE, Woodford FP. Maternal serum-alpha-fetoprotein measurement in antenatal screening for anencephaly and spina bifida in early pregnancy. Report of U.K. collaborative study on alpha-fetoprotein in relation to neural-tube defects. *Lancet.* 1977;1:1323-1332.

9. Eubanks JD, Cheruvu VK. Prevalence of sacral spina bifida occulta and its relationship to age, sex, race, and the sacral table angle: an anatomic, osteologic study of three thousand one hundred specimens. *Spine.* 2009;34:1539-1543.

10. Giza CC, Sankar R. Spina bifida. In: Yazdani S, McGee SA, Stiehm ER, eds. *Chronic Complex Diseases of Childhood: A Practical Guide for Clinicians.* Boca Raton, FL: Brown Walker Press; 2011:460-464.

11. Mili či G, Krolo I, Anti čević D, et al. Causal connection of non-specific low back pain and disc degeneration in children with transitional vertebra and/or Spina bifida occulta: role of magnetic resonance—prospective study. *Coll Antropol.* 2012;36:627-633.

12. van Tulder MW, Assendelft WJ, Koes BW, Bouter LM. Spinal radiographic findings and nonspecific low back pain. A systematic review of observational studies. *Spine*. 1997;22:427-434.

13. Avrahami E, Frishman E, Fridman Z, Azor M. Spina bifida occulta of S1 is not an innocent finding. *Spine*. 1994;19:12-15.

14. Laurence KM, Tew BJ. Natural history of spina bifida cystica and cranium bifidum cysticum. Major central nervous system malformations in South Wales. IV. *Arch Dis Child*. 1971;46:127-138.

15. Chaseling RW, Johnston IH, Besser M. Meningoceles and the tethered cord syndrome. *Childs Nerv Syst*. 1985;1:105-108.

16. Verhoef M, Barf HA, Post MW, van Asbeck FW, Gooskens RH, Prevo AJ. Secondary impairments in young adults with spina bifida. *Dev Med Child Neurol*. 2004;46:420-427.

17. Adzick NS, Thom EA, Spong CY, et al. A randomized trial of prenatal versus postnatal repair of myelomeningocele. *N Engl J Med*. 2011;364:993-1004.

18. Drake JM, Kestle JR, Milner R, et al. Randomized trial of cerebrospinal fluid shunt valve design in pediatric hydrocephalus. *Neurosurgery*. 1998;43:294-303.

19. National Institute of Neurological Disorders and Stroke. Chiari malformation page. http://www.ninds.nih.gov/disorders/chiari/chiari.htm. Accessed March 3, 2015.

20. Hayhurst C, Osman-Farah J, Das K, Mallucci C. Initial management of hydrocephalus associated with Chiari malformation Type I–syringomyelia complex via endoscopic third ventriculostomy: an outcome analysis. *J Neurosurg*. 2008;108:1211-1214.

21. Bowman RM, Mohan A, Ito J, Seibly JM, McLone DG. Tethered cord release: a long-term study in 114 patients. *J Neurosurg Pediatr*. 2009;3:181-187.

22. Spina Bifida Association. Spinal cord tethering health information sheet. http://www.spinabifidaassociation.org/site/c.evKRI7OXIoJ8H/b.8277207/k.6DCB/Spinal_Cord_Tethering.html. Accessed March 3, 2015.

23. Schoenmakers MA, Uiterwaal CS, Gulmans VA, Gooskens RH, Helders PJ. Determinants of functional independence and quality of life in children with spina bifida. *Clin Rehabil*. 2005;19:677-685.

24. Dik P, Klijn AJ, van Gool JD, de Jong-de Vos van Steenwijk CC, de Jong TP. Early start to therapy preserves kidney function in spina bifida patients. *Eur Urol*. 2006;49:908-913.

25. Blumchen K, Bayer P, Buck D, et al. Effects of latex avoidance on latex sensitization, atopy and allergic diseases in patients with spina bifida. *Allergy*. 2010;65:1585-1593.

26. Swaroop VT, Dias L. Orthopaedic management of spina bifida—part II: foot and ankle deformities. *J Child Orthop*. 2011;5:403-414.

27. Mercado E, Alman B, Wright JG. Does spinal fusion influence quality of life in neuromuscular scoliosis? *Spine*. 2007;32:S120-S125.

28. Mapstone TB, Rekate HL, Nulsen FE, Dixon MS Jr, Glaser N, Jaffe M. Relationship of CSF shunting and IQ in children with myelomeningocele: a retrospective analysis. *Childs Brain*. 1984;11:112-118.

29. Rose BM, Holmbeck GN. Attention and executive functions in adolescents with spina bifida. *J Pediatr Psychol*. 2007;32:983-994.

30. Holbein CE, Lennon JM, Kolbuck VD, Zebracki K, Roache CR, Holmbeck GN. Observed differences in social behaviors exhibited in peer interactions between youth with spina bifida and their peers: neuropsychological correlates. *J Pediatr Psychol*. 2014;40:320-335.

31. Schoenmakers M. *Functional Aspects of Spina Bifida in Childhood* [dissertation]. Utrecht, The Netherlands: University of Utrecht; 2003.

32. Bartonek Å, Saraste H, Knutson LM. Comparison of different systems to classify the neurological level of lesion in patients with myelomeningocele. *Dev Med Child Neurol*. 1999;41:796-805.

33. Oi S, Matsumoto S. A proposed grading and scoring system for spina bifida: Spina Bifida Neurological Scale (SBNS). *Childs Nerv Syst*. 1992;8:337-342.

34. Broughton NS, Menelaus MB, Cole WG, Shurtleff DB. The natural history of hip deformity in myelomeningocele. *J Bone Joint Surg Br*. 1993;75:760-763.

35. McDonald CM, Jaffe KM, Shurtleff DB. Assessment of muscle strength in children with meningomyelocele: accuracy and stability of measurements over time. *Arch Phys Med Rehabil.* 1986;67:855-861.

36. Kirshblum SC, Burns SP, Biering-Sorensen F, et al. International standards for neurological classification of spinal cord injury (revised 2011). *J Spinal Cord Med.* 2011;34:535-546.

37. Mahony K, Hunt A, Daley D, Sims S, Adams R. Inter-tester reliability and precision of manual muscle testing and hand-held dynamometry in lower limb muscles of children with spina bifida. *Phys Occup Ther Pediatr.* 2009;29:44-59.

38. Maynard FM Jr, Bracken MB, Creasey G, et al. International Standards for Neurological and Functional Classification of Spinal Cord Injury. American Spinal Injury Association. *Spinal Cord.* 1997;35:266-274.

39. Morrow MM, Hurd WJ, Kaufman KR, An KN. Shoulder demands in manual wheelchair users across a spectrum of activities. *J Electromyogr Kinesiol.* 2010;20:61-67.

40. Ottenbacher KJ, Msall ME, Lyon N, Duffy LC, Granger CV, Braun S. Measuring developmental and functional status in children with disabilities. *Dev Med Child Neurol.* 1999;41:186-194.

41. Msall ME, DiGaudio K, Rogers BT, et al. The Functional Independence Measure for Children (WeeFIM). Conceptual basis and pilot use in children with developmental disabilities. *Clin Pediatr.* 1994;33:421-430.

42. Danzer E, Gerdes M, Bebbington MW, Koh J, Adzick SN, Johnson MP. Fetal myelomeningocele surgery: preschool functional status using the Functional Independence Measure for children (WeeFIM). *Childs Nerv Syst.* 2011;27:1083-1088.

43. Simsek TT, Türküçüoglu B, Tezcan S. Examination of the relationship between body mass index (BMI) and functional independence level in children with spina bifida. *Dev Neurorehabil.* 2015;18:149-154.

44. Tsai PY, Yang TF, Chan RC, Huang PH, Wong TT. Functional investigation in children with spina bifida—measured by the Pediatric Evaluation of Disability Inventory (PEDI). *Childs Nerv Syst.* 2002;18:48-53.

45. Feldman AB, Haley SM, Coryell J. Concurrent and construct validity of the Pediatric Evaluation of Disability Inventory. *Phys Ther.* 1990;70:602-610.

46. Parkin PC, Kirpalani HM, Rosenbaum PL, et al. Development of a health-related quality of life instrument for use in children with spina bifida. *Qual Life Res.* 1997;6:123-132.

47. Padua L, Rendeli C, Rabini A, Girardi E, Tonali P, Salvaggio E. Health-related quality of life and disability in young patients with spina bifida. *Arch Phys Med Rehabil.* 2002;83:1384-1388.

48. Davies PL, Soon PL, Young M, Clausen-Yamaki A. Validity and reliability of the school function assessment in elementary school students with disabilities. *Phys Occup Ther Pediatr.* 2004;24:23-43.

49. Zwinkels M, Verschuren O, Janssen TW, et al. Exercise training programs to improve hand rim wheelchair propulsion capacity: a systematic review. *Clin Rehabil.* 2014;28:847-861.

50. Oliveira A, Jácome C, Marques A. Physical fitness and exercise training on individuals with spina bifida: a systematic review. *Res Dev Disabil.* 2014;35:1119-1136.

51. de Groot JF, Takken T, van Brussel M, et al. Randomized controlled study of home-based treadmill training for ambulatory children with spina bifida. *Neurorehabil Neural Repair.* 2011;25:597-606.

Acute Lymphoblastic Leukemia

Megan L. Freeland

A previously healthy 4-year-old boy presented to his pediatrician with a 2-month history of fever, fatigue and generalized weakness, joint pain, loss of appetite, and frequent bruising. A complete blood count (CBC) revealed an extremely low absolute neutrophil count (ANC), and bone marrow biopsy confirmed the diagnosis of acute lymphoblastic leukemia (ALL). Chemotherapy was initiated following a protocol that included dexamethasone, vincristine, and doxorubicin. Six weeks following his diagnosis, during the first cycle of the consolidation phase of chemotherapy, the patient was referred to outpatient physical therapy for evaluation, patient education, and treatment.

▶ What examination signs may be associated with ALL?
▶ What are the most appropriate examination tests?
▶ What are the examination priorities?
▶ What are the most appropriate physical therapy outcome measures for peripheral neuropathy?
▶ Describe a physical therapy plan of care based on each stage of treatment.
▶ Identify referrals to other team members important to this case.

KEY DEFINITIONS

ABSOLUTE NEUTROPHIL COUNT (ANC): Percentage of neutrophils present within total white blood cell (WBC) count; normal range is approximately 1.5 to 8.0; lower values indicate increasing neutropenic severity

CHEMOTHERAPY-INDUCED PERIPHERAL NEUROPATHY (CIPN): Adverse effect of several chemotherapeutic agents that results in damage to motor and sensory peripheral nerves of the feet and hands, typically in a stocking/glove distribution

COMPLETE BLOOD COUNT (CBC): Blood test that measures the number or amount of leukocytes, erythrocytes, and platelets as well as hemoglobin and hematocrit

NEUTROPENIA: Abnormally low number of neutrophils, leaving the individual at high risk for infection

STEM CELL TRANSPLANT (SCT): Complete and sustained replacement of an individual's blood cell lines with cells derived from donor stem cells

Objectives

1. Identify the signs and symptoms of ALL.
2. Identify valid and reliable outcome measures for peripheral neuropathy in this population.
3. Recognize the complications of cancer treatment.
4. Identify the signs and symptoms of adverse effects of chemotherapy that can be addressed through physical therapy intervention.
5. Design an appropriate physical therapy program for a child with ALL during the consolidation phase of treatment.

Physical Therapy Considerations

PT considerations during management of the child undergoing treatment for ALL:

▶ **General physical therapy plan of care/goals:** Closely monitor for and manage the signs/symptoms of chemotherapy-induced peripheral neuropathy (CIPN); maximize functional capacity, endurance, and functional mobility; optimize quality of life

▶ **Physical therapy interventions:** Patient and family education regarding ALL and appropriate expectations for mobility and participation, early signs and natural progression of CIPN, and importance of skin checks; strengthening exercises, dynamic balance activities, passive range of motion (ROM) and stretching exercises, fitting for solid ankle-foot orthoses (AFOs); endurance and flexibility training; monitor progress with appropriate outcome measures

▶ **Precautions during physical therapy:** Diligent attention to cleanliness and infection control due to significant immunocompromise; heart rate monitoring due to cardiotoxic effects of doxorubicin; physical supervision to enhance safety and prevent falls related to CIPN; activity modifications due to chronically low hemoglobin or platelet levels

▶ **Complications interfering with physical therapy:** Nausea and fatigue, which are heightened during periods of neutropenia; neuropathic pain and bone pain; inability to participate in exercise during active chemotherapy infusion or blood product transfusion; behavioral and mood changes

Understanding the Health Condition

Acute leukemia is the most common type of childhood cancer comprising nearly 30% of all cases. ALL is the most common type of leukemia in children, nearly five times more common than the next most prevalent form, acute myeloid leukemia (AML).[1-3] ALL is a disease of the bone marrow in which precursor lymphoid cells, or lymphoblasts, are arrested in an early stage of development and proliferate and overtake typical hematopoietic cells in the bone marrow. This results in a marked decrease in the production of normal bone marrow elements. ALL has an incidence of approximately 35 per 1 million children in the United States.[1,2,4] Incidence peaks between 2 and 3 years of age.[1,2] Over the past 30 years, survival rates have improved dramatically with the current 5-year survival rate at over 85%.[1,2,5]

Individuals with ALL present with signs and symptoms related to the decrease in production of normal marrow elements, including anemia, fatigue, fever, other signs of infection, and bone and joint pain. Diagnosis is made by CBC, peripheral blood smear, and bone marrow aspiration. Risk stratification is determined as low, standard, high, or very high risk based on initial WBC count, involvement of sanctuary sites (areas that are difficult to treat with systemic chemotherapy such as the central nervous system and testicles), cytogenetics, immune type, age at diagnosis, and response to initial treatment.[6]

The primary treatment for standard risk ALL is chemotherapy. Agents utilized in treatment vary with treatment centers and individual practitioners employ a wide variety of protocols. Two common chemotherapeutic agents in treatment protocols for ALL are vincristine and doxorubicin, both of which have significant dose-dependent adverse drug reactions (ADRs). Vincristine's dose-limiting ADR is CIPN, which typically follows a stocking/glove distribution, but may be isolated to either lower or upper extremities, and almost exclusively presents with bilateral involvement. The natural progression of CIPN starts with muscle cramping as one of the first indicators. Cramping then progresses to neuropathic pain, weakness and loss of deep tendon reflexes in ankle dorsiflexors and/or long finger flexors, and loss of sensation and eventual paralysis of ankle dorsiflexors and/or long finger flexors.[7-12] CIPN affects nearly all children receiving vincristine as part of the treatment for ALL.[7,8] The likelihood of CIPN increases with increasing drug dose, frequency, and total dose. Prognosis of CIPN is variable. While some children may experience symptoms for weeks or months, others will continue to struggle with

CIPN for years. One of doxorubicin's dose-limiting ADRs is cardiotoxicity that manifests as an exaggerated heart rate response to exercise and an increased life-time risk of congestive heart failure.[6,13] Acute cardiotoxicity is less common than the anticipated late effects. The degree of cardiotoxic ADRs is related to the child's age at exposure to doxorubicin and total dose.[14] Many children also receive glucocorticoids that result in symmetrical proximal muscle weakness. The steroid-induced myopathy typically resolves once the glucocorticoid is discontinued or dosage is reduced.[15]

Chemotherapy treatment for ALL can last for up to two years for girls and three years for boys due to the potential for the testes to be a sanctuary site and its associated adverse prognosis.[16] Chemotherapy treatment, which is typically performed on an outpatient basis, is traditionally divided into three phases: induction, consolidation/intensification, and maintenance. Induction, which typically lasts 4 to 6 weeks, is an extremely intense, high-dose cycle of chemotherapy intended to bring the child into complete remission. Consolidation/intensification lasts several months and is aimed at maintaining remission and may include radiation, depending on the protocol. The final stage of treatment continues for up to two years, typically consisting of low-dose chemotherapy to prevent recurrence of the disease. Chemotherapy is given in cycles that consist of three distinct periods: "chemo week," "neutropenic week," and "week of rest." Though medical professionals often refer to each phase as a "week," the actual length can vary. Each phase of chemotherapy treatment consists of several cycles. For example, a patient may be in consolidation phase, cycle 4. During a "chemo week," patients receive additional hydration and antiemetics with their chemotherapy. During the induction phase of chemotherapy, patients generally feel well and should be encouraged to participate in both functional mobility and exercise except during the active infusion of chemotherapy because of the extremely small risk of the chemotherapeutic agent spilling due to disrupted intravenous access. During the "neutropenic week," patients typically feel their worst. They frequently have an ANC of 0.0; they feel nauseous, weak, and fatigued, and complain of mucositis. Because of the high risk for infection at this time, patients presenting with a fever during this phase must be admitted to the hospital to address the potential for life-threatening infections. The "week of rest" usually results in a rebound in the child's ANC and, with it, a rebound in energy levels, strength, and participation in functional mobility.

Some children may require a hematopoietic stem cell transplant (SCT), or "bone marrow transplant." Modern transplants include stem cells from a variety of sources including peripheral blood, cord blood (blood from the umbilical cord), and bone marrow. Thus, it may be said that all bone marrow transplants are SCTs, but not all SCTs are bone marrow transplants. Candidates for SCT due to ALL include children who fail to attain remission with induction chemotherapy or those with relapsed disease. It is important to note that many children undergoing active treatment for any type of cancer demonstrate consistent symptoms of anemia with hemoglobin <8.0 g/dL and thrombocytopenia with platelet levels <20,000/µL. It is important for the physical therapist to discuss the risk/benefit ratio of intervention with the child's oncologist.[17-18] Most often, when the physical therapist closely monitors for adverse effects, the benefits of mobility far outweigh the risk of participation in modified physical therapy sessions for children who might otherwise remain sedentary.[19]

Physical Therapy Patient/Client Management

Management of the child with ALL requires a multidisciplinary approach with continual communication among all team members. The team for a child newly diagnosed with ALL may include a pediatric medical hematologist/oncologist, pediatric surgical subspecialist, radiation oncologist, physical therapist, occupational therapist, pediatric physiatrist, pediatric nurse practitioner, nurse specialists, social worker, child life specialist, psychologist, and dietician. The physical therapist works with all team members in addition to the patient and his family to obtain an overall assessment of his unique functional abilities and participation restrictions. The overall goal is to optimize participation, functional mobility, and quality of life throughout the course of treatment as well as monitor for the adverse effects of treatment that negatively impact functional mobility. Patient and family education is of paramount importance for the physical therapy plan of care. Physical therapy treatment may include stretching, strengthening, dynamic balance exercises, endurance training, and ongoing education of patient and family and potentially of administrators and educators at the patient's school. **Physical therapy intervention** is both feasible and beneficial at all stages of cancer treatment and in survivorship.[20-22]

Examination, Evaluation, and Diagnosis

Prior to evaluating the patient, the physical therapist must gather a variety of information regarding the patient's case as it relates to his physical therapy plan of care. This includes stage of chemotherapy treatment (induction, consolidation, or maintenance), chemotherapeutic agents included in that particular stage of the protocol, and where within the cycle the child is. Patients actively receiving chemotherapy should not engage in physical therapy due to the risk of intravenous access compromise and the potential for chemotherapy agent spill. Similarly, children receiving blood or platelet transfusion should not engage in active therapy due to the need for continuous monitoring of vital signs to detect any adverse reaction to the transfusion. Proactively timing physical therapy intervention around chemotherapy and blood product infusion with the help of the child's nurse will allow for optimal participation.

Obtaining a patient history, including the child's level of function and preferred activities prior to diagnosis, is extremely helpful in understanding his motivation for play and movement. It also helps establish a rapport with both the child and his family and guides the goal-setting process. A comprehensive assessment of the child with ALL includes strength, ROM, gait, functional mobility, dynamic balance, and endurance. The primary objective of the physical therapy examination is to determine the child's level of function and document the degree of physical impairments with particular attention to screening for the presence of CIPN.

Assessment of CIPN may be completed with the pediatric-modified total neuropathy score (ped-mTNS). The **ped-mTNS** is both valid and reliable for children with non-central nervous system cancer and shows correlation to functional limitations in this population.[23,24] The ped-mTNS is simple to complete and includes objective measures of bilateral gastrocnemius and soleus length, deep tendon reflexes, protective sensation (as measured by monofilaments), vibratory sense, and dorsiflexion strength. The physical therapist must carefully observe the posture of the foot and presence of arches from all angles in weightbearing and nonweightbearing positions to note whether changes occur with progression of neuropathy. Gait should be assessed over an increased distance because milder cases of CIPN become visually apparent only after some fatigue has set in. For this purpose, gait analysis in combination with the 6-minute walk test (6MWT) is ideal as the distance covered during this test might be long enough to identify any gait abnormalities such as tripping or stumbling. In addition, the 6MWT may be used to measure the child's endurance as it is a validated assessment of submaximal functional capacity for severely ill children.[25] To quantify functional mobility, the Timed Up and Go (TUG) test is valid and reliable in children with ALL.[26] Limitations in cardiovascular endurance for participation in play are commonly seen as a compounding result of potential doxorubicin-induced cardiotoxicity and general deconditioning due to inactivity related to the generalized adverse effects of treatment.[27]

The therapist should thoroughly assess attainment of age-appropriate gross motor milestones. Currently, a developmental assessment tool specific to the oncology population does not exist. Children undergoing treatment for ALL are typically not able to engage in full-scale extended developmental testing such as the Peabody Developmental Motor Scale, 2nd Edition (PDMS-2) due to decreased endurance. However, a shorter assessment such as the Bruininks-Oseretsky Test of Motor Proficiency, Short Form (BOTMP-SF) is reliable, valid, and generally well tolerated by this population.[28,29]

Tolerance for participation can be quantified using the Lansky Play Performance Scale/Karnofsky Performance Scale (Lansky/Karnofsky Scale), which was developed specifically to quantify performance in children with cancer. The Karnofsky scale is used to quantify activity for children aged 16 years and older,[29] and the Lansky scale is used for those younger than 16 years.[30] Both scales range from 100 ("normal, no complaints, no evidence of disease" or "fully active") for the Karnofsky and Lansky scales, respectively, to 10 ("moribund, fatal processes progressing rapidly" and "completely disabled, not even passive play"), respectively.[30,31]

Health-related quality of life (QOL) may be significantly improved by participation in physical therapy. By improving functional mobility and participation, interactions between the child and his peers, siblings, family, and community can be amplified. Participation in physical activities can impact a child's anxiety and perception of pain.[32] Health-related QOL can be quantified utilizing the PedsQL Cancer Module. The PedsQL Cancer Module is either an observer- (parent) or patient-reported measure that is valid and reliable for the assessment of health-related QOL for children with cancer.[33] The questionnaire consists of 27 questions in eight domains rated on a scale from 0 (never a problem) to 4 (almost always a problem). A lower score is correlated with a higher health-related QOL.

Due to the potentially severe immunocompromise that affects individuals diagnosed with ALL, the physical therapist must also pay significant attention to cleanliness, disinfection, and infection control of the treatment space, including all toys and equipment used. Treatment spaces should be free of carpet or porous upholstered surfaces to minimize potential risk for infection. If at all possible, children undergoing active treatment for ALL should be seen in a private space or the number of additional children in the treatment area minimized as much as possible.

Plan of Care and Interventions

Physical therapy interventions should address the impairments found on assessment and should additionally include education of both the parent and child regarding expectations and warning signs for adverse effects of treatment. Purposeful play is helpful, not only for improving strength, cardiovascular endurance, and functional mobility, but also for restoring or maintaining the child's confidence to play. Loss of confidence to participate in play is a common psychosocial complication of cancer treatment in children due to limited opportunities for free play, decreased endurance, and an inability to keep up and compete with peers.[19] Parent education regarding expectations for consistent participation in mobility, self-care, and out-of-bed play is essential to physical carry over and behavioral modification for children with ALL.

To allow for early detection, the medical team and caregivers should regularly monitor a child receiving chemotherapy that does not yet present with the signs and symptoms of CIPN. Although there is no evidence that physical therapy interventions can prevent or facilitate recovery from CIPN, these interventions may prevent long-term consequences of CIPN such as loss of ankle ROM. Incorporation of regular stretching of the calf muscles maintains ROM in the muscles and joints most profoundly affected by CIPN. Because children may rely on caregivers for stretching, caregivers should be educated in proper technique and maintenance of neutral positioning of the subtalar joint during stretching to optimally target the gastrocnemius/soleus complex. In addition, the child should be frequently challenged to attempt heel walking and to perform toe grasp activities. The therapist can propose that the family chooses a particular hallway or room as the "heel walking area" and that the child may enjoy cleaning his room by picking up objects with his toes. By incorporating these challenges into everyday tasks, it decreases the burden of performing a formal home exercise program on the family while still providing for necessary screening and carry over.

The child who is affected by CIPN eventually presents with ankle dorsiflexor weakness along the continuum from minimal weakness resulting in a mild foot slap to complete paralysis with foot drop and toe drag. At this time, **balance training, neuromuscular re-education, stretching, and gait training** become important. These children benefit from **solid AFOs** to prevent foot drop and improve safety in ambulation. In addition, AFOs help preserve the arches, prevent loss of dorsiflexion ROM, and limit pronation compensation in gait. Due to the loss of sensation, orthoses must be custom-molded and should be fully lined in foam to reduce the risk of pressure and skin breakdown that could quickly lead to a potentially fatal infection in an immunocompromised child. The physical therapist must underscore the importance of proper socks and footwear and frequent skin checks with both the patient and his family.

Children are most easily engaged in physical therapy through play and motivation for participation. Distraction from the "work" at hand is paramount when asking a chronically ill child to partake in physical therapy sessions. Table 20-1 shows a number of play-based activities, indications, and instructions for the

Table 20-1 SAMPLE PURPOSEFUL PLAY ACTIVITIES FOR A CHILD WITH CHEMOTHERAPY-INDUCED PERIPHERAL NEUROPATHY		
Activity	Indication(s)	Instructions
Bean bag toe grasp race	Weak foot intrinsic muscles, decreased dynamic balance, decreased endurance	Place bean bags around treatment area. Ask child to heel walk from one to another, pick up the bean bag with his toes, transfer it to his hand, then run to place the bean bag in the bucket at the "start."
Gross flexion in single limb stance with ring stack	Decreased dynamic balance, weak dorsiflexion	Place several rings (6 inches or larger) in a semi-circle around child. The child must flip the ring up and hook it on his foot. While maintaining ankle dorsiflexion so the ring does not fall, he must flex his hip and knee to place the ring on a cone in front of him.
Climbing in and out of a barrel or box	Decreased dorsiflexion ROM, decreased dynamic balance	Place puzzle pieces at bottom of large box or barrel that is approximately waist high for the child. Box should be large enough to allow a squat, but small enough to prevent quadruped. The child must climb in, squat down to pick up a puzzle piece, then stand and climb out to place the piece on the board.
Tricycle riding or scooter board propulsion	Decreased endurance, decreased strength	Additional resistance can be added with the therapist standing on the back of the tricycle or the child "towing" a scooter loaded with toys.
Jumping forward, backwards, down, sideways, and over	Decreased strength, decreased endurance, decreased dynamic balance	Present child with varying difficulty of obstacles, starting first with a simple line on the floor and progressing toward steps and hurdles of increasing height. Hand-hold assistance and close guarding may be necessary in early stages of peripheral neuropathy.
Nintendo Wii Fit™	Decreased dynamic balance	The balance board component of the Wii Fit™ can be used to visually track the child's center of mass. Ensure that the child is shifting his weight by moving his center of mass as opposed to simply moving the upper body since many children with CIPN will demonstrate this compensation.

preschool-aged patient in this case. Several or all of these activities may be incorporated into a single session based on the child's tolerance.

Yoga may also be incorporated into the treatment plan by therapists who are competent in this intervention. In both the inpatient and outpatient settings, yoga is feasible to perform with children diagnosed with cancer and has been documented to decrease pain, improve quality of life, and decrease cancer-related fatigue.[34-37]

Ideally, children should be monitored and referred to physical therapy throughout the course of their treatment as their physical function warrants. A continual link to physical therapy services throughout the duration of cancer treatment is essential to ensure monitoring of physical status. Due to the prolonged course of medical treatment and resultant prolongation of need for rehabilitation services, therapists must be mindful of using reimbursement resources wisely. Discharge planning should begin when the child can complete a 6MWT with an age-appropriate gait pattern and distance and complete jumps at age-appropriate distance and height utilizing appropriate musculature without orthoses or assistive devices. Discharge planning must be accompanied by patient and caregiver education regarding the late effects of cancer treatment and their impact on a child's functional mobility.

Evidence-Based Clinical Recommendations

SORT: Strength of Recommendation Taxonomy

A: Consistent, good-quality patient-oriented evidence
B: Inconsistent or limited-quality patient-oriented evidence
C: Consensus, disease-oriented evidence, usual practice, expert opinion, or case series

1. Participation in physical therapy during all stages of chemotherapy treatment and into survivorship is feasible and beneficial. **Grade A**

2. The ped-mTNS is a valid and reliable tool for measuring chemotherapy-induced peripheral neuropathy in children with non-central nervous system cancer. **Grade B**

3. Ankle-foot orthoses in combination with stretching, neuromuscular re-education, gait training, and strengthening are essential to the management of CIPN. **Grade C**

COMPREHENSION QUESTIONS

20.1 The dose-limiting ADR of the chemotherapeutic agent vincristine is

   A. Myopathy

   B. Peripheral neuropathy

   C. Cardiotoxicity

   D. Hypotension

20.2 Children undergoing treatment for ALL should be encouraged to:

A. Rest and conserve energy throughout treatment

B. Engage in play and exercise without modification

C. Engage in play and exercise with proper infection control measures in place

D. Engage in play and exercise with proper infection control measures in place and modification for symptoms as needed

20.3 Which of the following is *not* unique to the assessment of children with cancer?

A. Ped-mTNS

B. Lansky/Karnofsky scale

C. Bruininks-Oseretsky Test of Motor Proficiency, Short Form

D. PedsQL Cancer module

ANSWERS

20.1 **B.** Vincristine is known to cause neuropathy that typically follows a stocking/glove distribution, but may be isolated to either lower or upper extremities, and is almost exclusively bilateral. Cardiotoxicity is a common ADR of doxorubicin (option C). Myopathy is a common ADR of glucocorticoids (option A).

20.2 **D.** Children undergoing treatment for ALL benefit from participation in play and exercise and demonstrate improvements in quality of life, strength, and functional mobility.[35,36] Participation in physical therapy intervention has been documented as both feasible and beneficial at all stages of treatment and in survivorship.[20-23]

20.3 **C.** The Bruininks-Oseretsky Test of Motor Proficiency, Short Form is a developmental testing tool used to assess functional mobility in the general pediatric population. Outcomes of this assessment may be used to compare children diagnosed with cancer to their age-matched, typically developing peers.[28-29]

REFERENCES

1. Howlader N, Noone AM, Krapcho M, et al., eds. Childhood cancer. In: *SEER Cancer Statistics Review, 1975-2010*. Bethesda, MD: National Cancer Institute; 2013:Section 28.

2. Howlader N, Noone AM, Krapcho M, et al., eds. Childhood cancer by the ICCC. In: *SEER Cancer Statistics Review, 1975-2010*. Bethesda, MD: National Cancer Institute; 2013.

3. Margolin JF, Steuber CP, Poplack DG. Acute lymphoblastic leukemia. In: Pizzzo PA, Poplack DG, eds. *Principles and Practice of Pediatric Oncology*. 5th ed. Philadelphia, PA: Lippincott Williams & Wilkins; 2006.

4. Smith MA, Ries LA, Gurney JG, et al. Leukemia. In: Ries LA, Smith MA, Gurney JG, et al., eds. *Cancer Incidence and Survival Among Children and Adolescents: United States SEER Program 1975-1995*. Bethesda, MD: National Cancer Institute, SEER Program; 1999:NIH Pub. No. 99-4649.

5. Smith MA, Altekruse SF, Adamson PC, Reaman GH, Seibel NL. Declining childhood and adolescent cancer mortality. *Cancer.* 2014;120:2497-2506.

6. Shan K, Lincoff AM, Young JB. Anthracycline-induced cardiotoxicity. *Ann Intern Med.* 1996;125:47-58.

7. Vainionpaa L, Kovala T, Tolonen U, Lanning M. Vincristine therapy for children with acute lymphoblastic leukemia impairs conduction in the entire peripheral nerve. *Pediatr Neurol.* 1995;13:314-318.

8. Ramchandren S, Leonard M, Mody RJ, et al. Peripheral neuropathy in survivors of childhood acute lymphoblastic leukemia. *J Peripher Nerv Syst.* 2009;14:184-189.

9. Hausheer FH, Schilsky RL, Bain S, Berghorn EJ, Lieberman F. Diagnosis, management, and evaluation of chemotherapy-induced peripheral neuropathy. *Semin Oncol.* 2006;33:15-49.

10. Visovsky C, Daly BJ. Clinical evaluation and patterns of chemotherapy-induced peripheral neuropathy. *J Am Acad Nurse Pract.* 2004;16:353-359.

11. Cooper SL, Brown PA. Treatment of pediatric acute lymphoblastic leukemia. *Pediatr Clin North Am.* 2015;62:61-73.

12. Reinders-Messelink HA, Schoemaker MM, Hofte M, et al. Fine motor and handwriting problems after treatment for childhood acute lymphoblastic leukemia. *Med Pediatr Oncol.* 1996;27:551-555.

13. Hijiya N, Liu W, Sandlund JT, et al. Overt testicular disease at diagnosis of childhood acute lymphoblastic leukemia: lack of therapeutic role of local irradiation. *Leukemia.* 2005;9:1399-1403.

14. Dickerman JD. The late effects of childhood cancer therapy. *Pediatrics.* 2007;119:554-568.

15. Stubgen JP. Neuromuscular disorders in systemic malignancy and its treatment. *Muscle Nerve.* 1995;18:636-648.

16. Von Hoff DD, Layard MW, Basa P, et al. Risk factors for doxorubicin-induced congestive heart failure. *Ann Intern Med.* 1979;91:710-717.

17. Gerber LH, Vargo M. Rehabilitation for patients with cancer diagnoses. In: Delisa JA, Gans B, eds. *Rehabilitation Medicine: Principles and Practice.* 3rd ed. Philadelphia, PA: Lippincott-Raven; 1998.

18. James MC. Physical therapy for patients after bone marrow transplantation. *Phys Ther.* 1987;67:946-952.

19. Götte M, Kesting S, Winter C, Rosenbaum D, Boos J. Experience of barriers and motivations for physical activities and exercise during treatment of pediatric patients with cancer. *Pediatr Blood Cancer.* 2014;61:1632-1637.

20. Gohar SF, Comito M, Price J, Marchese V. Feasibility and parent satisfaction of a physical therapy intervention program for children with acute lymphoblastic leukemia in the first 6 months of medical treatment. *Pediatr Blood Cancer.* 2011;56:799-804.

21. Marchese VG, Chiarello LA, Lange BJ. Effects of physical therapy intervention for children with acute lymphoblastic leukemia. *Pediatr Blood Cancer.* 2004;42:127-133.

22. Robert RS, Paxton RJ, Palla SL, et al. Feasibility, reliability, and validity of the Pediatric Quality of Life Inventory™ generic core scales, cancer module, and multidimensional fatigue scale in long-term adult survivors of pediatric cancer. *Pediatr Blood Cancer.* 2012;59:703-707.

23. Gilchrist LS, Marais L, Tanner L. Comparison of two chemotherapy-induced peripheral neuropathy measurement approaches in children. *Support Care Cancer.* 2014;22:359-366.

24. Gilchrist LS, Tanner L. The pediatric-modified total neuropathy score: a reliable and valid measure of chemotherapy-induced peripheral neuropathy in children with non-CNS cancers. *Support Care Cancer.* 2013;21:847-856.

25. Nixon PA, Joswiak ML, Fricker FJ. A six-minute walk test for assessing exercise tolerance in severely ill children. *J Pediatr.* 1996;129:362-366.

26. Gocha Marchese V, Chiarello LA, Lange BJ. Strength and functional mobility in children with acute lymphoblastic leukemia. *Med Pediatr Oncol.* 2003;40:230-232.

27. Götte M, Kesting S, Winter C, Rosenbaum D, Boos J. Comparison of self-reported physical activity in children and adolescents before and during cancer treatment. *Pediatr Blood Cancer.* 2014;61:1023-1028.

28. Bruininks RH. *BOT-2: Bruininks-Oseretsky Test of Motor Proficiency, 2nd ed. Manual.* Pearson Assessments; 2005.

29. Venetsanou F, Kambas A, Aggeloussis N, Fatouros I, Taxildaris K. Motor assessment of preschool aged children: a preliminary investigation of the validity of the Bruininks-Oseretsky test of motor proficiency - short form. *Hum Mov Sci.* 2009;28:543-550.

30. Schag CC, Heinrich RL, Ganz PA. Karnofsky performance status revisited: reliability, validity, and guidelines. *J Clin Oncol.* 1984;2:187-193.

31. Lansky SB, List MA, Lansky LL, Ritter-Sterr C, Miller DR. The measurement of performance in childhood cancer patients. *Cancer.* 1987;60:1651-1656.

32. Evans S, Moieni M, Sternlieb B, Tsao JC, Zeltzer LK. Yoga for youth in pain: the UCLA pediatric pain program model. *Holist Nurs Pract.* 2012;26:262-271.

33. Varni JW, Burwinkle TM, Katz ER, Meeske K, Dickinson P. The PedsQL in pediatric cancer: reliability and validity of the Pediatric Quality of Life Inventory Generic Core Scales, Multidimensional Fatigue Scale, and Cancer Module. *Cancer.* 2002;94:2090-2106.

34. Thygeson MV, Hooke MC, Clapsaddle J, Robbins A, Moquist K. Peaceful play yoga: serenity and balance for children with cancer and their parents. *J Pediatr Oncol Nurs.* 2010;27:276-284.

35. Sadja J, Mills PJ. Effects of yoga interventions on fatigue in cancer patients and survivors: a systematic review of randomized controlled trials. *Explore (NY).* 2013;9:232-243.

36. Geyer R, Lyons A, Amazeen L, Alishio L, Cooks L. Feasibility study: the effect of therapeutic yoga on quality of life in children hospitalized with cancer. *Pediatr Phys Ther.* 2011;23:375-379.

37. Braam KI, van der Torre P, Takken T, Veening MA, van Dulmen-den Broeder E, Kaspers GJ. Physical exercise training interventions for children and young adults during and after treatment for childhood cancer. *Cochrane Database Syst Rev.* 2013 Apr 30;4:CD008796.

Cystic Fibrosis

Anne K. Swisher

The patient is a 13-year-old boy with cystic fibrosis (CF) who is a typically developing 7th grader. He was diagnosed via newborn screening and has been cared for
at a CF Care Center, seeing the team (including the physical therapist) every three
months, as recommended. He was hospitalized for the first time three months ago
for dehydration and electrolyte imbalance after playing in a soccer tournament on
a very hot day. This hospitalization frightened his parents. His current lung function is good (forced expiratory volume in one second [FEV_1] 90% of predicted),
but he is somewhat underweight (BMI-for-age 35th percentile) and short for
his age (40th percentile for height). His medical routine includes taking pancreatic enzymes with every meal and snack, nebulized mucolytic medication, and
inhaled antibiotics twice daily, as well as airway clearance via manual percussion
and vibration or oscillatory vest twice daily. However, he often skips treatments
due to "school starting too early in the morning" or "being too busy." He attends
middle school and is a good student. He has played for two years on a competitive
community soccer team, but he is concerned he may not make the school soccer
team because he is smaller than most of his classmates. He reluctantly admits to
becoming tired sooner than his teammates during practice. His teammates and
coach get concerned when he plays hard, as it makes him cough and turn very
red in the face. At his next quarterly visit to the CF Care Center, his parents ask
the physical therapist for advice regarding an exercise program to decrease his
exercise-related symptoms and improve his overall health.

► Based on his health condition, what do you anticipate will be the contributors
  to activity limitations?
► What are the examination priorities?
► What are the most appropriate tests and measures?
► What are the most appropriate physical therapy interventions?
► What precautions should be taken during physical activity?

KEY DEFINITIONS

PANCREATIC INSUFFICIENCY: Inadequate production or release of pancreatic enzymes into the digestive track; the major enzymatic insufficiency in most individuals with CF is in lipase, which is necessary for fat digestion

PULMONARY EXACERBATION: Episode of respiratory signs and symptoms (fever, increased cough and sputum production, fatigue, decreased exercise capacity, acute decline in pulmonary function tests) suggestive of an acute respiratory infection; typically treated with antibiotics and increased frequency of airway clearance treatments and often requires hospitalization

Objectives

1. Describe the multisystem effects of CF and how they impact exercise performance in a child.

2. Describe limitations to sports or exercise due to CF.

3. Develop an age-appropriate examination plan to assess a child with CF.

4. Discuss the information obtained through exercise testing in a child with CF and how the results inform the treatment plan.

5. Create a plan of care that integrates prevention of postural issues and maximizes exercise capacity for sport participation.

Physical Therapy Considerations

PT considerations during management of the physically active adolescent with CF after an acute pulmonary exacerbation:

▶ **General physical therapy plan of care/goals:** Appropriate airway clearance; improve exercise capacity through regular physical activity; maintain or improve flexibility and strength

▶ **Physical therapy interventions:** Patient and family education on appropriate airway clearance techniques; prescription of aerobic, strengthening, and flexibility exercises; education (in conjunction with the CF Care Center dietitian) on the impact of sports/exercise on nutritional needs; education of coaches about CF and considerations for sports

▶ **Precautions during physical therapy:** Monitoring of vital signs with exercise and signs/symptoms of exercise intolerance; impact of nutritional status on exercise capacity

▶ **Complications interfering with physical therapy:** Cough-related complications; time demands of CF care and impact on adherence to plan of care

Understanding the Health Condition

CF is a genetic disease affecting approximately 30,000 Americans and 70,000 people worldwide.[1] The disease is caused by a malfunction in the cystic fibrosis transmembrane regulator (CFTR) protein, which leads to the formation of abnormally thick, sticky mucus in the lungs, digestive tract, and reproductive tract.[1] Newborn screening blood tests are performed in all 50 states to diagnose CF early in life, since appropriate care by an interprofessional CF care team (including physical therapists) at a Cystic Fibrosis Foundation–accredited CF Care Center improves health and prolongs life.[2] Although the average age of death today due to respiratory failure is approximately 37 years old, it is thought that infants born with the disease today and cared for appropriately should have a normal lifespan. Although all people with CF have impaired CFTR function, there is great diversity in both genotypical and phenotypical presentations. Thus, each person should be managed based on his or her specific presentation.

People with CF typically develop respiratory infections and progressive obstructive disease (bronchiectasis) from mucus plugging of airways. Routine use of inhaled mucolytic agents (*e.g.*, Pulmozyme), specially formulated antibiotics (*e.g.*, Tobi), and bronchodilators is prescribed to prevent or slow the lung disease.[2] Airway clearance techniques are taught to all patients and should be performed daily to clear the abnormally thick, viscous secretions. There are many **airway clearance techniques** that can be used; all have been proven to be equally effective, if performed regularly and correctly.[3] Thus, it is important to match the technique(s) with the patient's situation (medical status, family support, independence). The options range from passive techniques such as manual percussion and vibration typically performed by parents, to active techniques such as active cycle breathing or autogenic drainage, which require the patient to perform a variety of breathing maneuvers and assess secretion movement within the chest. There are also a variety of devices, such as oscillatory vests (*e.g.*, Vest, SmartVest, inCourage) or positive expiratory pressure devices, with or without oscillation (*e.g.*, Acapella, PEP mask, TheraPEP, RC-Cornet). As care for people with CF has advanced, the most lethal complication (respiratory failure) is now uncommon in childhood. Recently, the development of a medication that improves CFTR function (Kalydeco) has shown promise to reverse the underlying airway dysfunction in some patients.[2] Very exciting research is ongoing in this area.

Pancreatic insufficiency is common in children with CF, causing them to be leaner and shorter than their peers. Due to malabsorption of fat and fat-soluble vitamins, people with CF are advised to consume at least 150% of the recommended daily caloric intake as well as supplemental pancreatic enzymes with consumption of fatty foods to aid absorption.[2] Daily ingestion of specially formulated vitamins is also essential for normal growth and health. Adults with CF often have impaired bone density, so it is important to encourage weightbearing exercise for children and adolescents with the disease to build their "bone bank" for the future.[2]

Multiple studies have shown that **physical activity and exercise** positively impact lung function, decrease pulmonary exacerbations and hospitalizations, and improve function, endurance and energy level, and quality of life for both children and adults with the disease.[4-9] Thus, it is currently considered part of standard CF care to encourage a physically active lifestyle. Indeed, many patients report regular physical activity and exercise to be critical in helping them participate in a normal life. It is truly seen that "exercise is medicine" for CF. However, CFTR malfunction in sweat glands means that people with CF lose more sodium and chloride through perspiration than their peers, and can become ill from electrolyte imbalance and dehydration.[2] Studies have indicated that adolescents with CF demonstrate an impaired muscular metabolic response to exercise, which may limit their maximal exercise capacity.[10-14]

Physical Therapy Patient/Client Management

An interprofessional team of experts, including physicians, nurses, dietitians, social workers, pharmacists, respiratory therapists, and physical therapists, manage the care of individuals with CF. These professionals work together to assess patient status at quarterly routine visits to a Cystic Fibrosis Foundation–accredited Care Center, and provide recommendations to optimize health throughout the lifespan. Patients who develop pulmonary exacerbations or other CF-related complications also receive this team care upon admission to the hospital. The goal of the CF care team is to achieve normal lung function and normal nutrition and growth, and to prevent CF-related complications. This requires that the team focus first and foremost on the patient and family and adapt recommendations to each unique circumstance. The care team, including the physical therapist, must be able to adapt to changes across the lifespan and disease course. The physical therapist in the CF Care Center focuses primarily on exercise issues, airway clearance (often in conjunction with the respiratory therapist), and neuromusculoskeletal issues such as breathing pattern or postural abnormalities.

Examination, Evaluation, and Diagnosis

During the interview with the patient and his family, the physical therapist recognized that this young man has an interest in sports and competition, but lacks awareness of how his CF impacts his abilities. At this age, many of his peers are experiencing growth spurts and other pubertal changes and he is concerned that he is small for his age. It is important for the physical therapist to understand the demands of this child's sport, including any specific playing position demands. As indicated by his history and FEV_1, his current CF lung disease is mild, and should not limit his exercise capacity.

Studies of individuals with CF have linked **higher aerobic capacity** with improved longevity[15] and **participation in regular aerobic exercise** has been shown to slow decline in pulmonary function.[16] The best way to assess his current aerobic capacity is to perform a cardiopulmonary exercise test to determine his maximal aerobic capacity and any abnormal exercise responses, such as oxygen desaturation or cardiac abnormalities. Most pulmonary function laboratories at CF Care Centers have the ability to perform these tests. One of the preferred exercise tests for children and adolescents with CF is the Godfrey cycle ergometer protocol.[17] After the exercise test, the physical therapist compares the child's performance to age-related norms. This information helps the physical therapist determine not only the child's relative aerobic fitness, but also whether ventilation or cardiac issues led to premature stoppage of a test. If a cycle ergometer is not available, the physical therapist can have the child perform an incremental shuttle walking test (the Modified Shuttle Walk test is ideal for this population)[18,19] to determine at what point the child stops progressive exercise. By assessing vital signs at the beginning and end of the test, the physical therapist can determine any abnormal exercise responses (*e.g.*, oxygen desaturation, excessive heart rate rise, blood pressure abnormalities) and/or coughing, which would indicate impaired airway clearance.

In addition to assessing maximal aerobic capacity, the physical therapist assesses muscular strength, particularly of the trunk and "core" muscles. Since CF can lead to an increased demand on these muscles to assist in ventilation and/or coughing, **weakness in the trunk muscles** can impair overall exercise performance.[20] The therapist can assess trunk muscle strength and endurance by having the child perform "plank" (side and/or prone positions), push-up, sit-up, or "superman" exercises. Weakness and/or poor endurance can be noted by the child's inability to hold the positions or observable asymmetries or muscle activation problems. Repetitions or hold times for these exercises can serve as useful outcome measures to document comparisons following a training program. The lung disease of CF leads to hyperinflation of the lungs and compensatory chest wall changes that impact flexibility. Thus, the physical therapist must assess shoulder girdle and chest wall mobility to ensure that no muscle imbalances exist. Common findings include tightness of anterior chest muscles, overstretched scapular retractors, forward head posture (leading to tightness of cervical extensors and more vertical alignment of sternocleidomastoid muscles), and excessive lumbar lordosis.[20]

To assess the patient's airway clearance ability, the physical therapist should ask the patient and family about the technique(s) currently used and the productivity of coughing. At this age, most patients are able to learn and perform methods of airway clearance that utilize different ventilatory volumes (*e.g.*, active cycle breathing, autogenic drainage, huff coughing). Aerobic exercise that causes the same ventilatory effects has been shown to be equally effective as more passive modes of airway clearance.[21] However, aerobic exercise is currently recommended as an *adjunct* to the routine airway clearance techniques prescribed for the patient.[3] Similar to other airway clearance techniques, the exercise must be performed daily to be of benefit. In addition, the child must be willing to expectorate the mobilized secretions, which can be distressing to children in a group environment. Exercise for 20 minutes at 60% of peak aerobic capacity has been found to improve water content in secretions and improve ease of expectoration.[22] Thus, aerobic exercise should be recommended as an important component of this patient's routine airway clearance techniques in addition to preparing him for physical activity and sports participation.

The therapist should also ask the patient and family about the child's heat intolerance or dehydration with sports and their understanding of how to manage these issues. The physical therapist, in conjunction with the CF Care Center dietitian, can develop a plan to minimize these risks, as well as strategies to obtain adequate healthy daily caloric intake to compensate for the additional demands of sports and exercise. While many parents are concerned that participation in exercise will cause their child to lose weight, they should be informed that exercise can stimulate appetite and if caloric needs are met, weight loss should not occur.

Plan of Care and Interventions

The plan of care for this child includes education in airway clearance techniques best suited to his current situation, an appropriate exercise prescription to address identified deficits in aerobic capacity, strength or flexibility exercises, and education of the family and coaches on the benefits of exercise and modifications that might be needed for the child with CF.

The physical therapist, in conjunction with the respiratory therapist, can instruct the child on the use of hand-held devices (e.g., Acapella, Flutter, RC-Cornet) or the use of breathing techniques (active cycle breathing or autogenic drainage and huff coughing) for airway clearance. The breathing techniques take more practice to learn so follow-up should be frequent during the learning process. These techniques can be combined with aerobic exercise training, thus improving time efficiency for a busy adolescent. In addition, as the patient performs moderate-to-vigorous physical activity, ventilatory patterns will naturally encourage secretion movement and easier clearance. Those physical activities that demand higher ventilatory flows have been shown to increase airway surface liquid in the lungs of adults with CF[22] and the impact of vigorous activities may loosen secretions from the airway walls, making expectoration easier.[8,22] The patient and family must understand, however, that some additional form of airway clearance besides aerobic exercise must be performed daily, as the abnormal secretions are produced continually. It is also important that the child is comfortable with a variety of techniques so that adherence to daily airway clearance is more likely (e.g., technique to use at home vs. on a sleepover, what to do if a device breaks, etc.).

At this age, stretching tight muscles and strengthening trunk muscles should resolve any identified postural imbalances and are important to prevent problems later in adulthood. Running, jumping, and ball games such as basketball or volleyball also involve significant impact forces that may help build or maintain bone density. Resistance training is also recommended for this age group,[23] provided that children are properly supervised and technique is emphasized over the amount of weight lifted.

The physical therapist should counsel the adolescent patient about the benefits of aerobic exercise as well as the potential dangers of performance-enhancing substances that may be available and commonly used by his peers. Participation in the same sports year-round should be discouraged, since this increases the risk of musculoskeletal injuries. Adolescents who express interest in extreme sports activities (e.g., high-intensity training programs) should be counseled to seek well-trained leaders who teach techniques safely and will not push them too quickly into high-level performance. The physical therapist needs to be aware of the popular exercise types and routines in general society and be prepared to analyze, along with the adolescent, the benefits and risks of participation. The physical therapist should also work with the adolescent to develop plans to resume higher-level exercise following pulmonary exacerbations or injuries.

Performing activities that increase ventilation, raise heart rate, and are perceived as moderately intense for 30 to 60 minutes daily can increase aerobic capacity. National guidelines for healthy children recommend 60 minutes of moderate-to-vigorous physical activity performed daily[24] and children with CF should also strive to meet this recommendation. This can be met by a variety of activities, and the physical therapist should aim for a balanced exercise program to complement this child's interest and involvement in soccer, while minimizing risk of overuse injuries. Ideal intensity for aerobic training effect in individuals with CF is similar to healthy persons (70%-85% of age-predicted maximal heart rate or 60%-80% of age-predicted maximal oxygen consumption).[25] At this level, training-related improvements in cardiovascular, pulmonary, and metabolic systems occur. However, the chosen intensity should be one that can be maintained for 20 minutes or more. Exercise intensity can be reliably measured in children with CF using the OMNI scale[26] or can be approximated by assessing the child's ability to carry on a conversation while still breathing somewhat harder.

Aerobic training effects have been equally demonstrated in boys and girls with CF[27] and are more pronounced in those patients who begin at a lower level of aerobic fitness.[28] The physical therapist should serve as a consultant to the family and sports coaches, educating them on the benefits of regular exercise and sports for children with CF and allaying fears about coughing or heat intolerance. As this adolescent's aerobic conditioning and strength improves, he should notice less retention of secretions in his airways and less fatigue with soccer practices and games. His heat intolerance and risk of dehydration should be managed jointly with the CF Care Center dietitian to plan for adequate sodium and water intake and healthy ways to increase caloric intake to compensate for higher level physical activities.

Adolescence is a challenging and exciting time for parents and emerging young adults. For adolescents with CF, puberty is often delayed and they may feel embarrassed by physically lagging behind their peers. In addition, physical activity levels drop dramatically in this age group,[29] particularly in girls with CF.[30,31] The unique concerns of CF, such as coughing, expectorating, flatulence (which often occurs during physical activity), and body image concerns, may make adolescents with CF even more likely to decrease their physical activity. Further, adolescents' behavior is influenced not only by family members but also strongly by their peers. If his peers are sedentary, the adolescent with CF may lack the desire to be physically active. For some adolescents, this may be a time of team sports or physically active hobbies that can help reinforce regular physical activity. However, adolescents who are smaller or have less muscular development than their peers may find that they are no longer able to keep up with the emerging demands of competitive team sports. Families need to continue to encourage outlets for vigorous physical activity as a routine part of CF care, just like taking prescribed medications and performing regular airway clearance. With counseling on physical activity choices that best fit the adolescent's interests and abilities, adoption and long-term adherence of a physically active lifestyle has been demonstrated.[32] Particularly for adolescent girls, participation in regular physical activity slows the decline in lung function and predicts long-term survival.[33]

Adherence to all CF care guidelines can be challenging at this time period, and the physical therapist needs to consider ways for the adolescent to have his own choice in types and timing of activities in order to maximize adherence. At least one study has found that free-choice physical activity participation was correlated with maximal aerobic capacity,[34] suggesting that the precise mode of physical activity may not be as important as the ability to choose an activity in which the adolescent will engage. Encouraging patients to view appropriate websites and online chat groups targeted to teens with CF may help them appreciate the value of physical activity. Many high-profile people with CF that can be seen or reached through these websites have highlighted the value of exercise and physical activity in maintaining their physical and emotional health through this sometimes difficult time of life (e.g., Boomer Esiason Foundation's website: http://www.esiason.org/ and Cystic Fibrosis Foundation's website: http://www.cff.org).

It is important that the physical therapist speak directly to the adolescent, ideally without the parents' presence, to establish rapport and openness to questions and concerns he may have about exercise, particularly "fad" or trendy programs, and to talk about the dangers of performance-enhancing substances. The physical therapist must be aware of both the positive and negative influences to which the adolescent may be exposed and talk frankly with the patient about these issues. The goal in this time period is to maintain physical activity as a desirable and positive reaction to having a chronic illness, offering exercise as something the adolescent can control.

The physical therapist should realize that healthy habits instilled at this age provide the child with the means to manage his CF for a long and productive life. As advances occur in the management of the medical issues of CF, this child should expect to live well into adulthood and have a strong, flexible body to allow all the options for mobility, exercise, and sports open to his peers. Most adults living successfully with CF credit daily physical activity and exercise as one of the most important ways they manage their disease. Convincing an adolescent to do anything can be challenging, but also rewarding, as the physical therapist bonds with the emerging young adult.

Evidence-Based Clinical Recommendations

SORT: Strength of Recommendation Taxonomy

A: Consistent, good-quality patient-oriented evidence
B: Inconsistent or limited-quality patient-oriented evidence
C: Consensus, disease-oriented evidence, usual practice, expert opinion, or case series

1. Active breathing techniques and devices for airway clearance are equally effective as manual techniques in individuals with cystic fibrosis. **Grade A**

2. Regular exercise training should be considered part of the routine management of CF. **Grade A**

3. Higher aerobic capacity is an important determinant of pulmonary function and lifespan in individuals with CF. **Grade A**

4. In adolescents with CF, identification and correction of postural and muscle imbalances (especially in the trunk) is critical because weakness can impair exercise performance. **Grade B**

COMPREHENSION QUESTIONS

21.1 A child with CF performs an incremental shuttle walking test in the clinic. At the end of the test, which of the following is an abnormal finding?

A. Pulse is 30 bpm higher than resting level

B. Rating of perceived exertion is "hard"

C. Systolic blood pressure is 20 mm Hg higher than resting level

D. Oxygen saturation is lower than resting level

21.2 Which of the following would *not* be a desirable result of an exercise training program for a child with CF?

A. Weight loss

B. Improved airway clearance

C. Improved quality of life

D. Improved functional capacity

21.3 Which of the following would be the *best* exercise to address typical postural abnormalities in an adolescent with CF?

A. Bicep curls

B. Scapular retraction exercises

C. Barbell squats

D. Straight leg raises

ANSWERS

21.1 **D.** Since exercise increases ventilation and mobilization of secretions, oxygen saturation at the end of an exercise exertion should be the same or higher than resting values. All other vital sign changes (increases in heart rate, systolic pressure, and RPE) are expected with a moderate exercise challenge and would not be different for a child with CF.

21.2 **A.** While all of the effects listed typically result from exercise training, children with CF need to increase their caloric intake to balance the expenditure with exercise. Most children with CF are normal weight or underweight and need to avoid weight loss that can occur with exercise. Fortunately, many patients find that regular exercise stimulates appetite and makes consumption of additional calories easier than those who are sedentary.

21.3 **B.** Due to obstructive changes in the lungs and hyperinflation, most patients tend to adopt a "forward shoulder" posture with tight anterior chest muscles and overstretched and weak scapular retractors. Therefore, exercises to strengthen the scapular retractors would best target this postural deficit. The other exercises would be good for an adolescent to perform as part of a general strengthening program.

REFERENCES

1. About CF: Causes, Signs and Symptoms of Cystic Fibrosis Web site. http://www.cff.org/AboutCF/. Accessed August 19, 2015.

2. Cystic Fibrosis Foundation: Therapies Web site. http://www.cff.org/treatments/Therapies/. Accessed August 19, 2015.

3. Flume PA, Robinson KA, O'Sullivan BP, et al. Cystic fibrosis pulmonary guidelines: airway clearance therapies. *Respir Care.* 2009;54:522-537.

4. Boas SR, Danduran MJ, McColley SA. Parental attitudes about exercise regarding their children with cystic fibrosis. *Int J Sports Med.* 1999;20:334-338.

5. Bradley JM, Moran F. Physical training for cystic fibrosis. *Cochrane Database Syst Rev.* 2008;Jan 23:CD002768.

6. Shoemaker MJ, Hurt H, Arndt L. The evidence regarding exercise training in the management of cystic fibrosis: a systematic review. *Cardiopulm Phys Ther J.* 2008;19:75-83.

7. Rand S, Prasad SA. Exercise as part of a cystic fibrosis therapeutic routine. *Expert Rev Respir Med.* 2012;6:341-352.

8. Wheatley CM, Wilkins BW, Snyder EM. Exercise is medicine in cystic fibrosis. *Exerc Sport Sci Rev.* 2011;39:155-160.

9. Dwyer TJ, Elkins MR, Bye PT. The role of exercise in maintaining health in cystic fibrosis. *Curr Opin Pulm Med.* 2011;17:455-460.

10. Selvadurai H, Allen J, Sachinwalla T, Macauley J, Blimkie CJ, Van Asperen PP. Muscle function and resting energy expenditure in female athletes with cystic fibrosis. *Am J Respir Crit Care Med.* 2003;168:1476-1480.

11. Swisher A. Not just a lung disease: peripheral skeletal muscle abnormalities in cystic fibrosis and the role of exercise to address them. *Cardiopulm Phys Ther J.* 2006;17:10-15.

12. deMeer K, Jeneson AJ, Gulmans VA, van der Laag J, Berger R. Efficiency of oxidative work performance of skeletal muscle in patients with cystic fibrosis. *Thorax.* 1995;50:980-983.

13. Lamhonwah A, Bear CE, Huan LJ, Kim Chiaw P, Ackerley CA, Tein I. Cystic fibrosis transmembrane conductance regulator in human muscle: dysfunction causes abnormal metabolic recovery in exercise. *Ann Neurol.* 2010;67:802-808.

14. Wells GD, Wilkes DL, Schneiderman JE, et al. Skeletal muscle metabolism in cystic fibrosis and primary ciliary dyskinesia. *Pediatr Res.* 2011;69:40-45.

15. Nixon PA, Orenstein DM, Kelsey SF, Doershuk CF. The prognostic value of exercise testing in patients with cystic fibrosis. *N Engl J Med.* 1992;327:1785-1788.

16. Schneiderman-Walker J, Pollock SL, Corey M, et al. A randomized controlled trial of a 3-year home exercise program in cystic fibrosis. *J Pediatr.* 2000;136:304-310.

17. Radtke T, Stevens D, Benden C, Williams CA. Clinical exercise testing in children and adolescents with cystic fibrosis. *Pediatr Phys Ther.* 2009;21:275-281.

18. Rogers D, Smith P, John N, Oliver W, Doull IJ. Validity of a modified shuttle walk test as a measure of exercise tolerance in paediatric CF patients. *J Cyst Fibros.* 2002;1:S22.

19. Cox NS, Fottett J, McKay KO. Modified shuttle test performance in hospitalized children and adolescents with cystic fibrosis. *J Cyst Fibrosis*. 2006;5:165-170.

20. Massery M. Musculoskeletal and neuromuscular interventions: a physical approach to cystic fibrosis. *J R Soc Med*. 2005;98:55-66.

21. Cerny F. Relative effects of bronchial drainage and exercise for in-hospital care of patients with cystic fibrosis. *Phys Ther*. 1989;69:633-639.

22. Dwyer TJ, Alison JA, McKeorgh ZJ, Daviskas E, Bye PT. Effects of exercise on respiratory flow and sputum properties in patients with cystic fibrosis. *Chest*. 2011;139:870-877.

23. van Doorn N. Exercise programs for children with cystic fibrosis: a systematic review of randomized controlled trials. *Disabil Rehabil*. 2010;32:41-49.

24. United States Department of Agriculture. My Plate. ChooseMyPlate.gov Web site. http://www.choosemyplate.gov/. Accessed August 19, 2015.

25. Williams CA, Benden C, Stevens D, Radtke T. Exercise training in children and adolescents with cystic fibrosis: theory into practice. *Int J Pediatrics*. 2010; doi: 10.1155/2010/670640.

26. Higgins LW, Robertson RJ, Kelsey SF, et al. Exercise intensity self-regulation using the OMNI scale in children with cystic fibrosis. *Pediatr Pulmonol*. 2013;48:497-505.

27. Gruber W, Orenstein DM, Braumann KM, Paul K, Huls G. Effects of an exercise program in children with cystic fibrosis: are there differences between females and males? *J Pediatr*. 2011;158:71-76.

28. Gruber W, Orenstein DM, Braumann KM. Do responses to exercise training in cystic fibrosis depend on initial fitness level? *Eur Respir J*. 2011;38:1336-1342.

29. Britto M, Garret JM, Konrad TR, Majure JM, Leigh MW. Comparison of physical activity in adolescents with cystic fibrosis versus age-matched controls. *Ped Pulmonol*. 2000;30:86-91.

30. Schneiderman-Walker J, Wilkes DL, Strug L, et al. Sex differences in habitual physical activity and lung function decline in children with cystic fibrosis. *J Pediatr*. 2005;147:321-326.

31. Selvadurai HC, Blimkie CJ, Cooper PJ, Mellis CM, Van Asperen PP. Gender differences in habitual activity in children with cystic fibrosis. *Arch Dis Child*. 2004;89:928-933.

32. Hebestreit H, Keiser S, Junge S, et al. Long-term effects of a partially supervised conditioning programme in cystic fibrosis. *Eur Respir J*. 2010;35:578-583.

33. Wilkes DL, Schneiderman JE, Nguyen T, et al. Exercise and physical activity in children with cystic fibrosis. *Paediatr Respir Rev*. 2009;10:105-109.

34. Hebestreit H, Kieser S, Rudiger S, et al. Physical activity is independently related to aerobic capacity in cystic fibrosis. *Eur Respir J*. 2006;28:734-739.

Hemophilia

Sarah Martyn

CASE 22

The patient is a 10-year-old boy with severe hemophilia A and history of a right elbow target joint. He is on a prophylaxis schedule three times per week (Monday, Wednesday, Friday) using recombinant factor VIII (rFVIII). The boy was playing at recess on a Tuesday afternoon when he jumped five feet from the jungle gym platform, landing on his feet. Before school ended for the day, he felt his left ankle tingling and it became increasingly warm, swollen, and painful. Recognizing this as a hemarthrosis, he went to the school nurse, who elevated and ace-wrapped his ankle. She also called his father, who notified the hemophilia treatment center (HTC) of the bleed to receive instructions on a plan of care. The boy's father came to the school and infused his son with rFVIII within two hours of the onset of symptoms. After dinner that evening, the pain and swelling had decreased. The boy had been reclined with his left leg elevated for several hours. Before bed, he received another dose of rFVIII as prescribed by the HTC hematologist. The next day, he used crutches around school to keep weight off his left foot. By the weekend, he progressed to walking without crutches, but he was not allowed back to normal play. On Monday, the boy went to his HTC for a follow-up appointment. No imaging was performed, but the physical therapist at the HTC noted pain-free limited left ankle range of motion (ROM). After the brief assessment by the HTC physical therapist, the hematologist made a referral to outpatient physical therapy for left ankle ROM and strengthening.

▶ Describe the most appropriate physical therapy interventions based on the acuity of a bleed in an individual with hemophilia.
▶ What are the possible complications related to hemophilia that would interfere with physical therapy interventions?
▶ What precautions should be taken during physical therapy examination and intervention?
▶ What laboratory values associated with hemophilia should the therapist review?
▶ Identify other medical team members important to this case.

KEY DEFINITIONS

HEMARTHROSIS: Bleeding into the intra-articular space

HEMOPHILIA TREATMENT CENTER (HTC): Comprehensive outpatient clinic that focuses on treating the whole person and his/her family through continuous supervision of all medical and psychosocial aspects of bleeding disorders

RECOMBINANT FACTOR VIII (rFVIII): Manufactured blood-clotting protein first introduced in the late 1980s used to treat hemophilia; now does not contain proteins derived from animals or humans[1]

TARGET JOINT: Joint with repeated bleeding (defined as three hemorrhages within six months) often leading to chronic synovitis[2]

Objectives

1. Define hemophilia.

2. Recognize the signs of an acute joint bleeding event (hemarthrosis).

3. Understand the medical management of hemophilia.

4. Understand the long-term effects of repetitive joint bleeds.

5. Recognize the potential risks of hemophilia.

6. Create an appropriate outpatient physical therapy program for a child with hemophilia who has sustained a joint bleed.

Physical Therapy Considerations

PT considerations for the young child with hemophilia and current joint bleed:

▶ **General physical therapy plan of care/goals:** Minimize or prevent the loss of ROM, strength, and aerobic capacity; minimize secondary impairments and maximize function, joint protection, and quality of life; prevent future bleeding episodes

▶ **Physical therapy interventions:** Patient/family education in the prevention and management of a hemophilic bleeding episode; weight management; safe activities for play; promote ROM to prevent contractures; exercises to maximize strength and balance for protection from injury and joint bleeding

▶ **Precautions during physical therapy interventions:** Joint protection, prevention of new bleeding episode, pretreatment with factor replacement prior to therapy session

▶ **Complications interfering with physical therapy:** New bleeding episode, pain, contractures

Understanding the Health Condition

Hemophilia is a bleeding disorder characterized by missing or defective clotting factor protein necessary for blood coagulation. Hemophilia A is a deficiency in factor VIII (FVIII) and hemophilia B is a deficiency in factor IX (FIX). Hemophilia is caused by an inherited X-linked recessive trait, meaning that almost all individuals with hemophilia are male. Because the defective gene is located on the X chromosome, daughters of men with hemophilia will be carriers of the gene, but sons of female carriers have a 50% chance of having hemophilia. Hemophilia can also be caused by a spontaneous mutation. The number of people with hemophilia in the United States is estimated to be 20,000.[3]

The timing of diagnosis can vary based on symptoms or known familial history of hemophilia. Initial signs of hemophilia may include neonatal head bleeds due to the use of delivery instruments, bleeding for a prolonged time after a blood draw, bleeding after circumcision, or excessive bruising. One-third of babies who are diagnosed with hemophilia have no known family members with the disorder.[4] Diagnosis is based on multiple blood tests. Clotting factor tests called factor assays assess the plasma levels of FVIII or FIX. Other frequently used diagnostic indicators include hemoglobin, activated partial thromboplastin time (APTT), prothrombin time (PT), and fibrinogen. FVIII and FIX are part of the intrinsic pathway of the clotting cascade; therefore, PT remains normal, yet the APTT is prolonged. For a person with hemophilia, the clotting cascade begins normally with vessel constriction. A plasma clotting protein initiates a platelet plug; however, the plug does not fully form, and bleeding resumes. Thus, the person with hemophilia does not bleed faster than someone without the disorder, but the bleeding occurs for *longer*.

Hemophilia is characterized as mild, moderate, or severe based on the amount of FVIII or FIX a person has. Whereas the person without hemophilia has 50% to 150% of normal factor activity in the blood, someone with mild hemophilia has 5% to 50% of normal factor activity and this is manifested by excessive bleeding following a trauma or surgery. Moderate hemophilia (factor levels 1%-5%) is typically characterized by excessive bleeding after minor trauma. A person with severe hemophilia (factor levels <1%) can have spontaneous bleeding without trauma.

To treat or prevent bleeding, the goal is to raise deficient FVIII or FIX levels. There are several intravenous products that contain the FVIII or FIX protein. These concentrates may be derived from human plasma or may be recombinant (derived from animal cells). A person with mild hemophilia is typically treated only prior to an invasive procedure or after significant trauma. Those with moderate hemophilia may also require treatment after a bleeding event that could occur after minor-moderate trauma. For a person with severe hemophilia, there are two types of intervention. The first is on-demand treatment, which is infusion of the clotting factor after a bleeding event. The second is prophylactic intervention, in which the factor is infused on a regular schedule to maintain plasma factor levels greater than 1% to prevent spontaneous bleeding. For an individual with severe hemophilia, this prophylaxis is considered the goal of therapy to preserve normal musculoskeletal function.[2,5] For an individual with any severity of hemophilia undergoing a surgical procedure, it is the standard of care for factor levels to be corrected to 100% to prevent excessive bleeding. Treatment is based on the factor's half-life, which varies somewhat for each person; FVIII has a half-life between 7.4 and 20.4 hours[6] and the half-life of FIX is about 18 hours.[7] Approximately 15% to 20% of people with hemophilia will develop an antibody to the recombinant factor, known as an inhibitor. To overcome an inhibitor, a person is given either a higher dose of the FVIII or FIX product, or a factor VII (FVII) product as a bypassing agent to complete the clotting cascade.

Even with treatment, individuals with hemophilia can experience excessive bleeding. This can occur internally (e.g., within the central nervous system, gastrointestinal tract, airways), externally (e.g., epistaxis, superficial cuts, gums), and into joints and muscles. The most common bleeding sites are into joints, specifically the elbows, knees, and ankles.[8] Recognition and treatment at the first sign of an acute bleed is imperative to minimize damage. Symptoms of a joint or muscle bleed include tingling (sometimes described as "prickling" or an "aura") or numbness (potential adverse effect from a compressed nerve), swelling, decreased ROM, tightness of skin, tachycardia, and hypotension. Ideally, the person should infuse with factor as soon as possible to aid in successful completion of the clotting cascade and halt bleeding. For a joint or muscle bleed, the affected joint should be rested (off-loading when appropriate), immobilized in a position of least pain (often the open-packed position), and compression applied. Writing down the bleeding episodes may help to identify trends in order to optimize risk reduction and treatment.

An acute joint or muscle bleed results in pain, swelling, and decreased ROM due to intra-articular blood.[9] Blood is deposited in the form of hemosiderin into the synovium, whose function is to resorb the material. Over time, the synovium hypertrophies and vascular projections (villi) grow on the synovial surface. To facilitate breakdown of excessive blood products within the joint, a dense capillary network develops beneath the synovium. The villi can become trapped and torn within the joint, severing subsynovial vessels and causing further bleeding. As this process occurs repeatedly in a single joint, the cycle can continue in spite of adequate factor level.[10] A single joint that is prone to such bleeding is known as a target joint.

A person who has experienced bleeding into joints or muscles over time may have joint malalignment, synovial hypertrophy, and/or contracture. Although physical therapy is a common and effective conservative intervention to improve strength, joint ROM, and submaximal activity, surgical intervention may be required.[11] Synovectomy (surgical removal of the hypertrophic joint lining) is an effective intervention that decreases pain and bleeding by 70% to 100%.[12] If conservative interventions fail to improve symptoms of chronic arthropathy, a total joint arthroplasty may be beneficial. Arthrodesis (surgical fusion of the joint) may be performed for individuals with advanced arthropathy of the ankle.

Pain is common in acute joint bleeds and chronic arthropathy. There are several precautions for medically managing pain in individuals with hemophilia. Aspirin is not recommended because it increases bleeding time.[13] Although the other non-steroidal anti-inflammatory drugs (NSAIDs) are effective analgesics, the risk for gastric bleeding is significant. Under close supervision, NSAIDs can be safe analgesics.[14] Acetaminophen does not alter bleeding time; however, due to its effects on the liver, it is used with caution, as factor proteins are produced in the liver.[15] Often, opioids are prescribed to relieve the pain of chronic arthropathy, but concerns of abuse and addiction must be recognized.

A child with hemophilia should seek life-long care at an HTC annually or biannually.[4] Here, the child is managed by a hematologist, nurse, social worker, physical therapist, and other providers specializing in the care of persons with hemophilia. HTCs are the standard models for delivery of comprehensive care to people with hemophilia and aim to improve quality of life and independence while lowering mortality and providing cost-effective care.

Physical Therapy Patient/Client Management

It is important to be in contact with the patient's HTC in order to obtain an in-depth history of recent bleeding episodes, target joints, and factor infusion schedule. The physical therapist works with the patient, family, and HTC team to maximize ROM, strength, and activity while minimizing bleeding. **During an acute joint or muscle bleed, it is important to allow the bleeding to stop and resorb while resting the affected area.**[16,17] An important guide is to allow active ROM only within the pain-free range as this process takes place. After this acute stage (ranging from a few days to months, depending on the joint integrity and individual's ability to clot), the overall goal is to maximize ROM, strength, and balance to progress activity.

For a patient on prophylaxis intervention, it is imperative to schedule physical therapy sessions on the days of factor replacement treatment to minimize the risk of a bleeding episode and maximize participation in therapy. A patient may require external bracing such as an ankle brace or high top sneakers to increase joint protection to assist with long-term joint preservation. A valuable role of the physical therapist is to educate the patient and family on appropriate exercise, maintenance of a healthy lifestyle, and joint protection. "Playing It Safe; Bleeding Disorders, Sports, and Exercise" is an excellent resource provided by the National Hemophilia Foundation for guidance and recommendations for general activity.[18]

Examination, Evaluation, and Diagnosis

Prior to evaluating the patient, the physical therapist needs to obtain information relevant to the patient's bleeding history, comorbidities, and factor treatment plan. Other important information is the current medication list and imaging results of the affected joint. It may be helpful to contact the physical therapist from the HTC for a more in-depth history. Obtaining a history of the patient's functional status prior to the joint bleed will help guide activities and goal setting.

Depending on the bleeding history, the person may have asymmetrical joints due to contractures, muscle tightness, synovial hypertrophy, chronic swelling, or decreased ROM. Gait dysfunction may also be apparent. It is important to assess ROM and strength around the joints in the involved and uninvolved extremity, balance, proprioception, gait, pain, functional mobility, and body mass index (BMI). Specific objective measures include active or active assisted ROM assessed within a pain-free range. For this 10-year-old boy, ankle ROM, including dorsiflexion, plantar flexion, inversion, eversion, and subtalar motion, should be measured via standard goniometry on the affected (left) side and unaffected side. Length of the gastrocnemius and soleus muscles should be measured with an extended knee and then again with a flexed knee to determine if there is tightness present from either the gastrocnemius crossing the ankle and knee joint, or the soleus crossing only the ankle joint.[19] Manual muscle testing using the 0 to 5 point scale can be used to compare strength in the affected limb to the contralateral limb. Strength throughout the affected limb should be assessed, especially if there have been prior joint or muscle bleeding events. For the child with an acute bleed, the therapist should only assess pain-free active ROM. After the bleed has resolved (as indicated by decreased pain, decreased swelling, decreased tightness, increased ROM, and increased ability to use the affected limb), full resistance may be applied.

Since walking is a functional daily task for children, the 6-minute walk test (6MWT) can be used as an appropriate outcome measure to assess everyday mobility.[20] The 6MWT is a submaximal functional aerobic capacity test commonly utilized for children with chronic conditions affecting the musculoskeletal system. For this test, the child walks as far as possible in 6 minutes. This test may be especially helpful since the child just returned to ambulating without crutches. It may be possible to determine how close he is to his baseline aerobic capacity, if his performance can be compared to a 6MWT performed by the physical therapist at the HTC.

The **Functional Independence Score in Hemophilia** (FISH) is a performance-based assessment tool that objectively measures an individual's functional mobility.[21] The FISH assesses eight activities: eating, grooming, dressing, chair transfer, squatting, walking, step climbing, and running. Each activity is graded based on the amount of assistance needed to complete the activity. A score of 1 indicates that the person is unable to complete the task or requires maximal assistance to complete the task. A score of 4 indicates independence and normal performance of the task. The highest score is 32. The FISH has excellent reliability (0.98) and good criterion validity as it correlates well with two frequently used assessments of functional ability, the Stanford Health Assessment Questionnaire and the Western Ontario and McMaster Universities Osteoarthritis Index (WOMAC).[21] There is a ceiling effect for those who have a high functional status. Although there is not yet a reported meaningful clinically important difference (MCID), the FISH has been shown to be responsive to changes in treatment after correction of joint deformities with a standardized response mean (SRM) of −1.93.

Plan of Care and Interventions

Understanding the timeline of recent events and bleeding history is essential in creating an appropriate plan of care. It is important for the therapist to note the date of the bleed and the present symptoms. Prior to outpatient physical therapy intervention, it is imperative that the joint or muscle bleeding has stopped (which may take days to weeks) and that the patient is properly medicated with factor replacement. Once the hematologist has referred a patient to outpatient physical therapy, the patient is past the acute bleeding phase and can progress with exercise. However, it is important to note whether the patient is on a factor replacement dosing regimen for physical therapy sessions. For example, some patients may take a prescribed prophylactic dose on physical therapy days, whereas others may only take factor during those physical therapy sessions that focus on gaining significant ROM. For further clarification of a patient's baseline status, contacting the HTC physical therapist is reasonable.

The primary interventions address the noted impairments in strength and ROM. Once the joint bleed has stopped, progressive resistance exercises should target the muscles that have been weakened and inhibited due to inflammation, pain, and disuse. Gentle stretching and pain-free ROM activities should be included to maximize functional ROM.

General activity and education involving weight management is an important aspect of joint protection. **In young males with hemophilia, BMI is a modifiable risk factor strongly related to ROM limitation.**[4,22] For all individuals, it is important for long-term joint health to maintain a healthy weight and activity level.[23]

Boys with severe hemophilia have lower dynamic strength and anaerobic power (as assessed by the Wingate anaerobic test) and are less active compared to boys without hemophilia.[24] It is important to address these deficits with strengthening and low-impact aerobic activities such as using an elliptical trainer, upper extremity ergometer, or swimming.

Children with hemophilia are also likely to have decreased bone mineral density (BMD) due to factors including decreased activity and increased bleeding/joint damage.[25] While decreased BMD contributes to osteoporosis, childhood use of prophylactic factor replacement may preserve BMD in those with severe hemophilia.[26] Therapists can address low BMD by stressing bone and including weight-bearing activities, as tolerated, to increase cellular bone growth. Incorporation of high impact activity (plyometrics, ballistic training) is typically avoided, especially for therapists newly practicing with this patient population.

Functional activities that focus on muscular co-contractions and joint stability are key to maintaining strength, balance, and protection of the joint. Balance activities such as those performed on an unstable foam pad (Airex pad), Bosu ball, or balance board, or exercises including single leg stance, squats, and proprioceptive neuromuscular facilitation (PNF) are appropriate. High stress activities such as jumping and kicking could be incorporated into the final phase of rehabilitation, if appropriate for the particular patient to return to desired activities.

The therapist must carefully consider the use of modalities in the individual with hemophilia. Ice should not be utilized because studies have demonstrated that cooling can reduce platelet and vessel wall function, prolong bleeding time, decrease platelet adhesion and aggregation, impair procoagulant enzyme activity, increase clotting times and clot formation times, and impair clot firmness.[27] The use of continuous ultrasound for therapeutic deep heat is also contraindicated because the increased blood flow would increase the tendency to bleed. Even on a pulsed setting, some heat is produced.[28] The Medical and Scientific Advisory Council (MASAC) does not recommend use of ultrasound in the hemophilia population for the resorption of blood.[29]

Hemophilia is a bleeding disorder characterized by a genetic deficiency in a factor protein necessary to clot blood. The most common site of bleeding is into a joint, causing deterioration, pain, and decreased function. However, injuries resulting in excessive bleeding may occur in any vascular area of the body with potentially life-threatening consequences. However, proper therapeutic intervention, physical therapy, and patient education can help those with hemophilia have a good quality of life and maintain active, healthy lifestyles.

Evidence-Based Clinical Recommendations

SORT: Strength of Recommendation Taxonomy
A: Consistent, good-quality patient-oriented evidence
B: Inconsistent or limited-quality patient-oriented evidence
C: Consensus, disease-oriented evidence, usual practice, expert opinion, or case series

1. During an acute joint or muscle bleed in a person with hemophilia, ROM should be avoided and rest should be promoted. **Grade B**

2. The Functional Independence Score in Hemophilia (FISH) is a reliable and valid performance-based assessment tool that objectively measures the functional mobility of an individual with hemophilia. **Grade B**

3. In persons with hemophilia, maintenance of a healthy weight has positive effects on joint health. **Grade B**

COMPREHENSION QUESTIONS

22.1 Hemophilia is:
   A. An inherited bleeding disorder
   B. Expressed in women more than men
   C. Associated with faster bleeding
   D. Is a bleeding disorder characterized by lack of clotting protein Factor VI or VII

22.2 The characteristics of a target joint are:
   A. Swelling and erythema
   B. Tachycardia and tightness
   C. Hypertrophy and contracture
   D. Tingling and weakness

22.3 Which of the following is true regarding management of an acute joint bleed in a person with hemophilia?
   A. Rest, ice, compression, elevation (RICE)
   B. Infuse with factor concentrate, rest, elevation, compression
   C. Early and aggressive ROM
   D. No intervention needed

ANSWERS

22.1 **A.** Hemophilia is a bleeding disorder characterized by a deficiency in the protein Factor VIII or Factor IX. It is an X-linked recessive trait mutation affecting about 20,000 men in the United States (option B). Men with hemophilia will pass the hemophilia gene, but it will not be expressed; however, any daughter of a man with hemophilia carries the gene and is known as an obligate carrier. The obligate carrier has a 1 in 4 chance of having a child with hemophilia, and a 1 in 4 chance of having a daughter who carries the gene. People with hemophilia do not bleed faster (option C), but rather longer than those without a blood clotting disorder.

22.2 **C.** A target joint has had multiple bleeds within a short period of time. The process of bleeding into a joint breaks down the components of the joint including the synovium and cartilage. Over time, the synovium overgrows to compensate, resulting in hypertrophy. When an acute bleed occurs, rest in a pain-free position is important. Over time, if ROM is not restored, a contracture can result. The clinical presentation of an *acute* joint bleed include: swelling and erythema (option A), tingling (option D), limited ROM, and tightness as well as tachycardia (option B) and hypotension.

22.3 **B.** It is imperative to infuse with factor at the first sign of a bleed. The days following a bleed require off-loading, rest, elevation, and splinting for compression and protection to assist with healing. Ice is not recommended as a primary means to assist blood coagulation (option A). During the acute phases of a joint bleed, ROM should be limited to pain-free range only (option C). It is important to treat every joint bleed (option D).

REFERENCES

1. Gomperts E, Lundblad R, Adamson R. The manufacturing process of recombinant factor VIII, recombinate. *Transfus Med Rev.* 1992;6:247-251.

2. Guidelines for the Management of Hemophilia. 2nd ed. World Federation of Hemophilia Web site. http://www1.wfh.org/publications/files/pdf-1472.pdf. Accessed December 15, 2014.

3. National Hemophilia Foundation. www.hemophilia.org. Accessed December 20, 2014.

4. Hemophilia. Centers for Disease Control and Prevention Web site. http://www.cdc.gov/ncbddd/hemophilia. Accessed December 20, 2014.

5. Tagliaferri A, Di Perna C, Rivolta GF. Secondary prophylaxis in adolescent and adult haemophiliacs. *Blood Transfus.* 2008;6:s17-s20.

6. van Dijk K, van der Bom JG, Lenting PJ, et al. Factor VIII half-life and clinical phenotype of severe hemophilia A. *Hematologica.* 2005;90:494-498.

7. Peters RT, Low SC, Kamphaus GD, et al. Prolonged activity of factor IX as a monomeric Fc fusion protein. *Blood.* 2010;115:2057-2064.

8. Raffini L, Manno C. Modern management of haemophilic arthropathy. *Brit J Haematol.* 2007;136:777-787.

9. Gilbert MS. Musculoskeletal complications of haemophilia: the joint. *Haemophilia.* 2000;6 (Suppl 1):34-37.

10. Mulder K, Llinás A. The target joint. *Hemophilia*. 2004;10(Suppl l4):152-156.

11. Mulivany R, Zucker-Levin AR, Jeng M, et al. Effects of a 6-week, individualized, supervised exercise program for people with bleeding disorders and hemophilic arthritis. *Phys Ther*. 2010;90:509-526.

12. Simpson ML, Valentino LA. Management of joint bleeding in hemophilia. *Exp Rev Hematol*. 2012;5:459-468.

13. Mielke CH. Comparative effects of aspirin and acetaminophen on hemostasis. *Arch Intern Med*. 1981:141:305-310.

14. Thomas P, Hepburn B, Kim HC, Saidi P. Nonsteroidal anti-inflammatory drugs in the treatment of hemophilic arthropathy. *Am J Hematol*. 1982;12:131-137.

15. Larson AM, Polson J, Fontana RJ, et al. Acetaminophen-induced acute liver failure: results of a United States multicenter, prospective study. *Hepatology*. 2005;42:1364-1372.

16. MASAC recommendations regarding physical therapy guidelines in patients with bleeding disorders. Physical therapy practice guidelines for persons with bleeding disorders: Joint Bleeds. MASAC document 204. www.hemophilia.org. Accessed December 30, 2014.

17. Joint Damage. Canadian Hemophilia Society. http://www://hemophilia.ca. Accessed December 30, 2014.

18. Playing It Safe; Bleeding Disorders, Sports and Exercise. National Hemophilia Foundation Web site. http://www.hemophilia.org/sites/default/files/document/files/PlayingItSafe.pdf. Accessed December 30, 2014.

19. Palmer M, Epler M. *Fundamentals of Musculoskeletal Assessment Techniques*. 2nd ed. Philadelphia, PA: Lippincott Williams & Wilkins; 2008.

20. Hassan J, van der Net J, Helders PJ, Prakken BJ, Takken T. Six-minute walk test in children with chronic conditions. *Br J Sports Med*. 2010;44:270-274.

21. Functional Independence Score in Hemophilia (FISH). World Federation of Hemophilia. http://www.wfh.org/en/page.aspx?pid=884. Accessed December 30, 2014.

22. Soucie JM, Cianfrini C, Janco RL, et al. Joint range-of-motion limitations among young males with hemophilia: prevalence and risk factors. *Blood*. 2004;103:2467-2473.

23. Body Mass Index Table 1. National Institute of Health. National Heart, Lung, and Blood. http://www.nhlbi.nih.gov/health/educational/lose_wt/BMI/bmi_tbl.htm. Accessed December 30, 2014.

24. Falk B, Portal S, Tiktinsky R, Weinstein Y, Constantini N, Martinowitz U. Anaerobic power and muscle strength in young hemophilia patients. *Med Sci Sports Exerc*. 2000;32:52-57.

25. Eid MA, Ibrahim MM, Aly SM. Effect of resistance and aerobic exercise on bone mineral density, muscle strength and functional ability in children with hemophilia. *Egypt J HumanMed*. 2014;15:139-147.

26. Khawaji M, Akesson A, Berntorp E. Long-term prophylaxis in severe haemophilia seems to preserve bone mineral density. *Hemophilia*. 2009;15:261-266.

27. Forsyth AL, Zourikian N, Valentino LA, Rivard GE. The effect of cooling on coagulation and haemostasis: should "ice" be part of treatment of acute haemarthrosis in haemophilia? *Haemophilia*. 2012;18:843-850.

28. Baker KG, Robertson VJ, Duck FA. A review of therapeutic ultrasound: biophysical effects. *Phys Ther*. 2001;81:1351-1358.

29. MASAC Recommendation Regarding the Use of Therapeutic Ultrasound to Aid in Blood Resorption ID 130. National Hemophilia Foundation. https://www.hemophilia.org/Researchers-Healthcare-Providers/Medical-and-Scientific-Advisory-Council-MASAC/MASAC-Recommendations/MASAC-Recommendation-Regarding-the-Use-of-Therapeutic-Ultrasound-to-Aid-in-Blood-Resorption. Accessed December 30, 2014.

Complex Regional Pain Syndrome

Katherine Fash

CASE 23

A previously healthy 16-year-old female developed right lower extremity and back pain two days after sustaining a right ankle sprain during soccer practice. The pain extended from her right lumbosacral region and right hip distally to her toes. The teenager initially reported to her primary care physician (PCP) with decreased skin temperature upon palpation and cyanosis in her right foot, right knee swelling, and allodynia in all painful areas. Her pain ranged from 4/10 to 10/10 on a visual analog scale (VAS). She could not report activities or events that aggravated or alleviated her pain. Following one week of unsuccessful home management including icing and heating the lumbosacral area, right hip, knee, and ankle as well as using over-the-counter pain relievers, she returned to her PCP. The PCP ordered blood tests to rule out infectious or active rheumatologic disease (*e.g.*, rheumatoid arthritis), which were all negative. Her PCP referred her to an orthopaedic surgeon. Radiographs and magnetic resonance imaging (MRI) studies were ordered for the lower spine, hip, knee, and ankle regions, and the results were unremarkable. The orthopaedic surgeon diagnosed the teenager with an ankle sprain and referred her to a rheumatologist. Based on the findings noted above, the rheumatologist diagnosed her with complex regional pain syndrome (CRPS) and referred the teenager to outpatient physical therapy. Since the onset of her symptoms one month ago, the teenager has missed 14 days of school due to pain and medical appointments. She has not participated in travel soccer or intramural basketball. She stands on her left foot only for showering and sits to dress herself. She does not allow the shower water to hit her right leg due to the pain it causes. The patient presented to her initial physical therapy evaluation ambulating with bilateral axillary crutches and nonweightbearing through her right leg.

▶ Based on the diagnosis of CRPS, what do you anticipate may be the contributing factors to her condition?
▶ What are the possible complications that may limit the effectiveness of physical therapy?
▶ What precautions should be taken during physical therapy examination and/or interventions?
▶ How might the patient's emotional condition affect rehabilitation?
▶ Identify referrals to other medical team members.

KEY DEFINITIONS

ALLODYNIA: Pain provoked by stimuli not usually considered painful

BRUININKS-OSERETSKY TEST OF MOTOR PERFORMANCE, SECOND EDITION (BOT-2): Standardized test that measures gross and fine motor function, as well as balance and coordination. Consists of eight subtests: (1) Fine Motor Control, (2) Fine Motor Integration, (3) Manual Dexterity, (4) Bilateral Coordination, (5) Balance, (6) Running Speed and Agility, (7) Upper-Limb Coordination, and (8) Strength. For each subtest, higher scores represent better performance. Scores from subtests are totaled together to measure the individual's total composite score, which can be compared to age- and sex-matched norms.

FUNCTIONAL DISABILITY INVENTORY (FDI): Self-report measure that asks individuals to rate how much physical "trouble" they experience when attempting to complete various functional activities due to pain. Activities are rated as: "No Trouble," "A Little Trouble," "Some Trouble," "A Lot of Trouble," or "Impossible." Ratings are given a number equivalent and added together for a final score that ranges from 0 to 60, with higher scores indicating higher levels of functional disability due to pain.

HYPERALGESIA: Increased sensitivity and excessive pain to noxious stimuli

SUDOMOTOR: Referring to autonomic nerves that stimulate activity of sweat glands

Objectives

1. Identify the signs and symptoms of CRPS.
2. Identify valid and reliable outcome tools to determine functional outcomes for this population.
3. Identify treatment interventions for a patient with CRPS.
4. Identify barriers to progress and determination of prognosis.
5. Determine the appropriate dose of physical therapy given the patient's impairments and functional limitations.

Physical Therapy Considerations

PT considerations for management of the individual with a new diagnosis of CRPS:

► **General physical therapy plan of care/goals:** Educate and empower the patient and family in all aspects of treatment; improve passive and active range of motion (ROM), strength, balance, agility, endurance, and functional strength; normalize gait; maximize physical function; improve tolerance to light and deep touch; improve quality of life; provide sports re-entry training, as indicated

► **Physical therapy interventions:** Patient and caregiver education regarding diagnosis and treatment; discussion of plan of care including appropriate level of intervention; education regarding prognosis, specifically that improvement depends on severity and duration of the individual's limitations, contributing factors, and compliance with interventions; reduce and/or eliminate physical accommodations being used due to pain; functional mobility, muscle strengthening, active and passive ROM, aerobic and anaerobic activities, agility and balance training, desensitization, sports re-entry

▶ **Precautions during physical therapy:** Supervision is required to ensure proper body mechanics during activities without use of the accommodations the individual has adopted due to pain. Selection and progression of interventions should be based on minimizing risk for overuse and orthopaedic injuries, especially in individuals with history of prolonged immobilization, sedentary lifestyle, altered body mechanics, dual diagnosis such as cardiac disease and fragile bones.

▶ **Complications interfering with physical therapy:** Decreased attendance to physical therapy sessions; decreased compliance with home exercise program (HEP) and recommendations to return to activity and participation level; lack of collaborative goals between patient and caregiver; psychological contributors to pain; orthopaedic or overuse injury

Understanding the Health Condition

CRPS is diagnosed based on clinical signs and symptoms of pain with neuropathic descriptors. According to criteria established by the International Association for the Study of Pain, CRPS is characterized by the presence of an initiating noxious event or cause for immobilization, continued pain, allodynia, or hyperalgesia with pain disproportionate to any inciting event, evidence at some time of edema, changes in skin blood flow, or abnormal sudomotor activity in the region of pain and the exclusion of medical conditions that would otherwise account for the degree of pain and dysfunction.[1] Depending on the symptoms and the physician making the diagnosis, other terms that have been used include: reflex sympathetic dystrophy (RSD), reflex neurovascular dystrophy (RND), amplified musculoskeletal pain syndrome (AMPS), chronic pain, or causalgia. The term CRPS is more widely used than RSD since only a subset of patients with presumed RSD respond therapeutically to sympathetic blockade.[1] CRPS has also been categorized as type I (no nerve involvement) or type II (nerve involvement). Diagnostic testing is frequently unremarkable and orthopaedic causes for pain have been ruled out. In chronic cases, osteopenia due to disuse and/or lack of weightbearing on the affected limb can be detected via a bone scan. Laboratory tests are not considered essential to arriving at the diagnosis of CRPS, but often confirm the clinical diagnosis when the test results are normal.

CRPS is a health condition affecting children and adults. The prevalence of CRPS is not well documented and the ranges tend to be large, which may reflect underdiagnosis of CRPS in certain populations. Overall, prevalence is higher in females (3:1).[1] In the United States, CRPS is diagnosed in 2% to 5% of the population following limb fractures[2] and 50,000 new cases are reported every year.[3] Annual incidence is 5.46 to 26.2 persons per 100,000 with 22% demonstrating long-term symptoms.[4]

Many consider the precise pathophysiology of CRPS unknown.[1,5] The **patho-physiological mechanisms** are likely multifactorial, involving both the peripheral and central nervous systems.[1,5] CRPS is thought to have both a sympathetically mediated peripheral component and a central nervous system (CNS) component. Individuals with CRPS present with impairment of sympathetic nervous system (SNS) function in target tissues manifested as decreased sympathetic outflow and increased adrenergic responsiveness in the areas of pain. This alteration in sympathetic function can be generalized (*i.e.*, not only affecting the painful region/s), which suggests impaired processing in the CNS.[1] Noted dysfunctions in patients with CRPS include altered cutaneous innervation after injury, central sensitization, peripheral sensitization, inflammation, altered sympathetic function, altered somatosensory representation of the affected area in the brain, genetic abnormalities, and psychophysiological interactions.[6] The degree to which each of these contribute to a specific individual's deficits varies.[6]

Specific risk factors for the development of CRPS have not been clearly defined. General triggers for the onset include injuries, illnesses, or stress. There is also no specific connection with the *severity* of the clinical presentation and that of the initial injury.[1] Onset is often linked to a history of immobilization, trauma, history of a medical or surgical procedure, or stress coupled with inadequate coping mechanisms. Frequently, patients diagnosed with CRPS also demonstrate psychological distress. The severity of CRPS is influenced by anxiety, depression, fear, decreased coping mechanisms, and anger.[5,7] The psychological distress can worsen as a result of increased immobilization and disuse that often occurs in patients with CRPS.

The most common history includes patient report of pain in a body area following minor trauma, illness, or even without incident. It is not uncommon for the patient to report "I just woke up one day with it" or "I am not sure when it started, but it got worse over time." Common symptoms include motor disturbances, burning deep somatic pain, hyperalgesia, allodynia, dysesthesia, and paresthesia. Autonomic nervous system (ANS) signs include cyanosis, mottling of the skin, hyperhidrosis (excessive sweating), edema, and change in temperature (often coldness) of the involved extremity. The pain and swelling are often disproportionate to the mechanism of injury.[8] CRPS should be suspected if there are regional pain and sensory changes that *exceed* the trauma or duration of typical healing time. A diagnosis of CRPS should also be considered if there is no known injury or illness coincident with the onset of symptoms, or if healing time is prolonged with high reported pain level after resolution of a precipitating illness.

Vasomotor and ANS changes common in children with CRPS include edema extending beyond the vicinity of joints that displays an inconsistent pattern and gives the skin a glossy and smooth appearance. Other vasomotor changes include cyanosis and/or a change in temperature or color compared to unaffected areas of the patient's body. For example, the affected extremity may appear blue, purple, red, or mottled and demonstrate increased sweating or abnormal hair growth.[1] Allodynia is common, and presents with varying borders. The severity of the allodynia greatly affects the individual's ability to accept touch or tolerate environmental factors such as wind and cold on the surface of the skin. Allodynia can affect participation in activities of daily living (ADLs) including dressing, clothing selection, and bathing.

The quality of the pain experienced by persons with CRPS ranges from achy to burning or stabbing. Patients are often unable to identify alleviating factors. Treatments that typically relieve pain caused by orthopaedic procedures (*e.g.*, ice or heat) may increase or have no effect on their pain. There is a considerable amount of variability in the progression and intensity of symptoms among patients. It is not uncommon for pain to "spread" from the original body location to other areas with no set pattern, especially when CRPS is untreated or the affected limb is immobilized.[7]

Historically, CRPS has been challenging to treat. With no definitively effective medical interventions, treatments have included a variety of pharmacologic therapies, immobilization of the affected body part, modalities (*e.g.*, ice, heat, transcutaneous electrical nerve stimulation [TENS]), sympathetic nerve blocks, surgeries including amputation,[9] physical therapy, aquatic therapy, behavioral modifications, and counseling. No single medication has been proven to be effective for all patients.[1] Medications that have been used include topical dimethyl sulfoxide, topical clonidine, oral glucocorticoids, oral analgesics, intravenous phentolamine, intravenous lidocaine, and intranasal calcitonin. Other treatments include sympathetic blockade with local anesthetics intended to reduce pain and improve peripheral blood flow and tissue perfusion. Sympathetic blocks have had variable degrees of success.[1,10,11] Since some patients experience pain relief without alteration of SNS function, the SNS may not be involved in the pathogenesis of CRPS in all individuals.

A multidisciplinary approach—including an individualized physical therapy treatment plan—has been considered the most effective treatment for CRPS.[4,8,12-15] The physical therapy plan of care should consist of interventions for desensitization, mobilization, edema control, muscle strengthening, progressive weightbearing, ROM, postural retraining, aerobic and anaerobic conditioning, and functional rehabilitation.[8,16,17] If individuals are fearful about their pain, they often adopt protective avoidance behaviors such as immobilization and decreased weightbearing through the painful limb, which will affect their functional mobility. Immobilization of the painful limb should be discontinued as soon as clinically appropriate and patient acceptance allows. Immobilization can take many forms including the use of wheelchairs, crutches, orthoses, and slings. More often, immobilization takes the form of decreased participation and activity levels (*e.g.*, not using stairs as frequently, limiting participation in sports activities, or not dressing in weightbearing positions). **Immobilization** can cause an exacerbation of symptoms including increased pain and loss of function. Typically, the longer the immobilization time, the longer the time required for recovery.[4,7,18,19]

Psychological assessment is recommended to identify the presence of any underlying or contributing factors to the pain so that they can be addressed. The duration of an individual's pain predicts the need for psychological intervention. Raja et al.[1] suggested that if pain associated with CRPS lasts more than two months, the individual should be evaluated by a psychologist. **Psychological interventions** are needed to address pain-related fear in children with CRPS because fear is a strong predictor of pain-related disability.[5] Treatment with the focus on improving coping mechanisms and motivation are necessary to increase participation in other treatments including physical therapy and HEPs.[4]

If not properly treated in a timely manner, CRPS causes disuse atrophy, deficits in muscle strength and ROM, increased edema, bone demineralization, and the possibility of contractures.[1,12] When diagnosis and treatment are provided in the early stages of CRPS, individuals are more likely to respond to intervention.[20] Other predictors of improved outcomes include younger age at time of injury and fewer school days missed during the first year following the precipitating injury.[18] Those younger than 11 years at the onset of symptoms of CRPS were more likely to return to sports.[18]

Children with CRPS may also be at elevated risk for multiple pain-related symptoms, emotional distress, and attention deficits.[21] When symptoms become chronic, prognosis for recovery and improvement is limited. Persistent or recurrent chronic pain in children can impact and disrupt the family unit due to persistent and recurrent distress, disability, and increased adult attention on the child in pain.[22] Parental distress, attention to the child's pain, and overprotectiveness have been associated with increased functional disability in children with chronic pain.[22] Young people with chronic pain often report sleep disturbances, disordered mood, appetite disruption, and depressed feelings.[12,23] Children with chronic pain are frequently absent from school due to difficulty concentrating, inability to sit for prolonged periods of time, and interpersonal challenges with other students due to their misunderstanding of the child's condition.[12]

Physical Therapy Patient/Client Management

Individuals with CRPS can be successfully managed in both inpatient and outpatient settings. An individualized approach including the dose of physical therapy must take into account the severity and chronicity of the child's symptoms. Management is multidisciplinary. In an inpatient setting, the medical team may include physicians, physical and occupational therapists, nurses, psychologists, social worker, and music or art therapists. In the outpatient setting, management is still multidisciplinary, though the healthcare providers may be limited to a physician, therapists, and a psychologist. The child and her family are an integral part of the team as their cohesiveness and compliance with the plan of care affects prognosis. The primary goal is for the child to regain function and resume her normal activity level through the development of an individualized treatment plan. The focus of treatment sessions should not be surrounding the discussion of pain.[4] Distraction techniques to avoid attention on pain assists in the patient's ability to functionally progress. It is useful to integrate the psychologist's recommendations into physical therapy sessions to address contributing environmental factors that may be limiting function and contributing to the child's pain. These may include addressing internal factors such as coping mechanisms and anxiety or external factors such as contributing social situations. Occupational therapy sessions address ADLs and fine motor deficits such as handwriting, typing, and self-grooming tasks. Physical therapy intervention focuses on gross motor needs and functional mobility, postural retraining, aerobic training, regaining ROM and functional strength, and eliminating compensations in the child's participation level. To address allodynia, desensitization with a variety of textures and stimuli should be incorporated throughout the day. This can be accomplished through tasks such as wearing fitted instead of loose clothing, wearing socks and shoes, and through interventions such as towel rubbing over the affected area or contrast baths of the involved extremity.[16,17,24] Physical therapy interventions are tailored to provide challenging activities to the specific patient. These activities could include progressive weightbearing through the painful extremity, handwriting, washing the painful limb, or maintaining a static position. The child should be able to complete each activity without accommodations provided for pain relief. Each person with CRPS will have a different baseline. The key to physical therapy intervention is getting the child to understand that pain when moving without accommodations is normal, and not an indicator to modify the activity if progression in physical therapy is occurring as noted by improvement in functional mobility. While pain intensity is assessed, pain does not improve significantly until after overall function improves. A child will typically be able to walk faster, accept more weight through the painful limb, and/or complete ADLs in the age-appropriate manner, prior to reporting a lower pain level. The ultimate goal is progressing from a baseline level of painful function to pain-free movement.

Examination, Evaluation, and Diagnosis

Prior to the examination, the physical therapist needs to review the patient's history of present illness and other medical history including any comorbidities or concurrent diagnoses. Identifying precautions is imperative to developing an appropriate plan of care. History includes previously trialed treatment interventions, challenging and difficult activities due to the pain, sleeping and eating difficulties, and any changes in participation level including at school, home, and social venues. It is important that the physical therapist builds a rapport and empowers the patient in her own treatment.

Examination of the teenager with a new CRPS diagnosis is not unique in many aspects. Physical assessment still includes ROM, manual muscle testing (MMT), functional strength, motor coordination, functional mobility, gait analysis, static and dynamic balance, agility and fluidity of movement. For the 16-year-old in this case, special attention must be paid to ROM, strength, and functional deficits in the right lower extremity. ROM would be measured both actively and passively in her hip, knee, and ankle. Strength is best assessed through observations of functional movement and MMT. Balance testing is particularly important for the patient that arrives to the clinic utilizing crutches for ambulation. Standing balance could be measured in pounds of pressure that she places on her affected limb and length of time she can hold the affected limb in a standing position. If the child with CRPS is able to demonstrate single leg stance equally bilaterally, the physical therapist can assess functional strength in higher-level activities such bilateral and single leg hopping, lunges, and single leg squat.

The physical therapy examination typically includes gross motor assessment via standardized tests such as the Bruininks-Oseretsky Test of Motor Performance Second Edition (BOT-2), baseline endurance assessment, and physical functioning outcomes using the FDI. To assess baseline endurance, any test utilizing the lower extremity (*e.g.*, treadmill, bicycle ergometer) would be prematurely terminated due to pain and thus would not be an accurate measure of aerobic fitness. For the individual with CRPS affecting the lower extremity, a more appropriate option would be an upper extremity ergometer. Once the child is able to bear full weight on the affected lower extremity and the protocol used is not terminated due to the pain of CRPS, a treadmill test could be used.

In this population, pain is often measured using the VAS. Pain assessment via the VAS should include pain at baseline, as well as the levels of greatest and least pain. Quantity and quality of pain should be documented as well as any identified aggravating and alleviating factors. It is not uncommon for a patient to state that "nothing" alleviates her pain. Movement, touch, and/or stress are often reported as aggravating factors. Qualitative descriptors can include achy, burning, stabbing, to highly descriptive statements such as "it feels like a hammer is constantly hitting my ankle" or "like someone is constantly standing on my foot." It is not uncommon for a patient to report 10 out of 10 pain, but express little emotion or concern that might be expected for someone with this stated level of pain. In addition, pain severity is often unrelated to the individual's level of functioning. For example, a patient who is able to walk without an assistive device may report 10 out of 10 pain in her affected limb. When the physical examination begins and as it progresses, the therapist asks the patient to verbalize when her pain increases. Throughout the examination, the therapist notes verbal pain ratings and qualitative reports as well as physical deviations or accommodations to normal movement. For example, when assessing gait, any deviations caused by pain including decreased stance time or step length should be assessed and noted. Other accommodations related to pain should be carefully observed and noted, including use of the upper extremities to complete a floor-to-stand transfer or any facial grimacing in response to MMT.

ROM, flexibility, and muscle strength should be assessed in all major joints, including the painful areas. During these measurements, the therapist does not solicit reports of pain, but rather focuses the patient on functional completion of each assessment. ROM deficits in areas that are not painful also need to be addressed due to faulty mechanics that can lead to overuse injuries during total body and closed chain treatment interventions.

The physical therapy assessment should identify limitations in activity and body functions due to pain and helps to formulate therapeutic goals. It also allows the physical therapist to identify the need for referral to other disciplines that should be involved in the patient's care.

Plan of Care and Interventions

The results of the physical therapy examination and evaluation guide the choice of interventions for children and adolescents with CRPS. Not every person requires direct physical therapy interventions to resolve symptoms. Some individuals follow physical therapy recommendations and return to normal activity without direct interventions, while others require further services to achieve progress and recovery. Preference is to have patients return to normal activities with the least amount of disruption to their daily life. For patients that are compliant with home recommendations such as completing a daily exercise regimen and eliminating any physical accommodations throughout the day due to pain, skilled physical therapy can be successful in an outpatient setting. The therapist should be aware that self-imposed physical accommodations can be varied and extensive. For example, the patient may avoid sleeping in her own bed to avoid walking up stairs, avoid bed covers touching the painful limb, or arrive late or leave early from school. Individuals with CRPS who do not progress with outpatient physical therapy require an inpatient or day hospital program with daily therapy sessions and a multidisciplinary approach. Regardless of setting, the focus of intervention remains on improving overall function and progressing to normal activity level and participation. Included in the physical therapy education and training are activities to improve function and participation each day despite the pain. While reassessments are important to ensure that no overuse or orthopaedic injury has occurred, all members of the treatment team must provide reassurance to the patient that the pain level does *not* reflect damage to the body. If psychological deficits such as decreased coping mechanisms begin to outweigh the patient's ability to participate in physical therapy, it may be important to address these needs prior to further physical therapy intervention.

For this 16-year-old female with right leg and back pain, interventions included progressive standing static and dynamic balance activities. Initially, interventions focused on progressing weightbearing in a functional manner and desensitization of the skin during treatment sessions with specific emphasis on carryover at home.[25] Activities started and progressed with: double limb stance with equal weightbearing to single limb stance, transfers of squatting to the floor and up and down off the floor, muscle strengthening in functional and closed chain positions, gait training, and ADL re-training. The therapist discontinued the teenager's use of the crutches quickly, since any form of immobilization prolongs recovery. Desensitization techniques for the right lower extremity included towel rubbing or brushing along the skin and contrast baths. Education provided to the patient and family emphasized focus on functional improvement, and not specifically on the reduction of pain because returning to normal function as quickly as possible has been shown to result in better management and resolution of symptoms.[16,17,19] The physical therapist prescribed an aerobic exercise program because exercise has been shown to be effective in treating childhood CRPS.[16,17,24] Sherry et al.[24] investigated the efficacy of an intensive exercise program in a study with 103 children with CRPS type I (mean age 13 years). They reported that more than 90% of the children who participated in a daily program that included 4 hours of aerobic exercise, 1 to 2 hours of aquatic therapy, and desensitization were symptom-free after the 6- to 14-day intervention period. Two years later, 88% of those followed were still symptom-free. Accommodations throughout the teenager's day were removed as quickly as possible including activity level at home, school, and social activities. Once she demonstrated normal functional strength and balance, gait pattern with proper push-off and weight acceptance onto the right lower extremity, and normal endurance, physical therapy interventions progressed to sports retraining. After this episode of outpatient physical therapy (2 times per week for 8 weeks), the patient reported no pain in her right leg or back. She was cleared to return to sports as determined in part by functional hop tests and achieving age-appropriate norms on the BOT-2.

Evidence-Based Clinical Recommendations

SORT: Strength of Recommendation Taxonomy

A: Consistent, good-quality patient-oriented evidence
B: Inconsistent or limited-quality patient-oriented evidence
C: Consensus, disease-oriented evidence, usual practice, expert opinion, or case series

1. The pathophysiological mechanisms of chronic regional pain syndrome (CRPS) are likely multifactorial, involving both the peripheral and central nervous systems. **Grade A**

2. In the individual with CRPS, immobilization of the affected limb prolongs recovery time. **Grade A**

3. Psychological interventions are needed to address pain-related fear in children with CRPS because fear is a strong predictor of pain-related disability. **Grade B**

COMPREHENSION QUESTIONS

23.1 Clinical presentation of an individual with CRPS would include all of the following *except*:
  A. Allodynia
  B. Motor disturbances
  C. Burning deep somatic pain
  D. Bruising

23.2 Individuals with CRPS typically have altered participation in all of the following *except*:
  A. School
  B. Leisure
  C. ADLs
  D. Eating

23.3 Which of the following is *not* a recommended treatment for a patient with CRPS?
  A. ROM
  B. Weightbearing
  C. Immobilization
  D. Desensitization

ANSWERS

23.1 **D.** Bruising is not included in the criteria for CRPS as defined by the International Association for the Study of Pain.

23.2 **D.** A person with CRPS can be limited in participation level for any normal daily activities including school, leisure, sports, or ADLs because of altered activity due to the pain.

23.3 **C.** Evidence indicates that immobilization of the affected limb in CRPS can actually cause an exacerbation of symptoms including increased pain and resulting loss of function.

REFERENCES

1. Raja SN, Grabow TS. Complex regional pain syndrome I (reflex sympathetic dystrophy). *Anesthesiology.* 2002;96:1254-1260.

2. Schlereth T, Birklein F. Mast cells: source of inflammation in complex regional pain syndrome? *Anesthesiology.* 2012;116:756-758.

3. Bruehl S, Chung OY. How common is complex regional pain syndrome-Type I? *Pain.* 2007;129:1-2.

4. Ek JW, van Gijn JC, Samwel H, van Egmond J, Klomp FP, van Dongen RTM. Pain exposure physical therapy may be a safe and effective treatment for longstanding complex regional pain syndrome type 1: a case series. *Clin Rehabil.* 2009;23:1059-1066.

5. de Jong JR, Vlaeyen JW, de Gelder JM, Patijn J. Pain-related fear, perceived harmfulness of activities, and functional limitations in complex regional pain syndrome type 1. *J Pain.* 2011;12:1-10.

6. Bruehl S. An update on the pathophysiology of complex regional pain syndrome. *Anesthesiology.* 2010;113:713-725.

7. Atkins RM. Complex regional pain syndrome. *J Bone Joint Surg Br.* 2003;85:1100-1106.

8. Ayling Campos A, Amaria K, Campbell F, McGrath PA. Clinical impact and evidence base for physiotherapy in treating childhood chronic pain. *Physiother Can.* 2009;63:21-33.

9. Bodde MI, Dijkstra PU, den Dunnen WF, Geertzen JH. Therapy-resistant complex regional pain syndrome Type 1: to amputate or not? *J Bone Joint Surg Am.* 2011;93:1799-1805.

10. van Eijs F, Geurts J, van Kleef M, et al. Predictors of pain relieving response to sympathetic blockade in complex regional pain syndrome type 1. *Anesthesiology.* 2012;116:113-121.

11. Meier PM, Zurakowski D, Berde CB, Sethna NF. Lumbar sympathetic blockade in children with complex regional pain syndromes: a double blind placebo-controlled crossover trial. *Anesthesiology.* 2009;111:372-380.

12. Clinch J, Eccleston C. Chronic musculoskeletal pain in children: assessment and management. *Rheumatology (Oxford).* 2009;48:466-474.

13. Ruggeri SB, Athreya BH, Doughty R, Gregg JR, Das MM. Reflex sympathetic dystrophy in children. *Clin Orthop Relat Res.* 1982;163:225-230.

14. Oerlemans HM, Oostendorp RA, de Boo T, van der Laan L, Severens JL, Goris JA. Adjuvant physical therapy versus occupational therapy in patients with reflex sympathetic dystrophy/complex regional pain syndrome type I. *Arch Phys Med Rehabil.* 2000;81:49-56.

15. Maneksha FR, Mirza H, Poppers PJ. Complex regional pain syndrome (CRPS) with resistance to local anesthetic block: a case report. *J Clin Anesth.* 2000;12:67-71.

16. Sherry DD. An overview of amplified musculoskeletal pain syndromes. *J Rheumatol Suppl.* 2000;58:44-48.

17. Bernstein BH, Singsen BH, Kent JT, et al. Reflex neurovascular dystrophy in childhood. *J Pediatr.* 1978;93:211-215.

18. Wilder RT, Berde CB, Wolohan M, Vieyra MA, Masek BJ, Micheli LJ. Reflex sympathetic dystrophy in children. Clinical characteristics and follow-up of seventy patients. *J Bone Joint Surgery Am.* 1992;74:910-919.

19. Maillard SM, Davies K, Khubchandani R, Woo PM, Murray KJ. Reflex sympathetic dystrophy: a multidisciplinary approach. *Arthritis Rheum.* 2004;51:284-290.

20. Quisel A, Gill JM, Witherell P. Complex regional pain syndrome: which treatments show promise? *J Fam Pract.* 2005;54:599-603.

21. Cruz N, O'Reilly J, Slomine BS, Salorio CF. Emotional and neuropsychological profiles of children with complex regional pain syndrome type-I in an inpatient rehabilitation setting. *Clin J Pain.* 2011;27:27-34.

22. Sieberg CB, Williams S, Simons LE. Do parent protective responses mediate the relation between parent distress and child functional disability among children with chronic pain? *J Pediatr Psychol.* 2011;36:1043-1051.

23. Palermo TM, Fonareva I. Sleep in children and adolescents with chronic pain. *Pediatr Pain Letter.* 2006;8:11-15.

24. Sherry DD, Wallace CA, Kelley C, Kidder M, Sapp L. Short- and long-term outcomes of children with complex regional pain syndrome type I treated with exercise therapy. *Clin J Pain.* 1999;15:218-223.

25. Kashikar-Zuck S, Flowers SR, Claar RL, et al. Clinical utility and validity of the Functional Disability Inventory among a multicenter sample of youth with chronic pain. *Pain.* 2011;152:1600-1607.

Post-Concussion Syndrome

Wendy Webb Schoenewald

CASE 24

Four weeks ago, a 10-year-old male was playing tag on the playground during recess when he slipped on mulch and hit his head on a pole. He was knocked unconscious for less than a minute and was taken to the school nurse. Her recommendations were that he should rest several days and not attend school. He quickly developed significant persistent headaches so his parents took him to the pediatrician. The pediatrician diagnosed a concussion and recommended that he be given a period of brain rest and not attend school until his headaches decreased. He was held from school for approximately three weeks and recently began half-day sessions, although he continued to have persistent headaches and balance difficulties. The pediatrician referred him to a concussion specialist who recommended physical therapy for vestibular rehabilitation for post-concussion syndrome. No brain computed tomography (CT) or magnetic resonance imaging (MRI) scans were performed. During the initial physical therapy examination, the child's chief complaints are of a headache that is constant in nature (6-8/10 on the numerical pain rating scale), difficulty reading for more than 15 minutes, poor concentration, and difficulty with balance during activities of daily living. His mother also reports that her son has demonstrated recent mood changes. He has no history of prior concussions, migraines, or learning disorders. Prior to this injury, the boy was an excellent fifth grade student and an avid reader. He is not active in formal sports, but plays the recorder and cello. His mother is extremely concerned about him falling behind in school because of his difficulty with reading as well as his inability to play the cello.

▶ What are the most appropriate examination tests?
▶ What are the examination priorities?
▶ What do you anticipate may be contributing factors to his condition?
▶ What are the possible comorbidities interfering with physical therapy?
▶ What are the most appropriate physical therapy outcome measures?
▶ Describe the physical therapy plan of care based on clinical findings.

KEY DEFINITIONS

BRAIN REST: Symptom-limited cognitive and physical rest recommended immediately after concussion to promote brain recovery and reduction of symptoms

CONCUSSION: Common features: (1) may be caused by a direct blow to the head, face, neck, or elsewhere with an "impulsive" force transmitted to the head; (2) typically results in rapid onset of short-lived impairment of neurologic function that resolves spontaneously; (3) may result in neuropathology changes, but largely reflects functional disturbance rather than structural injury; (4) symptoms that may or may not involve loss of consciousness. Resolution of symptoms typically follows sequential course; however, in a small percentage of cases, post-concussive symptoms may be prolonged.[1]

GAZE STABILITY: Ability to keep eyes stabilized on visual images while moving around the environment; involves several visual motor processes including the vestibuloocular reflex, smooth pursuit, and saccadic coordination

POST-CONCUSSION SYNDROME (PCS): Persistence of concussion symptoms beyond the typical 7- to 10-day period; criteria for diagnosis include postural instability, attention or memory deficits, and three or more of the following symptoms: fatigue, sleep disturbance, headache, dizziness, personality change, or irritability[2]

SACCADES: Involuntary rapid ballistic eye movements made to turn the eye toward an object in the periphery of the visual field

SMOOTH PURSUIT: Ability to track a moving object in the visual field; visual input from the retina contributes to the pursuit of an object and maintains the image on the fovea

SPURLING'S SIGN: Clinical test performed on patients with suspected cervical spondylosis or acute cervical radiculopathy; with patient seated, the therapist laterally flexes the patient's neck toward the symptomatic side and applies overpressure; a positive test is reproduction of the patient's symptoms

VESTIBULOOCULAR REFLEX (VOR): Three-neuron reflex connecting sensory information (angular head acceleration) from the semicircular canals of the vestibular apparatus to the oculomotor system to control eye movements when the head is moving; the VOR allows for gaze stabilization when the head is moving during functional tasks; disruptions of these neurons can cause oscillopsia (world appears unsteady or jumpy) and dizziness with head movements

Objectives

1. Identify the signs and symptoms associated with post-concussion syndrome (PCS).
2. Identify valid and reliable outcome tools to measure oculomotor, vestibular, balance and coordination, and aerobic exercise tolerance deficits in individuals with PCS.
3. Understand the complexity of multiple systems that need to be addressed in the treatment of children with PCS.

4. Design a physical therapy program for a child with PCS.

5. Provide education for the parents, the child, and the school academic team (*e.g.*, teachers, coaches, administrative staff) in symptom management.

Physical Therapy Considerations

PT considerations for management of the child with a diagnosis of PCS:

▶ **General physical therapy plan of care/goals:** Normalize visual motor and vestibular function; achieve normal dynamic balance; achieve increased cervical strength and cardiovascular conditioning; restore child to full academic level; return to extracurricular activities

▶ **Physical therapy interventions:** Patient education about concussion and postconcussion symptoms and management; exercises for visual motor and vestibular deficits; cardiovascular conditioning; coordination training; cognitive retraining; strengthening of cervical spine

▶ **Precautions during physical therapy:** Avoidance of overstimulation during rehabilitation that may trigger headaches, dizziness, and nausea and may delay recovery

▶ **Complications interfering with physical therapy:** Pre-existing conditions of anxiety and depression, amblyopia or eye alignment issues, learning disabilities, attention deficit hyperactivity disorder (ADHD)

Understanding the Health Condition

A concussion is a type of traumatic brain injury (TBI) caused by a bump, blow, or jolt to the head that causes mechanical forces to be transmitted to the brain, resulting in complex pathophysiological processes that affect brain function. These forces can be directly applied to the head or indirectly through the body, such as a whiplash-type injury where the resulting rotational acceleration forces cause the damage. A concussion is considered a mild TBI (mTBI) because it causes a brief change in mental status or consciousness that is usually not life-threatening, compared to a severe TBI in which there is an extended period of unconsciousness or memory loss after the injury.[3,4]

There are an estimated 3.8 million sports-related concussion injuries per year seen in the emergency departments in the United States.[2] However, this is an underestimate because children are often not seen in the emergency department for consultation after concussions. It is estimated that 65% of all concussions occur in children between 4 and 15 years of age. Fifty percent of these concussions are not sports related but are caused by falls, and 15% are caused by unintentional blunt trauma such as being hit by an object.[2,5]

Over the past decade, animal models and human studies have advanced our understanding of the pathophysiology of mTBI. After an acute injury to the brain, the metabolic needs of neurons are very high. Normally, neuronal mitochondria upregulate the production of adenosine triphosphate (ATP) to meet increased metabolic demands. However, the concussion injury produces a neurometabolic cascade that results in impaired mitochondrial function.[3] An additional problem is that the fuel which generates ATP—primarily glucose—is less available after a concussion because cerebral blood flow is decreased. This decrease in cerebral blood flow is more prolonged in the early adolescent population compared to adults.[4] Thus, at a moment of high metabolic brain demand, energy production and the availability of glucose for energy production are simultaneously decreased. This phenomenon has been termed the "metabolic mismatch phase" of concussion.[4] The concept of brain rest to promote healing in acute concussion management derives from the fundamental mismatch between increased cerebral metabolic needs and decreased availability of ATP. **Physical and cognitive rest immediately after concussion** is a cornerstone in concussion management to attempt to maintain equilibrium between energy needs and energy production of the brain tissue. If given sufficient time and energy to recover, the cells can restore intracellular function and remain viable and post-concussion symptoms should resolve.[3,4]

After concussion, the majority of children recover in 7 to 10 days from the initial injury, though approximately 10% to 15% of children have persistent symptoms beyond this period and develop PCS. A broad definition of PCS from the clinical criteria of the World Health Organization's International Classification of Diseases (ICD-10) includes three or more of the following symptoms: fatigue, sleep disturbance, headache, dizziness, concentration difficulty, or memory difficulties. In addition, postural instability is common in individuals with PCS.[2]

Signs and symptoms related to PCS are grouped into four categories. Somatic signs and symptoms include headache, nausea, vomiting, balance deficits, slowed reaction time, dizziness, sensitivity to light and sound, and blurred vision. Cognitive issues include difficulty concentrating, mental fogginess, and confusion. Sleep disturbances can present as sleeping more or less than usual, difficulty falling asleep, or generalized fatigue. Mood disruption can include increased irritability, sadness, increased emotional behavior, or depression. Functional deficits can present as balance, coordination, and exertion issues. In the pediatric population, loss of consciousness and dizziness is associated with prolonged recovery.[6] Headache and nausea as well as balance and visual problems are often evident immediately after injury. It is not uncommon though for many of the signs and symptoms to develop 24 to 48 hours after injury. Table 24-1 presents the common signs and symptoms associated with PCS.[1,6]

Comorbidities associated with prolonged recovery from a concussion include personal or family history of ADHD, dyslexia, learning disability, amblyopia (or other visual tracking disorders), mood disorders such as anxiety or depression, and history of migraine headaches. These comorbidities also limit tolerance to rehabilitation activities and progression of physical exercise.[5,6]

The use of neurocognitive assessment tools to provide information regarding cognitive baseline in athletes has been increasing. ImPACT (Immediate Post-Concussion Assessment and Cognitive Testing) is a widely used and validated computerized measurement that can be administered by physical therapists, athletic trainers, school nurses, or team physicians. It is recommended that the ImPACT

Table 24-1 SIGNS AND SYMPTOMS ASSOCIATED WITH POST-CONCUSSION SYNDROME	
Somatic and Functional	**Mood Disruption**
Headache Dizziness Nausea and vomiting Photophobia and phonophobia Blurred vision Balance deficits Slowed reaction times Poor coordination	Depression Anxiety Irritability Sadness Increased emotional behavior
Cognitive	**Sleep Disturbances**
Difficulty concentrating Memory issues Mental fogginess Confusion	Difficulty falling asleep Difficulty staying asleep Sleeping more or less than usual Generalized fatigue

be administered annually in athletes that engage in impact sports.[5,7] The ImPACT measures an individual's symptoms, attention span, nonverbal memory, verbal and visual memory, and processing speed and reaction times. If a concussion is suspected, the ImPACT is administered and results are compared to the baseline scores. Professionals can use the results to assess potential changes caused by a concussion and measure readiness for return to sport. Presently, baseline testing is performed in many high school sports programs. However, for the child who sustains a concussion outside of organized school or team sports, baseline test scores will not be available. When a baseline result is not available, the ImPACT can be readministered during recovery to measure improvement.[7,8]

Physical Therapy Patient/Client Management

Physical and cognitive rest, or brain rest, should be implemented in the acute stages of concussion. Though the duration should be individualized for each child, brain rest is often necessary for 3 to 10 days after the concussion. Until there is a decline in the initial concussive symptoms at rest, the individual should not do homework, read, text, or play video games.[6] Activities should be limited to those that do not trigger an immediate or delayed increase in symptoms. Activities such as listening to music or watching television may need to be individualized as these can cause symptoms in some children, but not in others. As symptoms reduce with rest, children are encouraged to begin engaging in light aerobic exercise such as walking or bicycling for 20 to 30 minutes as symptom intensity allows. The key is not to participate in any activities that worsen symptoms.[6,9] The child with PCS is generally referred to physical therapy after 2 to 3 weeks of rest when the symptoms have decreased.[9] Physical therapy management is part of a multidisciplinary approach. A key component is providing education to the parents and child in symptom management and frequent communication with the pediatrician or neurologist, teachers, and coaches. The physical therapist informs them of the child's impairments and the relationship between impairments and increased symptoms, his specific functional limitations, as well as his delayed recovery. Symptom management with physical and cognitive activities is important to facilitate recovery. Monitoring changes in headaches, dizziness, nausea, and/or visual symptoms with a verbal rating scale (0-10, in which 0 is "none" and 10 is "severe") can help set and modify the level of activity intensity the child can tolerate.[10,11] It is also important to work with the child's teachers, nurse, guidance counselor, coach, and, in this case, the music teacher. They should be an integral part of developing goals to progress the child toward return to academics, sports, and music. The implementation of cognitive rest is important in the school setting since attempting to continue normal cognitive workload while recovering from a brain injury can exacerbate and prolong symptoms and recovery.[10,12] Academic accommodations are recommended when children are allowed to return to school. These recommendations may include: (1) attending classes for limited periods of time; (2) listening to lectures, but not taking notes; and (3) limited test taking with additional time, if needed. In the transition back to the school setting, students should be given frequent breaks during the school day in the nurse's office to decrease overstimulation that commonly causes increased headaches and decreased cognitive abilities.[13] Physical therapy goals include reducing complaints of symptoms with physical and cognitive activities, improving gaze stability, achieving normal oculomotor tracking, improving static and dynamic postural control, and improving reading tolerance. The long-term goals are to transition the child to full academic coursework and to allow him to return to sport or chosen activities.[10] It is also important to educate the family about the risks involved with reinjury, second impact syndrome, and proper management, if subsequent head injuries occur. Repeated concussions can cause more severe symptoms and longer recovery periods. Second impact syndrome is a rare, often fatal, TBI that occurs when a repeat injury is sustained before symptoms of a previous head injury have completely resolved.[10,12,14,15]

Examination, Evaluation, and Diagnosis

It is important to have a thorough medical history intake that includes specific factors related to type of concussion injury, duration of loss of consciousness, neck pain associated with the injury, number of prior concussions, and comorbidities. There are four patient severity outcome measures that are helpful in guiding the examination: the verbal rating scale for ranking symptoms, the Post-Concussion Symptom Scale (PCSS), the ImPACT, and the Dizziness Handicap Inventory (DHI). The therapist starts by asking the child to verbally rate his baseline symptoms (0-10 scale, in which 0 is "none" and 10 is "severe") such as headache, dizziness, nausea, neck pain, and disequilibrium which can then be used to determine if subsequent assessments provoke symptoms, and to what extent.[11] The PCSS can also be used to measure concussion-related symptoms. The PCSS is a segment of the ImPACT and is used during the examination and treatment to rate symptoms. The PCSS is a 22-item scale that asks the individual to rate the severity of symptoms on a 7-point Likert scale (0 is "none"; 6 is "severe"). The total symptom score ranges from 0 to 132, with 132 indicating maximal severity of symptoms. More recent analysis shows that subsets of symptoms within the PCSS can be used by the physical therapist to develop an impression of the child's symptoms.[11,16,17] For example, Joyce et al.[17] found that in the pediatric population, females and individuals with anxiety disorders had higher scores than males on the cognition-, somatic-, and emotional-related items on the PCSS. To assess and rate dizziness and vestibular symptoms after concussion, the **DHI** can be used.[18] Additional questions about sleep issues, reading tolerance, and eye disorders (*e.g.*, amblyopia, strabismus) are also helpful in directing the examination. Inquiries should be made regarding the duration of absence and/or attendance to school, practices and sports, and the extent of any academic accommodations that have been instituted.[10]

The physical examination also includes an assessment of cervical spine range of motion, palpation of neck musculature, pain complaints, and signs of cervical cord compression tests (*e.g.*, Spurling's sign). A comprehensive upper quarter neurologic screening should be performed with attention to deficits in upper quarter strength. A screen is important to assess the need to incorporate a strengthening program which can be beneficial in preventing recurrence of injury.[12]

Further examination of the neurologic system includes specific assessment of cerebellar, vestibular, and visual motor systems. The cerebellar coordination examination includes the classic finger-nose-finger test to detect slowed reaction times and dysmetria. First, the therapist observes ocular alignment while the patient is seated. To detect for horizontal or vertical phoria (eye alignment deficits), the therapist administers the cover-uncover test in which the therapist asks the patient to focus on a given point and covers this eye. If the uncovered eye moves, strabismus is present. The therapist should also be aware that any pre-existing compensated ocular misalignment may be decompensated after a concussive injury and this finding is associated with protracted recovery.[2,6]

The Vestibular/Ocular-Motor Screening (VOMS) examination is a clinical screen that assesses smooth pursuit, horizontal and vertical saccades, near point of convergence distance, horizontal VOR, and visual motion sensitivity. The therapist examines smooth pursuits and abnormal nystagmus to investigate cranial nerve or central deficits. To do so, the therapist holds a finger approximately 20 to 24 inches from the child's eyes and then moves it horizontally back and forth repeatedly, slowly at first then progressively increasing the speed. The child's eyes should be able to follow the finger accurately and stop quickly as the target stops without abnormal eye movement. The therapist then repeats the test in a vertical pattern. Children with PCS may have difficulty with slow and fast tracking of the target and show saccadic intrusion (involuntary fast movement away from the desired target position followed by a secondary saccade or drift), jerky eye movements, or have symptoms of eyestrain and headache during this task.[6,12] During each test, the therapist asks the child to verbally rate change in dizziness, headache, and/or nausea on a numerical 0 to 10 scale.[6,11]

The next step in the VOMS is evaluating the accuracy of saccadic eye movements between targets. Saccades are assessed when the examiner holds two fingers apart horizontally (shoulder width apart) or vertically (placed chin and forehead distance apart), while the child is asked to repeatedly move his eyes horizontally or vertically from target to target with his head kept still. The therapist should perform the test for approximately 30 repetitions in each direction, and note how many repetitions the child can tolerate before stopping the test. During each test, the child is again asked to verbally rate changes in dizziness, headache, fogginess, and nausea. This test may increase eyestrain or headache. The child may have difficulty accurately reaching the target or maintaining the speed of the eye movement with repetition, or he may produce hypometric saccades (eye movements that undershoot the target). Difficulty in these tasks correlates with difficulty in classroom activities, such as looking from the computer to a whiteboard when taking notes or during reading activities.[13] These difficulties can also produce symptoms in sports in which running and focus on a moving ball are involved.[6,11]

Near point convergence (NPC) is the simultaneous inward movement of both eyes toward each other to maintain single binocular vision when viewing an object that is moving closer to the face. Convergence insufficiency is the inability to coordinate convergence of eyes within a physiological range (4-6 cm from the nose in children) and is a common deficit after a concussion, contributing to headache symptoms and cognitive difficulties.[2,13] It is measured by having the child fix his gaze on a pen with a letter on it. The therapist then moves the pen slowly toward his nose and measures the point at which the child complains of blurry and/or double vision. The therapist also notes whether there is any outward deviation of one eye during the test. After the test, the therapist asks the child to rate changes in dizziness, headache, and/or nausea. When testing NPC, abnormal findings include asymmetrical eye movement, blurred vision, headache, and/or NPC distance greater than age-expected norms.[6,11,19]

The sensitivity of the vestibular system is assessed with the VOR examination, which tests gaze stability, or the ability to maintain focus on a stationary object while the head or body is moving. The therapist asks the child to focus on a stationary target while repeatedly moving his head vertically approximately 20 times then repeating with horizontal head movements. Again, the therapist asks the child to rate any changes in dizziness, headache, fogginess, and nausea. Abnormal findings include blurry vision, dizziness, inability to stay focused on the target, increased headache, and/or symptoms of motion sensitivity. Another test of the VOR is called the head impulse test (head thrust test) in which the therapist applies a low-amplitude, high-acceleration vertical and/or horizontal rotation to the seated child's head while he is instructed to maintain his gaze on a stationary target. The test is considered abnormal if corrective saccades occur when the head is moved in a direction that the child does not predict.[6,12]

In children diagnosed with PCS, there is an increased risk of visual problems that are associated with verbal memory deficits and poor visual motor skills that affect academic performance. In a recent unpublished study by Master,[20] 69% of children examined after concussion were found to have visual problems, 55% had vestibular deficits, and 49% had both. Of the visual problems found, 51% showed accommodative disorder, 49% had convergence insufficiency, and 29% had saccadic dysfunction.[20] Table 24-2 presents a summary of the key physical examination and expected findings in individuals with PCS.

Table 24-2   PHYSICAL EXAMINATION OF THE CHILD WITH POST-CONCUSSION SYNDROME

Physical Examination Element	How to Perform Examination	Deficits Noted
Cerebellar coordination	Examiner moves finger horizontally and asks patient to touch finger and then his nose.	Slow reaction time, dysmetria
Nystagmus	Examiner moves finger horizontally in front of patient's eyes progressively more rapidly, stopping centrally.	Unable to visually track Beats of nystagmus at center of visual field
Smooth pursuits	Examiner moves finger horizontally and vertically in "H" pattern, then moves progressively more rapidly.	Unable to visually track Jerky or jumpy eye movements Provocation of headache, dizziness, eye fatigue, nausea (symptoms/signs rated on a 0-10 verbal rating scale)
Saccades	Examiner holds 2 fingers at shoulder-width and forehead-chin distance to test horizontal and vertical eye movements, respectively.	Unable to perform or can only perform a few repetitions before provocation of symptoms or signs (rated on a 0-10 verbal rating scale)
Gaze stability VOR	Patient fixes gaze on examiner's thumb while nodding horizontally and then shaking head vertically.	Unable to perform or can only perform a few repetitions before provocation of symptoms or signs (rated on a 0-10 verbal rating scale)
Convergence (NPC)	Patient watches a pen with a letter on it and tracks from arm's length distance while therapist brings it closer to nose.	Convergence insufficiency: letters become double at > 4-6 cm from the tip of nose. Note symptoms on 0-10 verbal rating scale
Balance	Tandem heel-toe gait forward and backward with eyes open and closed	Patient raises arms for stability, widens stance, and/or demonstrates extreme truncal swaying without normal righting
King-Devick test (eye movements, language, concentration)	Patient is asked to read single digit numbers displayed on 3 index-sized cards. Patient is timed on how quickly he can accurately read 5 lines of numbers. The time (in seconds) it takes for the patient to read each of the 3 pages is summed together for a total timed score and the number of errors is noted.	Number of errors and speed of reading numbers can be measured for individual and used for baseline and to show improvement. Headache, dizziness, nausea
Aerobic endurance: modified Balke treadmill test	Child walks on treadmill (3.3 miles/hr) for 2 minutes. 1% grade is added each minute until 15 minutes is reached. Test is terminated when symptoms reach 2 points above baseline on 0-10 verbal rating scale or 80% of maximal age-predicted HR for children.	Symptoms of headache and dizziness greater than a 2-point change on 0-10 verbal rating scale, while monitoring RPE Abnormal HR or BP response to exercise

Abbreviations: BP, blood pressure; cm, centimeters; HR, heart rate; NPC, near point convergence; RPE, rating of perceived exertion; VOR, vestibuloocular reflex.

Up to this point, the therapist has assessed the integrity of the cerebellar, visual, and vestibular systems using the tests within the VOMS examination. The King-Devick test was designed to evaluate impaired eye movements, language, concentration, and other correlates of suboptimal brain function after concussion in athletes.[8,21] It is also beneficial in assessing a child with PCS. During this one-minute test, the therapist asks the child to read single-digit numbers displayed on index-sized cards. There are a series of three cards that increase in complexity. The child is timed on how quickly he can accurately read five lines of numbers. The total time it takes to read the five lines on each of the three cards is added together for the score and the number of errors is noted. Traditionally, the results are used as a baseline test before the sports season. After a head trauma, any increase in the time to complete the test suggests a concussion has occurred.[21,22] In a study by Galetta et al.,[21] collegiate contact sport athletes scored a median time of 37.0 seconds on baseline tests and immediate post-concussion scores worsened by an average of 9.9 seconds. Abnormal findings include increased time to complete the task, increased headache symptoms, and difficulty with verbal fluency. The King-Devick test has been shown to correlate with deficits and improvements on the ImPACT neurocognitive testing scores, and could be used as a helpful sideline test for recognition of acute concussive injuries.[8,21]

After the oculomotor and cognitive tests have been administered, the therapist should assess dynamic movement control. The therapist can test dynamic balance by initially asking the child to tandem walk forward with his arms across his chest for ten steps, and then ten steps backward. This task should be observed for ability to maintain heel-toe pattern, instability with gait and raising arms, and presence of abnormal hip strategy or missteps. Then, the task can be made more difficult by repeating forward and backward tandem walking with the eyes closed for ten steps, again noting the child's ability to perform this task.[6,12] The Balance Error Symptom Scale (BESS) can be used to assess static balance and as a sideline concussion balance test. For the BESS, the child is asked to stand with feet together, single leg stance, and tandem stance with eyes closed on a firm surface and on a foam surface for 20 seconds in each position. Other balance measures such as the modified Clinical Test for Sensory Integration of Balance (CTSIB) or the Functional Gait Assessment (FGA) that are used in adults may provide good information in evaluation of children.[23]

A modified Balke treadmill test can be utilized to evaluate the cardiovascular health of individuals with concussion. Post-concussive patients often have difficulty tolerating aerobic exercise without symptoms of dizziness, imbalance, and headache. Aerobic exercise training may reduce concussion-related physiological dysfunction and symptoms by restoring autonomic balance and improving autoregulation of cerebral blood flow.[2,24] Leddy and colleagues[2] have proposed that prolonged PCS symptoms result from impaired autonomic function and that a gradual return to exercise can be used to treat the symptoms. Prior to performing a treadmill test, the therapist calculates the child's age-predicted heart rate maximum. For children and adolescents, the most accurate maximal heart rate (HRmax) prediction equation is $208 - (0.7 \times age)$.[25,26] The modified Balke protocol is performed on a treadmill at constant speed of 3.3 miles per hour for the initial two minutes. After each subsequent minute, a 1% grade incline is added until the test is completed at 15 minutes. The child's heart rate and blood pressure are monitored before and after the test and signs and symptoms of headache, dizziness, and nausea are again rated on the

0 to 10 verbal rating scale. Heart rate and rating of perceived exertion (RPE) are also monitored throughout the test. When the child's symptoms on the verbal rating scale increase more than two points from baseline or heart rate reaches 80% of age-predicted HRmax, the test is terminated. Modification of the test is sometimes necessary for children. In our clinic, the speed is lowered for smaller children to allow walking at a more comfortable walking pace. In addition, a pediatric RPE scale such as the OMNI may be used. The treadmill test is often not tolerated (or appropriate) on the initial visit and is usually completed on the second visit. The results of this test help the therapist design an aerobic program that meets the tolerance of the post-concussive child. The therapist can set a sub-symptom and/ or heart rate threshold of aerobic activity with the goal of 30 minutes of sustained aerobic exertion.[27,28] Because of motion sensitivity and exercise intensity on the treadmill, children are often started on a stationary bicycle and then progressed to treadmill walking and eventually to treadmill running or exercising on an elliptical machine, which causes more vertical displacement challenging motion sensitivity.[12]

In this case, the 10-year-old child presented four weeks after a concussion with complaints of persistent headache rating 6-8/10 during school. He had no comorbidities and reading tolerance was 15 minutes. On the DHI, he scored 30% (0% = normal), indicating frustration, restricted activity, concentration issues, and movement sensitivity. His score on the PCSS was 43/132, with the most severe complaints of balance issues, sensitivity to light and noise, and headaches. During the physical examination, the child demonstrated normal cerebellar coordination, convergence insufficiency at 12 centimeters, and abnormal saccades (tolerating eight repetitions vertically and six repetitions horizontally before increased headache complaints). His VOR tasks were normal in both directions, but his King-Devick score was abnormal at 66 seconds. He had difficulty maintaining single leg stance and was unable to tandem walk without severe ataxia in any of the four conditions. On the modified Balke protocol, he tolerated ten minutes before his heart rate elevated above target heart rate range and the test was terminated.

Plan of Care and Interventions

Physical therapy and vestibular rehabilitation should address the impairments found on examination with a problem-based approach. Individuals with PCS often have multiple areas of impairments. Symptom intensity often drives the therapist's decision of which deficits to initially address. It is important to know what the child has been doing before coming to a therapy session. For example, has the child had a full day of school or been at home resting? This may affect the intensity of the symptoms and exercise progression for that session. The therapist begins by educating the child and parent about how to use the verbal rating scale in the progression of exercise and activity. Using this scale, he rates his symptoms when he enters the clinic, and before, during, and after each exercise or activity. The therapist introduces exercises that do not trigger significant headache or dizziness symptoms. If an exercise increases symptoms, rest is allowed and symptoms are monitored for the time it takes for them to return to baseline. The general rule of thumb is that **symptoms are allowed to increase two points on the verbal rating scale** and should recover with a brief rest before beginning the next exercise. A symptom log is used to help monitor the intensity of the symptoms with differing tasks and recovery times needed to return to baseline. Progression of exercises is symptom driven. The child can be progressed to the next level of difficulty if symptoms are not increased more than two points on the verbal rating scale. Initially, the simplest exercise is given, such as a visual coordination task. As the child demonstrates minimal symptoms, the complexity of the task is increased, such as performing a visual task while balancing on a wobble board. Home exercises are based on those in which the child demonstrates the most significant deficits. It is recommended that home exercises be performed in short but frequent sessions throughout the day to challenge the nervous system, but allow for recovery.

The frequency of physical therapy sessions varies depending on the child's academic schedule and tolerance. If the child begins therapy before he has resumed school, he is often treated twice per week. The parents are educated on the detailed home exercise program (HEP) to improve the child's compliance. The therapist alerts the child and his parents that when he resumes school, the environmental stimulation and cognitive challenges in the classroom may increase his symptoms and therapy progression may need to be modified. When children are out of school for extended periods, home tutoring can be introduced, but tutors need to be educated on tolerance and dosage of schoolwork. As the child progresses, sessions are reduced to once weekly. The HEP is modified and coordinated to allow the student to complete homework. It is also important to interact with the child's academic coordinator to make sure that tests are modified, extra time is given, and classroom notes are provided. The child should be allowed to have breaks in the nurse's office to allow recovery and facilitate the best environment to learn.[10]

In treatment sessions, the child is initially encouraged to perform progressive aerobic exercise daily, with the intensity level adjusted depending on symptom intensity demonstrated on the modified Balke protocol treadmill test. Often, treatment sessions begin with aerobic exercise on a stationary bicycle or a treadmill. As symptoms improve, more difficult aerobic activity that also challenges balance and coordination such as elliptical stair climbing, treadmill running, or fitter slalom exercises can be introduced. The therapist should closely observe the child during these activities because autonomic dysfunction can present quickly during exertion, causing prolonged dizziness after stopping treadmill walking or running.[12]

Several types of exercises can be used to address the identified impairments of the visual motor system. "Eye swing" exercises address saccadic deficits (Fig. 24-1). For these, the child is asked to move his eyes between two targets placed approximately 12 inches apart within arm's length away. He is asked to repeat these "eye swings" back and forth for 20 repetitions between the targets in a horizontal direction and then repeat the same exercise in a vertical pattern. Accuracy of eye movements on the target and maintaining clear vision is important with the task. As the child's tolerance increases, the number of repetitions can be increased. Gaze stability exercises begin with a stationary target placed about arm's length distance away. This time, the child moves his head horizontally while keeping his eyes focused on the stationary target. This can be repeated vertically, beginning with 10 to 20 repetitions and progressing up to 60 seconds as tolerated. The Brock string exercise (Fig. 24-2) is designed to improve convergence and divergence, which

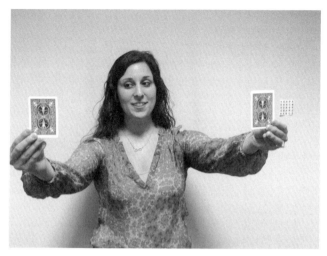

Figure 24-1. Patient performing eye swing exercise to improve saccadic eye movements.

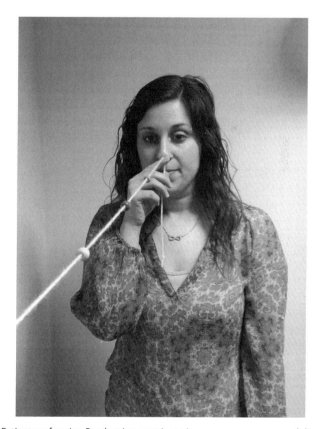

Figure 24-2. Patient performing Brock string exercise to improve convergence and divergence.

are common deficits post-concussion that can affect reading abilities and therefore academic status. The child is given a string approximately ten feet long with three beads placed along the string. The child holds one end of the string to his nose, while the other end is attached to a stationary object at about eye level. The patient is instructed to gaze from one bead to the next, first coming toward the nose and then away from the nose to the most distal bead, making sure to clearly focus on each bead for approximately three to five seconds. This can be repeated approximately three to five times, depending on complaints of associated headache or eyestrain (this is usually a difficult exercise to initially perform). The closest bead needs to be placed near to where the patient demonstrated difficulty converging on the initial examination.[12,18,29]

If the child had positive findings on the cervical examination, manual therapy, modalities, and cervical range of motion exercises can be used. Many exercises used to address impairments in the visual motor system may also be influenced by cervical spine stiffness that can limit treatment progression. Cervical muscles (upper trapezius, levator scapula, sternocleidomastoid, and suboccipital muscles) may be shortened. As the child progresses, strengthening exercises for the cervical muscles can be added to prevent future reinjury.[12]

Sensorimotor and balance deficits are addressed with stimulation of static balance reactions on varying surfaces such as tilt boards, wobble boards, and compliant surfaces. Activities can be progressed by adding more complex multiplanar balance tasks such as standing or squatting on a Bosu ball or moving in a slalom pattern on the ProFitter 3D cross trainer. Tandem walking is often challenging, especially backwards, or when performed with eyes closed or on foam surfaces. Generally, activities begin in linear patterns such as walking forward and backward and then progressed with 180° and 360° turns. Coordination tasks that correlate with sports-specific activities can also be introduced to challenge the balance system.[12,18]

When the child demonstrates tolerance for the above tasks, more functionally demanding tasks that incorporate visual tracking and hand-eye coordination to balance tasks can be added. For example, ball-tossing tasks or juggling can be used to facilitate normal saccadic eye movements. During the hand-to-hand tossing or up-and-down tossing, the eyes must track and follow the balls. This type of task can be varied in complexity by increasing the speed of the task, performing more difficult juggling patterns that involve bigger head and body movement, and using a smaller ball. When these activities are mastered, complexity can then be increased by adding walking while tossing a ball, and turning or spinning or standing on a compliant surface while catching a ball that is thrown in unpredictable patterns. Progressions can be developed that mimic specific sports or activities that would optimize the child's goal to return to play.

Cognitive challenges should be introduced when the patient tolerates these functional activities with minimal symptoms. First, the child performs a task that he has mastered, such as bouncing the ball in a three-pattern succession and walking. Next, the therapist asks him to perform a cognitive task, such as listing names in alphabetical progression while performing the mastered task. For some children, the ability to carry on a conversation and answer questions and continue to perform the task well is difficult; for others, listing or complex memory tasks are needed to challenge them. Math tasks such as serial sevens (counting backwards by 7 from 100) can be extremely difficult and affect coordination. Math and foreign language activities demand more attention and therefore are introduced in the later progression. It is important to create cognitive challenges that are age-appropriate and interesting to the child.[10,12]

As the child shows improvement and is cleared by the physician to return to sports practice, the intensity of the exercise program should progress to more dynamic exertion activities such as squatting, lunges, push-ups, free weights, dynamic plank exercises, core exercises with repetitive movement, and progressing to sprinting and hopping drills that increase strength, coordination, and improve reaction time.

With the current 10-year-old child, significant deficits were apparent in oculomotor, vestibular, and balance systems and these contributed to his headaches and difficulty reading. Interventions were initiated in the clinic and with a HEP to be performed 4 times per day, which included Brock string, eye swings, and VOR exercises. The child's interventions and progressions are described in Table 24-3. Table 24-4 summarizes the progression of exercises during 5 visits in a 4-week treatment period.

Table 24-3   EXERCISE PROGRESSION FOR VISUAL AND VESTIBULAR SYSTEMS FOR CURRENT CASE PATIENT

Exercise	Deficit Addressed	Progression
Brock string	Convergence	Move proximal bead closer to the nose Increase speed of task Increase duration of focusing or number of repetitions
VOR 1 (Target remains stationary and head moves)	Gaze stability	Increase speed of head movement Decrease size of target Change distance of target Perform while walking in all planes
VOR 2 (Head and eyes move in opposite directions)	Gaze stability	Increase speed of head movement Decrease size of target Change distance of target Perform while walking in all planes
Eye swings	Saccades	Add diagonal movement and complex patterns Use columns of numbers and letters as the stationary targets to focus on Recite the numbers or letters Increase speed of eye movement
Pencil push-ups	Convergence Divergence	Hold a pencil with words on it visible at arm's length then bring closer toward the nose until double vision occurs, then reverse to start position. Repeat 5 times, while keeping the words in focus. Increase speed of movement Decrease size of target

Table 24-4	PRESCRIBED EXERCISES AND PROGRESSION OVER FIVE SESSIONS FOR CURRENT PATIENT				
Exercise	Session 1	Session 2	Session 3	Session 4	Session 5
Aerobic conditioning	Education on performing light aerobic exercise daily	Modified Balke protocol treadmill test: 10 min with termination related to elevated heart rate associated with increased headache and dizziness	Treadmill walking for 15 min with increased speed and decreased use of upper extremity support	Fitter slalom with ski poles for 10 min Animal walks (inch worm, crab walk, kangaroo hops) for exertion and coordination: 2 × 20 ft each	Elliptical for 15 min Animal walks: added 3-legged puppy (using 2 hands and 1 leg to hop across floor)
Convergence exercise	Brock string with 3- to 5-sec focus on each bead; repeat 3 times	Brock string with focus on moving beads closer to increase vergence demand	Brock string with increased eye movement speed, increase duration to 60 sec, bead moved closer to vergence point	Pencil push-ups 2 sets of 5 reps	Continue pencil push-ups and Brock string
Vestibular exercise	VOR 1 in static stance for 30 sec × 2 repetitions horizontally and vertically	VOR 1 in static stance for 60 sec and perform walking while walking	VOR 1 on wobble board and perform walking with increased pace	VOR 2 added in static stance and walking	VOR 1 with step-ups VOR 2 while tandem walking
Visual motor tasks	Saccade eye swings 20 reps each, horizontally and vertically (1 rep is complete when eyes move back and forth to start position)	Eye swings: 40 repetitions	Saccade tower: patient reads out loud 2 vertical and horizontal lines of 20 letters and numbers	Perform saccades activity while standing on Bosu ball: up to 40 reps	Reps increased to 60-100

Sensory integration of balance	Wobble boards	Balance discs with squats	Added ball toss and catch while standing on discs Walking while wearing Chango Paws (1/2 balls strapped onto bottom of feet)	Walking with 180° turns and ball tossing while wearing Chango Paws
Dual task: motor or cognitive	Ball coordination task with 3 patterns to sequence while standing (e.g., bounce ball with left hand, toss to right, toss up with right hand and repeat)	Ball coordination task with 5 patterns to sequence Perform 3-sequence pattern while walking	Cognitive task added while walking (ABCs with names) Agility ladder with simple patterns	Add spins to tasks with ball, increase cognitive task (serial sevens) Agility ladder with more complex pattern
Functional tasks (HEP)	Playing cello with simple scales with time limits	Playing cello with songs from memory	Playing cello while reading simple music	Playing cello while reading new music

Abbreviations: min, minutes; reps, repetitions; sec, seconds.

Table 24-5 INITIAL AND DISCHARGE OUTCOME MEASURES FOR CURRENT PATIENT

Outcome Measure	Initial Evaluation	Discharge	Normal
Convergence measure	12 cm	3 cm	4-5 cm
King-Devick test	66 sec	61 sec	No norms published
PCSS	43/132	3/132	0/132
DHI	30/100	14/100	0/100
Reading tolerance	15 min	60 min	>60 min
Tandem walking	Ataxic in all 4 conditions	Stable in all 4 conditions	Stable in all 4 conditions

Abbreviations: cm, centimeters; min, minutes; sec, seconds.

In planning for discharge, the therapist should ensure that the family has been educated about the risk of reinjury. For discharge from physical therapy, the child should be able to resume his schoolwork without accommodations. It is important for the parent and school to continue to monitor his academic success, especially because oculomotor deficits were affecting his performance. If the child will be returning to playing sports, communication with the coaches and trainers should be completed, so that they understand the expectations of activity tolerance and can transition the child to practice and then games.[10,13]

Outcome data for this 10-year-old are presented in Table 24-5. He achieved normal values for the visual motor, vestibular, balance, and coordination tests. He was able to resume school for full days, was able to read for over one hour without headache, and resume playing the cello.

For the child with an atypical prolonged recovery of concussion symptoms lasting for more than 6 to 8 weeks, multidisciplinary management is recommended.[10] Often, vision therapy (as provided by an optometrist) is necessary for those children with persistent visual motor issues, headaches, and cognitive deficits. More detailed neurocognitive and psychological assessment may also be necessary in these individuals. The physical therapist may need to be the child's advocate to ensure that these secondary therapies are initiated.[12]

Evidence-Based Clinical Recommendations

SORT: Strength of Recommendation Taxonomy

A: Consistent, good-quality patient-oriented evidence
B: Inconsistent or limited-quality patient-oriented evidence
C: Consensus, disease-oriented evidence, usual practice, expert opinion, or case series

1. Physical and cognitive rest immediately after concussion decreases the likelihood of prolonged recovery and adverse effects. **Grade B**

2. The Dizziness Handicap Inventory (DHI) can be used to assess and rate dizziness and vestibular symptoms after concussion. **Grade B**

3. Physical therapy progression in the child with post-concussion syndrome should be symptom driven, allowing symptoms to increase only two points on the verbal rating scale and recovering with a brief rest before beginning the next exercise. **Grade C**

COMPREHENSION QUESTIONS

24.1 A thorough history of the concussed child is an important component of the examination and can be helpful in predicting an extended prognosis of recovery. Which comorbidity is *not* likely to indicate a more lengthy recovery?

A. ADHD

B. Migraines

C. Wearing prescription eyeglasses

D. Dyslexia

24.2 Convergence insufficiency is commonly found after concussion and can contribute to difficulties transitioning to the academic setting along with provoking headaches. Which of the following is a normal finding during convergence testing in children?

A. Blurred vision

B. Outward deviation of one eye

C. Near point convergence of 4-6 cm

D. Near point convergence of 8-10 cm

ANSWERS

24.1 **C.** Comorbidities associated with prolonged recovery from a concussion include personal or family history of ADHD, dyslexia, learning disability, mood disorders such as anxiety or depression, and history of migraine headaches. While amblyopia (or other visual tracking disorders) can prolong concussion recovery, there is no evidence to support that children who wear prescription eyeglasses will have a longer recovery from a concussion.

24.2 **C.** For children, normal near point convergence is 4-6 cm from the nose. When testing near point convergence, abnormal findings include asymmetrical eye movement (option B), blurred vision (option A), headache, and/or NPC distance greater than age-expected norms (option D).

REFERENCES

1. McCrory P, Meeuwisse WH, Aubry M, et al. Consensus statement on concussion in sport: the 4th International Conference on Concussion in Sport, Zurich, November 2012. *J Athl Train*. 2013;48:554-575.

2. Leddy JJ, Sandhu H, Sodhi V, Baker JG, Willer B. Rehabilitation of concussion and post-concussion syndrome. *Sports Health*. 2012;4:147-154.

3. Giza CC, Hovda DA. The new neurometabolic cascade of concussion. *Neurosurgery*. 2014;75:S24-S33.

4. Grady MF, Master CL, Gioia GA. Concussion pathophysiology: rationale for physical and cognitive rest. *Pediatr Ann*. 2012;41:377-382.

5. Borich MR, Cheung KL, Jones P, et al. Concussion: current concepts in diagnosis and management. *J Neurol Phys Ther*. 2013;37:133-139.

6. Master CL, Grady MF. Office-based management of pediatric and adolescent concussion. *Pediatr Ann*. 2012;41:1-6.

7. Darby DG, Master CL, Grady MF. Computerized neurocognitive testing in the medical evaluation of sports concussion. *Pediatr Ann*. 2012;41:371-376.

8. Tjarks BJ, Dorman JC, Valentine VD, et al. Comparison and utility of King-Devick and ImPACT® composite scores in adolescent concussion patients. *J Neurol Sci*. 2013;334:148-153.

9. Brown NJ, Mannix RC, O'Brien MJ, Gostine D, Collins MW, Meehan WP. Effect of cognitive activity level on duration of post-concussion symptoms. *Pediatrics*. 2014;133:e299-e304.

10. Master CL, Gioia GA, Leddy JJ, Grady MF. Importance of "return-to-learn" in pediatric and adolescent concussion. *Pediatr Ann*. 2012;41:1-6.

11. Mucha A, Collins MW, Elbin RJ, et al. A brief Vestibular/Ocular Motor Screening (VOMS) assessment to evaluate concussions: preliminary findings. *Am J Sports Med*. 2014;42:2479-2486.

12. Vidal PG, Goodman AM, Colin A, Leddy JJ, Grady MF. Rehabilitation strategies for prolonged recovery in pediatric and adolescent concussion. *Pediatr Ann*. 2012;41:1-7.

13. Halstead ME, McAvoy K, Devore CD, Carl R, Lee M, Logan K. Returning to learning following a concussion. *Pediatrics*. 2013;132:948-957.

14. Cantu RC, Gean AD. Second-impact syndrome and a small subdural hematoma: an uncommon catastrophic result of repetitive head injury with a characteristic imaging appearance. *J Neurotrauma*. 2010;27:1557-1564.

15. Weinstejn E, Turner M, Kuzma BB. Second impact syndrome in football: new imaging and insights into a rare and devastating condition. *J Neurosurg Pediatr*. 2013;11:331-334.

16. Kontos AP, Elbin RJ, Schatz P, et al. A revised factor structure for the post-concussion symptom scale: baseline and postconcussion factors. *Am J Sports Med*. 2012;40:2375-2384.

17. Joyce AS, Labella CR, Carl RL, Lai J, Zelko FA. The Postconcussion Symptom Scale: utility of a three-factor structure. *Med Sci Sports Exerc*. 2015;47:1119-1123.

18. Alsalaheen BA, Mucha A, Morris LO, et al. Vestibular rehabilitation for dizziness and balance disorders after concussion. *J Neurol Phys Ther*. 2010;34:87-93.

19. Scheiman M, Gallaway M, Frantz KA, et al. Nearpoint of convergence: test procedure, target selection, and normative data. *Optom Vis Sci*. 2003;80:214-225.

20. Master CL. Concussion increases risk for vision problems [American Academy of Pediatrics National conference. Abstract number 26430]. October 2014.

21. Galetta KM, Brandes LE, Maki K, et al. The King-Devick test and sports-related concussion: study of a rapid visual screening tool in a collegiate cohort. *J Neurol Sci*. 2011;309:34-39.

22. Galetta MS, Galetta KM, Mccrossin J, et al. Saccades and memory: baseline associations of the King-Devick and SCAT2 SAC tests in professional ice hockey players. *J Neurol Sci*. 2013;328:8-11.

23. Alsalaheen BA, Whitney SL, Marchetti GF, et al. Performance of high school adolescents on functional gait and balance measures. *Pediatr Phys Ther*. 2014;26:191-199.

24. Leddy JJ, Kozlowski K, Fung M, Pendergast DR, Willer B. Regulatory and autoregulatory physiological dysfunction as a primary characteristic of post concussion syndrome: implications for treatment. *NeuroRehabilitation.* 2007;22:199-205.

25. Machado FA, Denedai BS. Validity of maximum heart rate prediction equations for children and adolescents. *Arq Bras Cardiol.* 2011;97:136-140.

26. Mahon AD, Marjerrison AD, Lee JD, Woodruff ME, Hanna LE. Evaluating the prediction of maximal heart rate in children and adolescents. *Res Q Exerc Sport.* 2010;81:466-471.

27. Baker JG, Freitas MS, Leddy JJ, Kozlowski KF, Willer BS. Return to full functioning after graded exercise assessment and progressive exercise treatment of postconcussion syndrome. *Rehabil Res Pract.* 2012;705309.

28. Darling SR, Leddy JJ, Baker JG, et al. Evaluation of the Zurich guidelines and exercise testing for return to play in adolescents following concussion. *Clin J Sport Med.* 2014;24:128-133.

29. Alsalaheen BA, Whitney SL, Mucha A, Morris LO, Furman JM, Sparto PJ. Exercise prescription patterns in patients treated with vestibular rehabilitation after concussion. *Physiother Res Int.* 2013;18:100-108.

Congenital Limb Deficiency: Proximal Femoral Focal Deficiency

Colleen P. Coulter
Rebecca Grant
Brian Giavedoni

CASE 25

A 9.5-year-old male was diagnosed at birth with right proximal femoral focal deficiency (PFFD), Aitken B classification. Since 2 years of age, the patient has received orthotic interventions to equalize leg lengths for an anticipated leg length discrepancy of 20 cm. Based on his Aitken classification and absence of any other orthopaedic anomalies, his medical team initially proposed three treatment options: Syme amputation with knee fusion, Van Nes rotationplasty procedure with knee fusion, or limb lengthening operations staged over several years until he reached skeletal maturity. The patient's family chose the third option of staged limb lengthening. At 2 years of age, the initial treatment consisted of a shoe lift, which provided adequate compensation of the leg length discrepancy during gait. As he grew, the limb length discrepancy increased and the height of the right shoe lift was increased to equalize the limb lengths. However, the height required to equalize his leg length discrepancy created balance and coordination challenges during gait. At age 5 years, 10 months, the patient underwent his first limb lengthening procedure: a right femoral osteotomy and application of a unilateral external fixator. Following 6 months of lengthening, the external fixator was removed and a spica cast was applied for 8 weeks to allow for adequate bone healing. In this first lengthening, 5 cm of length was achieved. Shortly after cast removal, the patient developed a femoral bowing deformity that was treated with casting, followed by bracing and outpatient physical therapy. At age 7 years, he underwent subtrochanteric femoral osteotomy with valgus correction for varus flexion deformity and distal femoral osteotomy to correct for anterior bowing with placement of an external fixator for a second lengthening procedure. Eight months after application of the second external fixator, non-union occurred at the subtrochanteric pin site requiring a pin site allograft. Lengthening continued for 10 months with fixator removal at the end of this period. The patient's postoperative course was further complicated by a femur fracture through the regenerate site. Four months after the second lengthening, the therapist noted a 6-inch leg length discrepancy. The Limb Deficiency team at the children's hospital where the patient was receiving care met with the patient and his parents to review his surgical history and discuss future surgical prosthetic and orthotic options that would match their goals. After reviewing the patient's multiple complications that included four femoral fractures, non-union, continued limb length discrepancy, development of osteopenia, and restricted function, the patient and his parents indicated they were now open to future options of Syme amputation with knee fusion or rotationplasty. However, the patient's mother stated that she wanted to wait a year or so to give her son a break from surgery and requested that the team continue with conservative orthotic or prosthetic intervention. The goals of conservative treatment include equalizing the patient's limb length to protect the femur from further fracture and angular deformities and allowing increased activity without the fear of fracture. Since the initiation of limb lengthening, the patient's overall activity has been limited. He has been walking with a walker and a tall shoe lift on the right. He wants to begin participating in sports and other activities that are currently restricted due to increased risk of fracture with moderate to high impact activities. Therefore, the patient, his family, and the team have decided to proceed with an extension prosthesis that incorporates external knee hinges to allow flexion of the limb and clearance during swing phase of gait. Limb length was afforded by adding a pylon with a prosthetic foot (Fig. 25-1). Since receiving the extension prosthesis with the articulating knee, the patient has progressed to walking without an assistive device and participating in physical education class and recess at school. He has not had fractures or progression of femoral deformity. At 9.5 years of age, the patient and his parents have made the time-sensitive decision for definitive surgical correction of the limb length discrepancy—choosing the Van Nes rotationplasty with knee fusion over a Syme amputation with knee fusion. Rotationplasty offers below-the-knee function, while the Syme offers a knee disarticulation amputation functional level. The knee fusion stabilizes the proximal residual limb. The purpose of this physical therapy session is to initiate a plan of care that includes a brace to enable the patient to participate in age-appropriate chosen activities before the definitive surgical correction of his limb length discrepancy.

▶ Based on the patient's diagnosis, age, and past interventions, what factors should the medical team, patient, and patient's family take into consideration when making the decision for definitive surgical correction?

▶ Why is the definitive surgical decision time-sensitive?

▶ Why is it important to know the classification of the patient's PFFD?

▶ What are the physical therapy goals for limb lengthening, rotationplasty, and amputation?

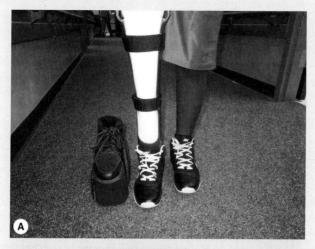

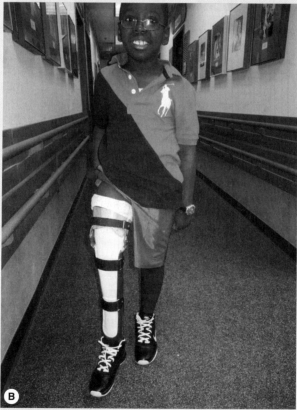

Figure 25-1. **A.** Child wearing an extension prosthesis that supports the entire right limb and incorporates an external knee joint to allow knee flexion and extension. The large shoe lift that was worn prior to the extension prosthesis is shown next to the extension prosthesis. While both equalize limb lengths, the extension prosthesis offers stability, controlled knee movement, and the ability to walk without an assisted device, which increased the child's activity. When wearing the shoe lift, the child required a walker and performed only limited activity. **B.** Child demonstrating the external knee joint of the extension prosthesis.

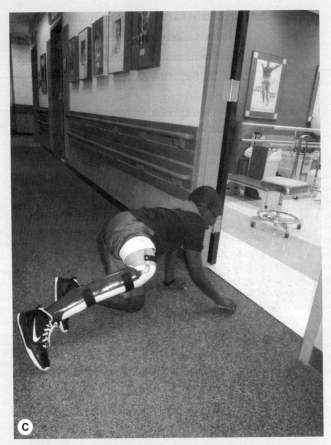

Figure 25-1. (*Continued*) **C.** Child transitioning from floor to stand wearing the extension prosthesis. Note that the external knee hinges are in alignment with the right anatomical knee. His right foot is incorporated into the lower section of the extension prosthesis. The height of the prosthesis is measured to equal that of the left uninvolved lower limb. To accommodate for the child's vertical growth, the prosthesis will be lengthened by adding height at the end of the prosthesis above the attachment of the prosthetic foot.

KEY DEFINITIONS

FEMORAL OSTEOTOMY: Surgical procedure to restore normal anatomy of the hip and provide optimal joint alignment[1]

LIMB LENGTHENING: Process of growing new bone and soft tissue through gradually lengthening the shortened limb; most common method is the application of an external fixator device that incorporates thin wires, thicker pins, and pins with screws to provide gradual distraction[2]

PROXIMAL FEMORAL FOCAL DEFICIENCY (PFFD): Rare congenital limb deficiency with hypoplasia or absence of the proximal femur[3]; exact cause is unknown, but is thought to be in utero maldevelopment of chondrocytes in the proximal femur with acetabular involvement[4]; clinical presentation varies from a short femoral segment with a normal acetabulum to short or absent femur and acetabulum[5]

ROTATIONPLASTY: Surgical procedure in which the tibia is rotated 180° so that the toes point posteriorly allowing the anatomical ankle to function as the knee in order to create a below-knee amputation level[5]

SYME AMPUTATION: Ankle disarticulation; in children with more significant presentation of PFFD, this procedure creates a functional above-the-knee amputation.[5]

Objectives

1. Identify the classifications of PFFD.

2. Identify surgical, prosthetic, orthotic, and physical therapy treatment options for equalizing leg length discrepancies.

3. Describe physical therapy goals preoperatively and postoperatively for the different surgical procedures aimed to equalize limb length.

4. Design an appropriate physical therapy program for a patient undergoing a lengthening procedure with an external fixator.

5. Develop an appropriate physical therapy program for a patient undergoing rotationplasty.

Physical Therapy Considerations

PT considerations for management of the child with PFFD:

▶ **General physical therapy plan of care/goals:** Equalize limb length by ongoing monitoring of limb length discrepancy with recommendations for appropriate height of shoe lift; support the development of symmetrical movements through physical therapy interventions and by equalizing limb lengths until definitive surgical decisions are made; increase strength of involved lower extremity and core musculature; during limb lengthening, increase range of motion (ROM) in joints above and below involved section of bone; maintain weightbearing precautions; increase independent functional mobility with assistive devices as indicated throughout each phase of intervention; promote participation in age-appropriate activities

▶ **Physical therapy interventions:** Patient and caregiver training on active and passive ROM to involved limb, bed mobility, transfers, use of assistive devices, exercises to improve strength and ROM, pin care, and scar management; pin and wound care during phases of external fixation; general strengthening and conditioning exercises; education on diagnosis and possible surgical, orthotic, prosthetic, and therapy interventions; patient and family education on home therapy program and precautions

▶ **Precautions during physical therapy:** Osteopenia, which increases risk of fractures; pin site infection; hypertrophic scarring; loss of ROM; muscle atrophy; increased risk of falls; decreased overall conditioning

▶ **Complications during physical therapy:** Fractures at lengthening site, pin site infection, emotional lability related to multiple surgeries, fear of movement and falls

Understanding the Health Condition

Proximal femoral focal deficiency (PFFD) is a rare congenital anomaly character-ized by failure of normal development of the proximal femur and hip joint. The clinical classification is defined by the degree of hip involvement and femoral short-ening.[6] There are several classification schemes for PFFD. The most commonly cited is the Aitken classification that classifies PFFD into four types: A, B, C, and D (Fig. 25-2). The femoral head is present in A and B, but absent in C and D. Types A and B are differentiated by the degree of femoral shortening and disconnection between the head and shaft of the femur, known as a pseudoarthrosis. The degree of acetabular dysplasia differentiates types C and D. Type D is the most severe form with significantly shortened femur and absent femoral head and acetabulum.[5] To compare the diagnosis of congenital short femur to that of PFFD, individuals with congenital short femur present with femoral shortening, but with normal hip development.[6]

Children with PFFD have unique physical characteristics that vary depend-ing on the severity of the condition. Characteristics include: shortened limb, thick bulbous thigh that has a ship's funnel appearance, abducted and flexed femoral seg-ment, and possibly a longitudinal deficiency of the fibula.[7] Associated impairments may include: knee instability with absence of the cruciate ligaments, genu valgus, fibula deficiency with talocalcaneal coalition and foot deformity, bilateral PFFD, and associated upper limb anomalies (Fig. 25-3).[5] Bilateral PFFD poses additional challenges for the child as well as the medical and surgical team.

The goal of surgical and prosthetic management for PFFD is to improve functional ambulation based on the degree of hip and knee stability, femoral shortening, and condition of the foot and ankle. Reconstruction of the hip joint with pelvic and femo-ral osteotomies may be possible in mild cases. Before considering limb lengthening or more definitive surgical interventions such as rotationplasty or Syme amputation,

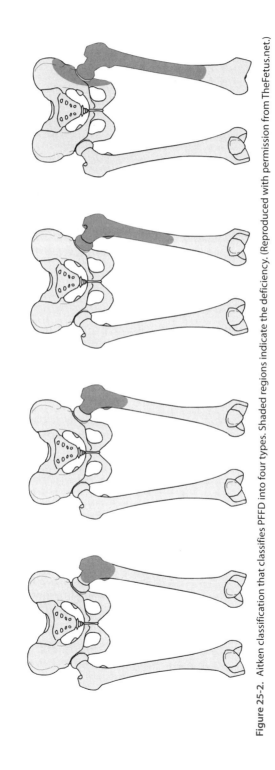

Figure 25-2. Aitken classification that classifies PFFD into four types. Shaded regions indicate the deficiency. (Reproduced with permission from TheFetus.net.)

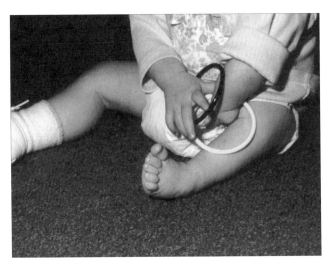

Figure 25-3. A 14-month-old female with left Aitken Type B PFFD and longitudinal deficiency of the fibula, complete. Note the associated left upper extremity longitudinal deficiency of the radius and ulna, incomplete, and carpal and metacarpal deficiencies.

achieving optimal hip alignment is recommended.[6] Therefore, a femoral osteotomy to obtain optimal hip alignment typically *precedes* the surgical options that address the limb length discrepancy. There are three main surgical options for individuals with PFFD: (1) femoral osteotomy with staged limb lengthenings; (2) femoral osteotomy, knee fusion, and Syme amputation (creating an above-knee prosthetic functional level; Fig. 25-4); and (3) femoral osteotomy with tibia rotationplasty (Fig. 25-5).

Prostheses and orthoses are used before and after surgery for PFFD.[5,7] Pre-operatively, shoe lifts with or without an ankle-foot orthosis (AFO) are used to equalize the limb length discrepancy. The higher the shoe lift, the heavier the shoe will be. Thus, an AFO is often prescribed to offer ankle stability for a young child with a significant length discrepancy that requires a shoe lift. Extension prostheses that incorporate the entire limb (containing the hip, knee, and foot) may be used. Whenever possible, the extension prosthesis should incorporate a knee joint to allow the patient to use knee function for crawling and walking and transitioning into and out of upright postures (Fig. 25-1C) and to obtain pelvic symmetry when walking or playing in kneeling and half-kneeling (Figs. 25-6 and 25-7). Last, orthoses are used for bracing of fractures. After a Syme amputation, a knee disarticulation prosthesis is used because the end of the child's residual limb is near or at the level of the contralateral knee, which necessitates an above-the-knee functioning prosthesis (Fig. 25-8). After a rotationplasty, a below-the-knee level prosthesis is made possible by using the anatomical foot and ankle to create a functional knee to power the prosthetic knee (Fig. 25-9).

The patient in this case was diagnosed with right PFFD, Aitken B classification, and absent cruciate ligaments creating both hip and knee instability. He underwent femoral valgus osteotomy to correct the hip deformity followed by two staged limb

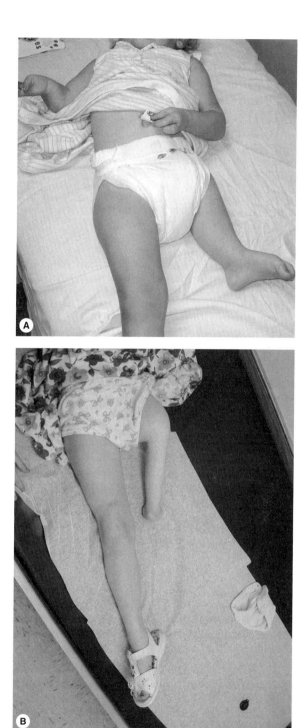

Figure 25-4. Young female with left Aitken Type C PFFD and associated bilateral upper limb deficiencies. **A.** Presurgery. **B.** 2 months after Syme amputation without knee fusion. The anatomical position of the left distal residual limb is at the level of the right knee offering the patient an above-the-knee prosthetic function. Note the classic physical characteristics of the left hip: flexion, external rotation, and adduction, and shaped like a "ship's funnel."

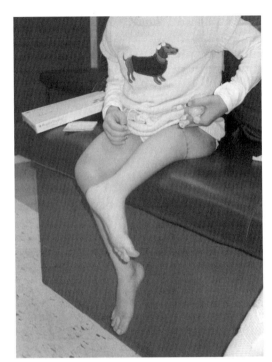

Figure 25-5. An 8-year-old female with left Aitken Type B PFFD 3 months after rotationplasty. Note the anatomical left ankle is at the level of the right knee and will function to control the prosthetic knee.

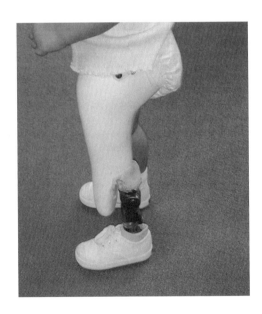

Figure 25-6. A 2-year-old female with left Aitken Type C PFFD wearing an extension prosthesis with a prosthetic knee. The leg length discrepancy was large enough to incorporate a prosthetic knee rather than using external knee hinges because the length offered adequate space.

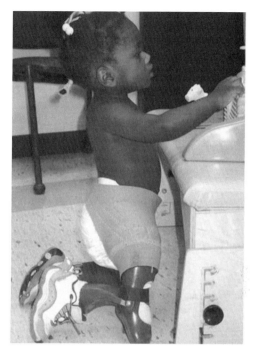

Figure 25-7. A 2.5-year-old female with Aitken Type C PFFD with an extension prosthesis that provides knee function by incorporating external knee hinges. By offering knee flexion, the child can assume tall kneeling and half-kneeling positions with control and balance and use her upper extremities for play.

lengthenings. Unfortunately, he had complications that prevented further lengthening, leaving a 6-inch limb length discrepancy and osteopenia. Deciding against additional limb lengthening surgeries, the family and patient instead chose to pursue a rotationplasty sometime in the future.

Fowler et al.[8] compared lower limb kinematics and kinetics in children diagnosed with PFFD following rotationplasty or Syme amputation. When tested at preferred and faster walking speeds, children with a 180° rotationplasty of the tibia demonstrated significantly improved prosthetic knee function during stance (*i.e.*, they were able to support a flexed-knee posture at both speeds) and produced greater knee-extensor moments at preferred speeds compared to the Syme group. The authors also compared compensations in the noninvolved limb. Those with the Syme amputation, knee disarticulation functional level demonstrated significantly greater compensations that included: stance phase vaulting, greater inappropriate ankle-power generation at both tested walking speeds, excessive hip-power absorption and generation at both speeds, and excessive knee-joint power generation at both speeds. The authors concluded that the **improved gait pattern noted in the subjects with rotationplasty should be a contributing factor when making surgical decisions for children with PFFD.**[8]

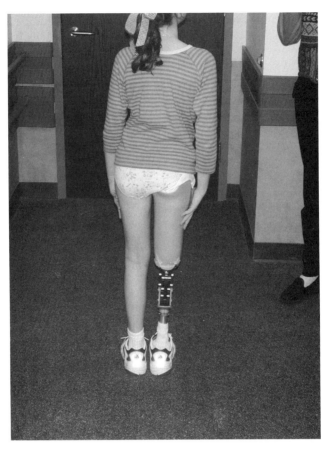

Figure 25-8. A 10-year-old female with Aitken Type B PFFD. At age 3, she underwent femoral osteotomy and then had a Syme amputation with knee fusion at age 4.

Physical Therapy Patient/Client Management

A child with PFFD requires a multidisciplinary team in a center specializing in the treatment of children with limb deficiencies. The resources and specializations of the institution will define the members of the team.[7] The Limb Deficiency team usually consists of an orthopaedic surgeon, prosthetist, orthotist, physical therapist, occupational therapist, nurse, social worker, and psychologist. The **physical therapist's role in all stages of treatment**—no matter the surgical procedure—is to evaluate the patient's functional limitations and to create a comprehensive treatment plan to improve all areas of impairment including balance, strength, ROM, sensation, and skin integrity. The plan of care will include gait training, wound care, pin site care during limb lengthening, edema control, strength training, stretching, and, most importantly, patient and family education. Throughout the episode of care, it is imperative for the physical therapist to consistently inform other members

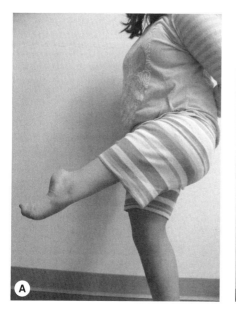
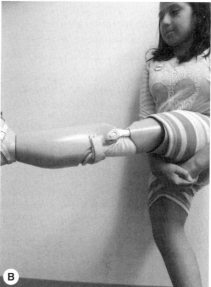
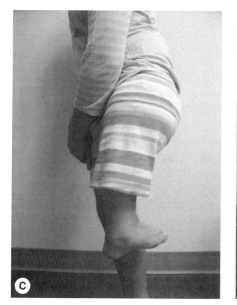
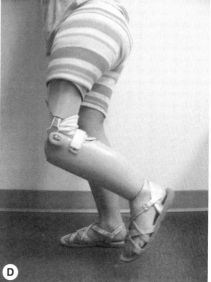

Figure 25-9. A 10-year-old female diagnosed with left PFFD Aitken C following rotationplasty of the left femur. **A.** Plantar flexion of the left anatomical foot controls prosthetic knee extension **B,** while dorsiflexion **C,** controls prosthetic knee flexion **D.**

of the medical team regarding the patient's functional gains as well as any setbacks related to skin integrity, contractures, and pain. Consistent and timely communication helps minimize obstacles and complications and promotes maximum functional gains for the patient.[9]

Examination, Evaluation, and Diagnosis

A thorough chart review prior to assessment should provide information regarding the classification and extent of the patient's limb deficiency, predicted leg length discrepancy at skeletal maturity, surgical procedures performed and any future procedures planned, complications of surgery, and weightbearing restrictions, if applicable. During the patient interview, the therapist should gain an understanding of the patient and family's short- and long-term goals and the decision making that has motivated them to pursue surgical lengthening. Whether the child has had a limb lengthening or rotationplasty procedure, the objective examination includes evaluation of strength, ROM, gait pattern, skin integrity, sensation of the lower extremities, posture, and limb length. Because limb lengthening can be a painful process, it is important for the therapist to be cognizant of the patient's pain level when performing assessments.[10]

Manual muscle testing on a 6-point scale (*i.e.*, 0-5) is a clinical standard method of isometric strength testing.[11] Strength testing of the trunk, hips, knees, ankles, and feet is important in creating an effective treatment plan and identifying those areas that will require particular attention during the course of treatment.

Goniometric ROM measurements are taken for both the involved and uninvolved extremities with particular focus on the hip, knee, and ankle because hip and knee contractures and pelvic and lumbar obliquities are very common during and after limb lengthening. It is important to differentiate between joint hypomobility and soft tissue and muscular shortening so that treatment methods are tailored accordingly.[10]

The therapist can assess gait with a variety of methods including video and observational analysis over level ground, a treadmill, uneven surfaces, and stairs. Radiographs will be taken at regular intervals throughout the limb lengthening process and the orthopaedic surgeon determines the weightbearing status. Typically during limb lengthening, patients are gradually progressed from partial weightbearing (PWB) to weightbearing as tolerated (WBAT) with careful monitoring of bone regeneration and consolidation by x-rays taken throughout the lengthening and consolidation phases.[12] Once the external fixator is removed, the patient will be nonweightbearing (NWB) on the operative limb until adequate bone consolidation has occurred. Both prior to and during lengthening, patients may use a rolling walker or axillary crutches in conjunction with a shoe lift for support during gait. In certain cases, an AFO may also be indicated to provide medial-lateral stability instead of a significant shoe lift.[10] To thoroughly assess gait pattern, the therapist should assess gait with and without the patient's assistive device/s (as weightbearing precautions allow). Any compensatory movement should be noted and an assessment of spinal mobility in static and dynamic standing should also be performed to better differentiate the causative factors of gait deviations.

After a limb lengthening procedure, the physical therapist should assess the skin integrity at the pin sites. Assessment of drainage, tissue formation, odor, and skin temperature are important measures to establish a baseline and monitor for infection during the course of treatment. The distal involved extremity should be consistently monitored for the presence of edema, neuropathy, and paresthesias.[10] Circumferential limb measurements are one method used to monitor for edema. Sensory testing for light touch, sharp/dull, and discrimination must be performed following surgical lengthening procedures because the repeated incisions, bony deformity, and fractures that occur during the lengthening process can affect the patient's neural feedback and sensation.[10,11]

The child's posture should be assessed in prone, supine, sitting, and standing with particular attention paid to obliquities and rotation noted in the spine, pelvis, shoulders, and upper extremities. Limb length can be assessed in one of three ways. First, the therapist can ask the patient to stand with blocks or orthotic lifts placed beneath the affected side until the pelvis is level. When this is achieved, the total height of the blocks or lift is measured. In children with hip and knee flexion contractures, this standing measurement method is inaccurate.[13] In an alternative method with the patient supine, the therapist measures the length of the lower extremity from either the anterior superior iliac spine (ASIS) to the medial malleolus or the ASIS to the lateral malleolus. Last, limb length can be measured via a scanogram, in which a radiograph is taken with a ruler parallel to the patient's legs so the length of the femur and tibia can be measured separately.

Since this child and his family chose the surgical option of femoral osteotomy with tibia rotationplasty to be performed at a future date, the physical therapist should be aware that the physical therapy literature is scarce on examination, evaluation, and interventions for patients who elect rotationplasty to correct the deformities and leg length difference in PFFD. Just as with the limb lengthening procedure, the physical therapist should have a thorough understanding of the specific surgical procedure and location of the rotational osteotomy. Depending on the surgeon, the patient may be placed in a body spica cast or a semi-rigid dressing for 6 to 8 weeks after surgery to stabilize the osteotomy at the site of the rotation.[14] Whether immediately after surgery or post-cast removal, the physical therapist should perform a thorough evaluation of the surgical incision, sensation, circulation, swelling, and active ROM. In rotationplasty, there is a risk for sensory compromise and hypersensitivity of the foot and ankle due to rotation of the neurovascular structures along with the bones. It is not uncommon for patients to have additional surgeries after the initial rotationplasty.[5,14] Massage and elastic bandage-wrapping of the involved limb are recommended for edema control and hypersensitivity.[9]

For optimal prosthetic fit and function, it is necessary to gain ankle and foot active and passive ROM as soon as possible after surgery. To functionally operate prosthetic knee flexion, 0° to 30° of ankle dorsiflexion and 50° to 60° of plantar flexion beyond neutral are required. The greater the plantar flexion ROM (*i.e.*, "ballerina foot"), the more streamlined the anatomical foot can be aligned within the prosthesis.[7,9,14] Strength of the anatomical foot, ankle, and toes powers the prosthetic knee. The physical therapist can instruct the patient in isometric strengthening exercises for the hip, ankle, foot, and toes at any time after surgery.[5,9] Once approved for weightbearing, prosthetic fitting is initiated. Fabricating a prosthesis for a child with rotationplasty requires a prosthetist that has knowledge, expertise, and skill in treating children with PFFD.

Plan of Care and Interventions

The plan of care focuses on: gait, flexibility, strength, and skin care to improve the patient's functional mobility and independence while minimizing secondary complications including contractures, infections, and fractures.[9,10,12] Important components of the physical therapy treatment plan include a comprehensive home program encouraging weightbearing, pain management strategies, pre-gait and gait training activities, and activities to improve strength and joint ROM.

Strengthening and ROM activities need to be developmentally appropriate and incorporate the patient's interests and account for weightbearing restrictions. Strengthening activities can include active assisted and isometric exercises as well as age-appropriate functional activities including negotiating playground surfaces and riding a bike as appropriate within clinical precautions. Additional activities may include propelling a scooter board while seated, negotiating an obstacle course, ascending/descending steps, using a therapy ball to increase core and trunk strength, and participating in supervised dynamic balance activities.[15]

Following fixator removal, contractures can persist and require conservative and/or surgical intervention. ROM is usually addressed most effectively with low-load prolonged stretching including bracing and splinting, if appropriate.[10,12,15] Physical therapists can use a variety of splints to address knee flexion contractures.[15] Bracing may be most effective after fixator removal because it is often difficult to cast at the knee while the patient is undergoing lengthening. Modalities including ice and electrical stimulation can be incorporated to assist in improving ROM and pain management.[15,16] Baker et al.[16] assessed knee ROM of 35 individuals (mean age 22 ± 12.8 years) who underwent limb lengthening. Measurements were taken preoperatively, immediately after surgical placement of Ilizarov external fixator before initiation of limb lengthening, during lengthening, and 6 and 12 months postsurgical removal of the external fixator. When assessing knee ROM, 76% of the range was lost immediately after surgery during the pre-lengthening period after application of the external fixator. Full knee ROM was achieved in 88% of the patients at 6 months post-fixator removal, 92% at 12 months, and 97% at 18 months. The authors concluded that physical therapy efforts should focus on the immediate postoperative period *before* initiation of limb lengthening to quickly recover joint motion and minimize anticipated muscle-related challenges during limb lengthening.

Gait training is unique with a patient following rotationplasty. Gait progression must follow weightbearing restrictions and patient's tolerance. Progression of weightbearing and initiation of prosthetic fitting after rotationplasty depends on bone healing of the osteotomy site. Following external fixator placement, patients typically are restricted to PWB for a short period of time and then progress to WBAT with an assistive device such as axillary crutches or a rolling walker for mobility (depending on the orthopaedic surgeon and patient's preferences). During the acute episode of care following placement of the external fixator, the physical therapist must work on normalizing components of the patient's gait such as heel-toe contact and knee extension during stance phase with the shoe lift donned.

Once the patient is cleared for full weightbearing or WBAT, the physical therapist can begin gait training over level ground or over a treadmill using a weight support harness to focus on appropriate trunk alignment and technique during the stance and swing phases. Due to the prolonged limb-lengthening period, additional gait training may be indicated because the patient may have become habituated to use an assistive device, shoe lift, and compensatory positions and movement patterns. Frequently, the patient will require minor adjustments to his shoe lift to maintain comfort as lengthening proceeds. It is essential for the therapist to regularly communicate with the orthotist and orthopaedic surgeon to make sure that all concerns are addressed during this period. Patients undergoing limb lengthening or post–limb lengthening also require continual monitoring and adjustment of orthotic devices, such as orthotic inserts or shoe lifts to encourage a normalized gait pattern.[9,10]

A unique and important aspect of physical therapy treatment in this patient population is pin care. Pin care includes the cleaning and dressing of the unilateral or Ilizarov fixator pin sites. Although the orthopaedic surgeon or wound team directs the method for pin care, the physical therapist often performs the wound care, depending on the facility's regulations.

The patient presented in this case is 9.5 years old and still has to face the pubertal challenges of growth and progressing limb length discrepancy. The rotationplasty will be scheduled during his summer break when he is 10 years old. Education to the patient and his family is imperative *before* the Van Nes rotationplasty procedure is scheduled. The plan of care should incorporate preoperative and postoperative evaluations. Timing of prosthetic fitting and gait training depends on the patient's bone healing and tolerance to touch and pressure that is required to wear a prosthesis. The therapist initiates gait training in the prosthesis by teaching the child how to move the prosthetic knee with the anatomical foot. Teaching him how to sit, kneel, and transition into upright positions is just as important as teaching him how to walk.[9] Gait training and upright activities should be age-appropriate and based on the child's wishes and desires. Assistive devices may be needed as the child gains proximal hip strength as well as the strength to power the prosthetic knee with the anatomical foot, ankle, and toes. Children with PFFD who have rotationplasty may demonstrate residual hip weakness regardless of the intensity of strengthening performed due to the degree of hip involvement from the severity of PFFD.

In a recent study, Akman et al.[3] investigated the **long-term effects of 12 patients who had rotationplasty due to PFFD** compared to age-matched controls who did not have PFFD or orthopaedic conditions. The researchers used well-established tools to measure quality of life, pain, posture and alignment, and movement efficiency. The authors concluded that there were no differences in overall health and well-being between the two groups, but found significant deficits in gait parameters and postural symmetry in the children that had rotationplasty. The authors concluded that regardless of the residual deficits in gait and posture, rotationplasty should be considered as a viable option for select children with unilateral PFFD.[3]

Evidence-Based Clinical Recommendations

SORT: Strength of Recommendation Taxonomy

A: Consistent, good-quality patient-oriented evidence

B: Inconsistent or limited-quality patient-oriented evidence

C: Consensus, disease-oriented evidence, usual practice, expert opinion, or case series

1. In individuals with PFFD, those who have rotationplasty demonstrate fewer gait compensations compared to those who have Syme amputation. In individuals with PFFD, the surgical option of rotationplasty surgery offers below the knee amputation level function compared to Syme amputation that provides above the knee amputation level function requiring a prosthetic knee. **Grade B**

2. Physical therapy plays an important role in the postsurgical management (*i.e.*, after limb lengthening, rotationplasty, or Syme amputation) of children with PFFD. **Grade C**

3. Rotationplasty is a viable surgical option for select children with PFFD. **Grade B**

COMPREHENSION QUESTIONS

25.1 The most common first intervention for a 14-month-old toddler with left Aitken Type C PFFD is:

A. Surgical amputation of the left foot with knee fusion

B. Shoe lift with AFO

C. Extension prosthesis with prosthetic knee

D. Femoral osteotomy with knee fusion

25.2 What is the most appropriate inpatient physical therapy intervention for a 6-year-old male immediately after limb lengthening and application of unilateral external fixator?

A. Active and active assisted hip, knee, and ankle ROM, bed mobility and transfers, and weightbearing to tolerance using assistive device

B. Bed mobility and transfers with nonweightbearing gait using assistive device. Hip, knee, and ankle ROM to be initiated one week after surgery during the first acute outpatient physical therapy session and following initiation of lengthening

C. Passive ROM only, bed mobility and transfers, and nonweightbearing 3-point gait

D. Active ROM within pain tolerance, bed mobility and transfers, nonweightbearing 3-point gait until patient is pain-free

ANSWERS

25.1 **C.** Equalizing limb lengths and offering the patient knee function is important for "normalizing" development. Equal limb lengths and knee function will allow the toddler to transition into and out of sitting and standing using prosthetic knee function. With equal limb lengths, movements can be more symmetrical with decreased compensations of circumduction and vaulting because the toddler can flex the prosthetic knee during transitions and when playing in tall and half-kneeling versus standing.

25.2 **A.** Literature supports the importance of early active and active-assisted ROM immediately after surgery even before initiation of limb lengthening. Early weightbearing to tolerance is important to promote bone healing. When the patient's pain is under control with or without medication, progression to full weightbearing can occur when the external fixator is in place. Once the external fixator is removed, the bone may not be fully consolidated, which necessitates partial weightbearing until the orthopaedic surgeon approves full weightbearing.

REFERENCES

1. Louahem M'sahah D, Assi C, Cottalorda J. Proximal femoral osteotomies in children. *Orthop Traumatol Surg Res*. 2013; 99:S171-S186.

2. Limb lengthening and deformity correction for adults and children. http://www.limblengthening. com. Accessed December 31, 2014.

3. Akman J, Altiok H, Flanagan A, et al. Long-term follow-up of Van Nes rotationplasty in patients with congenital proximal focal femoral deficiency. *Bone Joint J*. 2013;95-B:192-198.

4. Coskun G, Apaydin M, Varer M, Sarsilmaz A, Uluc E. Proximal femoral focal deficiency. *Eur J Rad Extra*. 2010;76:e99-e101.

5. Guidera K, Novick C, Marshall J. Femoral deficiencies. In: Smith DG, Michael JW, Bowker JH, eds. *Atlas of Amputations and Limb Deficiencies Surgical, Prosthetic and Rehabilitation Principles*. 3rd ed. Rosemont, IL: American Academy of Orthopaedic Surgeons; 2004:905-916.

6. Westberry DE, Davids JR. Proximal focal femoral deficiency (PFFD): management options and controversies. *Hip Int*. 2009;19:S18-S25.

7. Morrissy R, Giavedoni B, Coulter-O'Berry. The Child with a Limb Deficiency. In: Morrissy R, Weinstein S, eds. *Lovell and Winter's Pediatric Orthopaedics*. 3rd ed. Philadelphia, PA: Lippincott, Williams, and Wilkins; 2006:1329-1382.

8. Fowler EG, Hester DM, Oppenheim WL, Setoguchi Y, Zernicke RF. Contrasts in gait mechanics of individuals with proximal femoral focal deficiency: Syme amputation versus Van Nes rotational osteotomy. *J Pediatr Orthop*. 1999;19:720-731.

9. Coulter-O'Berry C. Physical therapy. In: Smith DG, Michael JW, Bowker JH, eds. *Atlas of Amputations and Limb Deficiencies Surgical, Prosthetic and Rehabilitation Principles*. 3rd ed. Rosemont, IL: American Academy of Orthopaedic Surgeons; 2004:831-840.

10. Simard S, Marchant M, Mencio G. The Ilizarov procedure: limb lengthening and its implications. *Phys Ther*. 1992;72:25-34.

11. American Physical Therapy Association. Guide to Physical Therapist Practice. *Phys Ther*. 1997;77:1163-1650.

12. Coglianese DB, Herzenberg JE, Goulet JA. Physical therapy management of patients undergoing limb lengthening by distraction osteogenesis. *J Orthop Sports Phys Ther.* 1993;17:124-132.

13. Leach J. Orthopedic conditions. In: Campbell S, Vander Linden D, Palisano R, eds. *Physical Therapy for Children.* St. Louis, MO: Saunders/Elsevier; 2006.

14. Gupta SK, Alassaf N, Harrop AR, Kiefer GN. Principles of rotationplasty. *J Am Acad Orthop Surg.* 2012;20:657-667.

15. Paley Advanced Limb Lengthening Institute. www.paleyinstitute.org. Accessed December 31, 2014.

16. Baker KL, Simpson AH, Lamb SE. Loss of knee range of motion in limb lengthening. *J Orthop Sports Phys Ther.* 2001;31:238-246.

Relapsed Clubfoot

Maureen Donohoe

A physical therapist is examining a 5-year-old boy who was born with bilateral idiopathic clubfeet. As an infant, his feet presented in forefoot adduction and hindfoot plantar flexion. He was treated conservatively with the Ponseti method with excellent results. He had weekly progressive serial casting for six of the first eight weeks of his life. At 8 weeks of age, bilateral percutaneous Achilles tenotomies were performed and he was casted for three weeks. At 11 weeks of age, he began wearing a foot abduction brace consisting of an adjustable length metal bar with footplates onto which a pair of boots is attached. The wearing schedule was 23 hours per day for the first six weeks and decreased to 18 hours per day for an additional six weeks. When the child wears the brace, the lower extremities are abducted and the feet are externally rotated. This position helps maintain the stretch created by the serial casting and tenotomy procedure. From the age of 6 months to 4 years, he has worn the foot abduction brace for 10 to 12 hours each night. The boy was able to stand on his own without holding onto an external surface by the age of 12 months and ambulated without assistance by 13 months. Six months prior to the physical therapy examination, he discontinued the use of the foot abduction brace. In the two months prior to the examination, he experienced a significant growth spurt and has been ambulating haphazardly and falling more frequently. His mother took him to see an orthopaedic surgeon, who felt his left foot was beginning to demonstrate clubfoot relapse. On the left, end range dorsiflexion and forefoot abduction were limited (both motions approximately 10° shy of neutral). On the right, dorsiflexion measured approximately 10° and forefoot abduction was roughly 15°. The plantar surface of the left foot was also "bean-shaped." The surgeon decided that the left lower extremity should be serial casted to improve alignment. Following completion of serial casting, the child was referred to physical therapy.

- ▶ What are the most appropriate examination tests?
- ▶ What are the examination priorities?
- ▶ What are the most appropriate outcome measures for range of motion (ROM), muscle strength, and gross motor skills for this age range?
- ▶ Describe a physical therapy plan of care based on the present level of function.
- ▶ Identify referrals to other team members.

KEY DEFINITIONS

FOOT ABDUCTION BRACE: Straight-laced shoes or boots connected via an attachment to a bar, allowing the lower extremities to be held in up to 70° of hip external rotation as well as 10° of ankle dorsiflexion

IDIOPATHIC CLUBFOOT: Foot deformity apparent at birth with no associated underlying diagnosis; foot has a high longitudinal arch associated with plantar flexed first ray, bean-shaped curved appearance with inability to correct forefoot to neutral from its adducted posture, and varus hindfoot that cannot be passively dorsiflexed to neutral.

PONSETI METHOD: Intervention for clubfoot correction involving a specific serial casting technique to realign the talus in the talocrural joint. After several above-knee casts, a percutaneous tendo Achilles lengthening procedure is performed to achieve full correction of the foot. After surgical realignment of the foot, the joint is casted for 3 weeks and then the child wears a foot abduction brace. Initially, the child wears the brace 23 hours per day for 3 months and then gradually reduces wear to 10 to 12 hours per day, up to the age of 5 years.

RELAPSED CLUBFOOT: Clubfoot that has previously been corrected (allowing forefoot abduction and hindfoot dorsiflexion past neutral), but has tightened through growth and change and can no longer achieve a neutral alignment

Objectives

1. Identify the signs and symptoms of a clubfoot.
2. Identify valid and reliable outcome measures to assess muscle strength and endurance in children with clubfoot.
3. Recognize gross motor deficits that may be associated with clubfoot.
4. Understand the medical treatments for clubfoot and their relevance to physical therapy management.
5. Design an appropriate physical therapy program for a child with relapsed clubfoot.

Physical Therapy Considerations

PT considerations during management of the child with relapsed clubfoot deformity:

▶ **General physical therapy plan of care/goals:** Improve ROM; improve great toe extension while first ray is held in neutral dorsiflexion; improve balance and strength; improve gait pattern; identify risk of clubfoot relapse; identify and address gross motor deficits as compared to age-matched peers

▶ **Physical therapy interventions:** Patient/family education regarding clubfeet and the risk of joint contracture development and asymmetrical muscle strength;

monitor progress with valid and objective outcome measures; therapeutic exercises to address muscular tightness and weakness; home program instruction

▶ **Precautions during physical therapy interventions:** Stress fracture prevention after serial casting; avoidance of high impact activities such as running, jumping, and hopping; identify and prevent compensatory strategies during higher level balance and weightbearing activities.

▶ **Complications interfering with physical therapy:** Stress fractures

Understanding the Health Condition

Idiopathic clubfoot is an equinovarus foot deformity of unknown origin that is present at birth. The hindfoot is positioned in plantar flexion and the forefoot is adducted beyond neutral alignment. The equinovarus position of the foot is a result of rotation of the talus medially on the calcaneus. Although the talus has no muscular attachments, many ligaments attach it to the bones surrounding it. As a result of the rotated talus, the fetal foot grows with a shortened longitudinal arch of the foot, also known as the medial column. This results in an elongation of the tissues on the lateral aspect of the foot, an area known as the lateral column. The elongated lateral column puts the fibularis muscles at a biomechanical disadvantage to work. The asymmetrical muscular pull (lengthened lateral muscles and shortened medial muscles) decreases the foot's ability to remain in a forefoot neutral alignment. Due to the medial rotation of the talus, the first ray tends to plantar flex and retract, and the base of the fifth metatarsal becomes prominent on the lateral surface of the foot.[1,2]

After initial correction of the clubfoot with the Ponseti method, it is recommended that the child wear a foot abduction brace for up to five years. This brace helps to hold the foot on stretch along the medial column of the foot. **Noncompliance with wearing the brace** is closely associated with recurrence of clubfoot deformity.[3-5] In a 2007 study with 51 babies with clubfeet, noncompliance was almost 50%. Those who did not adhere to the bracing protocol were five times more likely to have a relapse compared to children who regularly wore the brace.[6]

The **first indication of clubfoot relapse** is increased intoeing during stance phase of gait. Intoeing is noted with midstance that occurs through the lateral foot and increased weightbearing through the first ray during pushoff.[7-11] Intoeing will progress to early heel rise after initial foot contact. Eventually, if left untreated, there will be no heel strike during initial foot contact during gait.

In static standing, the child with a clubfoot may exhibit a foot flat posture with evidence of genu recurvatum because he must work to keep the foot flat on the floor in the absence of end range dorsiflexion.[11] Dynamically, squatting activities are limited because the child will have early heel rise with weight shift onto the uninvolved side into the squat position (Fig. 26-1). Persistent clubfoot can lead to secondary complications of weakness in the hip and the knee muscles due to compensatory strategies.

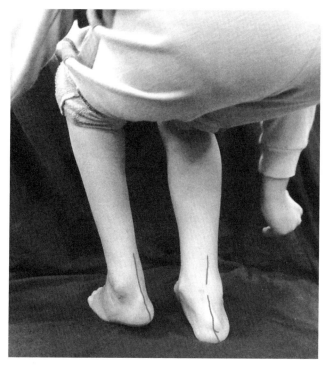

Figure 26-1. Child with left clubfoot squatting. Notice weight shift to the uninvolved right side and inability to maintain the foot flat on the involved side.

Physical Therapy Patient/Client Management

Physical therapy considerations during management of the child with clubfoot deformity include addressing body structures and function as well as how those limitations impact the child's participation. The deficits in ROM and strength can impact how a child performs gross motor skills when compared to typically developing peers.[12-16] Management of the child with relapsing clubfoot is improved using a multidisciplinary team approach. The team includes an orthopaedic surgeon, physical therapist, and orthotist. The physical therapist works with the patient, family, and team to provide objective assessment of the patient's specific functional abilities and impairments (*e.g.*, muscle strength, flexibility, and endurance). The overall goal is to maximize strength in order to help hold ideal alignment of the foot or to prepare the foot for a successful muscle transfer in the future, monitor change in status over time, and develop an appropriate physical therapy regimen that promotes optimal physical function and quality of life. Physical therapy treatments may include stretching, strengthening, higher-level balance skills, gait training, aerobic training, and ongoing education to the patient, family/caregivers, and possibly educators or administrators at the patient's school.

Examination, Evaluation, and Diagnosis

Prior to seeing the patient, the physical therapist needs to obtain information regarding the patient's current medical status and relevance to the physical therapy plan. If available, review of the medical chart will give information on course of treatment and radiographic information. If the chart is unavailable, a detailed parent and child interview should explore the child's birth history and past and current medical management of the clubfeet, as well as developmental milestones. Questions should include information regarding changes in function over the past few months and the goals of the child and his family. Baseline vital signs as well as distal pulses are part of a comprehensive initial examination.

The priorities of the examination are ROM and strength as they impact postural alignment. Formal testing for functional measures should be done to establish noted deficits compared to the lesser involved side as well as to typically developing peers. The objective examination begins with observation of gait. Evaluation of all phases of the gait cycle, especially the position of the feet during each stage, is essential. Various methods of gait assessment are helpful to the physical therapist.[7-10] The therapist can take a video of the child ambulating across a force plate and collect information about foot pressures.[2,11] Alternatively, the physical therapist may employ a low technology option such as having the child walk across brown paper with wet feet and document the alignment of the child's feet based on the footprint impressions. The Observational Gait Scale is a quick visual tool that requires no special equipment and yields objective measurements.[17] If the child wears orthoses, gait should be assessed with them on as well as in bare feet.

The child's posture and alignment should be assessed with attention to overall joint alignment, specifically at the knee and foot. The physical therapist observes the position of all aspects of the foot while the child is standing. The therapist should note whether the hindfoot is in varus (Fig. 26-2) with a plantar flexed first ray and/or if the great toe is in extension.[2,11]

ROM and flexibility should be thoroughly assessed. Limitations in children with clubfeet are most commonly seen in gastrocnemius and soleus muscles. Standard goniometry can be utilized to assess joint ROM. ROM is assessed bilaterally at the foot, ankle, knee, and hip with special attention to great toe extension, ankle dorsiflexion with knee flexed, ankle dorsiflexion with knee extended, and hamstring length. The degree of hindfoot varus or valgus can be measured in prone (Fig. 26-2) and in weightbearing (Fig. 26-3). The standard measurements for inversion and eversion are based on stabilization of the talus at the starting position. However, since the alignment of the talus is pathological in children with clubfoot, a more reliable and repeatable measure of forefoot flexibility is forefoot abduction and adduction. This measurement is performed in the frontal plane with the child in supine or sitting. The therapist measures abduction and adduction of the forefoot past neutral by aligning the stationary arm of the goniometer with the anterior tibia and the moving arm with the second ray of the foot.[2,18] Special tests, such as the Thomas test or prone knee flexion (for hip flexor tightness) and straight leg raise or popliteal angle (for hamstring tightness), should be performed to establish areas of asymmetry.

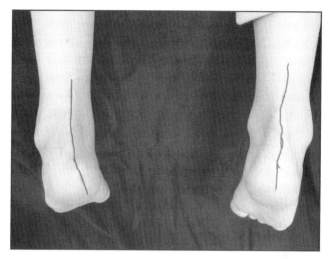

Figure 26-2. In prone position, the varus alignment of the left foot is still apparent in nonweightbearing.

During palpation of the foot and ankle, the therapist assesses the ability to passively attain a neutral hindfoot position and elevation of the first ray. For the child with relapsed clubfoot, single limb balance should not only be a timed outcome measure, but also an opportunity to evaluate the quality of the performance, since many strategies are used to substitute for mobility limitations at the ankle.[12] If the child wears orthoses, single limb balance should be assessed in and out of the braces. It is important for the physical therapist to assess wear patterns on the child's shoes, as they are typically asymmetrical. If orthoses are used to help manage the child's clubfoot deformity, the braces need to be assessed for fit, comfort, and control of the deformity.

If the child typically wears orthoses, functional skills should be assessed with these on. If the goal of therapy is to have the child transition away from wearing

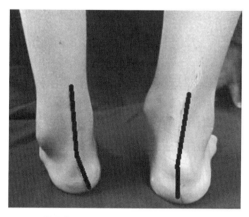

Figure 26-3. Varus alignment of left foot in standing position. The black lines start proximally on the Achilles tendon and run distally through the midpoint of the calcaneus.

Table 26-1 FUNCTIONAL MEASURES USED TO ASSESS FUNCTION IN CHILDREN WITH CLUBFOOT[20,21]				
Test	Purpose	Description	Time to Administer	Equipment Required
10-m walk test	Assess walking speed	Individual walks 10 m and is timed. This is performed for 3 trials and the average speed is recorded.	<5 min	Designated 10-m walk space Stopwatch
2-min walk test	Assess walking speed and distance	Individual walks for 2 min and the distance is measured.	<3 min	Area, such as a hallway, free of obstacles Stopwatch Tape measure or rolling measure
Timed Up and Go (TUG)	Assess mobility, balance, walking, and fall risk	Child starts in sitting position. Child is asked to stand, walk 3 m, turn around, and walk back to chair and sit down.	<3 min	Standard chair with arms Designated 3-m distance without obstacles Stopwatch
Single limb stance test	Assess ability to balance on one foot	With eyes open and hands on hips, child stands on one foot. Test ends when hands come off hips or foot touches ground.	<1 min	Stopwatch

orthoses, a baseline should include skills tested with and without orthoses. Table 26-1 shows common functional measures that physical therapists use in this population. Each of the measures takes less than five minutes to complete. To date, there are no normative data for these functional measures for individuals with clubfeet, but they have been used with typically developing children as well as children with Down syndrome and cerebral palsy. Based on the reliability and validity of these tools across multiple diagnoses, their use may be appropriate for the child with clubfoot.

To establish areas of delay as a result of the clubfoot, the therapist can administer the gross motor subsections of norm-referenced developmental tests. For example, the Peabody Developmental Motor Scales, Second edition (PDMS-2) is used to assess children birth to 5 years of age.[22] The gross motor assessment of the PDMS-2 includes three separate subsections (stationary skills, locomotion skills, and object manipulation). The stationary skills subsection assesses the child's balance skills and includes items that test the ability of the child to stand on one foot with hands on hips, and the ability to stand on tiptoes. The static and dynamic balance deficits exhibited by children with clubfeet may negatively impact these scores. In the locomotion skills section, special attention should be given to walking, running, walking on tiptoes, jumping, hopping, and skipping skills. In the object manipulation subsection, the ability to perform a step through pitch or to perform an age-appropriate kick of a ball may be negatively impacted by the clubfoot.

Last, muscle strength can be measured via manual muscle testing (MMT) using either the 6- or 11-point scales.[23]

Plan of Care and Interventions

During the examination, the physical therapist identified weakness in bilateral ankle dorsiflexors, including the anterior tibialis and fibularis muscles (left side weaker than right) and weakness in bilateral hip extensors and abductors (left side one muscle grade weaker than right). ROM limitations on the left side included: limited forefoot abduction and limited dorsiflexion, though dorsiflexion range was increased with the knee extended compared to with the knee flexed. When his left foot was held in end range dorsiflexion, his great toe could only extend to neutral. In a nonweightbearing posture, the child's first ray was in 40° of extension. The child could stand on his right foot for five seconds. However, when attempting to stand on his left foot, he was only able to briefly lift his right foot to clear his toes. He could hop twice on his right foot, but could not hop at all on his left foot. He was able to gallop leading with the left leg, but could not skip reciprocally. He was able to jump down from an 8-inch surface with his feet together. However, when jumping down from greater heights, he landed with more weight on the right foot than the left. When kicking a ball, he used a step-to pattern when kicking with his left foot. On stairs, he used a reciprocal pattern when ascending. When descending, he used a step-to pattern, leading with his left leg.

Physical therapy intervention should address these identified impairments. Therapeutic exercises are developed to address the muscular tightness on the medial side and weakness on the lateral side as they impact static and dynamic foot alignment. Muscle weakness is addressed through traditional active ROM activities, but children with clubfeet may also benefit from electrical stimulation for neuromuscular education.[24] Strengthening and stretching exercises should be done to the patient's tolerance. It is important to incorporate closed chain higher-level balance skills such as standing on one foot and hopping to help with developing rapid response of the muscles that were strengthened in open chain alignment.

Formal exercise protocols and physical therapy management for a relapsed clubfoot have not been published. However, the **French Physical Therapy method of clubfoot management** includes stretching, strengthening, and closed chain training that encompass the areas needed to support optimal alignment of the foot.[25] Originally designed as a nonsurgical approach to the treatment of clubfoot, the program entails daily stretching of shortened tissues, stimulation and strengthening of weakened muscles, and taping and splinting to maintain the positional correction of the child's affected foot.

Table 26-2 provides an example of an appropriate exercise program for a child attending physical therapy for clubfoot management. Special attention is necessary to train caregivers in stretching and strengthening activities. If the child is wearing the foot abduction brace at night, it is important to train the child to walk in the brace for two reasons. First, the ability to walk in the brace allows the child to get in and out of bed independently with the brace intact. Second, walking facilitates symmetrical weight shifts and balance on a daily basis at home.

Table 26-2	SAMPLE EXERCISE PROGRAM FOR A CHILD WITH A CLUBFOOT
Exercise	**Instructions**
Midfoot mobilization	Child sits in a chair or on edge of treatment table with his knee flexed. Therapist uses long axis distraction on each midtarsal joint. Anterior-posterior glides can be applied to mobilize joints prior to muscle stretching.
Stretch medial column of foot	Child sits in a chair or on edge of treatment table with his knee flexed. Therapist manually stretches midfoot by elongating soft tissue along longitudinal arch of the foot. Emphasis is placed on allowing first ray to dorsiflex.
Stretch hindfoot into dorsiflexion	Child sits in a chair or on edge of treatment table with his knee flexed. Therapist stabilizes the forefoot in neutral alignment and manually distracts calcaneus while guiding forefoot into dorsiflexion.
Stretch great toe into extension	Child sits in a chair or on edge of treatment table with his knee flexed. Therapist stabilizes first ray in dorsiflexed position and then passively extends the great toe.
Holding contraction at end range dorsiflexion	With child supine or sitting, therapist places foot in end range ankle dorsiflexion and then asks child to hold the position. If child uses toe extensors, or has an asymmetrical pull, therapist stops, repositions, and tries again.
Holding contraction at end range eversion	With child supine or sitting, therapist places foot in end range ankle eversion and then asks child to hold the position. If child cannot recruit ankle evertors, tapping and vibration can be used to help facilitate appropriate fibularis muscles. If the child recruits accessory muscles to hold alignment, the therapist should stop, reposition the ankle, and try again.
Resistive strengthening ankle dorsiflexors and evertors	Child sits in a chair or on edge of treatment table with his knee flexed. Child uses resistance bands appropriately positioned to strengthen ankle dorsiflexors or evertors.
Hamstring stretches	In supine, child's hip is flexed to 90° and the knee is extended until the child feels the muscle stretching. Stretch is held for at least 30 seconds.
Standing balance on one foot	Child initially works on standing on one foot in shoes with brace on and progresses to standing on one foot in bare feet. Changing the child's upper extremity position increases or decreases the balance challenge.
Squat with hand over foot support to maintain foot flat	From a standing position, child works to move into squatting position with feet flat on floor. Therapist works to support weight shift to more involved extremity. If the child does not have dorsiflexion to neutral, a heel wedge under the foot will help promote weightbearing through the heel.
Elliptical trainer	Work on weight shift and step-through pattern on an elliptical trainer (in forward and backward motions). This can be done with or without shoes. Therapist may need to provide support over the foot to maintain flat foot alignment throughout the entire cycle and to facilitate weight shift to allow symmetrical pattern on the equipment.
Stair ambulation	Child practices ascending and descending stairs slowly, without holding railing, if possible. Therapist may need to provide support over the foot to assist child in weight shift during descent.

Although children who have clubfeet often do not have significant delays in skills by the time they are school age, skills such as roller skating and riding a bicycle are sometimes challenging.[14,15] These balance and weight shift activities may need additional therapy interventions to address.

Evidence-Based Clinical Recommendations

SORT: Strength of Recommendation Taxonomy

A: Consistent, good-quality patient-oriented evidence
B: Inconsistent or limited-quality patient-oriented evidence
C: Consensus, disease-oriented evidence, usual practice, expert opinion or case series

1. Noncompliance with wearing the abduction foot brace is closely associated with recurrence of clubfoot deformity. **Grade B**

2. The first indication of clubfoot relapse is increased intoeing during stance phase of gait. **Grade A**

3. The French Physical Therapy method that includes daily stretching of short-ened tissues, stimulation and strengthening of weakened muscles, taping and splinting, and closed chain training can be used to help support optimal align-ment of the clubfoot. **Grade C**

COMPREHENSION QUESTIONS

26.1 Which of the following *best* describes the anatomic position of a clubfoot that is not completely corrected?

A. Elongated and plantarflexed first ray with dorsiflexion beyond 10°

B. Prominent base of the fifth metatarsal on palpation

C. Forefoot abduction beyond neutral and ability to squat with feet flat on floor

D. Retracted and plantar flexed first ray, forefoot adduction that does not cor-rect past neutral, and a prominent base of the fifth metatarsal on palpation

26.2 Which of the following is a common gait pattern with relapsing clubfoot?

A. Heel strike at initial contact and toe out through stance

B. Foot flat at initial contact, collapsing into pronation during stance phase

C. Early heel rise after initial contact with intoeing during stance phase

D. Steppage gait during swing phase

26.3 Which of the following would be an appropriate activity for the physical ther-apist to give a child with clubfeet as a home program?

A. Picking up a marble with the toes

B. Balancing on one foot

C. Heel raises

D. Standing on a slant board with heels down and knees in hyperextension

ANSWERS

26.1 **D.** A relapsed clubfoot has tightening of the structures along the medial aspect of the foot, resulting in the great toe being shortened through plantar flexion on the first ray. With the tight medial structures, it is hard to stretch the medial column of the foot beyond neutral forefoot abduction. As a result of the tight medial structures, the lateral column of the foot is elongated with the base of the fifth metatarsal becoming visibly prominent. The hindfoot becomes tight resulting in inability to keep feet flat on the floor when attempting to squat.

26.2 **C.** Although heel strike may be present at initial contact during gait, stance phase is marked by early heel rise on an internally rotated supinated foot. Although a child may use a variety of substitutions to assist with swing phase on the involved side, a steppage gait pattern (option D) is not typically present with a newly relapsing clubfoot.

26.3 **B.** Strategies for encouraging foot flat with control, such as standing on one foot, are helpful for a child who has a clubfoot. Marble pick-ups with toes (option A) and heel raises (option C) strengthen muscles that are already tight. Standing on a slant board with heels down but knees hyperextended (option D) limits the opportunity to effectively stretch the tight gastrocnemius and soleus muscles.

REFERENCES

1. Epeldegui T. Deformity of talus and calcaneous in congenital clubfoot: an anatomical study. *J Pediatr Orthop B.* 2012;21:10-15.

2. Gharehdaghi M, Alhaosawi M, Ariamanesh AS, Nejad A, Sandokji AM, Abdellsalam M. Hyperextension of the big toe at metatarsophalangeal joint (MTPJ): a sign of the undercorrection of cavus in idiopathic clubfoot in Ponseti method. *Iran J Child Neurol.* 2010;4:39-44.

3. Zhao D, Liu J, Zhao L, Wu Z. Relapse of clubfoot after treatment with the Ponseti method and the function of the foot abduction orthosis. *Clin Orthop Surg.* 2014;6:245-252.

4. Ramírez N, Flynn JM, Fernández S, Seda W, Macchiavelli RE. Orthosis noncompliance after the Ponseti method for the treatment of idiopathic clubfeet: a relevant problem that needs reevaluation. *J Pediatr Orthop.* 2011;31:710-715.

5. Boehm S, Sinclair M. Foot abduction brace in the Ponseti method for idiopathic clubfoot deformity: torsional deformities and compliance. *J Pediatr Orthop.* 2007;27:712-716.

6. Haft GF, Walker CG, Crawford HA. Early clubfoot recurrence after use of the Ponseti method in a New Zealand population. *J Bone Joint Surg Am.* 2007;89:487-493.

7. Church C, Coplan JA, Poljak D, et al. A comprehensive outcome comparison of surgical and Ponseti clubfoot treatments with reference to pediatric norms. *J Child Orthop.* 2012;6:51-59.

8. Gottschalk HP, Karol LA, Jeans KA. Gait analysis of children treated for moderate clubfoot with physical therapy versus the Ponseti cast technique. *J Pediatr Orthop.* 2010;30:235-239.

9. El-Hawary R, Karol LA, Jeans KA, Richards BS. Gait analysis of children treated for clubfoot with physical therapy or the Ponseti cast technique. *J Bone Joint Surg Am.* 2008;90-A:1508-1511.

10. Wicart P, Richardson J, Maton B. Adaptation of gait initiation in children with unilateral idiopathic clubfoot following conservative treatment. *J Electromyogr Kinesiol.* 2006;16:650-660.

11. Jeans KA, Karol LA. Plantar pressures following Ponseti and French physiotherapy methods for clubfoot. *J Pediatr Orthop.* 2010;30:82-89.

12. Zumbrunn T, MacWilliams BA, Johnson BA. Evaluation of a single leg stance balance test in children. *Gait Posture*. 2011;34:174-177.

13. Sala DA, Chu A, Lehman WB, van Bosse HJ. Achievement of gross motor milestones in children with idiopathic clubfoot treated with the Ponseti method. *J Pediatr Orthop*. 2013;33:55-58.

14. Kenmoku T, Kamegaya M, Saisu T, et al. Athletic ability of school-age children after satisfactory treatment of congenital clubfoot. *J Pediatr Orthop*. 2013;33:321-325.

15. Garcia NL, McMulkin ML, Tompkins BJ, Caskey PM, Mader SL, Baird GO. Gross motor development in babies with treated idiopathic clubfoot. *Pediatr Phys Ther*. 2011;23:347-352.

16. Andriesse H, Westbom L, Hägglund G. Motor ability in children treated for idiopathic clubfoot. A controlled pilot study. *BMC Pediatrics*. 2009;9:71-78.

17. Mackey AH, Lobb GL, Walt SE, Stott S. Reliability and validity of the observational gait scale in children with spastic diplegia. *Dev Med Child Neurol*. 2007;45:4-11.

18. Clarkson HM. *Musculoskeletal Assessment: Joint Motion and Muscle Testing*. 3rd ed. Baltimore, MD: Lippincott, Williams & Wilkins; 2012.

19. Oatis CA. Biomechanics of the foot and ankle under static conditions. *Phys Ther*. 1988;68:1815-1821.

20. Rehabilitation Measures Database. http://www.rehabmeasures.org. Accessed February 14, 2015.

21. Nicolini-Panisson RD, Donadio MV. Normative values for the Timed 'Up and Go' test in children and adolescents and validation for individuals with Down syndrome. *Dev Med Child Neurol*. 2014;56:490-497.

22. Tieman BL, Palisano RJ, Sudive AC. Assessment of motor development and function in preschool children. *Ment Retard Dev Disabil Res Rev*. 2005;11:189-196.

23. Kendall FP, McCreary EK, Provance PG. *Muscles: Testing and Function With Posture and Pain*. 5th ed. Baltimore, MD: Lippincott, Williams & Wilkins; 2005.

24. Gelfer Y, Durham S, Daly K, Shitrit R, Smorgick Y, Ewins D. The effect of neuromuscular electrical stimulation on congenital talipes equinovarus following correction with the Ponseti method: a pilot study. *J Pediatr Orthop B*. 2010;19:390-395.

25. Dimeglio A, Canavese F. The French functional physical therapy method for the treatment of congenital clubfoot. *J Pediatr Orthop: Part B*. 2012;21:28-39.

Joint Hypermobility Condition

Paula Melson
Stephanie Sabo

A 12-year-old female presents to outpatient physical therapy with reports of increasing pain in multiple joints. Her family notes that she has had intermittent joint pain for at least four years. During the past six months, the pain has spread to multiple joints and has increased in frequency and intensity. She also reports increasing difficulty with physical activities including walking for more than 10 minutes and she needs to stop frequently due to pain. The patient has participated in recreational soccer in the past; however, she has stopped due to increasing knee pain with running. She reports that her pain is worse in the evening, particularly after an active day and notes that painful areas include bilateral hips, knees, and ankles. She and her parents report symptoms of excessive fatigue at the end of the school day. She is often exhausted after school and wants to take a nap, which impacts the quality of her sleep at night. Her primary care physician (PCP) ordered radiographs of her knees and the results were normal. The PCP then referred the child to a pediatric rheumatologist. She was seen by the rheumatologist and diagnosed with hypermobility syndrome (joint hypermobility condition) and referred to physical therapy for evaluation and treatment.

▶ What examination signs might be associated with joint hypermobility condition?
▶ How would this child's contextual factors influence or change your patient/client management?
▶ Based on her health condition, what do you anticipate may be the contributors to activity limitations?
▶ What are the possible complications that may limit the effectiveness of physical therapy?
▶ What are the most appropriate physical therapy interventions?
▶ How might the patient's emotional condition affect rehabilitation?

KEY DEFINITIONS

AUTONOMIC DYSFUNCTION: Abnormal responses of the sympathetic and/ or parasympathetic nervous systems that can alter blood pressure, heart rate, digestion, and other functions

BEIGHTON SCALE: Screen for hypermobility in which a score of 5/9 or more is used to classify hypermobility.[1,2] However, in a comprehensive literature review it is noted that a score of 4/9 has also been used to classify hypermobility.[3] Scale includes five components: (1) forward flexion of the trunk with knees fully extended so that the palms of the hands rest flat on the floor (1 point); (2) hyperextension of the elbows >10° (1 point for each elbow); (3) passive extension of the little fingers >90° (1 point for each hand); (4) hyperextension of the knees >10°(1 point for each knee); (5) passive movement of the thumb to the flexor aspect of the forearm (1 point for each thumb)

COLLAGEN DEFICIENCY: Lower than normal levels or structurally abnormal collagen, the primary protein in human connective tissue; those with deficiency may experience decreased or delayed training effects on muscle and tendon and/or healing responses of connective tissues

EHLERS-DANLOS SYNDROME (EDS): Group of inheritable connective tissue disorders marked by abnormal collagen function; in the most common form of EDS (type III, hypermobile type), the major diagnostic finding is joint hypermobility

JOINT HYPERMOBILITY SYNDROME: Also known as hypermobility syndrome, joint laxity, Ehlers-Danlos syndrome, and/or benign joint hypermobility syndrome. For consistency, the term joint hypermobility condition will be used in this study, though it is becoming more widely accepted to use the term Ehlers-Danlos syndrome type III.[4]

KINESIOPHOBIA: Fear of movement, usually due to fear of inducing pain

POSTURAL ORTHOSTATIC TACHYCARDIA SYNDROME (POTS): Form of orthostatic intolerance that is characterized by an abnormally large increase in heart rate and syncope[5,6]

Objectives

1. Identify the characteristics of joint hypermobility.

2. Identify the potential impact joint hypermobility has on physical function and on quality of life.

3. Recognize the precautions and complications associated with treating an individual with joint hypermobility.

4. Describe key elements of physical therapy interventions in this population.

5. Design an appropriate physical therapy treatment plan for an individual with joint hypermobility.

Physical Therapy Considerations

PT considerations for management of the child with joint hypermobility condition:

▶ **General physical therapy plan of care/goals:** Increase muscle flexibility and strength; decrease pain; promote independence with pain management techniques; facilitate independence with joint protection and activity modification guidelines; facilitate independence with and adherence to home exercise program; improve postural alignment; increase core strength and stabilization; maximize neuromotor control and motor function

▶ **Physical therapy interventions:** Initiation of a therapeutic exercise program, beginning at a low intensity with slow progressions; joint protection including postural re-education and awareness to reduce stress on muscles and joints and limit pain and fatigue; controlled stretching; core and extremity strengthening; neuromuscular re-education

▶ **Precautions during physical therapy:** Monitor anxiety; minimize risk of joint subluxation and/or dislocation during exercise

▶ **Complications interfering with physical therapy:** Increased pain and joint stress with intensive physical therapy; collagen deficiency leading to increased risk of injury; abnormal response to exercise and position changes due to dysautonomia

Understanding the Health Condition

A joint hypermobility condition is not always identified as the primary diagnosis for which an individual presents to physical therapy. Hypermobility may be an underlying impairment identified when treating a variety of other impairments such as gross motor delays,[7-9] coordination difficulties,[10] fibromyalgia,[11,12] chronic fatigue syndrome,[13,14] or frequent and recurring injuries.[15]

Children and adolescents with joint hypermobility conditions often live with joint pain, fatigue, and poor tolerance to physical activity that significantly impacts their quality of life.[16] This population is often overlooked, yet has the potential to benefit from effective management by physical therapists.[17,18] Joint hypermobility is commonly found in the pediatric population, having been identified in 30% to 34% of school-aged children when assessed using a gross screening tool such as the Beighton scale (Fig. 27-1) without regard for associated symptoms.[1,2,19,20] Prior to puberty, there is no evidence of increased prevalence in females.[20,21] However, after puberty, the prevalence and degree of hypermobility increases in females and declines in males, possibly due to the hormonal changes that occur during puberty.[22]

Several comorbidities such as anxiety, headaches, postural orthostatic tachycardia syndrome (POTS), and gastrointestinal conditions have been identified that contribute to decreased function and quality of life. The potential impact of these comorbidities must be considered when planning effective physical therapy interventions. There are associated long-term effects of the joint hypermobility

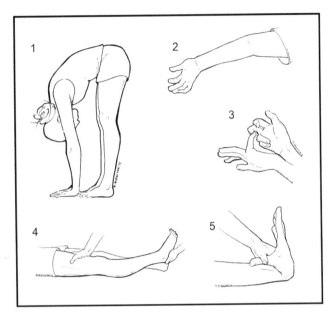

Figure 27-1. Illustration of the five components of the Beighton scale.

condition that, when addressed proactively during childhood, may have less detrimental impact on adult function and quality of life.[23]

Aside from the commonly reported symptom of pain, a major and under-recognized characteristic of joint hypermobility condition is fatigability. Proposed etiologies of the fatigue are biomechanical, cardiovascular, and central nervous system phenomena.[16] Patients may also experience other signs or symptoms including poor sleep,[5] headaches,[5,24] gastrointestinal dysmotility,[25] autonomic dysfunction, and POTS.[5,6] Thus, a multidisciplinary approach is needed to effectively address the complex needs of this patient population.[3,26-28]

Physical Therapy Patient/Client Management

Evidence supports the role of physical therapy as the primary intervention for joint hypermobility within the context of a multidisciplinary team.[17,18] A **modified, low-intensity approach to therapeutic intervention** that is progressed slowly and targets postural stability and endurance decreases pain, increases strength, and improves function.[15,29-31] Effective treatment should include chronic pain management, proprioceptive enhancement, postural awareness, and training for global muscle strength and endurance, core stability, and joint stabilization.[26,32-34] When initiating a therapeutic exercise program, intervention should begin at a low level and progress slowly. Interventions should address the whole child and not one joint or body region, and also consider the potential non-musculoskeletal manifestations of joint hypermobility conditions. Intervention should be customized and based on the individual's needs and goals.[28] When physical therapy is targeted to the specific needs and responses of the child or adolescent with joint hypermobility, it is possible to reverse the inevitable muscle imbalance that results from pain inhibition and kinesiophobia.[3] The approach should be holistic, patient-centered, specific, and aimed at giving the child the tools to independently manage the problem.[35-37] Therefore, it is incumbent upon the physical therapist to understand the specific needs of each client and to be equipped to provide effective services to this population. Beginning in childhood, a **proactive approach for joint protection, stabilization training, and body awareness** can facilitate management of pain and fatigue symptoms and potentially minimize long-term musculoskeletal deficits.[28,31,38-40] Without proper and timely interventions, pain and fatigue can progressively worsen over time and lead to chronic pain and functional impairments. Lack of intervention can result in significant decline in quality of life in children and adolescents with joint hypermobility when compared to their peers.[16,23,38]

Examination, Evaluation, and Diagnosis

The subjective interview should address the many potential factors that can impact quality of life. Pain history should include location, intensity, frequency, relationship to activity level, relief measures used by the patient, and exacerbating factors.[5] Pain can be present at any joint,[3] with the literature describing pain in the lower limbs, back,[30] temporomandibular joint,[41] and feet.[42,43] Many patients and families report fatigue,[5,16] difficulty with prolonged walking,[38] and challenges with age-appropriate physical activities, such as physical education classes or playing outside with peers. Families may also characterize the child or teen as being clumsy or having poor coordination.[44] It is important for the physical therapist to gather information regarding current activity modifications or limitations affecting school activities and activities of daily living (ADLs).[3] Headaches and poor sleep are also frequently reported in this population.[5,24]

There are several musculoskeletal complaints that may be reported by someone with hypermobility, including a history of subluxation or dislocation of joints,[30] clicking and/or popping in joints,[30] and fractures or other musculoskeletal injuries.[3] There may also be a history of prior musculoskeletal surgeries.[27] It is important to note that surgical interventions in this population may not have optimal outcomes due to abnormal connective tissue, prolonged postsurgical recovery, and deconditioning.[27]

The presence of recognized global signs and symptoms associated with a joint hypermobility condition should be discussed in the comprehensive subjective interview. These include anxiety and depression,[5,45,46] (pre)syncope, and/or POTS.[5,6] Cardiorespiratory complaints indicative of these conditions may include palpitations, chest pain, and/or shortness of breath. Gastrointestinal symptoms commonly include nausea, stomach ache, diarrhea, or constipation.[5,25,44] There is also a documented association between joint hypermobility and eosinophilic esophagitis (EE),[47] which is a chronic immune system disease with many manifestations including difficulty swallowing, intolerance to some foods, and upper abdominal pain.

There are a few factors revealed in the subjective history that may influence the readiness of the patient and her family to participate in physical therapy. Children and adolescents with joint hypermobility conditions may report a history of prior physical therapy intervention, often when the influence of hypermobility was not yet recognized, that made them feel worse or was not perceived as being effective.[48,49] The patient may fear similar experiences with another trial of physical therapy. If there is a family history of joint laxity or hypermobile conditions, the experiences of those family members may provide motivation to the patient to avoid some of the long-term problems that older family members might have experienced.[25,30]

Following completion of the subjective interview, the physical therapist should complete a comprehensive objective assessment. The physical therapist observes the child's standing and seated postural alignment. Commonly observed alignment deviations in children and adolescents with joint hypermobility conditions include rounded shoulders, forward head, scapular winging, anterior pelvic tilt, and increased lumbar lordosis.[3] In the lower extremity, the therapist might identify genu recurvatum, femoral inversion, calcaneal valgus, midfoot pronation, and hallux valgus.[3,42,43,50] Although many patients appear to have appropriate foot contour in nonweightbearing positions, collapse of the medial longitudinal arch in a weightbearing position is common and may be a contributing factor to pain and fatigue. An objective assessment of the foot and ankle for the current 12-year-old pre-teen would be useful. The Oxford Ankle Foot Questionnaire-Children, the Foot Posture Index, and the Lower Limb Assessment Scale demonstrate adequate intra-rater and inter-rater reliability in a healthy pediatric sample (7-15 years old).[50] When observing posture in the upper extremities, the physical therapist may note that the patient has a preference for weightbearing on hyperextended elbows and/or metacarpophalangeal (MCP) joints.

Following the static posture assessment, the physical therapist assesses functional mobility. The functional mobility assessment includes gait observation with specific emphasis on stance limb and pelvic/core stability.[38,40,51,52] Standardized manual muscle testing for strength often does not capture the full scope of deficits for patients with hypermobility related to muscular endurance and the quality of movements.[3] Therefore, objective assessment of strength and postural stabilization should be performed in both open and closed chain positions[53] with a focus on assessing the *quality* of movement.[54] Table 27-1 describes examples of methods physical therapists can use to assess the quality of movements and common deviations that are observed in individuals with hypermobility.

Due to muscular imbalances and joint laxity, individuals with joint hypermobility often lack dynamic muscular control.[55] If the therapist places the patient in a functional position and observes her ability to maintain neutral joint alignment for an extended time (*i.e.*, by a hold count), common deficits in muscular co-contraction[56] and proprioception are usually revealed.[57,58] In pediatric physical therapy, these deficits can be identified as gross motor or coordination deficits. However, assessment of motor competency through standardized testing may not be sensitive enough to capture the full impact that joint hypermobility has on musculoskeletal function and movement quality. It is important for the therapist to

Table 27-1 RECOMMENDED ACTIVITIES TO ASSESS QUALITY OF MOVEMENT		
Physical Activity	**Common Deficits**	**Recommended Corrections**
Single limb stance	Pelvic and trunk deviations, genu recurvatum, increased ankle modulation	Verbal and visual cues for neutral trunk and pelvis, cues to sustain neutral knee extension, practice activity with neutral, stable ankle[3]
Heel raises	Locking into extreme ranges of plantar flexion with inversion of ankles	Cues to raise heels in limited range with neutral ankle position, progressing from firm to less stable surfaces[3]
Bridging/buttock lift	Exaggerated trunk extension, poor core activation, pelvic instability	Cues to perform with neutral pelvic position, using core stabilizing muscles, without lumbar lordosis[3]
Mini-wall squat	Poor midrange knee control, locking into knee recurvatum when returning to stand	Consider initially using towel roll between knees. Practice controlled, eccentric partial squat to 30°-45° then controlled, concentric slide up the wall to neutral knee extension, avoiding locking into genu recurvatum[3]
Postural scapular activation	Scapular winging and exaggerated lumbar extension in seated and standing postures	Cues to isolate scapular stabilization while maintaining neutral trunk posture[3] and to limit compensatory shoulder elevation

remember that *repetition* of tasks often reveals deficits that may not be identified with one-time trials.[19]

A significant component of the objective examination for the patient with a joint hypermobility condition is palpation. The skin may present with a soft velvety texture, thin atrophic scarring, increased elasticity, and/or the presence of striae.[30,48,54] Assessment of mobility and laxity throughout the joints[32,58,59] often reveals an empty or boggy end feel.[54] The distribution of joints involved varies from patient to patient. However, common findings include: laxity or instability of the shoulder, scapula, wrist, thumb, and carpometacarpal (CMC) joints, hyperextension of bilateral knees, elbows, MCPs, and interphalangeal joints (IPs), and increased hip internal rotation and external rotation.[3]

Due to the muscular imbalances associated with joint laxity and hypermobility, it is recommended that the physical therapist perform additional targeted range of motion[31,35] and muscle flexibility measures.[31,55] Common findings in children with joint hypermobility conditions include *tightness* in the hamstrings, gastrocnemius, pectorals, and/or paracervical muscles.[3]

Plan of Care and Interventions

Therapeutic exercises should be developed to target antigravity postural stability, quality of neuromuscular control, and postural/muscular endurance. Postural alignment is an important aspect of physical therapy intervention. Postural re-education and awareness reduces stress on muscles and joints and can reduce pain and fatigue over time.[6] To reduce long-term detrimental effects on the musculoskeletal system, **joint protection** should be incorporated into all aspects of exercise and physical activity.[33,60,61] Evidence supports the safety and effectiveness of initiating low-intensity exercise and slowly progressing the level of difficulty, number of repetitions, length of hold counts, and range of movement required for the exercises.[17,18,49] Usually, exercise should be initiated in gravity-reduced positions for core training, then progressed to sitting and standing postures, and then further progressed through modified ranges of motion. Extremity strengthening should progress from proximal to distal, slowly increasing through modified ranges of motion. All activities should focus on facilitation of co-contraction and on quality of movement in both open and closed chain activities.[53] The assessment activities performed in Table 27-1 can also be used as therapeutic exercises to improve movement quality. Neuromuscular re-education can target movement efficiency and improve response to sudden, unanticipated external loads, balance, and proprioception. Verbal and tactile cues are often required to promote mid-range control throughout activities.[3] For example, when teaching an individual with joint hypermobility condition to perform a commonly prescribed exercise such as wall squats, it is essential that the therapist provides specific modification to the technique and cues. For this exercise, the therapist initially positioned the 12-year-old patient in this case with her back against the wall and a towel roll placed between her knees to promote neutral alignment of the knees. The therapist observes the patient practice controlled, eccentric squatting in a modified pain-free range (30°-45°). Then, the therapist shifted the focus to the concentric phase of the squat, cueing her to avoiding locking her knees into hyperextension (genu recurvatum). The therapist typically needs to provide both verbal and tactile cues to assist the patient with finding and sustaining neutral knee positioning throughout several repetitions. The goals of this specific activity are to facilitate proprioception, strength, and neuromuscular control in neutral alignment.

Physical therapists should consider the potential for subluxation or, in rare cases, dislocation of lax joints during exercise or activity. Patient tolerance to exercises is an important factor and should be considered with each step of treatment planning, using modifications as necessary. Besides physical complaints, persons with joint hypermobility may have an increased potential for anxiety and other psychosocial components.[45,62] Encouragement and support, as well as education regarding the condition and expected responses to intervention are vital components of physical therapy. Recognition of the slower response to intervention[48,49] and the **need for consistent and ongoing home exercise program completion**[30,34,36,49] plays a role in improving the patient's overall outcomes. A consultative model of physical therapy, where patients are seen periodically for reassessment to update the home exercise program and reinforce activity modifications, is often effective for this population. For some patients, an intensive model, with frequent visits over a short time period, can provide a knowledge boost regarding the proper form for exercises, therefore improving their overall level of reported pain and fatigue. Table 27-2 describes sample exercises that could be included in the plan of care for an individual with a joint hypermobility condition.

Table 27-2   EXERCISES FOR A PATIENT WITH A JOINT HYPERMOBILITY CONDITION

Exercise	Quality of Movement/Progressions
Hamstring stretching	In long sitting position on firm surface, with low back against upright support, maintain knees extended and ankles in neutral dorsiflexion (DF). Use towel roll under knees to partially relieve stretch for increased tolerance. Alternative: Stand on one leg with the opposite heel elevated on a step, maintain the elevated leg with knee straight, ankle DF to neutral and trunk upright (or slightly forward). Be sure patient keeps hips facing anteriorly to avoid compensatory rotation to either side.
Heel cord stretching	Facing wall, patient stretches gastrocnemius with attention to keeping toes straight ahead, heel flat on floor and back knee kept straight. Ensure patient is wearing supportive shoes and orthotics (if indicated) to avoid stretch through medial longitudinal arch of foot.
Abdominal isometrics	In hooklying, have patient contract transversus abdominis and maintain for 5 to 10 seconds. Be sure patient is not holding her breath. Progress by increasing time. Next progression is performance in conjunction with single extremity controlled movements.
Posterior pelvic tilt	In hooklying, tighten abdominal muscles and flatten back to the ground by rolling pelvis posteriorly. Progress this exercise to bridging.
Bridging	Perform posterior pelvic tilt (PPT), and then lift hips upward into neutral hip extension. Keep knees apart or keep towel roll between them, depending on stability. Provide verbal and manual cueing to encourage PPT, proper breathing techniques, and avoidance of excessive lumbar lordosis or hip hyperextension.
Isometric hip adduction	In hooklying, squeeze ball or towel roll between knees for 5 seconds. Progress first by increasing time. Next, progress by combining with bridging.
Resisted hip abduction	Resisted hip abduction in hooklying with resistive band for 3 to 5 seconds in minimal abduction. Verbal cueing to encourage slow eccentric control back to starting position. Progress by increasing time and gradual resistance through band color.
Mini wall squatting	Partial wall squats for lower extremity strengthening and core and postural stability through controlled eccentric lowering into modified range (30° to 45°) and concentric rising to neutral knee extension. Provide verbal cueing to control speed during lowering and rising to starting position, and to sustain upright symmetrical trunk. Continue cueing at end of cycle to maintain "soft knees" (neutral knee) position.
Scapular squeezes	Seated scapular retraction for 5 to 10 seconds. Verbal cueing needed to promote shoulder depression, scapular retraction, and upright posture during exercise. Also provide cues to limit shoulder shrugging and/or exaggeration of lumbar lordosis.
Modified heel raises	Static partial heel raises for increased ankle stability and proprioception. Can initiate with single handheld assistance, if needed to maintain balance. Verbal cueing to avoid locking out ankles into full plantar flexion and to sustain neutral eversion/inversion while holding for 5-10 seconds.

Evidence-Based Clinical Recommendations

SORT: Strength of Recommendation Taxonomy

A: Consistent, good-quality patient-oriented evidence
B: Inconsistent or limited-quality patient-oriented evidence
C: Consensus, disease-oriented evidence, usual practice, expert opinion, or case series

1. A modified, low-intensity approach to therapeutic intervention that is progressed slowly and targets postural stability and endurance decreases pain, increases strength, and improves function in individuals with joint hypermobility. **Grade B**

2. A proactive approach for joint protection, stabilization training, and body awareness can facilitate management of pain and fatigue symptoms and potentially minimize long-term musculoskeletal deficits. **Grade B**

3. To reduce long-term detrimental effects on the musculoskeletal system, joint protection should be incorporated into all aspects of exercise and physical activity. **Grade C**

4. It is recommended that a home exercise program be continuous, progressive, and performed as part of a daily routine to achieve maximum benefit and prevent return to pre-intervention status. **Grade C**

COMPREHENSION QUESTIONS

27.1 Which of the following statements is the *best* description of recommended physical therapy exercise guidelines for children and teens with joint hypermobility conditions?

A. The physical therapy plan of care includes a brief period of exercise intervention and focuses on the specific structure that causes the patient the most pain.

B. The physical therapy plan of care includes core strengthening, facilitation of co-contraction for joint stability, and proprioceptive training with slow progression of exercise intensity.

C. The physical therapy plan of care includes rapid progression of exercise intensity because persons with joint hypermobility respond quickly to physical training.

D. The physical therapy plan of care includes progression to high impact aerobic exercise.

27.2 Which factor has the *most* impact on the long-term response to physical therapy treatment in children and teens with joint hypermobility conditions?

A. Results of joint imaging

B. Ability of the patient and his/her family to play an active role in the management of the condition

C. Presence of kinesiophobia

D. Ability of the patient to attend twice weekly therapy sessions

27.3 For the 12-year-old girl presented in this case, the factors that *most* likely contributed to her recently declining tolerance to physical activity are:

A. Her training program in recreational soccer was not intense enough to build her tolerance to the sport.

B. She is so tired at the end of the school day that she cannot participate in physical activity.

C. The influence of pubertal maturation on joint laxity has been detrimental to her functional status.

D. She is probably no longer interested in playing soccer or other sports.

ANSWERS

27.1 **B.** Low-intensity, slowly progressing exercise programs should focus on each component in this description. The focus should be on overall mechanics and function since many joints are affected (option A). Persons with joint hypermobility conditions respond slowly to training and generally do not tolerate rapid progression of exercise programs (option C). Exercise programs include facilitation of joint protection. High impact aerobic activity may not be tolerated by this population (option D).

27.2 **B.** Joint hypermobility can be a complex, chronic condition that requires ongoing, intermittent management throughout childhood/adolescence. Imaging rarely plays a role in diagnostic or prognostic management of joint hypermobility conditions (option A). Kinesiophobia is often present in hypermobile persons who have experienced pain secondary to physical activity. However, this can be overcome with proper physical therapy management to slowly build strength, postural stability, endurance, and confidence (option C). Frequency of therapy varies from case to case and is based on current level of function, response to therapy, and ability to carry out a home exercise program effectively (option D).

27.3 **C.** Pubertal maturation has been shown to lead to increased joint laxity in females and many female adolescents experience an exacerbation of symptoms during this time. Intense physical training programs are often not tolerated during periods of significant joint pain. Recreational level soccer was likely a better choice for her than a more highly competitive program, although some adolescents can eventually tolerate higher-level programs (option A). Her fatigue likely contributes to her poor tolerance to physical activity, but does not explain why she has recently developed more pain and fatigue (option B). It is unlikely that poor motivation or interest would lead to the pattern of symptoms described in this case (option D). Her increased pain at the end of the day, after activity, even while not playing soccer, is typical of children and adolescents with joint hypermobility conditions.

REFERENCES

1. Beighton P, De Paepe A, Steinmann B, Tsipouras P, Wenstrup RJ. Ehlers-Danlos syndromes: revised nosology, Villefranche, 1997. Ehlers-Danlos National Foundation (USA) and Ehlers-Danlos Support Group (UK). *Am J Med Genet.* 1998;77:31-37.

2. Junge T, Jespersen E, Wedderkopp N, Juul-Kristensen B. Inter-tester reproducibility and inter-method agreement of two variations of the Beighton test for determining Generalised Joint Hypermobility in primary school children. *BMC Pediatr.* 2013;13:214.

3. Cincinnati Children's Hospital Medical Center Joint Hypermobility Team 2014. *Evidence-Based Clinical Care Guideline for Identification and Management of Pediatric Joint Hypermobility.* Cincinnati, OH: Cincinnati Children's Hospital Medical Center; October 21, 2014.

4. Tinkle BT, Bird HA, Grahame R, Lavallee M, Levy HP, Sillence D. The lack of clinical distinction between the hypermobility type of Ehlers-Danlos syndrome and the joint hypermobility syndrome (a.k.a. hypermobility syndrome). *Am J Med Genet A.* 2009;149A:2368-2370.

5. Hakim AJ, Grahame R. Non-musculoskeletal symptoms in joint hypermobility syndrome. Indirect evidence for autonomic dysfunction? *Rheumatology (Oxford).* 2004;43:1194-1195.

6. Gazit Y, Nahir AM, Grahame R, Jacob G. Dysautonomia in the joint hypermobility syndrome. *Am J Med.* 2003;115:33-40.

7. Bernie C, Maillard SM. The frequency of parent-reported motor coordination difficulties in children diagnosed with benign joint hypermobility syndrome. *Pediatric Rheumatology.* 2011;9 (Suppl 1):O35.

8. Davidovitch M, Tirosh E, Tal Y. The relationship between joint hypermobility and neurodevelopmental attributes in elementary school children. *J Child Neurol.* 1994;9:417-419.

9. Tirosh E, Jaffe M, Marmur R, Taub Y, Rosenberg Z. Prognosis of motor development and joint hypermobility. *Arch Dis Child.* 1991;66:931-933.

10. Kirby A, Davies R. Developmental Coordination Disorder and Joint Hypermobility Syndrome--overlapping disorders? Implications for research and clinical practice. *Child Care Health Dev.* 2007;33:513-519.

11. Karaaslan Y, Haznedaroglu S, Ozturk M. Joint hypermobility and primary fibromyalgia: a clinical enigma. *J Rheumatol.* 2000;27:1774-1776.

12. Ting TV, Hashkes PJ, Schikler K, Desai AM, Spalding S, Kashikar-Zuck S. The role of benign joint hypermobility in the pain experience in Juvenile Fibromyalgia: an observational study. *Pediatr Rheumatol Online J.* 2012;10:16.

13. Barron DF, Cohen BA, Geraghty MT, Violand R, Rowe PC. Joint hypermobility is more common in children with chronic fatigue syndrome than in healthy controls. *J Pediatr.* 2002;141:421-425.

14. Nijs J, Aerts A, De Meirleir K. Generalized joint hypermobility is more common in chronic fatigue syndrome than in healthy control subjects. *J Manipulative Physiol Ther.* 2006;29:32-39.

15. Briggs J, McCormack M, Hakim AJ, Grahame R. Injury and joint hypermobility syndrome in ballet dancers--a 5-year follow-up. *Rheumatology (Oxford).* 2009;48:1613-1614.

16. Voermans NC, Knoop H, van de Kamp N, Hamel BC, Bleijenberg G, van Engelen BG. Fatigue is a frequent and clinically relevant problem in Ehlers-Danlos Syndrome. *Semin Arthritis Rheum.* 2010;40:267-274.

17. Kemp S, Gamble C, Wilkinson S, et al. A randomized comparative trial of generalized vs targeted physiotherapy in the management of childhood hypermobility. *Rheumatology (Oxford).* 2010;49:315-325.

18. Pacey V, Tofts L, Adams RD, Munns CF, Nicholson LL. Exercise in children with joint hypermobility syndrome and knee pain: a randomised controlled trial comparing exercise into hypermobile versus neutral knee extension. *Pediatr Rheumatol Online J.* 2013;11:30.

19. Arroyo IL, Brewer EJ, Giannini EH. Arthritis/arthralgia and hypermobility of the joints in schoolchildren. *J Rheumatol.* 1988;15:978-980.

20. Remvig L, Kümmel C, Kristensen JH, Boas G, Juul-Kristensen B. Prevalence of generalized joint hypermobility, arthralgia and motor competence in 10-year-old school children. *Int Musculoskelet Med.* 2011;33:137-145.

21. Juul-Kristensen B, Kristensen J, Frausing B, Jensen D, Rogind H, Remvig L. Motor competence and physical activity in 8-year-old school children with generalized joint hypermobility. *Pediatrics.* 2009;124:1380-1387.

22. Quatman CE, Ford KR, Myer GD, Paterno MV, Hewett TE. The effects of gender and pubertal status on generalized joint laxity in young athletes. *J Sci Med Sport.* 2008;11:257-263.

23. Voermans NC, Knoop H, Bleijenberg G, van Engelen BG. Pain in ehlers-danlos syndrome is common, severe, and associated with functional impairment. *J Pain Symptom Manage.* 2010;40:370-378.

24. Rozen TD, Roth JM, Denenberg N. Cervical spine joint hypermobility: a possible predisposing factor for new daily persistent headache. *Cephalalgia.* 2006;26:1182-1185.

25. Zarate N, Farmer AD, Grahame R, et al. Unexplained gastrointestinal symptoms and joint hypermobility: is connective tissue the missing link? *Neurogastroenterol Motil.* 2010;22:e252-e278.

26. Bathen T, Hangmann AB, Hoff M, Andersen LO, Rand-Hendriksen S. Multidisciplinary treatment of disability in ehlers-danlos syndrome hypermobility type/hypermobility syndrome: a pilot study using a combination of physical and cognitive-behavioral therapy on 12 women. *Am J Med Genet A.* 2013;161A:3005-3011.

27. Castori M, Morlino S, Celletti C, et al. Management of pain and fatigue in the joint hypermobility syndrome (a.k.a. Ehlers-Danlos syndrome, hypermobility type): principles and proposal for a multidisciplinary approach. *Am J Med Genet A.* 2012;158A:2055-2070.

28. Celletti C, Castori M, La Torre G, Camerota F. Evaluation of kinesiophobia and its correlations with pain and fatigue in joint hypermobility syndrome/Ehlers-Danlos syndrome hypermobility type. *Biomed Res Int.* 2013;2013:580460.

29. Kerr A, Macmillan CE, Uttley WS, Luqmani RA. Physiotherapy for children with hypermobility syndrome. *Physiotherapy.* 2000;86:313-317.

30. Murray KJ. Hypermobility disorders in children and adolescents. *Best Pract Res Clin Rheumatol.* 2006;20:329-351.

31. Russek LN. Examination and treatment of a patient with hypermobility syndrome. *Phys Ther.* 2000;80:386-398.

32. Rombaut L, Malfait F, De Wandele I, et al. Muscle-tendon tissue properties in the hypermobility type of Ehlers-Danlos syndrome. *Arthritis Care Res (Hoboken).* 2012;64:766-772.

33. Booshanam DS, Cherian B, Joseph CP, Mathew J, Thomas R. Evaluation of posture and pain in persons with benign joint hypermobility syndrome. *Rheumatol Int.* 2011;31:1561-1565.

34. Ferrell WR, Tennant N, Sturrock RD, et al. Amelioration of symptoms by enhancement of proprioception in patients with joint hypermobility syndrome. *Arthritis Rheum.* 2004;50:3323-3328.

35. Simmonds JV, Keer RJ. Hypermobility and the hypermobility syndrome, part 2: assessment and management of hypermobility syndrome: illustrated via case studies. *Man Ther.* 2008;13:e1-e11.

36. Barton LM, Bird HA. Improving pain by the stabilization of hyperlax joints. *J Orthop Rheumatol*. 1996;9:46-51.

37. Lorig KR, Holman H. Self-management education: history, definition, outcomes, and mechanisms. *Ann Behav Med*. 2003;26:1-7.

38. Fatoye FA, Palmer S, van der Linden ML, Rowe PJ, Macmillan F. Gait kinematics and passive knee joint range of motion in children with hypermobility syndrome. *Gait Posture*. 2011;33:447-451.

39. Grahame R. Joint hypermobility syndrome pain. *Curr Pain Headache Rep*. 2009;13:427-433.

40. Greenwood NL, Duffell LD, Alexander CM, McGregor AH. Electromyographic activity of pelvic and lower limb muscles during postural tasks in people with benign joint hypermobility syndrome and non hypermobile people. A pilot study. *Man Ther*. 2011;16:623-628.

41. Ogren M, Faltmars C, Lund B, Holmlund A. Hypermobility and trauma as etiologic factors in patients with disc derangements of the temporomandibular joint. *Int J Oral Maxillofac Surg*. Sep 2012;41(9):1046-1050.

42. Berglund B, Nordström G, Hagberg C, Mattiasson AC. Foot pain and disability in individuals with Ehlers-Danlos syndrome (EDS): impact on daily life activities. *Disabil Rehabil*. 2005;27:164-169.

43. Gross KD, Felson DT, Niu J, et al. Association of flat feet with knee pain and cartilage damage in older adults. *Arthritis Care Res (Hoboken)*. 2011;63:937-944.

44. Adib N, Davies K, Grahame R, Woo P, Murray KJ. Joint hypermobility syndrome in childhood. A not so benign multisystem disorder? *Rheumatology (Oxford)*. 2005;44:744-750.

45. Bulbena-Cabré A, Pailhez G, Bulbena A. Joint hypermobility links with anxiety: history and present. *Int Musculoskel Med*. 2011;33:132-136.

46. Martin-Santos R, Bulbena A, Porta M, Gago J, Molina L, Duro JC. Association between joint hypermobility syndrome and panic disorder. *Am J Psychiatry*. 1998;155:1578-1583.

47. Abonia JP, Wen T, Stucke EM, et al. High prevalence of eosinophilic esophagitis in patients with inherited connective tissue disorders. *J Allergy Clin Immunol*. 2013;132:378-386.

48. Hakim A, Grahame R. Joint hypermobility. *Best Pract Res Clin Rheumatol*. 2003;17:989-1004.

49. Keer R, Grahame R. *Hypermobility Syndrome: Recognition and Management for Physiotherapists*. Edinburgh: Butterworth Heinemann; 2003.

50. Evans AM, Rome K, Peet L. The foot posture index, ankle lunge test, Beighton scale and the lower limb assessment score in healthy children: a reliability study. *J Foot Ankle Res*. 2012;5:1.

51. Galli M, Cimolin V, Rigoldi C, et al. Gait strategy in patients with Ehlers-Danlos syndrome hypermobility type: a kinematic and kinetic evaluation using 3D gait analysis. *Res Dev Disabil*. 2011;32:1663-1668.

52. Cimolin V, Galli M, Vismara L, et al. Gait pattern in two rare genetic conditions characterized by muscular hypotonia: Ehlers-Danlos and Prader-Willi syndrome. *Res Dev Disabil*. 2011;32:1722-1728.

53. Augustsson J, Thomee R. Ability of closed and open kinetic chain tests of muscular strength to assess functional performance. *Scand J Med Sci Sports*. 2000;10:164-168.

54. Simmonds JV, Keer RJ. Hypermobility and the hypermobility syndrome. *Man Ther*. 2007;12:298-309.

55. Pacey V, Nicholson LL, Adams RD, Munn J, Munns CF. Generalized joint hypermobility and risk of lower limb joint injury during sport: a systematic review with meta-analysis. *Am J Sports Med*. 2010;38:1487-1497.

56. Jensen BR, Olesen AT, Pedersen MT, et al. Effect of generalized joint hypermobility on knee function and muscle activation in children and adults. *Muscle Nerve*. 2013;48:762-769.

57. Rombaut L, De Paepe A, Malfait F, Cools A, Calders P. Joint position sense and vibratory perception sense in patients with Ehlers-Danlos syndrome type III (hypermobility type). *Clin Rheumatol*. 2010;29:289-295.

58. Mallik AK, Ferrell WR, McDonald AG, Sturrock RD. Impaired proprioceptive acuity at the proximal interphalangeal joint in patients with the hypermobility syndrome. *Br J Rheumatol.* 1994;33:631-637.

59. Rombaut L, Malfait F, De Wandele I, et al. Muscle mass, muscle strength, functional performance, and physical impairment in women with the hypermobility type of Ehlers-Danlos syndrome. *Arthritis Care Res (Hoboken).* 2012;64:1584-1592.

60. Checa A. Severe cartilage damage of the knee joint in two young women with hypermobility. *Rheumatol Int.* 2012;32:3661-3664.

61. Russek LN. Hypermobility syndrome. *Phys Ther.* 1999;79:591-599.

62. Smith TO, Easton V, Bacon H, et al. The relationship between benign joint hypermobility syndrome and psychological distress: a systematic review and meta-analysis. *Rheumatology (Oxford).* 2014;53:114-122.

Idiopathic Toe Walking

Lisa K. Kenyon
Ryan Borck

CASE 28

A 5-year-old boy was referred to an outpatient physical therapy clinic for management of concerns related to his toe walking. The child's medical history was obtained through an interview with his parents and a review of available records. The patient was born at 36 weeks of gestation following a pregnancy complicated by oligohydramnios. Delivery occurred via Caesarean section with a birth weight of 4 pounds 1 ounce. Supplemental oxygen was briefly required after birth, but the child did not require an extended hospital stay and was discharged home with his mother. No other significant medical history was reported and the child's general overall health was reportedly excellent. Early developmental milestones were achieved within typical timeframes. From the onset of independent ambulation at 11 months of age, he inconsistently exhibited a bilateral toe-walking pattern. When the parents mentioned the intermittent toe walking as a concern at well-child visits, the child's pediatrician assured them that the patient would "outgrow" his toe walking. At the 5-year well-child visit, he was toe walking 100% of the time, complained of intermittent pain over the dorsal aspects of his tarsal heads, and had recently started to trip and fall especially when negotiating stairs. With knee extended, bilateral passive ankle dorsiflexion measured $-10°$ in subtalar joint neutral.

▶ Why is this child toe walking?
▶ Is toe walking associated with developmental delays or other conditions?
▶ Which developmental domains should be screened in children who toe walk?
▶ What are the examination priorities?
▶ What are the most appropriate physical therapy interventions?

KEY DEFINITIONS

IDIOPATHIC TOE WALKING: Toe walking that persists after 2 years of age without a known neurological or medical diagnosis

NEURODEVELOPMENTAL TREATMENT: Therapeutic intervention approach developed to address posture and movement disorders. The approach encourages inhibition of atypical or abnormal movement patterns and facilitation of typical movement patterns to promote skill development.

OLIGOHYDRAMNIOS: Decreased amount of amniotic fluid during pregnancy

TOE WALKING: Gait pattern characterized by weight acceptance and weight-bearing on the forefoot throughout the stance phase of the gait cycle

Objectives

1. Identify appropriate tests and measures to be used in the physical therapy examination of a child with idiopathic toe walking.

2. Describe the process of differential diagnosis in cases of idiopathic toe walking.

3. Identify appropriate outcomes and physical therapy interventions for a child with idiopathic toe walking.

4. Discuss the efficacy of medical interventions commonly used to address toe walking.

5. Recognize when to refer a child with toe walking for additional medical evaluation and diagnostic testing.

Physical Therapy Considerations

PT considerations during management of the young child who presents with concerns primarily related to toe walking:

▶ **General physical therapy plan of care/goals:** Improve active and passive dorsiflexion range of motion (ROM); increase incidence of heel strike at initial contact during gait; attain age-appropriate gross motor skills

▶ **Physical therapy interventions:** Stretching of tight lower extremity muscle groups (especially ankle plantar flexors); gait training; strengthening of weak lower extremity and trunk muscles; use of orthoses and serial casting; home exercise program (HEP) development

▶ **Precautions during physical therapy:** Pain or spasms related to overstretching the ankle plantar flexors (especially in serial casts)

▶ **Complications interfering with physical therapy:** Secondary skin complications related to serial casting; skin breakdown from ill-fitting orthoses; pain in the feet or legs

Understanding the Health Condition

Toe walking is a term used to describe a gait pattern that is characterized by weight acceptance and weightbearing on the forefoot throughout the stance phase of the gait cycle (Fig. 28-1). Often considered to be a transient stage in the development of a normal gait pattern, toe walking is a commonly reported parental concern occurring in 7% to 24% of children who do not have cerebral palsy (CP).[1,2] In a study of children (8 months to 10 years) being seen for well-child visits, Accardo et al.[3] noted that toe walking was observed in 24% of the 163 children studied. When examined by age groups within the study, toe walking was present or had been noted previously by a parent in 35% of the infants (0-2 years), 19% of the preschoolers (2-6 years), and 22% of the school-age children (6-10 years).[3] In a cross-sectional prevalence study of 5.5-year-olds, Engström and Tedroff[4] found that 2.1% of the 1436 children were active toe walkers at the time of the study. An additional 2.8% of the children had previously toe walked and were considered to be inactive toe walkers. The authors also found that among children with a

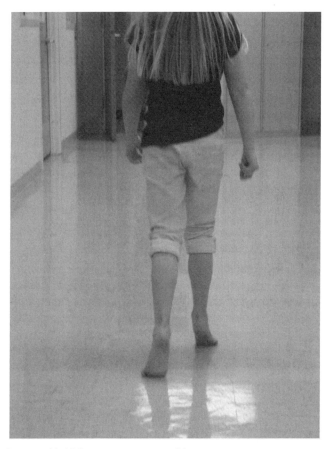

Figure 28-1. A 5-year-old girl demonstrates a toe-walking pattern.

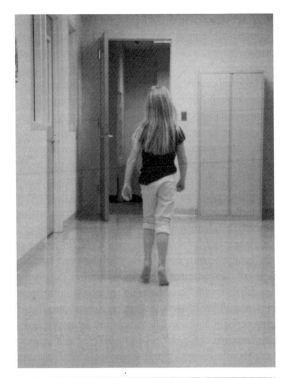

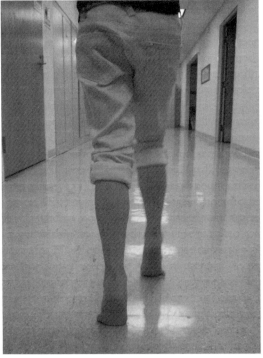

Figure 28-1. (*Continued*)

neuropsychiatric diagnosis or developmental delay, 41% were classified as active or inactive toe walkers.[4]

Given that heel strike at initial contact is consistently observed in typical gait by 18 to 24 months of age,[5,6] toe walking that persists after this age without a neurological or medical diagnosis is often diagnosed as idiopathic toe walking. First described by Hall et al.[7] in 1967 as congenital short tendo-calcaneus, idiopathic toe walking is defined as bilateral, persistent toe walking in the absence of other apparent etiologic abnormalities in a child older than 2 to 3 years.[2] Idiopathic toe walking is more commonly observed in boys than in girls[8,9] and often runs in families with a positive family history found in up to 34% of cases.[8]

Idiopathic toe walking is considered a diagnosis of exclusion because toe-walking behaviors are often associated with a wide variety of developmental and pathologic conditions including CP, muscular dystrophy, autistic spectrum disorders, tethered cord syndrome, diastematomyelia, schizophrenia, venous malformation of the posterior calf muscle, congenital/post-traumatic limb-length discrepancy, and myositis. Physical therapists must be able to recognize clusters of signs and symptoms that warrant referral for further medical evaluation and diagnostic testing. For example, signs related to upper motor neuron involvement such as a Babinski's sign, clonus, spasticity, or hyperreflexia should lead to a referral to rule out neuromuscular conditions including spastic diplegic CP. Although quantitative gait analysis can be used to clearly differentiate idiopathic toe walking from mild CP, children with idiopathic toe walking more often have the ability to ambulate with the typical heel-toe pattern upon verbal command than children with CP.[10] Due to the high prevalence of toe-walking behaviors in children with autism,[11,12] children who toe walk and also demonstrate difficulties in social interactions such as decreased eye contact, use of language, or symbolic/imaginative play should be referred to rule out an autistic spectrum disorder.

Developmental delays such as language disorders and sensory processing issues have been associated with toe-walking behaviors.[2,3,13-19] In a study with 13 children with persistent toe walking and normal neurologic examinations, Shulman et al.[13] found that 77% of the children had receptive or expressive language delays or both, 33% had fine motor delays, 40% had visuomotor delays, and 27% had gross motor delays. In an earlier study of 799 children who were referred for a developmental evaluation, the authors found that the frequency of toe walking increased as the severity of language impairment increased.[17] In the study of 163 children attending well-child visits, Accardo et al.[3] found that children who toe walked tended to have lower language quotients than those who did not toe walk. A number of authors have suggested a positive relationship between sensory processing dysfunction and idiopathic toe walking.[14,15,18,19] Research establishing this relationship, however, is limited. Recent studies by Len and Rao[14] and Williams et al.[15,19] suggest that vestibular and tactile processing abilities may be different in children who demonstrate idiopathic toe walking as compared to those with a typical gait pattern.

If conservative interventions fail to improve ankle ROM, if fixed ankle equinus contractures are present, or if toe walking reoccurs after a trial of nonsurgical management, **surgical lengthening of the triceps surae muscle-tendon complex or percutaneous lengthening of the Achilles tendon** is often considered.[2,20-22] Both surgical procedures are effective at lengthening the triceps surae muscle-tendon complex, increasing dorsiflexion in stance and swing phases of gait, and normalizing heel-toe gait in children with idiopathic toe walking.[2,20-22] While Achilles tendon lengthening has been shown to improve ankle kinematics without compromising triceps surae strength, plantar flexion *power* continues to be below normal even one year after surgery.[21] Some authors have suggested that over-lengthening is more likely to occur with surgical Achilles tendon lengthening.[2, 21] In long-term outcome studies that measure recurrence of toe walking and satisfaction of idiopathic toe-walking management procedures, surgical management seems to be more effective than nonsurgical interventions.[23]

Physical Therapy Patient/Client Management

The overall goals of physical therapy for the child with idiopathic toe walking center around improving active and passive ROM (especially in ankle dorsiflexion), increasing the incidence of heel strike during gait, and attaining age-appropriate gross motor milestones.

Examination, Evaluation, and Diagnosis

As part of the examination process, a complete history must be obtained including birth history, developmental history, medical history, family history of toe walking, and current and past interventions for toe walking.[24] Information about when the child started toe walking and the child's pattern of toe walking (consistent, intermittent, unilateral, bilateral) are also important factors. Other child-centered concerns should be explored including the possible presence of pain in the feet or legs and the possibility of other functional gait concerns such as stumbling or falling.[1,24,25] Tests and measures should include age-appropriate examinations of pain, muscle tone (including deep tendon reflexes and clonus), active and passive ROM, muscle length (especially of the ankle plantar flexors, hamstrings, and hip flexors), muscle strength, lower extremity alignment, and integumentary screening (especially for foot calluses, redness, etc.). Balance, posture, gait, and age-appropriate gross motor skills should also be assessed.

Developmental screening using tools such as the DENVER II[26] can be used to screen development across all functional domains. The DENVER II uses both parent observation and direct therapist observation to screen development in four areas (Personal-Social Skills, Fine Motor-Adaptive Skills, Language Skills, and Gross Motor Skills) in children ages 2 weeks to 6 years. The DENVER II is often preferred for developmental screening because it screens all major areas of development and can be administered and scored in 20 minutes or less. Since the majority of children who do not have developmental delays successfully pass the DENVER II, it has a very low false positive rate.[26] In light of the research demonstrating a positive correlation between idiopathic toe walking and sensory processing dysfunction, sensory processing should be screened. The Short Sensory Profile is a 38-item caregiver questionnaire designed to screen a child's ability to process sensory information in everyday situations. The tool was specifically designed for research and screening purposes and can be completed in 10 minutes.[27] Items on the Short Sensory Profile can help differentiate between typical performance, probable differences, and definite differences in a child's ability to process sensory information as a whole and in the following areas: Tactile Sensitivity, Taste/Smell Sensitivity, Movement Sensitivity, Under-responsive/Seeks Sensation, Auditory Filtering, Low Energy/Weak, and Visual/Auditory Sensitivity.[27]

Given that idiopathic toe walking is a diagnosis of exclusion, the **Toe Walking Tool**[28] may be helpful to differentiate between children who are true idiopathic toe walkers and children who toe walk as a result of a medical or developmental condition. The Toe Walking Tool is an easy-to-administer 28-item questionnaire composed of a series of questions and physical examination items.[28] Each item on the questionnaire falls into one of four sections: demographics, indicators of trauma, indicators of neuromuscular influence, or indicators of neurogenic influence. Questions include the presence or absence of factors such as premature birth, low birth weight, and the known existence of a medical or developmental condition associated with toe walking (*e.g.*, autism, CP, muscular dystrophy). Physical examination items include ankle and hamstring ROM, assessment of deep tendon reflexes, and observations of a child's movement. The tool is reliable and valid in children 4 to 8 years of age[28] and would be an appropriate tool to use in the examination of the 5-year-old boy in this case.

Plan of Care and Interventions

Early identification and intervention by a pediatric physical therapist may improve outcomes in children with idiopathic toe walking.[1,24] **Serial casting** is often used to address ROM deficits and improve gait in children who toe walk (Fig. 28-2).[8,24,29,30] In a study of 44 children with a diagnosis of idiopathic toe walking, 29 (66%) showed improvement in gait and clinician-determined outcomes such as improved ROM after serial casting.[8] Complications such as skin breakdown from casting were reported in only one subject.[8] Griffin et al.[29] also reported improved gait pattern (cessation of toe walking and normalized muscle activation patterns) in children with idiopathic toe walking after 6 to 8 weeks of casting. Brouwer et al.[30] observed that not only did children with idiopathic toe walking consistently walk in a normal heel-to-toe pattern after serial casting, but these improvements were also maintained for at least six weeks after casting. Use of botulinum toxin A (BTX-A) injections to the gastrocnemius-soleus complex in conjunction with serial casting has previously been suggested to improve outcomes.[31-34] However, a recent study of 47 children randomly assigned to serial casting only or serial casting in conjunction with BTX-A injections revealed no differences between the two groups.[33] Thus, the authors concluded that the addition of BTX-A injections prior to serial casting for idiopathic toe walking did not improve outcomes. A previous study by the same lead author found that while improvements in gait analysis were observed in children with idiopathic toe walking after a single injection of BTX-A performed in combination with an exercise program, the goal of ceasing to toe walk was only occasionally achieved over the course of the 12-month follow-up.[34]

Orthoses such as solid or articulating ankle-foot orthoses worn either at night or during the day may be useful in stretching the ankle plantar flexors and preventing excessive plantar flexion during gait.[2,24] Other possible interventions include stretching, strengthening of the anterior tibialis (and any other weak muscles), gait/treadmill training, and balance training.[2,24,35] Barret and Linn[35] reported success with neurodevelopmental treatment (NDT) techniques in combination with a behavior therapy technique in abolishing toe walking in a 9-year-old. In a 5-case series, Clark et al.[25] demonstrated that dorsiflexion limitations were reduced and heel-toe gait was improved (per parent report) following a motor control intervention.

Several authors recommend using passive ankle ROM as a guide to selecting interventions for the child with idiopathic toe walking.[8,24,30] Children with

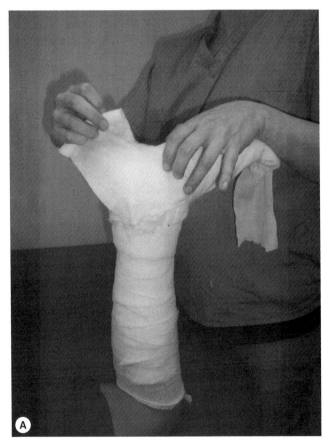

Figure 28-2. Application of serial cast to address ankle dorsiflexion ROM deficit in child with idiopathic toe walking. **A.** Application of cast padding over stockinette. Cast padding helps protect the skin.

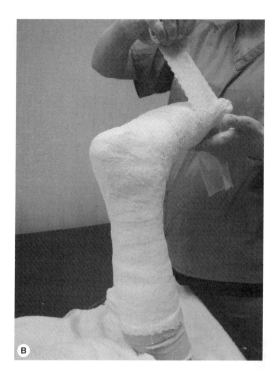

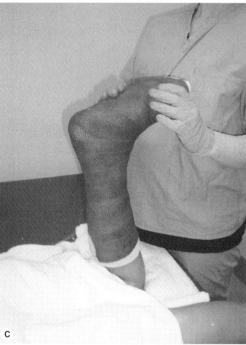

Figure 28-2. (*Continued*) Application of serial cast to address ankle dorsiflexion ROM deficit in child with idiopathic toe walking. **B.** Wrapping of the plaster layer that allows for more precise positioning of the foot and ankle in the cast. **C.** Application of the final fiberglass layer that helps protect the cast from damage and makes the cast lighter than if the cast were made entirely of the underlying plaster.

idiopathic toe walking who have 0° or less ankle dorsiflexion with the knee extended and the subtalar joint in neutral may benefit from serial casting with weekly cast changes.[8,24,30] For those who exhibit between 0° and 5° of ankle dorsiflexion, orthotic use, night splinting, and weekly physical therapy sessions may be best.[24,36] It is also important to recognize that in children with idiopathic toe walking, the amount of ankle dorsiflexion available in a nonweightbearing position may not correlate with the amount of ankle dorsiflexion actively used during gait.[37] In addition, some children with idiopathic toe walking may toe walk despite full passive and active ankle ROM.[24,33]

Evidence-Based Clinical Recommendations

SORT: Strength of Recommendation Taxonomy

A: Consistent, good-quality patient-oriented evidence
B: Inconsistent or limited-quality patient-oriented evidence
C: Consensus, disease-oriented evidence, usual practice, expert opinion, or case series

1. If conservative care for idiopathic toe walking fails, surgical lengthening of the triceps surae muscle-tendon complex improves ankle ROM and normalizes the gait pattern. **Grade B**

2. The Toe Walking Tool is a valid and reliable assessment to differentiate children who are true idiopathic toe walkers from children who toe walk as a result of a medical or developmental condition. **Grade B**

3. Early identification and nonsurgical interventions for idiopathic toe walking are critical for good outcomes. **Grade C**

4. Serial casting effectively improves ankle ROM and gait pattern in many children with idiopathic toe walking. **Grade B**

COMPREHENSION QUESTIONS

28.1 Which of the following statements regarding idiopathic toe walking is *most* accurate?

   A. Most elementary-age children will grow out of the behavior independent of management.

   B. Children with idiopathic toe walking may have delays in language skills or language disorders.

   C. Idiopathic toe walking typically presents as an asymmetrical condition.

   D. Idiopathic toe walking is more commonly observed in girls.

28.2 Which of the following examination findings is *most* suggestive of a non-idiopathic origin for toe-walking behaviors?

A. The presence of a plantar flexion contracture

B. Toe walking that occurs >75% of the time

C. Presence of spasticity in the gastrocnemius muscle

D. A report of pain in the feet or legs

28.3 A 15-month-old boy is referred for a physical therapy examination due to concerns related to his intermittent toe walking. Other than the occasional toe-walking pattern, the examination does not reveal any significant findings. What is the *most* appropriate physical therapy recommendation?

A. Refer. The child potentially has cerebral palsy or other underlying medical condition that is resulting in the toe-walking behavior.

B. Keep. Ongoing physical therapy sessions are needed to address the child's toe walking.

C. Monitor. Toe walking prior to the age of 2 years is a commonly reported gait deviation.

D. Keep and refer. The child requires intervention to address his toe walking and requires medical evaluation and testing to determine if an underlying medical condition is resulting in the toe-walking behavior.

ANSWERS

28.1 **B.** Children with idiopathic toe walking are more likely to have difficulties with language skills than children who do not toe walk. Elementary school-aged children who toe walk are not likely to outgrow the behavior (option A). Idiopathic toe walking almost always presents bilaterally (option C) and occurs more frequently in boys than in girls (option D).

28.2 **C.** Spasticity is not associated with idiopathic toe walking and is suggestive of upper motor neuron involvement. Children with idiopathic toe walking may have a plantar flexion contracture (option A), exhibit a high frequency of toe-walking behaviors (option B), and/or report pain in the feet or legs (option D).

28.3 **C.** In children younger than 24 months, toe walking is a commonly reported gait deviation. Monitoring the child is thus the most appropriate course of action. Only if toe walking persists beyond 2 years of age or if significant examination findings beyond the toe walking are found (such as ROM deficits), other options should be considered. The examination did not reveal any significant findings that would suggest the need to refer the child to rule out a condition such as CP (options A and D). The examination also did not reveal any findings that warrant regularly scheduled, on-going physical therapy intervention (option B).

REFERENCES

1. Sobel E, Caselli MA, Velez Z. Effect of persistent toe walking on ankle equinus. Analysis of 60 idiopathic toe walkers. *J Am Podiatr Med Assoc.* 1997;87:17-22.

2. Oetgen M, Peden S. Idiopathic toe walking. *J Am Acad Orthop Surg.* 2012;20:292-300.

3. Accardo P, Morrow J, Heaney MS, Whitman B, Tomazic T. Toe walking and language development. *Clin Pediatr.* 1992;31:158-160.

4. Engström P, Tedroff K. The prevalence and course of idiopathic toe-walking in 5-year-old children. *Pediatr.* 2012;130:279-284.

5. Sutherland DH, Olshen R, Cooper L, Woo SL. The development of mature gait. *J Bone Joint Surg.* 1980;62:336-353.

6. Burnett CN, Johnson EW. Development of gait in childhood. II. *Dev Med Child Neurol.* 1971; 13:207-215.

7. Hall JE, Salter RB, Bhalla SK. Congenital short tendo calcaneus. *J Bone Joint Surg Br.* 1967;49:695-697.

8. Fox A, Deakin S, Pettigrew G, Paton R. Serial casting in the treatment of idiopathic toe-walkers and review of the literature. *Acta Orthop Belg.* 2006;72:722-730.

9. Stricker SJ, Angulo JC. Idiopathic toe walking: a comparison of treatment methods. *J Pediatr Orthop.* 1998;18:289-293.

10. Westberry DE, Davids JR, Davis RB, de Morais Filho MC. Idiopathic toe walking: a kinematic and kinetic profile. *J Pediatr Orthop.* 2008;28:352-258.

11. Rinehart NJ, Bradshaw JL, Breeton AV, Tonge BJ. A clinical and neurobehavioural review of high-functioning autism and Asperger's disorder. *Aust N Z J Psychiatry.* 2002;36:762-770.

12. Barrow WJ, Jaworski M, Accardo PJ. Persistent toe walking in autism. *Child Neurol.* 2011;26:619-621.

13. Shulman LH, Sala DA, Chu ML, McCaul PR, Sandler BJ. Developmental implications of idiopathic toe walking. *J Pediatr.* 1997;130:541-546.

14. Len AY, Rao S. Sensory processing dysfunction in children with idiopathic toe-walking. *Pediatr Phys Ther.* 2013;25;112.

15. Williams C, Tinley P, Curtin M. Is idiopathic toe walking a symptom of sensory processing dysfunction? *J Foot Ankle Res.* 2011;4(S1):59.

16. Engström P, Van't Hooft I, Tedroff K. Neuropsychiatric symptoms and problems among children with idiopathic toe-walking. *J Pediatr Orthop.* 2012;32:848-852.

17. Accardo P, Whitman B. Toe walking: a marker for language disorders in the developmentally disabled. *Clin Pediatr.* 1989;28:347-350.

18. Montgomery P, Gauger J. Sensory dysfunction in children who toe walk. *Phys Ther.* 1978;58:1195-1204.

19. Williams C, Tinley P, Curtin M. Idiopathic toe walking and sensory processing dysfunction. *J Foot Ankle Res.* 2010;3:16-22.

20. McMulkin ML, Baird GO, Caskey PM, Ferguson RL. Comprehensive outcomes of surgically treated idiopathic toe walkers. *J Pediatr Orthop.* 2006;26:606-611.

21. Hemo Y, Macdessi SJ, Pierce RA, Aiona MD, Sussman MD. Outcome of patients after Achilles tendon lengthening for treatment of idiopathic toe walking. *J Pediatr Orthop.* 2006;26:336-340.

22. Jahn J, Vasavada AN, McMulkin ML. Calf muscle-tendon lengths before and after Tendo-Achilles lengthenings and gastrocnemius lengthenings for equinus in cerebral palsy and idiopathic toe walking. *Gait Posture.* 2009;29:612-617.

23. Eastwood DM, Menelaus MB, Dickens DR, Broughton NS, Cole WG. Idiopathic toe-walking: does treatment alter the natural history? *J Pediatr Orthop B.* 2000;9:47-49.

24. Le Cras S, Bouck J, Brausch S, Taylor-Haas A. Cincinnati Children's Hospital Medical Center: Evidence-based clinical care guideline for Management of Idiopathic Toe Walking. http://www.

cincinnatichildrens.org/service/j/anderson-center/evidence-based-care/occupational-therapy-physical-therapy/. Guideline 040, pp. 1-17. Accessed October 9, 2014.

25. Clark E, Sweeney JK, Yocum A, McCoy SW. Effects of motor control intervention for children with idiopathic toe walking: a 5-case series. *Pediatr Phys Ther*. 2010;22;417-426.

26. Frankenburg WK, Dobbs J, Archer P, Bresnick B, Maschka P, Edelman N. *Denver II Training Manual*. Denver, CO: Denver Developmental Materials; 1992.

27. McIntosh DN, Miller LJ, Shyu V, Dunn W. Overview of the Short Sensory Profile (SSP). In: Dunn W, ed. *The Sensory Profile: Examiner's Manual*. San Antonio, TX: Psychological Corporation; 1999:59.

28. Williams CM, Tinley P, Curtin M. The Toe Walking Tool: a novel method for assessing idiopathic toe walking children. *Gait Posture*. 2010;32:508-511.

29. Griffin PP, Wheelhouse WW, Shiavi R, Bass W. Habitual toe-walkers. a clinical and electromyographic gait analysis. *J Bone Joint Surg Am*. 1977;59:97-101.

30. Brouwer B, Davidson LK, Olney SJ. Serial casting in idiopathic toe-walkers and children with spastic cerebral palsy. *J Pediatr Orthop*. 2000;20:221-225.

31. Jacks LK, Michels DM, Smith BP, Koman LA, Shilt J. Clinical usefulness of botulinum toxin in the lower extremity. *Foot Ankle Clin*. 2004;9:339-348.

32. Gormley ME, Herring GM, Gaebler-Spira DJ. The use of botulinum toxin in children: a retrospective study of adverse reactions and treatment of idiopathic toe-walking. *Eur J Neurol*. 1997;4(Suppl 2): S27-S30.

33. Engström P, Bartonek A, Tedroff K, Orefelt C, Haglund-Åkerlind Y, Gutierrez-Farewik EM. Botulinum toxin A does not improve the results of cast treatment for idiopathic toe-walking: a randomized controlled trial. *J Bone Joint Surg Am*. 2013;95:400-407.

34. Engström P, Gutierrez-Farewik EM, Bartonek A, Tedroff K, Orefelt C, Haglund-Akerlind Y. Does botulinum toxin A improve the walking pattern in children with idiopathic toe-walking? *J Child Orthop*. 2010;4:301-308.

35. Barrett RP, Linn DM. Treatment of stereotyped toe-walking with overcorrection and physical therapy. *Appl Res Ment Retard*. 1981;2:13-21.

36. Gourdine-Shaw MC, Lamm BM, Herzenberg JE, Bhave A. Equinus deformity in the pediatric patient: causes, evaluation, and management. *Clin Podiatr Med Surg*. 2010; 27:25-42.

37. Stott NS, Walt SE, Lobb GA, Reynolds N, Nicol RO. Treatment for idiopathic toe-walking: results at skeletal maturity. *J Pediatr Orthop*. 2004;24:63-69.

Femoroacetabular Impingement

Jessica Laniak

A healthy 12-year-old female soccer goalie presented to a primary care physician with intermittent anterior hip and groin pain after her completed season. At first, she only had pain when kicking and punting with her dominant right leg. Now, she is having anterior hip and groin pain with all weightbearing activities. She denies any signs and symptoms of fever, malaise, or rash. Her primary care physician referred her to a physical therapist with a diagnosis of "hip flexor strain." Because her pain had not changed after two weeks of physical therapy, she was sent to a pediatric orthopaedist who confirmed the therapist's findings of limited right hip flexion and internal rotation (IR) and pain with palpation of the anterior inferior iliac spine and pubic symphysis. After a single-photo emission computerized tomography (SPECT) scan, the orthopaedist diagnosed her with an anterior inferior iliac spine avulsion fracture and pubic symphysis avulsion fracture. The scan also demonstrated increased uptake at the right femoral head and acetabulum. Per physician recommendation, the patient rested for an additional eight weeks and then went to another physical therapist for evaluation. The physical therapist suspected that the patient had femoroacetabular impingement (FAI) and determined that she was appropriate for a physical therapy plan of care.

▶ What examination signs may be associated with this diagnosis?
▶ What are the most appropriate examination tests?
▶ What are the possible complications that may limit the effectiveness of physical therapy?
▶ What are the most appropriate physical therapy interventions?
▶ Describe a physical therapy plan of care based on both immediate intervention and return to sport.
▶ Identify when it would be appropriate to refer to other medical team members.

KEY DEFINITIONS

CAM IMPINGEMENT: Increased diameter of cam or egg-shaped femoral head with undercoverage of the acetabulum

FEMOROACETABULAR IMPINGEMENT (FAI): Decreased hip range of motion (ROM) due to altered alignment of the femoral head and acetabulum

PINCER IMPINGEMENT: Increased bony coverage by the acetabulum over a typically developed femoral head, which results in a deeper socket

Objectives

1. Identify the signs and symptoms of FAI.
2. Determine the differential diagnoses that should be considered with FAI.
3. Develop appropriate impairment and functional limitation physical therapy interventions for an adolescent with FAI.
4. Progress the plan of care for return-to-sport performance.

Physical Therapy Considerations

PT considerations for the active adolescent athlete with FAI:

▶ **General physical therapy plan of care and goals:** Improve hip ROM, strength, mobility, and flexibility impairments; enhance core and lower extremity neuromuscular control; maximize function and return to sport

▶ **Physical therapy interventions:** Education to patient and family on biomechanics and course of physical therapy; manual therapy to hip and joints related to lower extremity function to improve biomechanics; lower extremity stretching; core and lower extremity strengthening; exercises to promote neuromuscular control, functional strength, and proprioception of the lower extremity; gait training (walking and running); return-to-sport interventions; education on prevention of overuse and on fitness maintenance, when appropriate for discharge

▶ **Precautions during physical therapy:** Monitor for unremitting pain that could indicate progression of bony abnormality or systemic disease; avoid impact activities until able to progress to return-to-sport activities

▶ **Complications during physical therapy:** Progressing avulsion fractures or development of new stress fractures; acetabular labral pathology; lumbar spine radiculopathy; sacroiliac joint dysfunction; depression due to psychosocial stress

Understanding the Health Condition

Femoroacetabular impingement (FAI) is a biomechanical diagnosis that describes altered joint kinematics of the ball and socket joint of the hip. Diagnostic imaging enables descriptions of the shape of the femoral head and acetabulum and the congruency between the two. A cam impingement describes when the femoral head is enlarged, but still convex in shape, so that it can sit in the acetabulum. A pincer impingement describes when the rim of the acetabulum is extended and causes "overcoverage" of a typically developing femoral head. Currently, FAI is a diagnosis of exclusion and needs to be more fully assessed, especially within the pediatric population. The ball and socket joint is susceptible to congenital defects or traumatic injuries that can mimic signs and symptoms of FAI and these conditions should be ruled out before the diagnosis of FAI is made.[1] Also, if the individual has a history of altered development of the hip joint, it is likely that he/she will have an increased risk of developing FAI later in life, even if the abnormal development has been successfully treated.[2]

Infants are often screened for congenital hip dysplasia. This is especially true with infants who are diagnosed with congenital muscular torticollis, are female, are first born, or were in a breech presentation at time of birth.[3] In infancy, hip dysplasia can be diagnosed with ultrasound to determine whether the cartilaginous femoral head is properly located in the acetabulum or if it is indeed subluxed or dislocated. To screen for hip dysplasia in infants, physical therapists use the Ortolani test and Barlow maneuver. The Ortolani test involves moving the lower extremities into a flexed position and then abducting and externally rotating the hips. A relocation of a dislocated hip will occur with a palpable "clunk." The Barlow maneuver dislocates an unstable hip by bringing the hip back from this position into flexion and adduction. In infants with hip dysplasia, it is common to intervene with a Pavlik harness to keep them in a frog-leg position to allow the femoral head to develop a round shape and stay in the acetabulum. If this is unsuccessful, closed or open reductions of the hips may be required. If children continue to have dislocations beyond the age of 2 years, femoral or pelvic osteotomies followed by spica casting to maintain hip alignment may be required. With hip dysplasia, the shape of the acetabulum may be affected and the femoral head and epiphysis are at risk for poor anatomical development. FAI can be a late sequela of poorly managed congenitally dysplastic hips as this would disrupt the anatomical alignment of one or both of the sides of the joint.[4]

Other congenital diagnoses that can affect normal hip joint development are coxa vara or coxa valga. With these diagnoses, the femoral head and neck angle of inclination is altered. The normal angle of inclination between the femoral head and neck is 120°.[5] Coxa vara creates a 90° angle between the femoral head and neck, thereby forcing the acetabulum to become deeper to seat the femoral head and creating the weightbearing surface on the superior border of the femoral head and acetabular rim. This would create a pincer impingement alignment.[6] In contrast, coxa valga creates a more obtuse angle between the femoral head and neck and therefore a more vertical orientation of the femoral head in the acetabulum. This would create a cam impingement alignment.[6] With either of these conditions, the femoral head and acetabulum will have a developmentally altered alignment that can lead to FAI alignment.[7] These two congenital anomalies can be treated surgically with femoral or acetabular osteotomies.

For pediatric patients presenting with hip pain or difficulty weightbearing, two additional diagnoses must be considered. In pre-adolescent and adolescent age groups, a slipped capital femoral epiphysis (SCFE) and Legg-Calve-Perthes (LCP) disease both involve collapse of the femoral head. SCFE is a disorder in which the proximal femoral epiphysis in the femoral head slips off of the femoral neck, usually in an anteromedial direction. SCFE is most common in males between 10 and 16 years old and is usually an acute or acute-on-chronic presentation without history of trauma.[8] With SCFE, it is very common for the individual to complain only of knee pain.[9] On clinical examination, the patient typically presents with loss of hip IR and adduction and excessive external rotation. Severity and progression of the slippage of the proximal femoral epiphysis is measured via radiographs or magnetic resonance imaging (MRI) scans. Most individuals undergo bilateral femoral head pinning, even if only one side is involved because a small percentage of individuals with unilateral SCFE will develop a contralateral slip later in life.[10]

The second condition associated with femoral head collapse is LCP disease. LCP is a childhood disorder associated with avascular necrosis of the femoral head, usually idiopathic in nature. Blood flow disruption occurs in the medial circumflex artery and results in a flattening of the proximal femoral head. Upon diagnostic imaging with MRI, the femoral head appears "moth-eaten" and is measured in severity by the amount of the lateral femoral head that presents in line with the acetabular rim.[11] The typical presentation of an individual with LCP is a child 3 to 12 years old with a history of limping or Trendelenburg gait and hip pain. However, these children tend to be very active and try to perform normal tasks despite their impairments.[12] In LCP, hip IR and abduction are limited. Although diagnostic imaging can demonstrate significant abnormalities, children with this diagnosis are often treated with a period of nonweightbearing (to decrease compressive forces on the femoral head), lower extremity strengthening in an open kinetic chain alignment, and aquatic physical therapy.[13] After such clinical management, LCP disease is self-healing in one to three years.[13] Despite appropriate management of LCP and SCFE to remedy collapse of the femoral head, altered joint biomechanics during the treatment and rehabilitation stages can negatively affect ongoing development of the acetabulum due to abnormal weightbearing. The alignment of the femoral head and acetabulum changes as the child develops, which may lead to FAI later in life.[14-17]

If all congenital and traumatic differential diagnoses have been ruled out, the pediatric orthopaedist evaluates diagnostic imaging of the hip and pelvis to determine the anatomical alignment and to rule out other intra-articular injuries. The most common orthopaedic diagnoses affecting children—especially children involved in sports—are femoral neck stress fracture and acetabular labral pathology. Symptoms of femoral neck stress fracture are usually deep hip pain with weightbearing and during sport. These stress fractures are common in female endurance athletes presenting with the female athlete triad of decreased energy availability (with or without disordered eating), menstrual dysfunction, and low bone mineral density.[18] Acetabular labral pathology presents with complaints of intra-articular clicking and catching. Typically, individuals with this pathology regularly perform hip motions to the excess of ROM (*e.g.*, dancers) or perform excessive rotation of the acetabulum on the femur with pivoting and cutting (*e.g.*, soccer and basketball players).[19] The clinical presentation of acetabular labral pathology is similar to that of FAI and can be ruled out with an MRI or magnetic resonance angiogram (MRA).[1]

Once a diagnosis of exclusion is made that points toward FAI, medical management is either conservative (physical therapy) or surgical (femoral or acetabular osteotomies or hip resurfacing).[20] Due to the open physis in the femoral head in skeletally immature individuals, hip resurfacing techniques are usually not surgical options.[21] Therefore, the most common surgical interventions are arthroscopic osteotomies. For a cam impingement, the femoral head is shaved down to be more congruent with the typically developing acetabulum. If there is a significant chondral lesion in the femoral head due to altered weightbearing surfaces, this may be addressed with microfracture (drilling into the cartilage of the hip). For a pincer impingement, the acetabular rim is surgically trimmed. Often, there is also an acetabular labral tear that needs to be debrided or repaired.

Physical Therapy Patient/Client Management

Management of the pediatric patient with FAI could be via direct access or via referral from an orthopaedist, rheumatologist, or primary care physician. In states where direct access is permitted for physical therapists, it is common for the physical therapist to be the first to evaluate athletic children and young adults. Although the physical therapist may be the first clinician to identify the biomechanical features of FAI, referral to an orthopaedist or other physician is necessary to obtain diagnostic imaging to rule out other intra-articular pathologies (*e.g.*, acetabular labral tear, femoral neck stress fracture) especially due to the young age of the patient and characteristics of the pain onset. In the absence of a labral tear or other chondral lesion that requires more immediate surgical intervention, physicians frequently refer patients to physical therapy for conservative management prior to considering surgical options. A rheumatologist may also refer an individual, if the rheumatologist has ruled out juvenile arthritis, avascular necrosis, or infectious etiology of acute onset. If the patient with FAI is not demonstrating improvements with physical therapy in 4 to 12 weeks,[22-24] it is imperative that the physical therapist know when it is appropriate to refer back to a physician. The physical therapist will likely be treating a patient with FAI who is still involved in a sport. The therapist must facilitate collaboration with the physician, patient/family, athletic trainer, and coach to develop appropriate training. This will involve audience-appropriate education regarding the biomechanics of the hip joint, impairment level interventions, and timetable for return to sport.

Examination, Evaluation, and Diagnosis

Most of the suspicion for FAI comes from actively listening to the patient's history and subjective complaints. The patient typically describes a localized hip pain that began as an anterior or anteromedial hip/groin pain with activity. The pain pattern often migrates to a deep hip pain and the patient may grasp around the lateral anterior and posterior femoral head and describe the pain as "inside of her hip."

This is called the "C sign."[20] The patient often describes athletic activity that aggravates the pain. Repetitive extremes of hip ROM especially with flexion, such as a soccer goalie punting, or excessive closed chain hip rotation and pivoting are common painful activities. Careful attention should be made to inquire about congenital hip issues or previous trauma to the lumbar spine, pelvis, or hip. The patient likely will not have pain with stretching of contractile tissue that can be palpated because the described pain is intra-articular.[25] Often, patients note pain with flexion and IR and may report having a feeling as though the hip is stuck or restricted from going through more ROM. Two systematic reviews[26,27] and a case study[22] have noted that the combination of historical report of groin pain, clicking, and tight hip flexors on the Thomas test is common in FAI or labral pathology.

The typical arthrokinematics of a ball and socket joint must be considered during assessment of the hip's available ROM. The normal roll and glide of the femoral head in the acetabulum should allow for improved hip flexion and IR with a posterior glide and for improved hip extension and abduction with an anterior glide. However, with cam and pincer misalignments in FAI, the femoral head and acetabulum are contacting prematurely, usually at the inferomedial acetabular rim with flexion and IR. Thus, on examination, the individual with FAI has decreased hip flexion and IR ROM as well as pain reproduction. Flexion of the hip may be more limited with the knee flexed because the hamstrings are not on tension and will not be drawing the pelvis or femoral head posteriorly. Rotation can be measured in supine (with the hip flexed to 90°) or prone (Craig's or Ryder test).[5] In prone, normal hip IR is approximately 40°. However, any asymmetry in the Ryder test contributes to the diagnostic picture of FAI. If the therapist suspects FAI, the flexion-adduction-internal rotation (FADDIR) test should be performed. The FADDIR test is positive (commonly called an anterior impingement sign) when pain is reproduced with the hip in maximum flexion, adduction, and IR with the patient supine. Although this position can reproduce the patient's pain, this may be due to FAI as well as other intra-articular lesions such as an acetabular labral tear. Decreased hip extension may be present secondary to pain as the femoral head moves anteriorly in the acetabulum. The therapist should also assess for pelvic rotation[28] by checking for asymmetry of the anterior superior iliac spine (ASIS) and posterior superior iliac spine (PSIS) on each side to determine if the acetabulum is restricting motion to create the impingement. Last, the therapist should perform a lumbar screen before continuing with the hip examination to determine whether there is any contribution from this area and to provide further information regarding the flexibility of the two-joint hip muscles (e.g., iliopsoas, hamstrings).

Muscle strength can be tested by manual muscle tests and functional tests. In individuals with FAI, significant weakness is notable in the gluteus muscles. Hip abduction and extension are weak and can be painful, whereas hip flexion and external rotation are usually strong and painless. From a brief gait assessment, the therapist may note a Trendelenburg sign in stance phase on the involved lower extremity. Functional measurements include lateral step-downs and squats. With the patient standing on her involved limb, a positive Trendelenburg sign is often noted during a lateral step-down. In this closed kinetic chain activity, the lower extremity forces the acetabulum to rotate on a fixed femur during hip flexion. During the lateral step-down (or unilateral or double limb squat), the physical therapist may observe the patient shifting her weight away from the involved side or increasing knee flexion (versus hip flexion) on the involved side due to altered kinematics in the hip. It is also important to assess core muscle strength, specifically that of the transversus abdominis and obliques because they help stabilize the lumbopelvic mechanics that may be compensating for the hip affected by FAI.[29] Sahrmann[30] describes a good core strength assessment for transversus abdominis and obliques. For endurance testing of these muscles, functional tasks such as prone planks can be used.

There are several diagnostic special tests for FAI. In a meta-analysis of 21 studies, Tijssen et al.[27] evaluated the diagnostic accuracy of 18 tests for FAI and labral pathology. Although multiple articles utilized similar tests (though often under different names), the most frequently evaluated tests in the studies were the FADDIR test (also known as the anterior impingement test), flexion-abduction-external rotation (FABER) test, and a resisted straight leg raise. For the FABER test, the patient is supine and the involved leg in flexed into a figure 4 position with the ankle resting on the contralateral knee. A positive FABER sign is typically pain reproduction in the hip or an increased distance of the knee from the table as compared to the contralateral side.[20] Tijssen et al.[27] concluded that there were no tests that provided good overall diagnostic accuracy and a significant recommendation could not be made due to the poor quality of the studies. In 2013, Reiman et al.[31] performed a systematic review with meta-analysis of 14 articles that examined the diagnostic accuracy of hip physical examination tests. For the diagnosis of FAI, labral, or intra-articular pathology, these authors found that the FABER test (used in three studies) had sensitivity ranging from 42% to 81% and specificity ranging from 18% to 75%. For the FADDIR test (used in six studies), sensitivity ranged from 59% to 100% and specificity ranged from 4% to 75%. Thus, both of these recent systematic reviews have concluded that **most clinical diagnostic tests for FAI have weak diagnostic utility**. Philippon et al.[20] and Frank et al.[32] summarized their criteria for assessing FAI. In these reviews, the authors proposed the use of a *combination* of diagnostic tests and concluded that positive FADDIR, FABER, and hip dial tests are suggestive of FAI. These authors characterized the FABER test as being positive when both the knee height of the involved lower extremity is greater than 4 cm off of the table as compared to the uninvolved side and pain is provoked. For the hip dial test, the patient is supine with knees extended. The therapist places a quick external rotation moment distally by rolling the leg out laterally. If the patient's limb does not rebound back to a place of relative hip IR or neutral alignment, as compared to the uninvolved side, the hip dial test is considered positive.

Plan of Care and Interventions

The first goal for this 12-year-old patient with FAI is to restore as much ROM to the hip joint as possible. **For a cam impingement, mobilizations of the posterior hip capsule may be used to improve hip ROM.**[33] With the patient in supine and the right (involved) hip flexed to 90°, the therapist can provide Grade III-IV mobilizations with a slight lateral distraction and anterior to posterior glide. If more distraction is required to improve mobility of the hip, the therapist may use a mobilization belt. If the therapist found that the pelvis was anteriorly rotated (by assessment of ASIS and PSIS symmetry), muscle energy techniques[34] or pelvic mobilizations can be performed to help align the acetabular portion of the FAI alignment. For this patient, the muscle energy technique (MET) to correct a right anterior pelvic rotation would be activation of the hamstring muscles and hip extensors on the right side and the hip flexors on the left side. This technique could be taught as part of a home exercise program if the patient was unable to maintain her pelvis in a neutral alignment between sessions. To mobilize the pelvis, the therapist could perform a manipulation in the figure 4 position as with a lumbopelvic rotation on the ipsilateral side.

It is important to regain muscle flexibility, especially in the hip flexors that may be pulling the femoral head forward in the acetabulum. A modified Thomas test stretching position would be appropriate to stretch the iliopsoas on the involved side. Piriformis stretching is also important because the posterior hip muscles can be shortened due to the anterior displacement of the femoral head in the acetabulum.[35]

For soccer players, core stabilization assists in trunk stability for cutting and pivoting maneuvers.[36,37] In individuals with FAI, altered trunk mechanics may both contribute to and compensate for the injury pattern in FAI.[38,39] Thus, for the current young soccer player with FAI, core strengthening and stabilization exercises should be included in the plan of care to assist in lumbopelvic alignment, postural correction, and support of the lower extremity. The evaluative techniques outlined by Sahrmann[30] can also be used as interventions to combine isometric exercises for the abdominal muscles with a progression of lower extremity movement patterns to retrain the neuromuscular control of the lumbopelvic complex. Activities such as planks, side planks, and oblique exercises also strengthen core musculature.[40]

Based on the patient's pain acuity level, it may be necessary to begin strengthening the hip abductors and extensors in a single plane. However, progression should advance to more functional strengthening in closed kinetic chain for the hip rotators, hip extensors, and quadriceps to begin neuromuscular retraining of the lower extremity. For example, with the patient in the quadruped position, the therapist can ask the patient to extend or rotate her hip without using trunk or pelvic rotation. The therapist provides verbal and tactile cues to help the patient maintain lumbar stability and posture. In this way, the therapist can correct a Trendelenburg sign and facilitate co-contraction of the hip abductors and extensors to specifically retrain the gluteus muscles in their function as hip stabilizers.[35,41]

The therapist needs to educate the patient and her family about the FAI diagnosis and necessary activity modification. It is important for the athlete with an acute pain presentation to take time off from sport to decrease inflammation and pain and to avoid compensatory gait patterns from developing. Activities of daily living that involve hip flexion (*e.g.*, tying shoelaces, climbing stairs) should be modified to avoid pain. Gait retraining is imperative to decrease the Trendelenburg gait presentation, even if the patient must be nonweightbearing on her involved lower extremity in the acutely painful stage.[42] Few studies have determined the success rate of conservative management. However, the available literature suggests

4 to 12 weeks of conservative management before surgical intervention should be considered.[22,23,42]

Once the patient is not painful and has normalized hip biomechanics, return-to-sport progression can begin. To return to soccer, this patient will first have to perform lower impact activities such as running and double-leg jumping before performing cutting, pivoting, and unilateral hopping. In 2012, Bizzini et al.[43] proposed a functional battery of tests for athletes returning to soccer after an anterior cruciate ligament tear, which mimics the demands after a course of rehabilitation for FAI. A **functional hop test** involving repeated unilateral hops is appropriate to determine power and symmetry of landing mechanics for return to sport.[44] A Yo-Yo test and a repeated shuttle-sprint ability test would also be appropriate to determine cutting and pivoting for return to sport. Finally, if a patient has been able to perform all of these tasks pain-free, sport-specific drills can be included. Since this patient is a soccer goalie, diving for a ball, long kicks, and lateral agility tests would be appropriate for her to perform in order to prepare for re-entry to sport.

Evidence-Based Clinical Recommendations

SORT: Strength of Recommendation Taxonomy

A: Consistent, good-quality patient-oriented evidence
B: Inconsistent or limited-quality patient-oriented evidence
C: Consensus, disease-oriented evidence, usual practice, expert opinion, or case series

1. Individual clinical diagnostic tests for femoroacetabular impingement (FAI) have higher sensitivity than specificity, but overall they have weak diagnostic properties. **Grade B**

2. For a cam impingement, mobilizations of the posterior hip capsule may improve hip ROM by allowing the femoral head to move closer to the neutral axis on the acetabular surface. **Grade C**

3. A functional hop test to determine strength and power development as well as landing technique and neuromuscular control can be used to help determine readiness to return to sport for the athlete with FAI. **Grade C**

COMPREHENSION QUESTIONS

29.1 With FAI, the range of motion loss typically involves:

A. Hip flexion and abduction
B. Hip flexion and internal rotation
C. Hip extension and abduction
D. Hip extension and external rotation

29.2 Hip mobilizations for addressing the _____ capsule should be Grade ____
to increase ROM.

A. Anterior capsule; I-II

B. Anterior capsule; III-IV

C. Posterior capsule; I-II

D. Posterior capsule; III-IV

ANSWERS

29.1 **B.** Hip flexion and internal rotation are limited in patients with FAI and patients typically complain of pain and discomfort when performing these active motions.

29.2 **D.** Grade III-IV mobilizations at the posterior capsule stretch the capsular and ligamentous structures and may provide the necessary accessory mobility to improve hip flexion and internal rotation range of motion. Grade I mobilizations only unweight supporting surfaces and grade II mobilizations take up the slack that exists in the joint capsule to reduce pain, but neither of these grades would decrease joint capsule tightness or increase range of motion.

REFERENCES

1. Giordano BD. Assessment and treatment of hip pain in the adolescent athlete. *Pediatr Clin North Am.* 2014;61:1137-1154.

2. Sangal RB, Waryasz GR, Schiller JR. Femoroacetabular impingement: a review of current concepts. *R I Med J.* 2014;97:33-38.

3. Loder RT, Skopelja EN. The epidemiology and demographics of hip dysplasia. *ISRN Orthop.* 2011;2011:238607.

4. Nakahara I, Takao M, Sakai T, Miki H, Nishii T, Sugano N. Three-dimensional morphology and bony range of movement in hip joints in patients with hip dysplasia. *Bone Joint J.* 2014;96-B:580-589.

5. Lowes LP, Sveda M, Gajdosik CG, Gajdosik RL. Musculoskeletal development and adaptation. In: Campbell SK, Palisano RJ, Orlin MN, eds. *Physical Therapy for Children.* 4th ed. St. Louis, MO: Elsevier Saunders; 2012:175-204.

6. Wright AA, Naze GS, Kavchak AE, Paul D, Kenison B, Hegedus EJ. Radiological variables associated with progression of femoroacetabular impingement of the hip: a systematic review. *J Sci Med Sport.* 2015;18:122-127.

7. Beck M, Kalhor M, Leunig M, Ganz R. Hip morphology influences the pattern of damage to the acetabular cartilage: femoroacetabular impingement as a cause of early osteoarthritis of the hip. *J Bone Joint Surg Br.* 2005;87:1012-1018.

8. Loder RT, Skopelja EN. The epidemiology and demographics of slipped capital femoral epiphysis. *ISRN Orthop.* 2011;2011:486512.

9. Georgiadis AG, Zaltz I. Slipped capital femoral epiphysis: how to evaluate with a review and update of treatment. *Pediatr Clin North Am.* 2014;61:1119-1135.

10. Baghdadi YM, Larson AN, Sierra RJ, Peterson HA, Stans AA. The fate of hips that are not prophylactically pinned after unilateral slipped capital femoral epiphysis. *Clin Orthop Relat Res.* 2013;471:2124-2131.

11. Kim HK, Wiesman KD, Kulkarni V, et al. Perfusion MRI in early stage of Legg-Calve-Perthes disease to predict lateral pillar involvement: a preliminary study. *J Bone Joint Surg Am.* 2014;96:1152-1160.

12. Hailer YD, Haag AC, Nilsson O. Legg-Calve-Perthes disease: quality of life, physical activity, and behavior pattern. *J Pediatr Orthop.* 2014;34:514-521.

13. Arkader A, Sankar WN, Amorim RM. Conservative versus surgical treatment of late-onset Legg-Calve-Perthes disease: a radiographic comparison at skeletal maturity. *J Child Orthop.* 2009;3:21-25.

14. Millis MB, Lewis CL, Schoenecker PL, Clohisy JC. Legg-Calve-Perthes disease and slipped capital femoral epiphysis: major developmental causes of femoroacetabular impingement. *J Am Acad Orthop Surg.* 2013;21(Suppl 1):S59-S63.

15. Murgier J, Reina N, Cavaignac E, Espie A, Bayle-Iniguez X, Chiron P. The frequency of sequelae of slipped upper femoral epiphysis in cam-type femoroacetabular impingement. *Bone Joint J.* 2014;96-B:724-729.

16. Bali K, Railton P, Kiefer GN, Powell JN. Subcapital osteotomy of the femoral neck for patients with healed slipped capital femoral epiphysis. *Bone Joint J.* 2014;96-B:1441-1448.

17. Ramachandran M, Azegami S, Hosalkar HS. Current concepts in the treatment of adolescent femoroacetabular impingement. *J Child Orthop.* 2013;7:79-90.

18. Rauh MJ, Barrack M, Nichols JF. Associations between the female athlete triad and injury among high school runners. *Int J Sports Phys Ther.* 2014;9:948-958.

19. Nawabi DH, Bedi A, Tibor LM, Magennis E, Kelly BT. The demographic characteristics of high-level and recreational athletes undergoing hip arthroscopy for femoroacetabular impingement: a sports-specific analysis. *Arthroscopy.* 2014;30:398-405.

20. Philippon MJ, Patterson DC, Briggs KK. Hip arthroscopy and femoroacetabular impingement in the pediatric patient. *J Pediatr Orthop.* 2013;33(Suppl 1):S126-S130.

21. Bloomfield MR, Erickson JA, McCarthy JC, et al. Hip pain in the young, active patient: surgical strategies. *Instr Course Lect.* 2014;63:159-176.

22. Reiman MP, Stovak M, Dart BR. Femoroacetabular impingement in a high school female athlete. *J Orthop Sports Phys Ther.* 2011;41:982.

23. Hunt D, Prather H, Harris HM, Clohisy JC. Clinical outcomes analysis of conservative and surgical treatment of patients with clinical indications of prearthritic, intra-articular hip disorders. *PM R.* 2012;4:479-487.

24. de Sa D, Cargnelli S, Catapano M, et al. Femoroacetabular impingement in skeletally immature patients: a systematic review examining indications, outcomes, and complications of open and arthroscopic treatment. *Arthroscopy.* 2015;31:373-384.

25. Dutton M. Patient/client management. In: Dutton M, ed. *Dutton's Orthopaedic Examination, Evaluation, and Intervention.* 3rd ed. New York, NY: McGraw Hill Medical; 2012:151-191.

26. Burgess RM, Rushton A, Wright C, Daborn C. The validity and accuracy of clinical diagnostic tests used to detect labral pathology of the hip: a systematic review. *Man Ther.* 2011;16:318-326.

27. Tijssen M, van Cingel R, Willemsen L, de Visser E. Diagnostics of femoroacetabular impingement and labral pathology of the hip: a systematic review of the accuracy and validity of physical tests. *Arthroscopy.* 2012;28:860-871.

28. Ross JR, Nepple JJ, Philippon MJ, Kelly BT, Larson CM, Bedi A. Effect of changes in pelvic tilt on range of motion to impingement and radiographic parameters of acetabular morphologic characteristics. *Am J Sports Med.* 2014;42:2402-2409.

29. Harris-Hayes M, Sahrmann SA, Van Dillen LR. Relationship between the hip and low back pain in athletes who participate in rotation-related sports. *J Sport Rehabil.* 2009;18:60-75.

30. Sahrmann SA. Exercises to correct movement impairment syndromes. In: Sahrmann SA, ed. *Diagnosis and Treatment of Movement Impairment Syndromes.* Philadelphia, PA: Mosby, Inc; 2002:401-447.

31. Reiman MP, Goode AP, Hegedus EP, Cook CE, Wright AA. Diagnostic accuracy of clinical tests of the hip: a systematic review with meta-analysis. *Br J Sports Med*. 2013;47:893-902.

32. Frank JS, Gambacorta PL, Eisner EA. Hip pathology in the adolescent athlete. *J Am Acad Orthop Surg*. 2013;21:665-674.

33. Hengeveld E, Banks K. The hip complex. In: *Maitland's Peripheral Manipulation*. 4th ed. New York, NY: Butterworth-Hernemann; 2005:495-486.

34. Dutton M. The sacroiliac joint. In: Dutton M, ed. *Dutton's Orthopaedic Examination, Evaluation, and Intervention*. 3rd ed. New York, NY: McGraw Hill Medical; 2012:1367-1399.

35. Bedi A, Thompson M, Uliana C, Magennis E, Kelly BT. Assessment of range of motion and contact zones with commonly performed physical exam manoeuvers for femoroacetabular impingement (FAI): what do these tests mean? *Hip Int*. 2013;23:S27-S34.

36. Borghuis AJ, Lemmink KA, Hof AL. Core muscle response times and postural reactions in soccer players and nonplayers. *Med Sci Sports Exerc*. 2011;43:108-114.

37. Imwalle LE, Myer GD, Ford KR, Hewett TE. Relationship between hip and knee kinematics in athletic women during cutting maneuvers: a possible link to noncontact anterior cruciate ligament injury and prevention. *J Strength Cond Res*. 2009;23:2223-2230.

38. Byrd JW. Femoroacetabular impingement in athletes: current concepts. *Am J Sports Med*. 2014;42:737-751.

39. Huxel Bliven KC, Anderson BE. Core stability training for injury prevention. *Sports Health*. 2013;5:514-522.

40. Ambegaonkar JP, Mettinger LM, Caswell SV, Burtt A, Cortes N. Relationships between core endurance, hip strength, and balance in collegiate female athletes. *Int J Sports Phys Ther*. 2014;9:604-616.

41. Selkowitz DM, Beneck GJ, Powers CM. Which exercises target the gluteal muscles while minimizing activation of the tensor fascia lata? Electromyographic assessment using fine-wire electrodes. *J Orthop Sports Phys Ther*. 2013;43:54-64.

42. Wall PD, Fernandez M, Griffin DR, Foster NE. Nonoperative treatment for femoroacetabular impingement: a systematic review of the literature. *PM R*. 2013;5:418-426.

43. Bizzini M, Hancock D, Impellizzeri F. Suggestions from the field for return to sports participation following anterior cruciate ligament reconstruction: soccer. *J Orthop Sports Phys Ther*. 2012;42:304-312.

44. Myers BA, Jenkins WL, Killian C, Rundquist P. Normative data for hop tests in high school and collegiate basketball and soccer players. *Int J Sports Phys Ther*. 2014;9:596-603.

Anterior Cruciate Ligament Rupture: Postoperative Management

Alyson Filipa
Mark V. Paterno

CASE 30

A 9-year-old skeletally immature male presents to a physical therapy clinic for his first postoperative visit five days after ACL reconstruction due to a left anterior cruciate ligament (ACL) tear. He injured himself while at football practice when one of his teammates collided with him resulting in a knee valgus mechanism injury. At the time, the patient reported hearing a "pop," noted immediate swelling, and had subsequent episodes of his knee giving way. Prior to injury, the patient was an active child who participated regularly in recreational football and baseball, in addition to regular free play. Magnetic resonance imaging (MRI) confirmed the clinical diagnosis of an acute, mid-substance rupture of the ACL with subchondral bone bruising of the lateral femoral condyle with no concomitant meniscal or articular cartilage damage.

▶ What factors need to be considered before choosing a non-operative or operative treatment plan following an ACL injury in a skeletally immature individual?
▶ What are the most appropriate physical therapy interventions if an operative treatment plan is implemented?

KEY DEFINITIONS

ALL EPIPHYSEAL, PHYSEAL-SPARING SURGICAL TECHNIQUE: ACL graft and fixation are entirely confined to the region of the knee between the femoral and tibial epiphysis with no violation of either the femoral or tibial growth plates

CLOSED KINETIC CHAIN (CKC): Lower limb is in contact with the ground when progressive resistance exercises are performed

LOWER QUADRANT: Musculature related to the core, hip, knee, and ankle

OPEN KINETIC CHAIN (OKC): Lower limb is not in contact with the ground when progressive resistance exercises are performed

SKELETALLY IMMATURE: Plain films of the knee and wrist reveal "wide open" growth plates (epiphysis still present) confirming that the individual is still growing; "wide open" has yet to be operationally defined in the literature, but is generally used to describe a child with significant residual growth left compared to someone who is nearing skeletal maturity.[1,2]

Objectives

1. Understand the rationale of using surgical versus non-surgical management for a skeletally immature child who has an ACL tear.

2. Understand potential complications of surgical and non-operative routes after ACL injury in skeletally immature individuals.

3. Discuss different surgical options for the skeletally immature child who has an ACL tear and advantages and disadvantages of each.

4. Identify appropriate interventions for the skeletally immature individual that has undergone postoperative management of an ACL injury.

Physical Therapy Considerations

PT considerations for management of the skeletally immature child after surgical reconstruction of an ACL tear:

▶ **General physical therapy plan of care/goals:** Decrease pain and effusion; increase lower quadrant muscular strength and knee range of motion (ROM); improve functional stability, neuromuscular control, and body mechanics

▶ **Physical therapy interventions:** Patient education regarding functional anatomy and injury pathomechanics; modalities and manual therapy to decrease pain and effusion; muscular flexibility exercises; OKC and CKC progressive resistance exercises to increase muscular strength, activation, and endurance capacity of the lower quadrant; balance and proprioception interventions; neuromuscular control and body mechanics interventions; progressive return-to-impact activities and sport-specific activities with criterion-based progression

▶ **Precautions during physical therapy:** Monitor all activities to ensure no episodes of knee giving way; address precautions or contraindications for exercise to prevent anterior shear forces at the tibiofemoral joint on the graft (limit OKC knee extension in the range of 30° to full knee extension); consider long-term outcomes for overall joint health (*e.g.*, early osteoarthritis) when making decisions regarding activities that are safe for the patient to recreationally participate in if family decides on non-operative care until skeletally mature

Understanding the Health Condition

Annually, over 200,000 ACL ruptures occur in the United States.[3] The majority of these were thought to occur in skeletally mature individuals. However, the incidence of ACL rupture in skeletally immature athletes has increased over the past 20 years.[4-10] Recent evidence suggests this increase is primarily due to increased sports participation by skeletally immature individuals.[4,9,11]

Management of ACL injury in skeletally immature individuals has evolved in recent years, but remains controversial. Historically, non-operative management following ACL injury was the standard of care and included activity modification to limit pivoting and cutting maneuvers, physical therapy, and the use of a functional performance brace.[3,4,12] Surgical management was avoided due to fear of secondary growth complications related to surgical disruption of the tibial or femoral growth plates. Violating the growth plate was feared to result in either growth arrest of that segment or growth malalignment.[10] Often, this plan of care resulted in persistent instability and resultant secondary joint injuries[13,14] such as meniscal or chondral damage.[8,15] Because both ACL injury and meniscal injury are risk factors for early development of osteoarthritis,[16,17] **non-operative management** may predispose these younger individuals to progressive joint degeneration and long-term disability.[18,19]

The potential for further joint injury prompted a shift from non-operative management to surgical management of ACL injuries in skeletally immature individuals. Recently, authors have suggested an algorithmic approach to surgical decision making based on the anticipated remaining growth of the child.[20] However, surgical ACL reconstruction in this patient population is not without risk. Of primary concern is the potential disruption of the immature epiphyseal growth plates (Fig. 30-1), or physes, of the tibia and femur.[10,14] Histological studies, primarily in animals, have demonstrated that violation of the physis with a bone tunnel can result in altered growth.[8] In a recent study by Kocher et al.,[10] 140 orthopaedic surgeons were surveyed regarding their standard of care with skeletally immature athletes with ACL deficiency. More than 11% of surveyed surgeons reported a growth plate complication following ACL reconstruction in a skeletally immature patient. Often, this was related to fixation across the physis or placement of a bony bar across this region. A high rate of growth arrest was also seen in animal models from the "tenodesis" of a soft tissue graft passing through or over the growth plate with fixation in the metaphysis, even in the absence of a bony bar.[21] Thus, Kocher et al.[10] recommended proceeding with caution with ACL reconstruction in a skeletally immature patient.

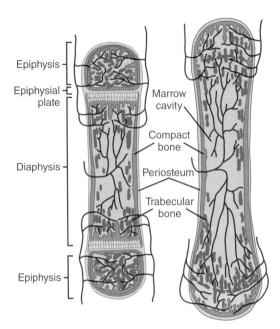

Figure 30-1. Anatomical representation of a long bone, with skeletally immature bone on the left. The epiphyseal plate (growth plate) is very proximal to the joint. The location of the epiphyseal plate in the distal femur and proximal tibia are at risk for injury due to the location of tunnel drilling during an adult ACL reconstruction procedure. (Reproduced with permission from Barrett KE, Barman SM, Boltano S, Brooks HL. *Ganong's Review of Medical Physiology*. 24th ed. New York: McGraw-Hill; 2012. Figure 21-9.)

To decrease the risk of damaging the growth plate, surgeons have developed **modified ACL reconstruction techniques** to provide stability to the joint, while minimally invading the physis.[22] Initial attempts focused on extra-articular procedures that attempted to minimally violate one or both growth plates with a soft tissue graft (*i.e.*, tendons without any bony components, such as a hamstring graft) or avoid the growth plate completely with a non-anatomic placement of the graft. These procedures were referred to as "over the top" procedures that did not involve tunnels drilled through the femur. Rather, the soft tissue graft was brought around the posterior portion of the lateral femoral condyle and then over the top of the lateral femoral condyle as it moved anteriorly to its extra-articular attachment site.[10,12,23] Most recently, Anderson[24] reported a **new all epiphyseal, physeal-sparing surgical technique** that attempts to approximate the normal anatomy of the ACL without interrupting either the tibial or femoral growth plate because the graft and fixation are entirely confined to the epiphysis.

Rehabilitation following surgical reconstruction in skeletally mature patients has been described extensively in the current literature[25-27] and rehabilitation guidelines that are accepted practice in adults are often applied to skeletally immature patients. The unique surgical procedure and considerations of the skeletally immature patient (including protection and preservation of future long bone growth and preservation of knee homeostasis) and the psychosocial aspects of a pediatric patient require the development of more age-appropriate rehabilitation guidelines.

The literature in this area is scarce, demonstrating that the physical therapy profession is in the preliminary stages of shaping the most appropriate rehabilitation guidelines for this patient population.

Physical Therapy Patient/Client Management

When considering the postoperative management of the skeletally immature ACL patient, the therapist cannot simply apply adult ACL guidelines because this may result in inadequate management of key impairments. For the skeletally immature patient, the therapist must emphasize a slower progression of weightbearing during the acute phase of rehabilitation, early protection of the knee joint with potential use of a postoperative knee brace, delayed progression of impact activities, decreased use of external loads, increased use of home-based functional exercises, and delayed return to pivoting sports (after 9-12 months) compared to the adult ACL-reconstructed population.[28,29]

Examination, Evaluation, and Diagnosis

Intraoperative findings confirm the medical diagnosis of an isolated ACL tear and determine whether there is any additional knee pathology. Based on these initial postoperative evaluation findings, the patient will present with specific impairments, including, but not limited to: loss of knee ROM, lower extremity weakness, and gait abnormalities. These impairments result in functional limitations with activities of daily living (ADLs), recreational activities, and activities related to schoolwork.

The initial postsurgical examination needs to encompass gathering the patient's impairments. Each should be continually reassessed and addressed throughout the episode of care until resolution. Postsurgically, the patient's knee ROM, effusion, strength, gait, balance, and proprioception are assessed. To subjectively monitor the patient's progress, it is recommended that the International Knee Documentation Committee (IKDC) subjective outcome survey[24] and an age-appropriate quality-of-life measure, such as the Pediatric Quality of Life Questionnaire,[30,31] be used throughout therapy and at the time of discharge.

Later, more performance-based testing is necessary to help guide clinical decision making as the patient nears the return-to-sport phase of his rehabilitation. Suggested measures of function include an objective strength test using an isometric (initially) or isokinetic dynamometer (later). To protect the healing graft, initial isometric testing should not occur until 12 weeks after surgery. Isometric strength assessment in adults and children has good test-retest reliability with interclass coefficients ranging from 0.81 to 0.94.[32,33] Isokinetic testing has been shown to be a reliable assessment of knee flexion and extension strength in children.[32] Isokinetic testing should be done throughout therapy until the patient has less than a 10% side-to-side strength deficit.[34] Physical performance measures of functional capacity can be measured with hop tests.[17,35] Hop tests have good (test-retest) reliability in non-impaired individuals and those with ACL reconstruction (ACL-R).[36-40] The therapist should also evaluate the patient's ability to perform agility-based drills, based on the specific sport he is returning to in order to determine if proper body mechanics without compensatory strategies are noted during more sport-specific movements.

Balance and postural stability must be assessed. When possible, postural stability can be objectively assessed using a force plate or dynamic force platform (*e.g.*, Biodex Stability System SD) prior to the patient returning to sports. A stabilometer is a platform that can provide varying levels of stability. It can be used to objectively assess average postural stability during a designated period of time. It is one example of an objective and quantitative method for evaluating postural stability.[13,41,42] Performance on these postural stability assessments has been shown to be deficient for up to 9-12 months following ACL-R.[43,44] Deficits in postural stability after ACL-R has been identified as a predictor of future ACL injury and return to sports.[45] Myer et al.[46] demonstrated that young patients must demonstrate sufficient postural stability as measured by a mean of <3° of deflection away from a level position on the stabilometer prior to return to sport. If these deficits persist, the individual may be at increased risk of future ACL injury. If this equipment is not available, other objective clinical tests of balance, such as the Star Excursion Balance Test can be used to assess the patient's level of balance and stability.[47]

The goal of ACL-R is to restore mechanical knee stability by restoring "near-normal" knee anatomy. Throughout the postoperative course, the physical therapist should assess the integrity of the repair of the knee joint, which can be assessed using a Lachman examination of anterior/posterior (AP) knee laxity, a pivot shift examination, or a computerized arthrometer.

Altered limb growth due to epiphyseal plate injury is a risk of ACL-R in a skeletally immature patient. In order to validate the appropriate placement of the graft away from the physes and ensure no residual growth abnormalities or malalignments, the patient may need further radiographic evaluation by the surgeon at subsequent follow-up visits. At 3 months after surgery, MRI can be used to ensure that the location of the femoral and tibial tunnels in relation to the growth plates is appropriate and confirm the absence of any growth plate injury. Clinically, symmetrical lower extremity limb growth can be tracked through bilateral leg length assessment at 3-month intervals from the date of surgery to 1 year after surgery. These measurements allow for early detection of altered or angulated growth in the involved lower extremity.

Plan of Care and Interventions

Currently, there is limited research on **specific ACL reconstruction rehabilitation programs in skeletally immature individuals.** In a clinical commentary by Moksnes et al.,[29] a proposed treatment algorithm was presented in which the skeletally immature ACL patient is progressed through a 4-stage program that focuses on regaining knee ROM, neuromuscular control, and muscle strength. In a case study, Greenberg et al.[28] implemented a protocol that was based on known ACL healing characteristics and surgeon expertise in the adult population with an 8-year-old that resulted in the patient ultimately returning to sport.

When considering the postoperative management of the skeletally immature patient, the application of adult ACL guidelines may be inappropriate. The acute phase of rehabilitation after ACL-R is focused on management of postoperative effusion, pain, loss of motion, and loss of muscle activation. In adults, this phase may last several weeks. In contrast, for the skeletally immature ACL patient, this phase may need to be prolonged to address common postsurgical impairments and more precautionary measures may need to be taken, such as utilizing an immobilizer[28] and limiting weightbearing[28,29] to help enforce activity modifications in the active child to help protect the healing tissue. Whereas partial weightbearing may be initiated immediately after surgery in adults, nonweightbearing may be recommended for 2 to 4 weeks after ACL-R in skeletally immature patients. In the acute and subacute phases of rehabilitation, there also needs to be an increased emphasis on neuromuscular control of terminal knee extension to normalize ADLs.[29] Later, a high emphasis on proper neuromuscular control with plyometric activities is needed to safely progress the patient from double-leg jumps to single-limb hops.[29] Finally, neuromuscular exercises that focus on maintaining functional stability of the knee is needed as a secondary prevention measure prior to full return to activity or sports.[29] Abnormal movement patterns, such as increased valgus during jumping and landing tasks (Fig. 30-2), are known to increase stress on the ACL.[41] The

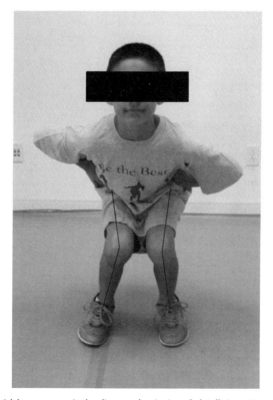

Figure 30-2. High-risk lower extremity landing mechanics in a skeletally immature male. Note the bilateral increased knee valgus when landing from a jump. This abnormal movement pattern increases stress on the ligamentous stabilizers of the knee and is considered a predictive factor for ACL injury.

Table 30-1   SIMILARITIES AND DIFFERENCES BETWEEN ADULT ACL-R AND SKELETALLY IMMATURE ACL-R

	Skeletally Immature ACL-R[28,29]	Adult ACL-R[25-27]
Early stages of rehabilitation	Increased focus to allow for adequate healing and joint protection Develop proper neuromuscular control prior to progression to more advanced exercises Consider OKC exercise in limited knee ROM	May progress faster with more autonomy given to patient to follow joint protection guidelines
Exercise interventions	Supervised rehabilitation with focus on return of knee ROM, muscular strength of lower extremity, and emphasis on neuromuscular control	Focus on return of knee ROM Strength training of core, hip, knee, ankle Balance/proprioception/neuromuscular control exercises and plyometrics Specific return-to-sport activities
End stages of rehabilitation	Slower progression toward running/jumping to reduce impact on physis Emphasize functional stability of knee joint and progress toward technical mastery of high risk movement patterns	Can be more aggressive if proper mechanics demonstrated with techniques
Timed vs. criterion-based progressions	Focus on criterion-based progression, with necessary consideration for potentially extended graft healing time	Increased emphasis on criterion-based progression
Bracing	Recommended	Physician preference, though less commonly used
Average time to return to sport	9-12 months	6 months

development of proper alignment during these tasks is critical to ensure safe return to pivoting and cutting activities. In order to address all impairments and allow a successful, safe, and more slowly progressed recovery, the physical therapist must consider that the young athlete may require additional cueing to optimize technique, more visits, and a longer duration of therapy.[28,29] Table 30-1 presents a summary of principles gathered from current evidence to highlight the differences in postoperative rehabilitative management of the adult and the skeletally immature patient after ACL-R.

Evidence-Based Clinical Recommendations

SORT: Strength of Recommendation Taxonomy

A: Consistent, good-quality patient-oriented evidence
B: Inconsistent or limited-quality patient-oriented evidence
C: Consensus, disease-oriented evidence, usual practice, expert opinion, or case series

1. For skeletally immature children, surgical management of anterior cruciate ligament tears is still controversial, but ACL reconstruction may help prevent future meniscus and articular cartilage pathology. **Grade C**

2. "Over the top" or all epiphyseal ACL reconstruction procedures help restore knee stability without violating the growth plate in skeletally immature children; however, only the all epiphyseal procedure restores normal anatomy of the knee. **Grade B**

3. Physical therapy rehabilitation programs for ACL reconstruction in skeletally immature individuals may result in increased knee ROM, neuromuscular control, and muscle strength sufficient to allow returning to sport. **Grade C**

COMPREHENSION QUESTIONS

30.1 Which statement is *true* when considering postsurgical physical therapy rehabilitation management for the skeletally immature ACL-R individual?

A. A knee immobilizer is not recommended, an increased emphasis on neuromuscular control is recommended, and rehabilitation will take the same amount of time as an adult prior to full return to sport.

B. A knee immobilizer is recommended, an increased emphasis on neuromuscular control is recommended, and rehabilitation will be longer prior to full return to sport compared to an adult.

C. A knee immobilizer is recommended, an increased emphasis on balance is recommended, and rehabilitation will be longer prior to full return to sport compared to an adult.

D. A knee immobilizer is not recommended, an increased emphasis on neuromuscular control is recommended, and rehabilitation will be longer prior to full return to sport compared to an adult.

30.2 Which surgical procedure restores the normal anatomy of the ACL, while sparing the femoral and tibial epiphysis?

A. An over-the-top procedure

B. An all epiphyseal, physeal-sparing surgical technique

C. A bone-patellar-bone autograft

D. There is no surgical procedure that has been shown to accomplish this.

ANSWERS

30.1 **B.** A knee immobilizer is recommended to assist in protecting the healing tissue and assist in modifying the child's activity. An increased emphasis on neuromuscular control is recommended to promote terminal knee extension to normalize ADLs. The duration of rehabilitation will be longer, and it will take longer to return to full activity (9-12 months).

30.2 **B.** The all epiphyseal, physeal-sparing surgical technique restores normal anatomy of the ACL while sparing the femoral and tibial epiphysis.

REFERENCES

1. Meller R, Kendoff D, Hankemeier S, et al. Hindlimb growth after a transphyseal reconstruction of the anterior cruciate ligament: a study in skeletally immature sheep with wide-open physes. *Am J Sports Med.* 2008;36:2437-2443.

2. Streich NA, Barie A, Gotterbarm T, Keil M, Schmitt H. Transphyseal reconstruction of the anterior cruciate ligament in prepubescent athletes. *Knee Surg Sports Traumatol Arthrosc.* 2010;18:1481-1486.

3. Bales CP, Guettler JH, Moorman CT, 3rd. Anterior cruciate ligament injuries in children with open physes: evolving strategies of treatment. *Am J Sports Med.* 2004;32:1978-1985.

4. Fehnel DJ, Johnson R. Anterior cruciate injuries in the skeletally immature athlete: a review of treatment outcomes. *Sports Med.* 2000;29:51-63.

5. Kocher MS, Garg S, Micheli LJ. Physeal sparing reconstruction of the anterior cruciate ligament in skeletally immature prepubescent children and adolescents. Surgical technique. *J Bone Joint Surg Am.* 2006;88(Suppl 1 Pt 2):283-293.

6. Lipscomb AB, Anderson AF. Tears of the anterior cruciate ligament in adolescents. *J Bone Joint Surg Am.* 1986;68:19-28.

7. McCarroll JR, Rettig AC, Shelbourne KD. Anterior cruciate ligament injuries in the young athlete with open physes. *Am J Sports Med.* 1988;16:44-47.

8. Shea KG, Apel PJ, Pfeiffer RP. Anterior cruciate ligament injury in paediatric and adolescent patients: a review of basic science and clinical research. *Sports Med.* 2003;33:455-471.

9. Shea KG, Pfeiffer R, Wang JH, Curtin M, Apel PJ. Anterior cruciate ligament injury in pediatric and adolescent soccer players: an analysis of insurance data. *J Pediatr Orthop.* 2004;24:623-628.

10. Kocher MS, Saxon HS, Hovis WD, Hawkins RJ. Management and complications of anterior cruciate ligament injuries in skeletally immature patients: survey of the Herodicus Society and The ACL Study Group. *J Pediatr Orthop.* 2002;22:452-457.

11. Micheli LJ, Metzl JD, Di Canzio J, Zurakowski D. Anterior cruciate ligament reconstructive surgery in adolescent soccer and basketball players. *Clin J Sport Med.* 1999;9:138-141.

12. Kocher MS, Garg S, Micheli LJ. Physeal sparing reconstruction of the anterior cruciate ligament in skeletally immature prepubescent children and adolescents. *J Bone Joint Surg Am.* 2005;87:2371-2379.

13. Dorizas JA, Stanitski CL. Anterior cruciate ligament injury in the skeletally immature. *Orthop Clin North Am.* 2003;34:355-363.

14. Utukuri MM, Somayaji HS, Khanduja V, Dowd GS, Hunt DM. Update on paediatric ACL injuries. *Knee.* 2006;13:345-352.

15. McCarroll JR, Shelbourne KD, Porter DA, Rettig AC, Murray S. Patellar tendon graft reconstruction for midsubstance anterior cruciate ligament rupture in junior high school athletes. An algorithm for management. *Am J Sports Med.* 1994;22:478-484.

16. Hawkins R, Misamore G, Merritt T. Follow up of the acute nonoperated isolated anterior cruciate ligament tear. *Am J Sports Med.* 1986;14:205-210.

17. Aichroth PM, Patel DV, Zorrilla P. The natural history and treatment of rupture of the anterior cruciate ligament in children and adolescents. A prospective review. *J Bone Joint Surg Br.* 2002;84:38-41.

18. Lohmander LS, Ostenberg A, Englund M, Roos H. High prevalence of knee osteoarthritis, pain, and functional limitations in female soccer players twelve years after anterior cruciate ligament injury. *Arthritis Rheum.* 2004;50:3145-3152.

19. von Porat A, Roos EM, Roos H. High prevalence of osteoarthritis 14 years after an anterior cruciate ligament tear in male soccer players: a study of radiographic and patient relevant outcomes. *Ann Rheum Dis.* 2004;63:269-273.

20. Jia G, Takayama Y, Flanigan DC, et al. Quantitative assessment of mobile protein levels in human knee synovial fluid: feasibility of chemical exchange saturation transfer (proteinCEST) MRI of osteoarthritis. *Magn Reson Imaging.* 2011;29:335-341.

21. Edwards TB, Greene CC, Baratta RV, Zieske A, Willis RB. The effect of placing a tensioned graft across open growth plates. A gross and histologic analysis. *J Bone Joint Surg Am.* 2001;83-A:725-734.

22. Kaeding CC, Flanigan D, Donaldson C. Surgical techniques and outcomes after anterior cruciate ligament reconstruction in preadolescent patients. *Arthroscopy.* 2010;26:1530-1538.

23. Kocher MS, Hovis WD, Curtin MJ, Hawkins RJ. Anterior cruciate ligament reconstruction in skeletally immature knees: an anatomical study. *Am J Orthop.* 2005;34:285-290.

24. Anderson AF. Transepiphyseal replacement of the anterior cruciate ligament in skeletally immature patients. A preliminary report. *J Bone Joint Surg Am.* 2003;85-A:1255-1263.

25. Shelbourne KD, Klootwyk TE, Wilckens JH, De Carlo MS. Ligament stability two to six years after anterior cruciate ligament reconstruction with autogenous patellar tendon graft and participation in accelerated rehabilitation program. *Am J Sports Med.* 1995;23:575-579.

26. Shelbourne KD, Nitz P. Accelerated rehabilitation after anterior cruciate ligament reconstruction. *Am J Sports Med.* 1990;18:292-299.

27. Wilk KE, Arrigo C, Andrews JR, Clancy WG. Rehabilitation after anterior cruciate ligament reconstruction in the female athlete. *J Athl Train.* 1999;34:177-193.

28. Greenberg EM, Albaugh J, Ganley TJ, Lawrence JT. Rehabilitation considerations for all epiphyseal ACL reconstruction. *Int J Sports Phys Ther.* 2012;7:185-196.

29. Moksnes H, Engebretsen L, Risberg MA. Management of anterior cruciate ligament injuries in skeletally immature individuals. *J Orthop Sports Phys Ther.* 2012;42:172-183.

30. Kaeding CC, Aros B, Pedroza A, et al. Allograft versus autograft anterior cruciate ligament reconstruction: predictors of failure from a MOON prospective longitudinal cohort. *Sports Health.* 2011;3:73-81.

31. Spindler KP, Huston LJ, Wright RW, et al. The prognosis and predictors of sports function and activity at minimum 6 years after anterior cruciate ligament reconstruction: a population cohort study. *Am J Sports Med.* 2011;39:348-359.

32. Merlini L, Dell'Accio D, Granata C. Reliability of dynamic strength knee muscle testing in children. *J Orthop Sports Phys Ther.* 1995;22:73-76.

33. Pincivero DM, Lephart SM, Karunakara RA. Reliability and precision of isokinetic strength and muscular endurance for the quadriceps and hamstrings. *Int J Sports Med.* 1997;18:113-117.

34. Schmitt LC, Paterno MV, Hewett TE. The impact of quadriceps femoris strength asymmetry on functional performance at return to sport following anterior cruciate ligament reconstruction. *J Orthop Sports Phys Ther.* 2012;42:750-759.

35. Noyes FR, Barber SD, Mangine RE. Abnormal lower limb symmetry determined by function hop tests after anterior cruciate ligament rupture. *Am J Sports Med.* 1991;19:513-518.

36. Levy BA, Dajani KA, Morgan JA, Shah JP, Dahm DL, Stuart MJ. Repair versus reconstruction of the fibular collateral ligament and posterolateral corner in the multiligament-injured knee. *Am J Sports Med.* 2010;38:804-809.

37. Wright R, Spindler K, Huston L, et al. Revision ACL reconstruction outcomes: MOON cohort. *J Knee Surg.* 2011;24:289-294.

38. Quatman CE, Paterno MV, Wordeman SC, Kaeding CC. Longitudinal anterior knee laxity related to substantial tibial tunnel enlargement after anterior cruciate ligament revision. *Arthroscopy.* 2011;27:1160-1163.

39. Garrett WE, Kaeding CC, ElAttrache NS, et al. Novel drug OMS103HP reduces pain and improves joint motion and function for 90 days after arthroscopic meniscectomy. *Arthroscopy.* 2011;27:1060-1070.

40. Reinke EK, Spindler KP, Lorring D, et al. Hop tests correlate with IKDC and KOOS at minimum of 2 years after primary ACL reconstruction. *Knee Surg Sports Traumatol Arthrosc.* 2011;19:1806-1816.

41. Harrison EL, Duenkel N, Dunlop R, Russell G. Evaluation of single-leg standing following anterior cruciate ligament surgery and rehabilitation. *Phys Ther.* 1994;74:245-252.

42. Miller T, Kaeding CC, Flanigan D. The classification systems of stress fractures: a systematic review. *Phys Sportsmed.* 2011;39:93-100.

43. Paterno MV, Hewett TE, Noyes FR. The return of neuromuscular coordination after anterior cruciate ligament reconstruction. *J Orthop Sports Phys Ther.* 1998;27:94.

44. Paterno MV, Hewett TE, Noyes FR. Gender differences in neuromuscular coordination of controls, ACL-deficient knees and ACL-reconstructed knees. *J Orthop Sports Phys Ther.* 1999;29:A-45.

45. Paterno MV, Schmitt LC, Ford KR, et al. Biomechanical measures during landing and postural stability predict second anterior cruciate ligament injury after anterior cruciate ligament reconstruction and return to sport. *Am J Sports Med.* 2010;38:1968-1978.

46. Myer GD, Paterno MV, Ford KR, Quatman CE, Hewett TE. Rehabilitation after anterior cruciate ligament reconstruction: criteria-based progression through the return-to-sport phase. *J Orthop Sports Phys Ther.* 2006;36:385-402.

47. Gribble PA, Hertel J, Plisky P. Using the Star Excursion Balance Test to assess dynamic postural-control deficits and outcomes in lower extremity injury: a literature and systematic review. *J Athl Train.* 2012;47:339-357.

Medial Epicondyle Apophysitis (Little League Elbow)

Chad Cherny
Mark V. Paterno

CASE 31

The patient is an 11-year-old right hand dominant male that presented to an outpatient physical therapy clinic with complaints of medial elbow pain. The patient began to have pain with repetitive throwing during baseball, in which he participates as a catcher and shortstop. He states the onset of pain was acute and began with one throw and then increased with additional repetitions and increased velocity. At the time of the evaluation, the patient stated he was only able to throw three to five times before the onset of pain, which continued to increase with repetition. Over time, the patient noted he experienced a decrease in velocity and accuracy as his pain increased. Mechanically, he noted the greatest pain occurred during a progression from maximum shoulder external rotation (ER) to ball release. He reports that his pain can persist into the next day after throwing in practice or a game. He reports no numbness or tingling in the upper extremity. In an attempt to relieve symptoms, the patient has been using ice and anti-inflammatory medication.

▶ What is the most appropriate conservative management plan?
▶ Prior to return to throwing, what is an appropriate progression of activity to prevent recurrence of pain and functional limitations?

KEY DEFINITIONS

APOPHYSITIS: Inflammation surrounding the bony outgrowth on a bone on which a muscle or muscle group attaches[1]

EPIPHYSEAL PLATE: Cartilaginous disc between the metaphysis and epiphysis from which skeletal bone growth occurs[2]

LITTLE LEAGUE ELBOW: Apophysitis of the medial epicondylar growth plate in young baseball players and overhead athletes[3,4]

Objectives

1. Outline the pathoanatomic differences between an apophysitis injury and an avulsion injury.

2. Understand nonoperative management of apophysitis and avulsion injuries of the elbow.

3. Describe the role of the posterior shoulder and scapular stabilizing musculature in the reduction of medial elbow pain.

4. Outline an appropriate progression of interventions to allow an athlete to return to overhead throwing sports following an upper extremity injury.

Physical Therapy Considerations

PT considerations during management of the young baseball player with medial epicondyle apophysitis, or little league elbow:

▶ **General physical therapy plan of care/goals:** Decrease pain and inflammation; identify current functional status; improve muscle activation patterns; improve strength and endurance of upper extremity (UE) and scapular stabilizers; advance core strength and proximal stability; improve throwing mechanics

▶ **Physical therapy interventions:** Patient education regarding injury pathomechanics; flexibility exercises to target restricted mobility; resisted exercise to optimize muscle activation; strength and endurance exercises to target identified deficits in the UE, scapular stabilizers, back, and core; perturbation training and rhythmic stabilization to improve dynamic stability and control; modalities to decrease pain and effusion

▶ **Precautions during physical therapy:** Monitor all exercise to ensure proper technique and mechanics during exercise performance to avoid development of abnormal compensatory patterns during activity or return-to-throwing program.

▶ **Complications interfering with physical therapy:** Tendency for young growing athletes to return to prior abnormal throwing mechanics despite the need to appropriately adapt to progressing physical maturation and growth

Understanding the Health Condition

Overuse injuries in the pediatric athletic population have increased with the growth of sports specialization and year-round participation in a single sport.[5-8] With approximately 25 to 40 million children participating in team sports annually, up to 30% or 18 million young athletes will seek medical attention for injury related to sport participation.[7-11] In the overhead athlete, shoulder and elbow injuries are the most common, accounting for up to 26% of the total number of injuries that occur annually in this population.[3,7,10,12] Medial epicondyle apophysitis, more commonly referred to as Little League elbow, is a common injury in the adolescent overhead throwing athlete. An estimated 17% to 40% of baseball players between the ages of 9 and 15 years experience elbow pain, with up to 8% of those having an overuse related injury.[3,10-13]

The overhead throwing motion is a high-risk movement for the developing arm. During the throwing motion, high levels of stress are placed through the UE. Biomechanically, the throwing motion can be broken down into six distinct phases, which include wind-up, early cocking, late cocking, acceleration, deceleration, and follow-through.[10,12,14-16] Three phases of overhead throwing (early cocking, late cocking, and acceleration) can place valgus and distraction forces on the medial elbow.[10,12,14-16] During deceleration and follow-through, the posterior shoulder muscles must function eccentrically to decelerate the arm. Often, young athletes do not have sufficient strength, endurance, or proper mechanics to tolerate these forces repetitively over a prolonged period of time, which leads to stress at the medial physis (Fig. 31-1).

The medial elbow is often a location of injury in the overhead pediatric athlete due to the open physis. Pediatric athletes are more susceptible to suffer physeal rather than ligamentous injuries because the physis is weaker than the surrounding ligaments.[3,7,11-13,17,18] Anatomically, the proximal insertion of the wrist flexor and pronator muscle groups attaches distal to the medial epicondylar physis. During the throwing motion, the physis is put under repetitive traction due to contractile forces of the flexor and pronator groups.[3,11,12,17-19] The repetitive nature of throwing may lead to mechanical separation, inflammation, and pain (*i.e.,* apophysitis) at the medial epicondyle apophysis.[3,7,11,12,17-19] This repetitive microtrauma to the physis in conjunction with inadequate recovery between episodes of throwing may lead to progression of symptoms and decreased ability to participate in throwing activities without pain.[12,14,17-19]

In addition to an apophysitis injury, adolescent athletes involved in overhead throwing may also incur a more severe injury to the medial elbow. A single, more forceful contraction of the flexor mass, in addition to a valgus elbow position may lead to an avulsion fracture.[7,11,13,14,18] An avulsion fracture involves a displacement of the medial epicondyle with respect to the humerus and is classified into one of two categories. A Woods type I fracture is an avulsion that involves the entire ossification center and typically occurs in an athlete that is less than 15 years of age.[13] A Woods type II fracture is usually seen in an athlete with a closed or nearly closed growth plate and involves a small bony fragment that avulses from the medial

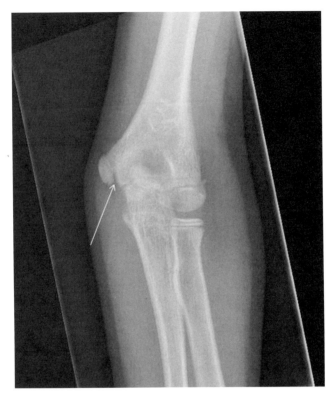

Figure 31-1. Radiograph of the elbow of an 11-year-old young male. Arrow indicates abnormal medial epicondyle physis.

epicondyle.[13] Management of medial epicondyle avulsion injuries varies based on the severity of fragment displacement. Athletes with isolated apophysitis injuries are treated conservatively with activity modification. These athletes are encouraged to rest for up to four weeks without throwing activity.[13,17,18] In contrast, avulsion injuries of less than 2 mm of displacement are typically treated with a short period of immobilization.[11,13,17,18] An avulsion fracture with greater than 2 mm but less than 10 mm of displacement may be treated with immobilization or may require an open reduction, internal fixation (ORIF). Displacement of greater than 10 mm requires ORIF for anatomic reduction.[11,13,17,18] In all athletes with a fragment displacement of greater than 2 mm, stability of the ulnar collateral ligament (UCL) must also be assessed. Improper healing of the bony fragment may affect the ligament's ability to handle loads and stabilize the elbow during throwing activity.[11,13,17,18]

Outcomes following medial elbow injury depend on several factors. Pathoanatomic changes as well as secondary impairments will affect the patient's ability to return to activity. Pathoanatomical changes can be related to structural changes within the bone and secondary effects on the surrounding ligaments and other static stabilizing structures. Involvement of the epiphyseal growth plate of a bone inherently creates risk of growth arrest. Premature closure of the growth center may result in a shortening of the limb or increased varus angulation of the arm. Athletes with injuries that include displacement of the medial epicondyle may also have resultant damage of the UCL. Healing of the fragment in an altered location can change the static and dynamic stability of the elbow, which may increase the risk of further injury to the athlete.[11] **Decreased throwing activity after the injury** may also affect long-term outcomes. When the physeal plates are open during adolescence, adaptive changes may occur to the throwing arm of the athlete. One of these changes involves the rotation of the humerus on the proximal humeral physis.[20-22] Humeral retroversion refers to the increased ER of the humeral shaft on the humeral head. This rotation allows for increased ER of the shoulder during the throwing motion without increased stress to the anterior shoulder and medial elbow.[20-22] If an athlete is unable to throw due to modifications placed on his activity level after the injury, the time in which this external rotation adaptation can occur is reduced and may limit the overall motion the athlete could have attained if not for the injury and subsequent activity modification. For this reason, limiting the amount of time the athlete is unable to safely participate in overhead sports should be a primary goal in the rehabilitation program.

With respect to secondary impairments, loss of mobility and strength can affect outcomes after medial elbow injury. Loss of elbow extension range of motion (ROM), particularly after a prolonged immobilization, can limit function with activities of daily living and work and recreational activity in the future. However, up to a 20° loss of elbow extension can often be tolerated in baseball players without a significant impact on function.[23,24] In terms of muscle performance, loss of strength and endurance following injury can limit an athlete's ability to regain strength symmetry and safely return to overhead activity.

Physical Therapy Patient/Client Management

Initial management by a physician typically includes a thorough clinical exam and imaging studies to assist in the diagnosis and determination of the severity of the injury.[13,17,18,25] Radiographs are often used to assess the integrity of the epiphyseal plate and determine if widening or displacement has occurred. If significant widening or displacement has occurred, the physician may order additional imaging studies, such as an MRI to assess the alignment and displacement of the fragment and the integrity of the ulnar collateral ligament. This can assist in surgical decision making.[3,13] Following diagnosis, a referral to physical therapy to address pain, edema, and functional limitations that the patient may be experiencing may be appropriate. The physical therapist needs to maintain communication with the physician to appropriately limit and restrict activity to allow healing and to safely advance the patient back to his pre-injury level of function.

Examination, Evaluation, and Diagnosis

A diagnosis of medial epicondyle apophysitis in the young overhead athlete is not uncommon.[3,11,13] The patient who presents with this diagnosis often reports a history that includes an increase in intensity of repetitive overhead throwing activities. The mechanism of the change in intensity can be related to the amount of throwing, distances being thrown, and/or a change in position played. Typically, the athlete is able to provide a history of when and how long the pain has been occurring. Onset of pain may be reported as either chronic with a slow progression of increasing pain with throwing or as more acute with ongoing pain reported after a single throw. The individual frequently reports that the intensity of the pain resulted in a need to discontinue throwing. The athlete typically reports point tenderness at the medial epicondyle with potential radiation of pain proximally along the biceps tendon and anterior shoulder, and distally along the medial aspect of the forearm.[13,14] The pain often occurs during the late cocking, acceleration, and deceleration phases and tends to be activity dependent, with pain reducing or intermittently resolving with rest.[3,24] The patient in this case reported increased pain with more repetitive throwing and with an increase in distance thrown. From a performance perspective, he also noted a decrease in velocity and control with his throws. During the subjective evaluation, the physical therapist should inquire about previous history of pain or injury in the involved elbow or shoulder, back, or hip. Prior history of pain or injury in other body regions may give insight into any compensatory mechanics that may be occurring as well as areas that may need to be addressed during the examination and rehabilitation. To help determine the mechanism of injury, necessary rehabilitation, and projected time to return to play, the therapist also needs to understand the patient's specific athletic exposures such as current practice schedule, games per week and per year, and all positions played.

The examination should focus on palpation of the target tissues as well as a more global assessment of potential impairments in ROM, strength, and functional mobility.[24-26] This will provide the physical therapist with a complete assessment of the individual and potential contributory factors to the patient's pathology. **Palpation of the medial elbow anatomy** is best completed in a dynamic fashion because tenderness to palpation may vary based on the position of the UE. Pain usually increases if the arm is placed in external rotation since this places a valgus load through the elbow (much as it would during the throwing motion). The therapist should also be aware that the athlete might try to compensate with the shoulder during palpation in order to prevent this stress to the elbow. In addition to the valgus position of the elbow during a throwing motion, the wrist is likely to move into an extended position that increases the tension of the flexor mass as it inserts to the medial epicondyle. Due to the passive and dynamic tensioning of the medial elbow that can increase sensitivity to palpable tenderness, the therapist should palpate the medial elbow in several different UE positions and document the sensitivity in each position. Assessment of ROM should include the elbow as well as the proximal and distal joints. Deficits in shoulder mobility may alter overhead throwing mechanics and contribute to medial elbow joint stress. The assessment of strength should also include a global determination of strength around the elbow as well as around the surrounding joints. In particular, the shoulder muscles and scapular stabilizers (trapezius, rhomboids, levator scapulae, and serratus anterior) must be assessed for strength and endurance because dynamic control of the shoulder during throwing depends on the ability of the scapula to stabilize during the throwing motion. If the young athlete does not have sufficient strength and endurance to tolerate the deceleration forces incurred during throwing over a prolonged period of time, increased stresses at the medial physis will persist. Special tests to assess overall UE stability (*e.g.*, O'Brien's test, biceps load test, lateral scapular slide test) should be performed because current elbow pain may be the result of compensations from a previous shoulder injury. During the exam, the therapist should note impairments and limitations, where and when pain is reproduced, and the similarity of each complaint of pain to the pain that occurs during overhead throwing.

Plan of Care and Interventions

Physical therapy interventions for a patient with medial epicondyle apophysitis must address identified impairments in the shoulder complex and the entire UE since impairments anywhere along the chain may have contributed to the present injury. **Early intervention** to correct dysfunctional muscle patterns, mechanical faults, and impaired strength and endurance of posterior shoulder, scapular stabilizing, and core musculature is recommended to improve proximal stability of the UE to reduce the stress and loading that goes through the elbow during the throwing motion.

The patient in this case presented with impaired strength and mobility of the involved UE. He demonstrated weakness in the right rotator cuff (RTC), scapular stabilizers, and wrist flexors and extensors that needed to be addressed prior to a full return to overhead activity. Since he initially experienced elbow pain with both passive and active external rotation of the shoulder on the involved side, active strengthening at the elbow was avoided to allow healing to occur. During this time, exercises to improve shoulder and scapular strength and endurance were started because these exercises avoided stress to the medial elbow. Initially, isometric exercises were used to focus on activation and neuromuscular control of the RTC and scapular stabilizing musculature. Since the patient was able to activate the RTC muscles and scapular stabilizers in a static position, he was progressed to more dynamic activities including seated arm raises into flexion, abduction, and scaption. These exercises were performed with the patient seated with his arm extended over a plinth. This allowed the patient to work in an advantageous length-tension curve of the muscle while still having the plinth available for rest if pain or fatigue increased. Once he was able to maintain correct form, these exercises were progressed by adding hand-held weights and resistance bands. To begin joint loading of the UE and shoulder, a standing wall push-up was added. This exercise was progressed by asking the patient to lift one hand off the wall, which requires increased contralateral stability through contraction of the RTC muscles and scapular stabilizers (Fig. 31-2). Progression of this exercise may include a lift-off with rotation of the UE into ER (Fig. 31-3), rhythmical horizontal abduction/adduction with a resistance band, and wall walks with the resistive band keeping hands at shoulder width.

During this progression of dynamic shoulder exercises, the therapist also started addressing the identified forearm weakness. Wrist and forearm exercises consisted of an isometric towel squeeze and resisted wrist flexion and extension, and ulnar and radial deviation to neutral with resistive bands. All of these exercises were

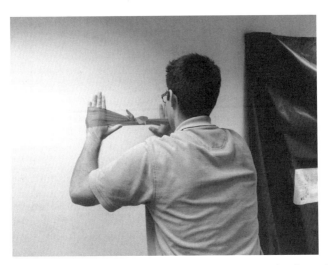

Figure 31-2. Resisted scapular lift-off from a wall push-up position. Patient's hands are placed shoulder-width apart inside a resisted band loop. Therapist provides cues for patient to retract and depress medial scapular border. Once patient demonstrates proper form, one hand is lifted from wall. Patient begins without a hold and progresses to a hold as endurance improves. Exercise promotes stability of support hand while opposite limb moves.

restricted to pain-free ranges, progressively advancing through the full ROM compared to the uninvolved side.

When the patient demonstrated proper form and control with the current exercise program, he was progressed to more unsupported activity to challenge the endurance of the RTC and scapular stabilizers while moving the UE into positions that mimic those necessary during the throwing motion. This can be done through

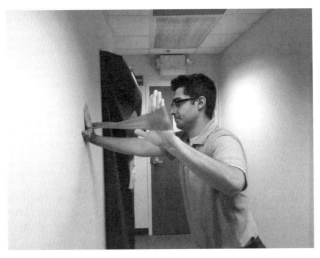

Figure 31-3. Scapular lift-off with external rotation. Exercise is performed in the same position as the resisted scapular lift. However, the UE is rotated externally when lifted from the wall in order to activate the RTC muscles.

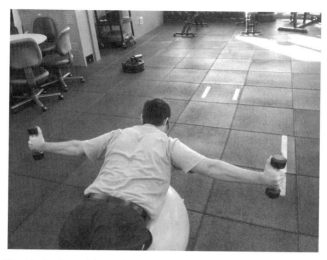

Figure 31-4. Shoulder horizontal abduction over stability ball.

exercises with free weights or resistive bands based on the resistance the patient is able to control while maintaining the correct form. Initially, exercises with static holds were performed to focus on increasing endurance of the scapular stabilizers and RTC required to meet the demands placed on the musculature during overhead activity (Figs. 31-4, 31-5, 31-6). When the patient demonstrated appropriate strength, endurance, and ability to maintain form with the static holds, the therapist progressed him to more dynamic activities. Standing shoulder flexion, scaption, and abduction of the shoulder were introduced, with the therapist providing cues to retract the scapulae prior to elevation or overhead activity. Resisted band exercises included shoulder internal rotation (Fig. 31-7) and external rotation

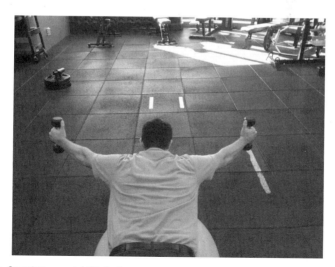

Figure 31-5. Scaption over stability ball.

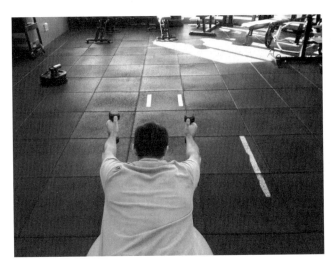

Figure 31-6. Shoulder flexion over stability ball.

(Fig. 31-8) at the 90/90 position of the UE (90° shoulder abduction and 90° elbow flexion).

To improve stability around the elbow, strength and endurance exercises of the wrist flexors and extensors were advanced. The therapist added wrist flexion and extension as well as supination and pronation with appropriate resistance that the patient was asked to perform until fatigue. Band exercises were progressed until the patient achieved full elbow and wrist ROM. Resistance was advanced provided he remained pain-free and was able to maintain proper form.

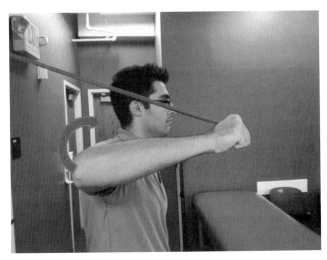

Figure 31-7. Resisted internal rotation. Arrow indicates the direction that patient pulls band to activate shoulder internal rotators. Axis of pull is far above patient's head to allow for full shoulder external rotation.

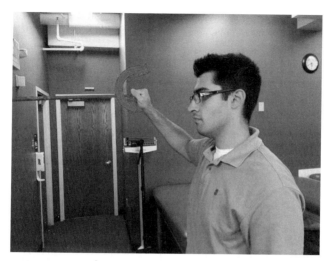

Figure 31-8. Resisted external rotation. Arrow indicates the direction that patient pulls band to activate shoulder external rotators. Axis of pull is initially placed at height of hand in 90/90 position. This position allows limits on ROM that may be necessary based on patient's tolerance. As patient progresses, axis may be lowered to allow greater ROM and increased resistance throughout ROM.

Core strength and stability were also addressed throughout the rehabilitation program since core musculature plays important roles in stabilization and force production in overhead throwing motion. Early exercises focused on activation of abdominal and paraspinal muscles to increase stability. As the patient demonstrated the ability to activate these muscles, he was challenged with balance and therapy ball exercises in conjunction with unsupported overhead activity to mimic the stability required during throwing motion.

Prior to the initiation of a return-to-throwing program, the patient entered a prefunctional phase to prepare for the forces placed on the arm during throwing. The goal of this phase is to increase the velocity of the arm in an unsupported pattern to assess the patient's ability to resume throwing. During this phase, the patient may begin releasing a medicine ball into a plyopitch trampoline from a kneeling position. To do this, the patient is in a tall kneeling position with his non-dominant leg flexed at the hip and knee at 90° and the involved (dominant) shoulder held at 90° abduction and the elbow flexed to 90°. The therapist instructs the patient to maintain this position while internally rotating the glenohumeral joint. As the arm moves through this motion, the patient releases the medicine ball into the plyopitch trampoline. The therapist also added ball drops while prone on a plinth (Fig. 31-9), which was progressed to lying prone on a stability ball. A throwing progression using a towel (Fig. 31-10) is also useful because it allows the patient to begin increasing the arm speed while still having resistance or drag created by the towel during the throwing motion. These exercises increase use of the posterior shoulder and scapular stabilizers to decelerate the UE rather than relying primarily on use of the biceps or wrist flexors and extensors, thus reducing the stress to the medial elbow.

At approximately six weeks of physical therapy, the patient was able to demonstrate appropriate strength, endurance, and form during the exercises. Thus, the

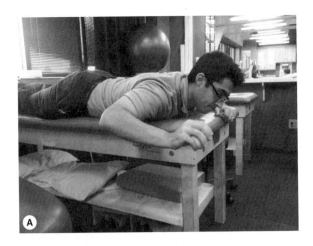

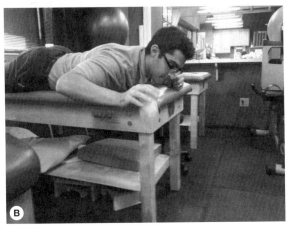

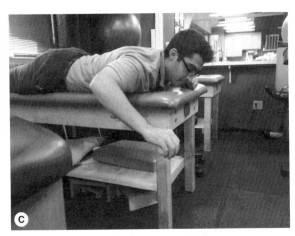

Figure 31-9. Prone ball drop series. This exercise uses acceleration and deceleration in a shortened ROM to focus on neuromuscular re-education during the throwing motion. **A.** Starting position. Patient positioned prone on plinth with involved right elbow placed over edge of plinth. Involved UE is placed at 90° abduction and 90° ER. The wrist is maintained in neutral or slight extension. **B.** Initial action phase when ball is released. **C.** Patient moves UE into IR and catches the ball.

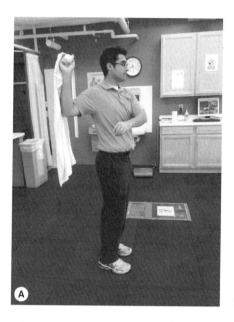

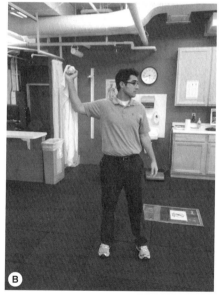

Figure 31-10. Towel throw progression. **A.** Patient faces forward to focus on initial arm position, trunk rotation, and follow-through. Use of the LEs is limited to require use of trunk musculature to generate force. **B.** Side facing without step. The therapist observes for correct arm position while the patient uses his trunk and left arm to assist with force generation during acceleration and force attenuation during deceleration much the same way the muscles would be used in a game. By limiting the step, the patient is not fully generating the forces produced while throwing and thus provides less stress to the involved right shoulder and elbow. This is a good position to assess patient's tolerance to increased force production during the throwing motion.

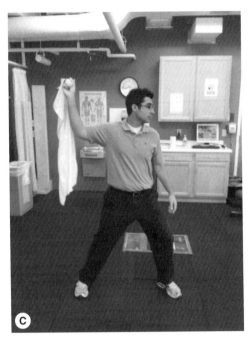

Figure 31-10. (*Continued*) Towel throw progression. **C.** Side facing with step for integration of lower extremity into throwing motion. This position allows for the patient to increase forces by using the LEs, which best mimics the speed and force generation of throwing a baseball. Therapist pays special attention to deceleration and follow-through phases to assess ability of posterior shoulder, scapular stabilizers, and back musculature to slow the arm. Once the patient is able to perform this exercise correctly and pain-free, he is ready to progress to a return-to-throwing program.

therapist progressed him to a return-to-throwing program that consisted of a proper warm-up, specific throwing program with distances and repetitions, and cool-down focusing on stretching and icing of the shoulder and elbow. The throwing program should take into account the needs of the athlete as well as unique characteristics of the sport. The specific throwing program utilized for this patient represents a modification of traditional throwing programs used with older adolescents and adults (Fig. 31-11).[27-29] It was chosen because this athlete did not play on a regulation field. For the 11-year-old baseball player, the distances to the bases, outfield wall, and pitcher's mound are all reduced. As a result, an age-appropriate throwing program was developed based on modifications from programs developed for older athletes who play on full-size fields.[28,29] Once the patient was able to demonstrate pain-free completion of a throwing program, he was advanced back to a pitching program that progressed the number of pitches as well as type of pitches.[28] The return-to-pitching program was adjusted in duration to not exceed the maximum number of recommended pitches per the patient's age. At about the 12-week mark, the patient was allowed to resume position play because he was pain-free with all active ROM, met the strength goals, and had completed the long-toss program without pain. Although he had begun a return-to-pitching program, his season was coming to an end and he decided to wait until next season to return to pitching.

Little League Interval Throwing Program

Guidelines

1. Throwing should be performed every other day.
2. Proper warm-up needs to be performed before throwing. This includes stretching and any other pre-throwing activity recommended by therapist or coach.
3. Throwing is to be done at 75%-80% of maximal effort.
4. Focus on proper throwing mechanics.
5. Apply ice to shoulder and/or elbow for 15-20 minutes following throwing.
6. Perform each step 2-3 times. If able to complete without increased symptoms, progress to next step. Each step should take approximately 1 week to complete; each phase should take approximately 2 weeks to complete.
7. If pain or soreness occurs while throwing, follow Soreness Rules or contact physical therapist for further instruction.

Warm-up

1. Jogging 5 min at 50%-60% of maximal effort (*i.e.,* "break a sweat")
2. Shoulder stretching
3. Towel throws
4. Warm-up throwing:
   a. 20-foot distance, with focus on form/mechanics/follow-through
   b. Throws should be made with an arc.
   c. Athlete is allowed to take a step with throws.

Soreness Rules

1. If no soreness occurs and you are able to make all throws, advance to next step as indicated.
2. If soreness occurs during warm-up, but soreness is gone by end of warm-up, repeat previous step. If soreness occurs during this throwing session, take 2 days off and drop down one step on next throwing day.
3. If soreness continues for 1 hour past throwing session or into next day, take additional day off and repeat most recent throwing session.
4. If soreness occurs during warm-up and continues through first 15 throws, stop throwing and take 2 days off. Resume throwing at one step lower.

Figure 31-11. Return-to-throwing program for pediatric athletes that do not participate on regulation fields (Little League interval throwing program).[27-29]

Little League Interval Throwing Program	
30 ft Phase	**45 ft Phase**
Step 1: Warm-up throwing 30' (20 throws) Rest 10 min Warm-up throwing 30' (20 throws)	**Step 3:** Warm-up throwing 45' (25 throws) Rest 10 min Warm-up throwing 45' (25 throws)
Step 2: Warm-up throwing 30' (20 throws) Rest 10 min Warm-up throwing 30' (20 throws) Rest 10 min Warm-up throwing 30' (20 throws)	**Step 4:** Warm-up throwing 45' (25 throws) Rest 10 min Warm-up throwing 45' (20 throws) Rest 10 min Warm-up throwing 45' (20 throws)
60 ft Phase	**90 ft Phase**
Step 5: Warm-up throwing 45' (25 throws) Rest 10 min Warm-up throwing 60' (20 throws)	**Step 7:** Warm-up throwing 45' (15 throws) 60' (20 throws) Rest 10 min Warm-up throwing 90' (15 throws)
Step 6: Warm-up throwing 45' (25 throws) Rest 10 min Warm-up throwing 60' (25 throws) Rest 10 min Warm-up throwing 60' (20 throws)	**Step 8:** Warm-up throwing 45' (15 throws) 60' (20 throws) Rest 10 min Warm-up throwing (45') 90' (25 throws) Rest 10 min Warm-up throwing 45' (15 throws)

Figure 31-11. (*Continued*)

Evidence-Based Clinical Recommendations

SORT: Strength of Recommendation Taxonomy

A: Consistent, good-quality patient-oriented evidence
B: Inconsistent or limited-quality patient-oriented evidence
C: Consensus, disease-oriented evidence, usual practice, expert opinion, or case series

1. In adolescent overhead athletes, long periods of decreased throwing activity may have detrimental effects on UE range of motion. **Grade B**

2. In individuals suspected of having medial epicondyle apophysitis, palpation of medial elbow anatomy is best completed in a dynamic fashion because tenderness to palpation may vary based on the position of the UE. **Grade C**

3. To reduce stress and loading through the elbow during the throwing motion, early intervention to correct dysfunctional muscle patterns, mechanical faults, and impaired strength and endurance of the posterior shoulder, scapular stabilizing, and core musculature is recommended. **Grade C**

COMPREHENSION QUESTIONS

31.1 During which phase of the throwing motion is the *most* stress placed along the medial elbow?

A. Early cocking

B. Late cocking

C. Deceleration

D. Follow-through

31.2 A 9-year-old baseball pitcher is referred to an outpatient physical therapy clinic with the diagnosis of Little League elbow. The family states he has been pitching one time per weekend and will pitch 60-70 pitches per game and then play the remaining games at third base or shortstop. His pain has been increasing over the past month and now he rates it at a 6/10 with baseball and 4/10 at other times. He wants to return to baseball as soon as possible. The initial home exercise program should consist of which of the following?

A. Balance exercises focusing on single limb stance

B. Return-to-throwing program for total arm strength

C. Core stabilization and control exercises

D. Progressive strengthening exercises for the scapular stabilizers

ANSWERS

31.1 **B.** During the late cocking phase, there is a medial distraction force that places high stress to the anterior band of the ulnar collateral ligament. This force combined with the rapid change to internal rotation of the humerus at the beginning of the acceleration phase leads to the most stress placed on the medial elbow.

31.2 **D.** Scapular stabilizers provide stability to the shoulder girdle while helping to maintain the arm in the overhead position and decelerate after the throw. During the throwing motion, the scapula provides a stable base for the humerus to rotate within the glenoid. If the scapula upwardly rotates too early or too late, the humerus is placed in a position that may lead to other pathologies such as rotator cuff impingement or biceps tendonitis. In order for the athlete to maximize function, the stability of the scapula and strength and endurance of the surrounding musculature need to be addressed *early* in the rehabilitation process.

REFERENCES

1. Prentice WE, Arnheim DD. *Arnheim's Principles of Athletic Training: A Competency-Based Approach.* 12th ed. Boston, MA: McGraw-Hill; 2006.

2. Erkonen WE, Smith WL. *Radiology 101: The Basics and Fundamentals of Imaging.* 2nd ed. Philadelphia, PA: Lippincott Williams & Wilkins; 2005.

3. Benjamin HJ, Briner WW Jr. Little league elbow. *Clin J Sport Med.* 2005;15:37-40.

4. Gomez JE. Upper extremity injuries in youth sports. *Pediatr Clin North Am.* 2002;49:593-626.

5. Brenner JS; American Academy of Pediatrics Council on Sports Medicine and Fitness. Overuse injuries, overtraining, and burnout in child and adolescent athletes. *Pediatrics.* 2007;119:1242-1245.

6. DiFiori JP. Evaluation of overuse injuries in children and adolescents. *Curr Sports Med Rep.* 2010;9:372-378.

7. Gill TJ, Micheli LJ. The immature athlete. Common injuries and overuse syndromes of the elbow and wrist. *Clin Sports Med.* 1996;15:401-423.

8. Hawkins D, Metheny J. Overuse injuries in youth sports: biomechanical considerations. *Med Sci Sports Exerc.* 2001;33:1701-1707.

9. Adirim TA, Cheng TL. Overview of injuries in the young athlete. *Sports Med.* 2003;33:75-81.

10. Keeley DW, Hackett T, Keirns M, Sabick MB, Torry MR. A biomechanical analysis of youth pitching mechanics. *J Pediatr Orthop.* 2008;28:452-459.

11. Magra M, Caine D, Maffulli N. A review of epidemiology of paediatric elbow injuries in sports. *Sports Med.* 2007;37:717-735.

12. Lyman S, Fleisig GS, Waterbor JW, et al. Longitudinal study of elbow and shoulder pain in youth baseball pitchers. *Med Sci Sports Exerc.* 2001;33:1803-1810.

13. Kijowski R, Tuite MJ. Pediatric throwing injuries of the elbow. *Semin Musculoskelet Radiol.* 2010;14:419-429.

14. Kocher MS, Waters PM, Micheli LJ. Upper extremity injuries in the paediatric athlete. *Sports Med.* 2000;30:117-135.

15. Wilk KE, Reinold MM, Andrews JR. Rehabilitation of the thrower's elbow. *Clin Sports Med.* 2004;23:765-801.

16. Escamilla RF, Andrews JR. Shoulder muscle recruitment patterns and related biomechanics during upper extremity sports. *Sports Med.* 2009;39:569-590.

17. Cain EL Jr, Dugas JR, Wolf RS, Andrews JR. Elbow injuries in throwing athletes: a current concepts review. *American J Sports Med.* 2003;31:621-635.

18. Osbahr DC, Chalmers PN, Frank JS, Williams RJ, Widmann RF, Green DW. Acute, avulsion fractures of the medial epicondyle while throwing in youth baseball players: a variant of Little League elbow. *J Shoulder Elbow Surg.* 2010;19:951-957.

19. Kelly AM, Pappas AM. Shoulder and elbow injuries and painful syndromes. *Adolesc Med.* 1998;9:569-587.

20. Borsa PA, Laudner KG, Sauers EL. Mobility and stability adaptations in the shoulder of the overhead athlete: a theoretical and evidence-based perspective. *Sports Med.* 2008;38:17-36.

21. Meister K, Day T, Horodyski M, Kaminski TW, Wasik MP, Tillman S. Rotational motion changes in the glenohumeral joint of the adolescent/Little League baseball player. *Am J Sports Med.* 2005;33:693-698.

22. Reagan KM, Meister K, Horodyski MB, Werner DW, Carruthers C, Wilk K. Humeral retroversion and its relationship to glenohumeral rotation in the shoulder of college baseball players. *Am J Sports Med.* 2002;30:354-360.

23. Safran MR. Elbow injuries in athletes. A review. *Clinical Orthop Relat Res.* 1995:257-277.

24. Frostick SP, Mohammad M, Ritchie DA. Sport injuries of the elbow. *Br J Sports Med.* 1999;33:301-311.

25. Klingele KE, Kocher MS. Little league elbow: valgus overload injury in the paediatric athlete. *Sports Med.* 2002;32:1005-1015.

26. Wilk KE, Arrigo CA, Andrews JR. Current concepts: the stabilizing structures of the glenohumeral joint. *J Orthop Sports Phys Ther.* 1997;25:364-379.

27. Axe MJ, Snyder-Mackler L, Konin JG, Strube MJ. Development of a distance-based interval throwing program for little league athletes. *Am J Sports Med.*1996;24:594-602.

28. Reinold MM, Wilk KE, Reed J, Crenshaw K, Andrews JR. Interval sport programs: guidelines for baseball, tennis, and golf. *J Orthop Sports Phys Ther.* 2002;32:293-298.

29. Axe M, Hurd W, Snyder-Mackler L. Data-based interval throwing programs for baseball players. *Sports Health.* 2009;1:145-153.

NOTE: Page numbers followed by *f* or *t* indicate figures or tables, respectively.